AF720395

Clinical Handbook of Psychiatry

Clinical Handbook of Psychiatry

Edited by Mason Baker

STATES
ACADEMIC PRESS
www.statesacademicpress.com

States Academic Press,
109 South 5th Street,
Brooklyn, NY 11249, USA

Visit us on the World Wide Web at:
www.statesacademicpress.com

© States Academic Press, 2022

This book contains information obtained from authentic and highly regarded sources. Copyright for all individual chapters remain with the respective authors as indicated. All chapters are published with permission under the Creative Commons Attribution License or equivalent. A wide variety of references are listed. Permission and sources are indicated; for detailed attributions, please refer to the permissions page and list of contributors. Reasonable efforts have been made to publish reliable data and information, but the authors, editors and publisher cannot assume any responsibility for the validity of all materials or the consequences of their use.

ISBN: 978-1-63989-111-5

Trademark Notice: Registered trademark of products or corporate names are used only for explanation and identification without intent to infringe.

Cataloging-in-Publication Data

Clinical handbook of psychiatry / edited by Mason Baker.
p. cm.
Includes bibliographical references and index.
ISBN 978-1-63989-111-5
1. Psychiatry. 2. Medicine and psychology. 3. Mental health. 4. Psychology, Pathological. I. Baker, Mason.
RC438 .C55 2022
616.890 09--dc23

Table of Contents

Preface ... IX

Chapter 1 **A Reconciliation for the Future of Psychiatry: Both Folk Psychology and Cognitive Science** ... 1
Daniel D. Hutto

Chapter 2 **Unraveling Executive Functioning in Dual Diagnosis** ... 13
Judith C. L. M. Duijkers, Constance Th. W. M. Vissers and Jos I. M. Egger

Chapter 3 **Circadian Rhythms and Mood Disorders: Are the Phenomena and Mechanisms Causally Related?** ... 22
William Bechtel

Chapter 4 **Factor Analysis of the Brazilian Version of UPPS Impulsive Behavior Scale** ... 32
Cristina Y. N. Sediyama, Ricardo Moura, Marina S. Garcia, Antonio G. da Silva, Carolina Soraggi, Fernando S. Neves, Maicon R. Albuquerque, Setephen P. Whiteside and Leandro F. Malloy-Diniz

Chapter 5 **Beyond Scientism and Skepticism: An Integrative Approach to Global Mental Health** ... 37
Dan J. Stein and Judy Illes

Chapter 6 **Causality in Psychiatry: A Hybrid Symptom Network Construct Model** ... 41
Gerald Young

Chapter 7 **What is Constructionism in Psychiatry? From Social Causes to Psychiatric Classification** ... 56
Raphael van Riel

Chapter 8 **Cognitive Neuroscience and Causal Inference: Implications for Psychiatry** ... 69
Nadine Dijkstra and Leon de Bruin

Chapter 9 **Executive Functions in Children Who Experience Bullying Situations** ... 78
Wandersonia Medeiros, Nelson Torro-Alves, Leandro F. Malloy-Diniz and Carla M. Minervino

Chapter 10 **Explanatory Pluralism and the (Dis)Unity of Science: The Argument from Incompatible Counterfactual Consequences** ... 87
Victor Gijsbers

Chapter 11 **Predicting Medical Students' Current Attitudes Toward Psychiatry, Interest in Psychiatry, and Estimated Likelihood of Working in Psychiatry** ... 97
Ingeborg Warnke, Alex Gamma, Maria Buadze, Roman Schleifer, Carlos Canela, Bernd Strebel, Tamás Tényi, Wulf Rössler, Nicolas Rüsch and Michael Liebrenz

Chapter 12 **Risky Decisions in a Lottery Task are Associated with an Increase of Cocaine Use** ... 110
Amrei Wittwer, Lea M. Hulka, Hans R. Heinimann, Matthias Vonmoos and Boris B. Quednow

Chapter 13 **Psychological Disorders and Ecological Factors Affect the Development of Executive Functions** ... 121
Rafika Zebdi, Louise Goyet, Charlotte Pinabiaux and Bahia Guellaï

Chapter 14 **Brain Oscillatory Correlates of Altered Executive Functioning in Positive and Negative Symptomatic Schizophrenia Patients and Healthy Controls** ... 127
Barbara Berger, Tamas Minarik, Birgit Griesmayr, Renate Stelzig-Schoeler, Wolfgang Aichhorn and Paul Sauseng

Chapter 15 **Against Explanatory Minimalism in Psychiatry** ... 141
Tim Thornton

Chapter 16 **Executive Function is Selectively Impaired in Old Age Bipolar Depression** ... 150
Leonardo Caixeta, Vânia L. D. Soares, Renata T. Vieira, Cândida D. Soares, Victor Caixeta, Sandra B. Ferreira and Tales A. Aversi-Ferreira

Chapter 17 **Enhancing Executive Function and Neural Health in Bipolar Disorder through Reasoning Training** ... 155
Erin E. Venza, Sandra B. Chapman, Sina Aslan, Jennifer E. Zientz, David L. Tyler and Jeffrey S. Spence

Chapter 18 **Balancing Automatic-Controlled Behaviors and Emotional-Salience States: A Dynamic Executive Functioning Hypothesis** ... 166
Bruno Kluwe-Schiavon, Thiago W. Viola, Breno Sanvicente-Vieira, Leandro F. Malloy-Diniz and Rodrigo Grassi-Oliveira

Chapter 19 **Executive Dysfunctions: The Role in Attention Deficit Hyperactivity and Post-traumatic Stress Neuropsychiatric Disorders** ... 178
Lía Martínez, Edward Prada, Corina Satler, Maria C. H. Tavares and Carlos Tomaz

Chapter 20 **Working Memory Training and CBT Reduces Anxiety Symptoms and Attentional Biases to Threat** ... 193
Julie A. Hadwin and Helen J. Richards

Chapter 21 **The Relationship between Sleep Complaints, Depression, and Executive Functions in Older Adults** ... 204
Katie M. de Almondes, Mônica V. Costa, Leandro F. Malloy-Diniz and Breno S. Diniz

Chapter 22 **Disentangling Working Memory Functioning in Mood States of Bipolar Disorder** ... 212
Carolina Soraggi-Frez, Flávia H. Santos, Pedro B. Albuquerque and Leandro F. Malloy-Diniz

Chapter 23 **The Geriatric Forensic Psychiatry Rotation at University of Chicago: Utilization and Educational Benefit of a Subspecialty Rotation in Psychiatric Residency Training** **230**
Carolyn Shima, Sanford Finkel, Deborah Spitz and Amanda I. Goldstein

Permissions

List of Contributors

Index

Preface

Psychiatry is a medical specialty that deals with the diagnosis, prevention and treatment of mental disorders. These mental disorders may include maladaptations related behavior, cognition, mood and perception. The initial psychiatric assessment of a person generally starts with mental state examination and a case history. Psychological tests and physical examination may also be conducted. Occasionally, neurophysiological techniques and neuroimaging are used. In current practice, a combination of psychotherapy and psychiatric medication is used for psychiatric treatment. But contemporary practice also includes several other modalities such as community reinforcement, assertive community treatment and supported employment. Depending on the severity, treatment may be delivered on an inpatient or outpatient basis. Such selected concepts that redefine psychiatry have been presented in this book. It brings forth some of the unexplored aspects of this field. The aim of this book is to serve as a resource guide for students and experts alike and contribute to the growth of the discipline.

This book unites the global concepts and researches in an organized manner for a comprehensive understanding of the subject. It is a ripe text for all researchers, students, scientists or anyone else who is interested in acquiring a better knowledge of this dynamic field.

I extend my sincere thanks to the contributors for such eloquent research chapters. Finally, I thank my family for being a source of support and help.

Editor

1

A Reconciliation for the Future of Psychiatry: Both Folk Psychology and Cognitive Science

*Daniel D. Hutto**

Faculty of Law, Humanities and the Arts, School of Humanities and Social Inquiry, University of Wollongong, Wollongong, NSW, Australia

Edited by:
Derek Strijbos,
Radboud University, Netherlands

Reviewed by:
Philip Gerrans,
University of Adelaide, Australia
Rachel Valerie Cooper,
Lancaster University, UK

***Correspondence:**
Daniel D. Hutto
ddhutto@uow.edu.au

Philosophy of psychiatry faces a tough choice between two competing ways of understanding mental disorders. The folk psychology (FP) view puts our everyday normative conceptual scheme in the driver's seat – on the assumption that it, and it only, tells us what mental disorders are (1). Opposing this, the scientific image (SI) view (2, 3) holds that our understanding of mental disorders must come, wholly and solely, from the sciences of the mind, unfettered by FP. This paper argues that the FP view is problematic because it is too limited: there is more to the mind than FP allows; hence, we must look beyond FP for properly deep and illuminating explanations of mental disorders. SI promises just this. But when cast in its standard cognitivist formulations, SI is unnecessarily and unjustifiably neurocentric. After rejecting both the FP view, in its pure form, and SI view, in its popular cognitivist renderings, this paper concludes that a more liberal version of SI can accommodate what is best in both views – once SI is so formulated and the FP view properly edited and significantly revised, the two views can be reconciled and combined to provide a sound philosophical basis for a future psychiatry.

Keywords: philosophy of mind, narrative therapy, cognitive neuroscience, philosophy of psychiatry, philosophy of cognitive science

> There are more things in heaven and earth, Horatio, than are dreamt of in your philosophy.
> *Hamlet* Act I, Scene 5, 167–8

FOLK PSYCHOLOGY RULES

How should we best understand, categorize, and treat mental disorders? A familiar answer in philosophical circles is that any approach to mental health must always operate with reference to the normative features that define our folk psychological (FP) understanding of mind. Call this the FP view of mental disorders and psychiatry. Its driving assumptions are that FP, and only FP, conceptually defines what it is to have a mind because FP, and FP alone, supplies the necessary and sufficient mark of the mental, emphasizing its essentially rational character. On the standard, narrow reading, FP plays this governing role precisely because it is understood to be the commonsense theory or conceptual scheme that reveals how mental states – typically assumed to be propositional attitudes – interact in the rational production of behavior and action.

Graham (1), a staunch spokesperson for the FP view, advances a theory of mental disorder according to which we have no choice but to make reference to reason and rationality when understanding such phenomena because such features "help to constitute and define distinctively mental activity such as believing, hoping, desiring, deciding, thinking and the like" [(1), p. 7].

The main idea behind this vision is that FP supplies the only normative standard of what minds are and how they operate. Hence, only against FP's standard is it even possible to detect and demarcate mental disorders. Mental disorders arise when things go awry with us at some level, when in some important sense, a person fails to live up to or systematically violates the standards of rationality that characterize our everyday folk psychological ways of thinking. There may be various mental and non-mental causes of such failures. But, simply put, FP is the necessary reference point of what a normatively defined well-functioning mind looks like and what its rational characteristics are. Disordered minds, by comparison, are less than flourishing minds that fail to meet that normative standard.

Even though proponents of the FP view accept that perfect rationality is a notoriously slippery notion that evades precise analysis they insist, nonetheless, that, "rationality is essential to mindedness" [(1), p. 12]. Moreover, it is assumed that rationality is only something exhibited by whole persons and not by the operations of their subpersonal parts. Putting all of this together, in standard formulations, the FP view holds that we have no choice but to understand minds by making use of FP concepts, which apply to persons whose intentional attitudes exhibit an inherent rationality.

> Thinking of intentional attitudes (beliefs, desires, and so on) as presupposing the rationality of persons makes it clear that we persons are purposive or goal directed in behavior and that how we act or behave depends on our purposes or reasons for acting [(1), p. 120].

Graham (1) dubs this the rationality-in-intentionality (RIT) thesis for short. RIT takes rationality to be the hallmark of the mental – one that sets the mental forever apart from all other kinds of phenomena, and this is what makes the mental irreducibly autonomous.[1] The autonomy of the mental thesis can be understood in more or less realistic terms. Yet in all versions the root idea, subscribed to by all fans of the FP view, is this: propositional attitudes can only be ascribed, or only have life, when they stand in appropriate kinds of holistically and normatively defined rational relations. Mental phenomena exist if and only if the relevant forms of rationality are in place: viz. they live in the space of reasons. This is allegedly why when rationality is absent, we must switch to another scheme for understanding the relevant phenomena; in such cases, a move to non-mental concepts and explanatory schemes becomes necessary precisely because minds, properly understood, are fading or absent.

The crucial assumption of the FP view is that it is the job of philosophy of mind to reveal and articulate the essential contours of our commonsense understanding of the mind – which are assumed to be *the only* bona fide conception of mind.[2] The standard view is that this can only be achieved by means of some kind of conceptual analysis or radical interpretation [see, e.g., Ref. (5)].

With these assumptions about the essential characteristics of minds in place, the FP view of mental disorders firmly opposes what, by its lights, is its only possible rival, a scientifically orientated, non-mentalistic FP-eliminativist approach – one that looks solely to neuroscience to discern "the best understanding of and treatment for mental disorder" [(1), p. 6]. A purely brain-based approach to mental disorders is oxymoronic from the perspective of those who hold that FP defines the mental; such an approach might tell us much about non-mental disorders of various kinds, but it could not be a starting point of inquiry into psychiatry because it misses out the mental altogether. Despite insisting on this point, fans of the FP view do not deny that neuroscience can play a part in the larger business of psychiatry. They do insist, however, that the part the brain sciences can play is always and everywhere secondary, servile, and subservient. Crucially, the FP view of psychiatry "does not relinquish the theory (of mental disorders) to, but deploys, brain science" [(1), p. 9].

Although clearly incompatible with a purely scientific, eliminativist vision of psychiatry, the FP view is compatible with making explanatory use of a range of scientific findings. The sciences of the mind have something important to add to the story so long as they take their direction from FP when it comes to understanding and classifying mental disorders on the basis of possible causes. There is no contradiction to be found in such a cooperative enterprise for those who think FP defines the mind: but this is so only as long as it is accepted that FP must always remain in the driver's seat when coordinating any such combined efforts [(1), p. 11].[3]

The logic is straightforward. Mental disorders – on the FP view – only ever show up as disturbances within the space of reasons. Even so, there can be non-mental causes of mental disorders. We can think of such causes as arational, non-mental disorder influences that, to use Graham's apt phrase, "gum up" "the rational works" [(1), p. 160]. Non-mental factors – the influences of brain and behavior – can interfere with and upset our rationally constrained mentality. Accordingly, non-mental factors can contribute to and help explain the occurrence of mental disorders – and this can happen even if the non-mental mechanisms in question are in perfect order and are operating just as they should.[4]

All in all, the FP view insists on a particular understanding of the explanatory relations that can hold between the mental and the

[1]The FP view endorses the irreducibility claim about the mind, which Davidson championed long ago: "The reason mental concepts cannot be reduced to physical concepts is the *normative* character of mental concepts" [(4), p. 46].

[2]Those who take the autonomy thesis seriously – whether in strongly realist or more interpretationist renderings – maintain that an FP understanding of mind plays an absolutely essential role in defining what minds are and, hence derivatively, what *mental* disorders are. Accordingly, "the mind *qua* mind puts its inscription on the sources of a disorder. We cannot recognize a mental disorder without uncovering that mark" [(1), p. 11]. It is because of the need for benchmarking against the mark of the mental – which can only be done *via* FP – that "no conceptually regimented and normatively informed theory of mental disorder can be devised without taking philosophy of mind seriously" [(1), p. 1].

[3]Thus in line with this, Graham (1) argues that going the FP-governed way ought not to encourage one to endorse the DSM atheoretical method of classifying and characterizing mental disorders.

[4]For example, Graham (1) illustrates the latter point vividly by reminding us that, "an addict … does not possess a broken brain" (p. 179). The reason this can be so, Graham (1) claims, is because, "The brain, in general, is not hard-wired for personal prudence. Neural activity may systematically underwrite unwise behaviors without exemplifying a breakdown or something wrong or damaged in its wetware or machinery" (p. 178).

non-mental when it comes to making sense of mental disorders. Neuroscience can help us to understand, for example, the condition of the unwilling addict because reference to brute arational neural mechanisms can help "*to explain* why addicts suffer from relapse in spite of themselves" [(1), p. 179, emphasis added]. Non-mental mechanisms – whether malfunctioning or not – feature in the larger story of specific mental disorders because they may explain what interferes with the rational works. Telling the right story about such non-mental influences is complicated by the fact that there can be "different hypotheses about the irruptive role of a-rational neurobiological/neurochemical mechanisms into the space of reasons" [(1), p. 178].

Speaking on behalf of the FP vision of psychiatry, Graham (1) sees no difficulty in asserting that, "even though mental disorders are not brain disorders, neuroscience helps to illuminate *their nature*" [(1), p. 13, emphasis added]. How should we understand this claim? It deserves attention for, as just noted above, the FP view holds that the essence of *mental* disorders can only be understood with reference to what occurs in the space of reasons. Accordingly, explanations that cite non-mental goings-on from outside that space can only shine a light on the nature of mental disorders if we distinguish the *essential* characteristics of the latter from explanations that tell a fuller story about their *actual* natures (or, more likely, how non-mental mechanisms make an actual but effective difference in particular cases).

This requires drawing a distinction between the *essence* of mental disorders and their *actual* natures. A standard way to do this is to take a leaf out of the analytic playbook of commonsense functionalism (6–8). Analytic functionalists hold that our everyday folk theories or practices conceptually define what minds are, fully and completely. On this score, the so-called sciences of the mind reveal nothing about the essential features of minds. *Prima facie*, this may seem extreme. However, adopting this view is entirely compatible with the idea that the sciences can discover much about how mental phenomena are, *as a matter of fact*, instantiated in the actual world – hence, the sciences can discover much about their *actual nature*. They can do so once FP tells "empirical inquiry what to look for" [(2), p. 51]. If we distinguish the essential and actual characteristics of mental phenomena and, relatedly, mental disorders, it becomes possible to understand how the sciences can assist with an understanding of the nature of mental disorders on the FP view. *Pace* Locke, on this vision, it is the scientists of mind, not the philosophers of mind, who must do the under-laboring.

PSYCHIATRY IN THE SCIENTIFIC IMAGE

The FP view of psychiatry has some fierce critics. It has been accused of presenting an unjustifiably restrictive vision of the role the sciences of mind play in mental health. Advancing the idea that psychiatry needs to be grounded entirely in the cognitive sciences, Murphy (2) is the foremost defender of the scientific image (SI) view of psychiatry. He and his friends see the FP view as unacceptable because it denies the sciences of the mind a free hand in revealing the essential character of mental phenomena. That restriction, SIers hold, results in an unwarranted fettering of psychiatric explanations and classifications [(2), p. 48, 51].

Adherents of the SI view are self-styled progressives. They insist that psychiatric explanation and nosology should not be regimented by, or beholden to, commonsense intuitions or assumptions. Psychiatric explanations, they hold, require no guidance, warrant, or mandate from FP. Proponents of the SI view insist that the future of the mental health field depends on fully embracing the sciences of the mind. The core assumption is that the sciences provide the requisite tools for a free inquiry into the nature of mental disorders. Moreover, the scientific work is to be conducted without requiring any appeal to commonsense notions of the mind, as filtered and understood through philosophy.

In place of the FP vision of psychopathology, Murphy (2) sets out his stall for a revisionary objectivism about the nature of mind. Accordingly, the bid is to discover what minds are through the development of a pragmatic and open-ended, scientifically driven conceptual framework, one that is revisable in practice and one that rests on testing out a series of empirical bets about mental phenomena.[5] Crucially, the scientific investigations Murphy envisages would not be shackled by FP's oversight. On the SI vision, to truly explain and classify normal and abnormal minds, we must look to our best cognitive sciences and to those alone.[6]

An immediate consequence of embracing the SI view is that it open up the scope of what we might think of as the mental and how we might think of it, quite considerably. By implication, the same goes for mental disorders. For example, given that perception is a paradigmatically mental phenomenon, it turns out that, on the SI view, blindness – however counterintuitive it may seem – counts not just as a disorder of the visual system but as a *mental* disorder [(2), p. 54, 55–57]. Murphy is happy to bite this and other, similar bullets. The justification is simple: violating a few folk intuitions is a small price to pay if going the purely SI way puts psychiatry on a "sounder footing" [(2), p. 11].

This is all very well and good as a sort of SI position statement but what justifies taking the SI path? Why suppose that SI might reveal new and deeper facts about how minds operate and how they can go wrong?[7] Why not hold that the sciences of the mind do whatever good work they do by functioning in exactly the way the FP view says they do – viz. by supplying "the empirical application of our pre-theoretic folk concepts" [(2), p. 50]?

The most straightforward and compelling answer is that there is surely more to the mental than dreamed of by FP. This conclusion is hard, if not impossible, to resist if FP characterizes the mental wholly in terms of the propositional attitudes and how

[5] In pressing for this future vision of mental health as wholly grounded in science, Murphy (2) laments that much contemporary psychiatry actively shies away from theory (as exemplified in the avowed theory-neutrality of the DSMs). Against the diagnostic descriptivism of the DSMs, he maintains that psychiatry must aim to find out how things "really are" with mental disorders and what underlies them. The only way psychiatry can do this, and thus secure its future, would be to take advantage of and actively contribute to developments in the cognitive sciences.

[6] A psychiatry cast in the scientific image must assume that, "what counts as normal human nature is decided by a variety of disciplines that comprise the cognitive and biological sciences" [(2), p. 11].

[7] Murphy (2) is certainly right that there is a real and urgent need for psychiatry to address the issues that lie at the heart of the debate between FP and SI views. For the troubling fact is that, "psychiatry as it stands is not a particularly mature or successful enterprise" [(2), p. 10].

they rationally inter-relate. For on any such a rendering, there is every reason to believe that

> mind has an existence and substantive character that *goes well beyond*, and is independent of our best common-sense interpretative practices. Hence knowing the truth about the mind requires *a great deal more* than informed reflection on those practices. In fact, it requires cognitive science [(9), xiv, emphases added].

A full understanding of all that is mental cannot be limited to FP characterizations alone. There are many aspects of mind – even quite ordinary, everyday ones – such as the complex ways that perceiving and acting interact – upon which FP, as construed above, has simply nothing to say. Such examples multiply. There are many forms and aspects of mentality that can only be understood by engaging in modes of inquiry that go beyond interrogating FP as traditionally conceived. FP casts no light on the properties and dynamics of basic minds [for an extensive discussion, see Ref. (10)].

Call this the "More to the Mind than FP" objection. It strikes at the core assumptions of the official FP view. Notably, however, even if the "More to the Mind than FP" objection defeats or should make us suspicious about the FP view, it does not, by itself, justify adopting the pure SI vision. For even if there is "More to the Mind than FP," it does not follow that our understanding of minds, and by implication mental disorders, can *only* and *wholly* be supplied by the sciences of the mind.

In the end, because FP is not the whole story about minds, it will be argued that going the SI way is best – but only if SI is carefully qualified. Why so? Because FP is part of the story of the mental: arguably, important aspects of human minds can only be understood in FP terms. This can be so even if FP assumptions about the mind should not be the basis for or otherwise restrict our investigations into the fundamental nature of minds. Before attempting to show how to marry these ideas in Section "Keeping FP in the Picture," the next two sections raise important doubts about standard cognitivist formulations of the SI view and their inherent neurocentrism.

A CERTAIN IRONY

The SI view is open to understanding the mind in new ways that go beyond FP. Despite the essential openness of the SI view, some of its most prominent proponents have tried to foreclose on certain possibilities. Based on assumptions about what the best explanations in the cognitive sciences will look like, some campaign for a neuro-based cognitivist version of the SI view. For example, under SI's auspices, Murphy offers a defense of the idea that, "psychiatry is a branch of medicine dedicated to uncovering the *neurological basis* of disease entities" [(2), p. 10, emphasis added].[8] For him, going the SI way paves the way for adopting the medical model of psychiatry such that the work of psychiatry becomes that of tracing "abnormalities in behavior and cognition to specific *causal factors that are realized in brain* tissue" [(2), p. 13, emphasis added].

In Murphy's mind, adoption of the SI view leads naturally to firmly recommending a merger of psychiatry and clinical neuropsychology.[9] He is supremely confident that a purely neuro-based approach will dominate the future of psychiatry. This is evinced by his commitment to neurocomputationalism, input–output functionalism, modules, and so on. But why assume that the brain's the thing? Retort: Who seriously doubts it? Murphy tells us that, "After all, *everyone knows that* psychological phenomena, like all human behavior, are *rooted in* brain processes" [(2), p. 9, emphasis added]. How should we interpret the "everyone knows that" operator in this statement and what epistemic backing does it have? There are several possibilities.

The first is to go "Folk Analytic." Perhaps we can appeal to folk intuitions about the mind to justify talk about what everyone knows about the brain basis of minds. Clearly, this is a non-starter for SIers. The SI view precludes making any appeal to hypothesized folk theories and the intuitions they sponsor in order to explain the epistemic credentials of "everyone knows" talk. Folk intuitions can give no backing to SI friendly claims about what everyone knows; hence, they cannot help justify the claim that cognition is wholly caused by and realized in the brain as opposed to having a wider and non-exclusively neural basis. Put simply, to adopt the SI view of psychiatry is to forego making appeals to folk intuitions in order to defend claims about "what everyone knows" about the mental. Call that Murphy's Law. Murphy too must abide by it.

The second way to go might be to appeal to consensus in this matter in the philosophy of cognitive science. Classical cognitivist approaches to cognition promote a brainbound account of cognitive processes by adopting a representationalist and internalist account of the vehicles of cognition. If everyone in the field agrees that cognition is always and everywhere content involving and that the vehicles of mental content are neural, then this would justify claiming that "everyone knows" neurocentrism to be true. The best cognitive explanations of behavior can, in effect, "throw away the world" and focus solely, and solipsistically, on the properties that supervene on the current internal neural states of cognizers (11–14).

SIers would be justified in saying that psychiatry ought to take an exclusive interest in brains if classical cognitivism were true. The trouble, for Murphy and followers, is that classical cognitivism may not be true, and – as things stand – it is far from a safe bet to assume that it is. More to the point, looking at the state of the philosophy of cognitive science, it can be safely said that classical cognitivism is *not known* to be true. There are deep-seated,

[8] Murphy's (2) defense is admittedly qualified because he admits there are limits to our understanding when it comes to naturalizing and mechanizing central reasoning processes such that it may turn out that a proper scientific understanding of the latter might never be attainable.

[9] Such a merger, he holds, is "necessary to develop the broadest and most fertile approach to understanding psychopathology" [(2), p. 12]. In saying this, he does not promote a crude reductionism. He does not assume that neuropsychology offers molecular explanations or that its explanations are somehow more fundamental. Nevertheless, he holds, neuropsychological explanations have a privileged status: they provide a special understanding that affords unique possibilities for intervening upon and treating mental disorders.

on-going philosophical debates about the character of cognition and the reach of cognitive processes – and these debates are far from being conclusively settled.

Murphy is well aware of these debates and their import. His official word on the matter in 2006 was to note that, "Some pictures of the mind stress embodiment very heavily … Others prescind from details of our embodiment to stress a more purely computational theory of the mental … what counts as the mental depends in part on who is right in these debates" [(2), p. 64]. Despite this acknowledgment, Murphy thinks there is really no doubt that the sciences of mind will stick to providing explanations in terms of brain-based, semantic representations. This he takes to be a settled issue – even if, in the end, the hypothesized brain-based representations in question turn out not to have contentful properties of the FP sort.[10]

However, what exactly are the defining properties of representations, as defined solely by the sciences of the mind, without any reference to the kinds of content understood by FP? How should we understand the disagreements between representationalist and non-representationalist if we do not appeal to some notion of content as supplied by FP or some other agreed upon non-FP theory (15)? And without agreement about the defining properties of representations understood in non-FP terms – which might be supplied if we had a well-developed non-FP theory of content – how are we to decide where the boundaries of mind and cognition lie? How are we to determine whether – in the end – the best explanations of sciences of the mind will be given in terms of "inputs" and "outputs" that are purely neural as opposed to involving extraneural factors too (16)?

Against this backdrop, Murphy's confidence in an exclusively representationalist and neuro-focused future for psychiatry will seem, at best, premature – and at worst, it will look like a groundless pledge of allegiance. For the fact is there is no agreement in the philosophy of cognitive science that supports the idea that everyone knows – at least, not yet – that psychological phenomena are rooted or realized exclusively in brain processes.

But wait. Surely, we are looking for consensus in the wrong place. The fact that philosophers – of the mind or otherwise – disagree about important topics is hardly news. Perhaps there is yet another, more properly scientific consensus that we can appeal to in order to make good on the "everyone knows" claim. Doesn't a quick glance at the current agreement in the theoretical commitments of actual scientists of the mind secure its truth? The great bulk of scientists of the mind do talk of neural and mental representations in free and easy ways these days. Does it follow that they are committed to a cognitivist take on mental representations of the sort described above – one that would justify neurocentrism? Establishing that would require serious and detailed interpretative work: it would need to be shown that the representational talk of scientists has all of the relevant commitments and that it is more than nominally unified. It is far from obvious that this is the case. One major problem is that no unified theory of representation currently exists. Worse still, if we look at the current state of cognitive science there does not seem to be a single, settled story to tell about which theoretical tools – representational or non-representational – are primary or the best ones to use when it comes to understanding cognition and explaining intelligent activity. We seem to be living in a mixed economy. If this is right, then there is not an existing scientific consensus SIers can point to in order to justify the claim that "everyone knows" cognition to be brainbound.

On top of this, even if such a current consensus did exist – even if all good cognitive scientists turned out to be representationalists in the relevant sense – more work would be needed in order to determine whether the entities and properties they posit now will stand the test of time. It is always possible that even if all cognitive scientists are currently committed to neural representations still, it might turn out that something with different properties will best explain the relevant phenomena. Cognitive science is, after all, an unfinished business. Hence, even if today's scientists did have common commitments that would justify adopting neurocentrism, we might still worry that any such contingent fact would not provide a secure basis for making firm predictions about the future of psychiatry. The official story is that not long ago cognitivism replaced old school behaviorism, right? Science is shifty – but in a good way. The SI view should surely embrace that.

At this stage of the game, there seems to be no obvious justification for fans of the SI view to reject the idea that psychiatry might look beyond the brain when it comes to understanding, explaining, and treating psychopathological disorders. Indeed, there are positive reasons for thinking that it is fruitful to look beyond the brain when it comes to understanding mental phenomena (16). Notably, since looking beyond the brain does not entail ignoring the brain, adopting such a liberal SI view is perfectly in line with a modified version of Murphy's assertion that "we are animals with a biology including a brain that is [part of] the foundation of our mental life" [(2), p. 10].

Still, it might be thought that the foregoing liberal assessment is too blithe, quick, and programmatic. Aren't there good grounds for thinking that cognitive science will remain deeply committed to cognitivism and neurocentrism, even if in the final reckoning, it deviates in some matters of detail from the classical versions of those views? Aren't there special reasons for favoring cognitivism – reasons that we can identify here and now – that would justify neurocentrism and thus rule out more radical and extensive possibilities for understanding the nature and extent of cognition. That seems to be the line of several prominent defenders of cognitivist variants of the SI view (2, 3).

COGNITIVE BRIDGE WORK?

In defending their predictions about the rightful dominance of an SI-based medical model, Murphy and Smart (17) make it clear that this future is to be secured by *cognitive* neuroscience

[10] Thus, in a forthcoming paper, Murphy writes, "The question whether science makes use of representational systems isn't really open to doubt any longer: many areas of psychology and neuroscience take for granted the existence of semantic interpretations of internal states of some cognitive system. The assumption that inputs and outputs to and from components of the brain represent distal features of the world has been part of neuroscience since the nineteenth century. What is open to doubt is whether representation, as used in the sciences of mind, has the properties that philosophers have found in intentional content, as presupposed by folk psychology. I am not taking a stand on that … " (Murphy D. *Brains and Beliefs* (Unpublished)).

and not merely some brutal brain science. What makes cognitive neuroscience special, they maintain, is that it posits subpersonal information-processing mechanisms that are at once both causal–mechanical and intentional in character. It is because it blends the cognitive with the neural that cognitive neuroscience has unique explanatory power: it, alone, allows for an integrated scientific story to be told about minds.

Looking exclusively at what goes on in brains is apparently justified because of the depth and unity cognitive neuroscientific explanations can provide. Gerrans (3) makes this case in great detail.[11] He argues that cognitive neuroscience understands, "persons as complex, hierarchically-organized information-processing systems implemented in neural wetware" [(3), p. 16].[12] Seeing persons as brain based, in turn, allegedly confers peculiar advantages because it puts us in a position, for example, to "show how *facts* identified and explained by disciplines operating at 'levels' such as molecular neurobiology or neuroanatomy *can explain* psychological and phenomenological level *facts* that give delusion its clinical profile" [(3), p. 20, emphases added].[13] What makes having a cognitive theory pitched at the subpersonal information-processing level so uniquely valuable is that it is needed to "*bridge the gap* between neurobiological and personal level explanation" [(3), p. 21, emphasis added].

Integrated explanations of the promised kind are said to be unavailable, in principle, to the isolationist FP view: this is precisely because to adopt the latter's "space of reasons" idea enforces an absolute distinction between the intentional and the mechanical.

To see what makes cognitive theory so appealing, it is worth getting clear about what exactly the FP view allegedly cannot do. Gerrans (3) accuses its proponents of operating with a disunified framework – one in which mechanisms are assumed to make only a causal difference to cognitive goings-on in a way that debars them from being properly explanatory (p. 15, 20). For example, Gerrans characterizes the FP view as being committed to the idea that organic damage might "*play a causal role* in introducing the drastic change in psychological structure but *plays no explanatory role*" [(3), p. 27, emphases added]. Does it make sense to think the explanatory space could carve up in the way Gerrans suggests? Can we distinguish between something's playing a merely causal versus a properly explanatory role? How should we understand this distinction?

As discussed in Section "Folk Psychology Rules," proponents of the FP view clearly allow that mental phenomena can be explained by what goes on in non-mental mechanisms. The FP view may be limited in that it is not interested in, or simply fails to provide, very detailed stories about the non-mental causal contributions of implementation mechanisms in information-processing terms. But it cannot be faulted for ruling out, or making it impossible to tell, such deeper explanatory stories. So this alone cannot be what makes its rival, the cognitivist view, special.[14]

Apparently, what makes cognitive theory special is that it brings something else – something quite unique – to the table. It regards the mind as a complex information-processing system – one that is organized in a hierarchical way, with a variety of interacting processes playing specific roles and where some of these diverse processes are responsible for the supervision of others in the system. Understanding the mind through the lens of cognitive theory allegedly provides a peculiar sort of intelligibility – one that allows theorists to go beyond the telling of merely "difference making" causal stories. The cognitive theory allows us to see how everything fits together in a systematic way; it bridges the gaps and enables explanations at many different scales and levels to be integrated by detailing how information flows from level to level and what role particular processes play in the wider cognitive economy [(3), p. 48, see also 32, 53, 79, 103].

From this vantage point, it is easy to see the attraction of having a broader vision of the mind that seeks to understand the roles played by various forms of cognitive activity, how various aspects of mind relate to and interact with one another, and how specific disturbances in those relations and interactions can lead to mental disorders with signature profiles.

This much is welcome. Yet friends of cognitivist SI, such as Gerrans (3), go further than this: they suggest that only cognitive neuroscience has what it takes to do the required integrating work. As Gerrans (3) says, "the *essential idea* of cognitive neuropsychiatry is that without a cognitive theory the problem identified by autonomy theorists ... *cannot be*

[11] Gerrans (3) follows Murphy's lead of treating the SI view as best seen through the lens of a "minimalist cognitivism" (p. 18). Like Murphy, he sees that the future of mental health resides with brain sciences of the cognitive variety. He too regards psychiatry "as *a branch of cognitive neuroscience* by employing cognitive models that do not abstract away from, but are sensitive to, details of neural implementation" [(3), p. 37].

[12] On this vision, "personhood is a cognitive phenomenon constituted by the fact that personal-level phenomena, such as feelings, beliefs, emotions and desires arise at the highest levels of a cognitive processing hierarchy whose nature can be described and explained" [(3), p. 21]. Human cognition is thus "a complex hierarchy of computational processes performed by neural circuitry" [(3), p. 30].

[13] Motivating this proposal, with a Parthian shot at the perceived limits of the FP view, Gerrans (3) stresses that, "collecting and collating correlations between neural, phenomenological and cognitive properties of the delusional mind is useful but we need a theoretical approach that *fits all this information together*" (p. 14). It is here that we meet the idea that the tools of cognitive neuroscience are uniquely well suited to integrating "evidence from different disciplines about the way the mind configures itself in response to incoming information according to the way neural mechanisms influence cognitive processing" [(3), p. 14].

[14] There is great potential for confusion and conflation about just what the FP view and cognitive theory might, respectively, have to offer in terms of deeper explanations. As Section "Folk Psychology Rules" made clear, the FP view allows that we can go to a different level of description in order to get deeper explanations of mental disorders. Remarkably, in some places, Gerrans (3) talks in ways that suggest cognitive theory is wholly at peace with the FP view's suggestion that underlying neural mechanisms only ever explain by describing implementing mechanisms of cognitive phenomena. As he writes: "It is normal practice *to explain phenomena* such as amnesia or macular degeneration in terms of the way neural circuits *implement the cognitive processes* involved in memory or perception. This suggests that the way to explain psychology and phenomenology in terms of neurobiology is via a cognitive theory" [(3), p. 15, emphasis added]. If this were the whole story, it would be hard to distinguish what cognitive theory could offer that is really different from what the FP view offers. Yet, there are reasons to think this is neither the whole story about what cognitive theory has to offer nor the right one. In an unpublished paper, Murphy (forthcoming) upbraids Gerrans for talking about explanations of mental disorders by appeal to implementation mechanisms. By Murphy's lights, such talk is just an unfortunate hangover of the philosophical tendency to mix up analytic functionalism with cognitive psychology.

solved. The gap between neurobiology and psychology will be *unbridgeable*" [(3), p. 36]. Hence, "there *must be* an explanatory relationship between neuroscience and folk psychology" [(3), p. 33, emphasis added]. These are very strong, philosophically "musty" claims – and they are not self-evidently true.[15] We might well doubt that cognitive neuroscience *per se* is best placed to provide the desired integrating theoretical vision, especially in light of the concerns raised about Murphy's neurocentrism in the previous section.

What might persuade us that a brain-based cognitive theory is necessary to bridge the putative gaps? Allegedly, that cognitive neuroscience supplies special means for understanding the links between various mental phenomena. It can do so, again allegedly, precisely because it endorses a vision of the neurally housed mind "organised as a hierarchical system ... which *uses representations* of the world and its own states to control behaviour" [(3), p. 47, emphasis added]. The claim is that cognitive theory posits neural representations that perform a variety of cognitive tasks and that once we understand how information flows between such representations, we will be in a position to provide complete and satisfying explanations of mental disorders in ways which make the links between subpersonal to personal-level cognitive phenomena intelligible. Thus, Gerrans (3) observes of this general strategy that, ultimately, supplying the correct account of what drives specific delusions requires accounting for "the way the brain encodes information acquired in experience and then reconstructs representations of that information when subsequently cued" (p. 33).

It seems that the central posits of cognitive theory – information and representation – provide the perfect theoretical glue for integrated explanations. Cognitive neuroscience promises to show how there can be relevant connections between various cognitive activities in a way that does not just cite correlations or brute causal relations. Instead, cognitive neuroscience alone proves to be genuinely explanatory of mental disorders because it alone *makes intelligible* multilevel interactions across various scales and levels.

Allegedly, cognitive neuroscience alone can achieve this feat because it is wedded to a representational theory of mind that assumes cognition to be at root both mechanical and intentional. Importantly, cognitive theory seems to provide us a new mark of the mental – not "rationality-in-intentionality" cast as person-level phenomena, to be sure. Instead it offers us a "content-in-intentionality" or CIT mark of the mental.[16] For those who accept something like CIT, even though the cognitive is regarded as quite a mixed bag that reaches across the so-called subpersonal and personal levels it is also united by the intelligible relations that are instantiated through the processing of informational and representational content in ways that define minds.

Some philosophers hold that cognitive scientists are committed to essentially characterizing minds in information-processing terms. This is, of course, not news. We frequently hear that

> cognitive science ... has as its subject matter capacities like memory, perception, attention, language processing and reasoning. The concepts that cognitive sciences *take to be essential* for understanding their domain include information, representations, and algorithms [(19), p. 74, emphasis added].

Let us suppose, for the sake of argument, that Shapiro (19) is right in thinking that working cognitive scientists take themselves to use and need these kinds of conceptual tools. Would this help fans of the cognitivist SI view to justify the claim that cognitive neuroscience operates with unique explanatory tools that give it special gap-closing powers?

Would assuming CIT make cognitive neuroscience ideally well placed to provide gap-bridging solutions? One reason for thinking so is that CIT seems to imply the existence of something like a neurally based space of reasons. To posit a space of reasons mark II would be to assume that there exists a cognitive level at which various mental phenomena do not just brutally interact but intelligibly inter-relate because they communicate by trafficking in contentful information and representations. Content would, on this picture, be the shared common coin traded by all cognitive phenomena. The CIT picture seems to make it possible to understand cognitive relations in explanatorily illuminating ways that do not reduce to the giving of merely brutal, causal explanations.

Let us imagine that cognitive neuroscience posits a neural space of reasons, ala CIT, and embraces internalism about the vehicles of various mental contents. If so (assuming the above analysis is correct), it would follow that cognitive neuroscience would have utterly special resources for bridging the sort of gaps of which Gerrans (3) speaks. All that would have to be done to seal the deal would be to show in detail how the cognitive neuroscience, as imagined above, could use those resources to in fact close such gaps. Doing all of this would be an effective way of motivating an exclusively neurocentric version of the SI view.

Before assessing whether cognitive neuroscience, so construed, really has what it takes to close the said gaps, it is important

[15] For example, elsewhere, Gerrans speaks of the "*necessary* role of cognitive theory in linking the neurobiological and phenomenological levels of explanation" [(3), p. 18, emphasis added]. Methodologically speaking, it is strange that Gerrans (3) makes appeal to such general and wholesale philosophical justifications, for when pinning his philosophical colors to the mast he clearly tells us that: "*Murphy is right*. Our best understanding of the mind comes from understanding cognitive architecture. However that argument *cannot be established a priori for all mental phenomena*. The best we can do is construct, revise and, ultimately, unify case-by-case explanations" [(3), p. 14, emphases added]. This fits better with his more retail defenses of cognitive theory, such as when he claims that the "cognitive theory of visuo-motor control embedded in the overall architecture of cognitive control ... is *required to explain* why high levels of activity in these regions produce loss of a sense of agency" [(3), p. 18, emphasis added], or when he tells us that "schizophrenic symptoms *can only be explained* in representational terms" [(3), p. 18].

[16] A CIT, intentionality-in-mechanism vision of the cognitive, is clearly in tune with the idea that, "The whole thrust of cognitive science is that there are sub-personal contents and sub-personal operations that are truly cognitive in the sense that these operations can be properly *explained only in terms of these contents*" [(18), p. 27, emphasis added].

to be clear about the source of the alleged need to do so. Notably, if there are any such explanatory gaps to bridge, then the need to bridge them is motivated by purely philosophical, not scientific, considerations. Without doubt, scientists and psychiatrists seek rich explanations of the roots of mental disorders. Providing such explanations would require going beyond FP and delving deeply into the sciences of the mind. However, crucially, providing such explanations is not the same as, nor does it require, bridging the putative intelligibility gaps – those that hold, e.g., between neurobiology and folk psychology and with which Gerrans (3) is concerned. Seen in this light, it becomes clear that Gerrans (3) seeks to motivate an exclusively cognitive neuroscientific take on SI by getting us to take seriously the need to address explanatory requirements of a distinctively philosophical kind.

The great irony is that elsewhere SIers reject the need to address such intelligibility demands as illegitimate. Compare the alleged need to make sense of the interactions between cognitive phenomena across levels by appeal to representational contents with the alleged need to make sense of the connections that hold between propositional attitudes in terms of rationality. If Gerrans (3) is right, cognitive theory can help us to make intelligible how various subpersonal cognitive phenomena inter-relate. How might it do this? By rendering the relations between cognitive phenomena intelligible. How? Not in RIT terms that explain how personal-level propositional attitudes relate rationally, to be sure, but in CIT terms that explain how neural representations relate contentfully.

It should now be easy to see why it would be a problem for SIers to advance this type of line. Any attempt to motivate a neurocentric cognitivist SI view by arguing that cognitive neuroscience alone can bridge otherwise unintelligible explanatory gaps requires being sensitive to the very sort of philosophical concerns that the SI view itself casts into doubt. Must there be some common feature (if not rationality then content) that is shared by all mental phenomena and which unifies them and explains how they intelligibly inter-relate? SIers say "No": They question the demand that "personal-level phenomena can only be explained in terms of other personal-level phenomena" [(3), p. 21]. This being the case, surely, we are also well within our rights to question whether there is a legitimate need for a unifying cognitive theory that makes intelligible how various cognitive phenomena intelligibly inter-relate in special, more-than-merely causal ways. As the old proverb reminds us, what's sauce for the goose is sauce for the gander.

And there is something else to consider. We might doubt that on close scrutiny appeals to information and representation could play the unifying and integrating roles that would satisfy the identified gap-bridging needs, if we were to take such needs seriously. The fact is that apart from bearing the names "cognitive," "representational," or "informational" nothing in so-called current cognitive theory deeply unifies all the various cognitive phenomena in terms of their importantly and interestingly diverse properties or roles.

Consider Gerran's claim that, "a scientist explaining some discrepant evidence *is doing the same thing* as the oculomotor system controlling the trajectory of a limb" [(3), pp. 46–7, emphasis added]. Is this credible? Undoubtedly, there may be some mileage in taking this route and drawing loose analogies for certain purposes. But a developed theory would be needed to back up any such claim if taken in a serious and literal way.[17]

To illustrate the point consider what Gerrans (3) has to say about the activation-information-mode (AIM) model of dreaming, which focuses on the flow of information within and between components of a control hierarchy. In discussing that model, he holds that the "*intrinsic cognitive properties* of these components *are preserved through transitions from mode to mode*. What changes are the interactions between these components" [(3), p. 79, emphases added].

Usually, in this sort of context, cognitive theorists upgrade talk of the flow of information to talk of the flow of informational content. Content, they hold, is what survives changes in mode and process. Canonically, the content of a mental state is determined by what it is about and how it represents the world to be. Now, if information processing literally involves the trading of contents that would make it easier to justify claiming that scientists and information-processing systems basically do the same cognitive work. Moreover, if content were the common coin that is always traded in some form, everywhere in the cognitive economy, it would be clear why there would have to be, and how there could be, intelligible relations holding between the many and various cognitive phenomena.

The trouble with this gambit is that it raises a host of unanswered questions. Just what is informational content anyway? What intrinsic cognitive properties does it have? Where does it get them? How can content be preserved through changes? How can it make a difference to cognition? How does it relate to representational content? Is it a kind of objective commodity? Does it make sense to say that we can take different perspectives – e.g., subjective and objective – toward it [as Ref. (3) appears to assume – see, e.g., p. 17]?

Cognitive theorists can avoid these tricky questions by sticking to an understanding of information in scientifically

[17]In the text surrounding this claim, Gerrans (3) makes clear that he is drawing on assumptions that predictive coding accounts of perception have made popular to support the idea that visual systems and scientists "do essentially the same thing." Predictive coding accounts understand cognition as a matter of making active inferences in continuous effort to minimize prediction error. But whether we should think of visual systems as really making contentful inferences at all, and whether if they do, they do so in anything like the way that scientists do, are highly contentious topics of current debate [for reasons why we ought to prefer a non-contentful reading of predictive processing, see Ref. (20, 21)]. For this reason, it might seem safer for cognitivists to advance a weaker claim about what makes these phenomena essentially the same. It might be argued that scientists and visual systems are essentially alike because they both use representations even though visual systems use different kinds of representation than scientists do. The idea here is that there is no requirement that visual systems and scientists need to operate with the same kinds of content in order to qualify as representational systems. While it is technically correct to go this way it raises afresh the question of what unifies and intelligibly relates these two cognitive phenomena if not the fact that they both involve manipulations of content of the same kind. The point is that without full details, it is far from clear why we should accept that vision and scientific theorizing – which appear to be quite disparate cognitive activities – are essentially alike.

respectable terms – those of covariance and correspondence. That is perfectly fine, but then it is difficult to justify claims that basic information processing is content involving in a way, which would license drawing a strong analogy with the theoretical activity of scientists.

This is just one example of a disunity objection to the integrationist picture. To make a full dress case against such a vision would require a much longer discussion [(10), esp. ch. 4]. For our purposes, it suffices to note that anyone offering a bridge building, unifying cognitive theory must answer the sorts of questions raised above. *Prima facie*, it seems they will only be able to do so with the backing of a well-developed naturalistic theory of content.

To highlight why such a theory is needed, consider a different set of cases. In many of the explanations that Gerrans (3) offers of delusions the "felt" aspect of the phenomenon in question turns out to be a pivotal factor. The phenomenological and emotionally charged aspects of our experience apparently matter to and help explain some of the strong tendencies we have when responding to, interpreting, and accounting for our situations. Yet, as is notoriously well known, we currently lack anything like a workable theory that shows how we are to understand such qualitative phenomena in purely information processing or representational terms. Once again, it looks like disunity rather than unity is the word of the day.

Things are even more puzzling if we consider the roles imaginings are meant to play in the integrative explanations on offer by cognitive theorists, such as Gerrans (3). For example, he holds that simulative activity generates imaginings that can be incorporated in a wider cognitive economy. By this, he means that imaginings can be the basis for action (including mental action). Despite the fact that imaginings are influential and we often act on them, they are cognitively interesting and distinct because they lack many of the properties of canonical propositional attitudes, such as belief [(3), p. 18].

On this score Gerrans (3) tells us that

> Imagination uses the mind's cognitive resources, such as perceptual, doxastic and emotional processing to create simulations. It thus inherits the intentional structure of these counterpart processes. However *qua* simulations *imaginative states do not have congruence conditions*. [(3), p. 105].

The basic claim, which is plausible enough is that imagination deploys specialized neural circuitry to "construct and manipulate *representations which have representational contents but no congruence conditions*" [(3), p. 114, emphasis added]. Gerrans (3) is concerned to show that simulative imagining can figure in and make a difference to one's thinking without the content of such imaginings being believed.

Yet, since most theorists hold that mental content requires some kind of correctness or congruence condition, it is puzzling in what sense imaginations can be said to have representational content if they lack such conditions altogether in the way Gerrans (3) proposes. What remains if you subtract congruence conditions from a mental representation? Gerrans's (3) answer is intentional structure. But it is not clear what exactly puts the intentionality in this structure for cognitivists if not the existence of mental representations with congruence conditions.[18]

Let us be clear. A simulative account of imaginings is attractive for many reasons [(23), ch. 4]. However, it is far from clear that imaginings without congruence conditions are best understood as any kind of mental representation for precisely the reasons stated above (20, 22). But even if this proves possible it would remain unclear how a simulative account of the imagination that emphasized the lack of congruence conditions could contribute to a unified cognitive theory of minds.

Our capacity for producing narratives – often quite spectacular ones – is yet another place in which it is important to recognize that interesting forms of cognition have special properties that break the standard representationalist mold. Gerrans (3) proposes that particular forms of delusional thinking arise from signature breakdowns in the usual interactions between cognitive systems. These breakdowns in turn prompt patterns of default thinking that take the form of experientially charged imaginative episodes. Default thoughts of this stripe provide raw material that can be woven together into what are, for those in the grip of a delusion, spectacular and hypersalient narratives. Importantly, such default thoughts "are subjectively adequate responses to experience constructed as narrative elements or fragments" [(3), p. 101].

The basic idea is that when operating in the default mode, we assemble first pass, coherent stories. Yet even when these stories are internally coherent, they are not always subjected to critical epistemic scrutiny. According to Gerrans (3) when unsupervised by decontextualized systems, the products of default thinking are not scrutinized for consistency or veridicality; they are not evaluated against "competing narratives for accuracy or utility" [(3), p. 77].

This is hardly surprising since the great bulk of narratives do not aim at truth. Although narratives all share certain basic structural properties, we must look to the contexts in which we use a given narrative in order to determine its semantic properties. Thus, as Goldie (24) points out "Fictional narratives do not aspire to be true, whereas real life narratives do. A narrative is fictional not in virtue of its content being false, but in virtue of its being narrated, and read or heard, *as part of a practice of a special sort*" (pp. 152–3, emphasis added). Thus fictional narratives, offered up as fictions, invite "the audience to imagine or make believe that what is being narrated actually happened, even when it is known that it did not. Thus the question of reference and of truth simply does not arise within the 'fictive stance'" [(24), pp. 152–3]. For these reasons, Goldie concludes that, "reference and truth have no application in fiction, but do have application in historical and everyday explanation" [(24), p. 154]. Different kinds of narratives exhibit different kinds of semantic

[18]When thinking about what might be leftover in such a subtraction, it is useful to consider Gerrans's (3) claim that, "different cognitive processes have *different computational properties* that enable them to meet their congruence condition. These *properties provide the intentional structure of representations* produced by different cognitive processes. For example, the representations produced by the visual system are 3D coloured scenes derived by processing spectral and luminance information" [(3), p. 105, emphases added]. However, once no correctness conditions are in play, it is not clear in what sense the residual structures ought to be thought to bear representational content or even what it means to say that they do (22).

properties, and we understand these differences if we are alert to the roles that these different kinds of narratives play in our lives and thinking.

A crucial contrast becomes evident if we compare the uncritical use of narratives that do not aim at truth with the intense critical scrutiny of beliefs and claims that do. In the most serious cases, the latter are subject to the norms of scientific testing, where we seek to fix what we believe only "according to standards of consistency and empirical adequacy" [(3), p. 13]. Put simply, some forms of cognition do have representational contents and do play roles in our cognitive economy that make them subject to epistemic norms which simply do not apply to other forms of cognition. Other forms of cognition lack these features. Our so-called default thoughts – those generated when our minds are wandering or in screensaver mode are a prime example. They do not involve any "attempt to confirm an empirical hypothesis" [(3), p. 76].

Although the above analysis only scratches the surface, the important thing to note is that the detailed explanations Gerrans (3) offers of the complexities of delusional thinking gain their power by focusing on the way diverse cognitive phenomena (e.g., feeling, imagining, and narrating) interact in virtue of their special cognitive roles and properties. Contrariwise, these explanations gain nothing from making the additional cognitivist assumption that all mental phenomena are united because they are, somehow, representational in character.

To tell a convincing explanatory story about minds and how they can become disturbed in particular ways, we need to recognize the important diversity of mental phenomena rather than insisting on a cognitivist account that downplays those differences in favor of fulfilling a philosophically motivated demand for unity. We can relinquish CIT and its problematic intelligibility requirement, recasting the integrating cognitive theory in far less ideologically demanding ways than do the friends of cognitivist SI. This does not mean we should give up on understanding how various mental phenomena interact or that we should not seek to understand the roles they play in the larger cognitive economy. It simply means that we can make sense of the relevant interactions and relations between mental and other phenomena without insisting that informational and representational content are needed to account for the intelligibility of such relations.

Only if we fully free ourselves from the constraints of FP-based philosophical suppositions about what is necessary for something to count as a properly cognitive phenomena does it become possible to concoct accounts of cognition that are truly unconstrained by FP thinking about the basic nature of minds. Interestingly, radically enactivist approaches that lay stress on the importance of interactions over contentful representations as the common coin of the cognitive looks well placed to pick up the explanatory burden (10). This is especially so if it is accepted that "what needs to be explained here is not just the causal interactions among neurons but *the way those interactions* enable cognitive processes and experiences" [(3), p. 30].[19]

KEEPING FP IN THE PICTURE

Only once the siren songs of an exclusively brain-focused future vision for psychiatry are silenced can the ground for a suitably open-minded and philosophically uncontaminated rendering of the SI view be laid. This closing section shows that when modestly formulated in the way suggested above, the SI view can make peace with an unimperialistic vision of FP.

Consider, once again, Gerrans's (3) plausible suggestion that narrative-based and theory-based explanations differ in important ways because they answer to different epistemic standards. Thus, to understand the delusional mind requires understanding how these modes of cognition interact or fail to interact in particular conditions.

Let us assume that Gerrans's (3) answer is along the right lines. Let us assume, for example, that those under the sway of specific delusions do indeed construct stories as opposed to rationally evaluated beliefs in order to make sense of such episodes. We might wonder, assuming they are not natural-born narrators, how they come to be able to weave such stories? We might be interested to know why a given kind or genre of story rather than another is more compelling to some populations rather than another? Or, why – upon experiencing an underlying mismatch between what-is-felt and what-was- anticipated-would have-and-should-have-been-felt – the narratives of deluded people unfold in one standard variant rather than another. The thing to notice is that in order to explain and understand key features of delusional narratives and the narrative practices that enable their generation requires looking at socioculturally and not purely neural factors [for extended arguments along these lines, see (23, 25–27)]. This is especially the case when it comes to understanding the distinctive kinds of norms relevant to the sorts of cognitive activity that differentiate narrative from scientific practices.

The point is that understanding the relevant norms requires looking beyond the brain (27). Only outside the skull of individuals do we find what we need for making sense of normative features of the cognitive phenomena that need explaining. Yet it is also when we look to certain public practices that we come by the resources for adopting a softer take on FP and its role in therapy. Certain kinds of treatment urge us to make best use of tools already available within cultures – such as incorporating traditional narrative practices into therapy – in order to respond to those in need.

There are compelling reasons to agree with Gerrans (3) that our foremost ways of making sense of ourselves and others are grounded in explanations that are not theoretical but narratively based. Such explanations function, primarily, as normalizing explanations. In giving them, any of a number of explanatorily relevant factors might be cited (e.g., facets of X's character, X's mood, X's larger projects, the content of this or that propositional attitude of X, and so on). Crucially, like historical explanations, these folk psychological explanations are not general and abstract but take the form of narratives that emphasize details that are personal and particular.

[19]Enactivists, of course, encourage multi-stranded investigations, involving explanations that are pitched at various "levels" and "scales." Gerrans (3) acknowledges this. Taking the case of vision as a prime example, he emphasizes the need for theories that seek to simultaneously investigate different levels of cognitive activity and how they integrate. Yet here he notes, "Even enactive theorists of vision who disagree with Marrians nonetheless debate with them about the causal relevance of mechanisms at different levels" [(3), p. 43].

Consider an idealized test case. Imagine a person suffering from a psychiatric condition that is brought on by a cascade of factors rooted in neural causes. Imagine that the condition can be wholly and successfully addressed by a perfectly targeted neuroscientific intervention. Even in this imagined case – one that best favors a purely neurocentric vision of psychiatry in terms of diagnosis explanation, and treatment – it is plausible there would be a need for the person to achieve a rehabilitating self-understanding. Graham (1) captures this point when he says:

> to mend or heal from a disorder in a self-respecting and dignified manner requires discovering a positive or purposeful place for past and present episodes of disorder in the … course of a person's life … [this] often consists of dealing with conflicting interpretations of one's past … [(1), p. 14].

The take-home lesson is that even in ideal cases in which targeted neural inventions might wholly relieve specific conditions we should not typically expect psychiatric therapy to boil down to a simple business of eradicating "disease" in the way a narrowly construed medical model can suggest.

Murphy (2) appears prepared to acknowledge that there is a need for psychiatry to go beyond the brain, at least in some cases. In this vein, he states clearly that, "there are important roles for non-scientific thinking about the methods of psychiatry" [(2), p. 47].[20]

Importantly, even for those who press for a more thorough brain-based vision of psychiatry, there need be no conflict between endorsing both an SI view of the field and recognizing the need and importance of non-scientifically focused therapies.[21] When it comes to therapy, a cautious pluralism seems to be the appropriate stance: it appears we need a variety of approaches if we are to improve the situation of individuals. Individual therapeutic requirements need to be assessed on a case-by-case basis. What matters is that a pluralist approach is always possible – and typically desirable – when it comes to treatment. As Murphy (2) rightly stresses, "Even if we have established that a symptom is best explained in terms of one main causal factor, such as neurotransmitter abnormality, it does not follow that treatment must be directed at directly manipulating that causal factor" [(2), p. 369].

This is all well and good, but Murphy (2) is almost completely silent about which non-scientific approaches and forms to therapy might be usefully brought to bear. And it is here that folk psychological narrative practices are likely to play a central role. This is because narratives are the familiar, everyday medium through which most of us readily evaluate and reflect upon our reasons, attitudes, and situations (24). Reviewing and recasting our narratives, with the assistance of others, is not only a way of making sense of our lives in new and fresh ways it can open up possibilities for living them differently[22]. Narrative practices afford such new possibilities precisely because they provide a means for thinking afresh about "who we are" based on richer understandings of our peculiar situations by revisiting our possible pasts and reimagining our possible futures.

Understanding FP as a kind of narrative practice in this way connects perfectly with the ambitions of narratively based therapies that seek to use so-called "talking cures" to empower people in the construction of a viable "future trajectory rather than achieving past accuracy" [(1), p. 14]. FP, as a special kind of narrative practice, is a possible object of philosophical and scientific study in a way that is wholly compatible with the modest rendering of the SI view argued for in the previous section. The views are compatible because FP, construed as a narrative practice, is not to be understood as a general theory embedded in that practice from which a philosophically discernable mark of the mental that defined mental disorders is to be sourced.[23]

CONCLUSION

There are excellent reasons to resist a forced choice between standard format FP and SI views of psychiatry. On the one hand, in its original variant, the FP view attempts to provide a definitive mark of all that is properly mental, which is imperialistic and isolationist. On the other hand, the SI view, at least when formulated in its popular cognitivist version, is unjustifiably and potentially unhelpfully overly narrow and neurocentric. Consequently, adopting either of these views of psychiatry in their standard forms threatens to leave us with an ideological vision of psychiatry's future that is too extreme and too limited. A better way forward is to salvage what is best from heavily edited versions of the familiar versions of the FP and SI views on the market, combining what remains to best effect.

Ultimately, the arguments presented here have been pitched at a quite general level, whereas to make good on this plan for reconciliation in a wholly convincing manner requires more detailed philosophical work on case studies in ways, which it

[20] Crucially, however, Murphy (2) insists that it is important to "distinguish between supplementing and replacing the medical model" (p. 367).

[21] Narrative therapy is, for example, neither scientifically focused nor scientifically based. It uses special techniques in order to provide the tools for empowering people, enabling them to exercise their agency in wider and more positive ways. Narrative therapy, although very much in the mould of "talking cures," is thus unlike more familiar psychoanalytic approaches to therapy in that it does not seek to divine and understand past causes of current trauma. Nevertheless, there seems no reason to discount narrative therapy as a bone fide therapy given that it is has been used successfully to help people deal better with a wide range of psychiatric and traumatic conditions, including asthma, anorexia, bulimia, and depression.

[22] Hutto DD, Gallagher S. Re-authoring narrative therapy: opening the way for future developments. *Philos Psychiatr Psychol* (Forthcoming).

[23] Whether FP should be understood as a narrative practice as opposed to, and distinct from, a theory of mind remains a controversial matter of dispute in the literature. It would take too much space to attempt to settle the issue or detail all the consequences of going one way rather than the other, in this paper. Extended arguments for treating FP as a narrative practice that does not reduce to theory can be found in Ref. (23, 25–28, Hutto DD, McGivern P. Updating the story of mental time travel: narrating and engaging with our possible pasts and futures. In: Altshuler R, Sigrist MJ, editors. *Time and the Philosophy of Action*. London: Routledge (Forthcoming)).

has not been possible to provide in this paper. But if the above arguments are sound, then the ambitions of this paper will have been realized and the ground will have been laid for those future, follow-up endeavors.

AUTHOR CONTRIBUTIONS

The author confirms being the sole contributor of this work and approved it for publication.

FUNDING

This work was supported by the Australian Research Council Discovery Project, Embodied Virtues and Expertise (DP: 1095109); the Marie-Curie Initial Training Network, TESIS: Towards an Embodied Science of InterSubjectivity (FP7-PEOPLE-2010-ITN, 264828); and the (Ministerio de Economía e innovación) Spanish DepartÂment of Economy and Innovation: Agency, Normativity and Identity: the Presence of the Subject in Actions (FFI-2011-25131).

REFERENCES

1. Graham G. *The Disordered Mind: An Introduction to Philosophy of Mind and Mental Illness.* London: Routledge (2009).
2. Murphy D. *Psychiatry in the Scientific Image.* Cambridge, MA: MIT Press (2006).
3. Gerrans P. *The Measure of Madness.* Cambridge, MA: MIT Press (2014).
4. Davidson D. Problems in the explanation of Action. In: Smart JJC, Pettit P, Sylvan R, Norman J, editors. *Metaphysics and Morality: Essays in Honour.* Oxford: Blackwell (1987). p. 35–49.
5. Davidson D. *Inquiries into Truth and Interpretation.* Oxford: Clarendon Press (1984).
6. Lewis DK. How to define theoretical terms. *J Philos* (1970) **67**:427–46. doi:10.2307/2023861
7. Lewis DK. Psychophysical and theoretical identifications. *Australas J Philos* (1972) **50**:249–58. doi:10.1080/00048407212341301
8. Jackson F. *From Metaphysics to Ethics.* Oxford: Oxford University Press (1998).
9. Carruthers P. *The Opacity of Mind: An Integrative Theory of Self-Knowledge.* Oxford: Oxford University Press (2011).
10. Hutto DD, Myin E. *Radicalizing Enactivism.* Cambridge, MA: MIT Press (2013).
11. Stich S. Autonomous psychology and the belief-desire thesis. *Monist* (1978) **61**(4):699–718. doi:10.5840/monist197861446
12. Fodor JA. Methodological solipsism considered as a research strategy in cognitive science. *Behav Brain Sci* (1980) **3**:63–73. doi:10.1017/S0140525X00001771
13. Hohwy J. *The Predictive Mind.* Oxford: Oxford University Press (2013).
14. Hohwy J. The self-evidencing brain. *Noûs* (2014). doi:10.1111/nous.12062
15. Rowlands M. Arguing about representation. *Synthese* (2015). doi:10.1007/s11229-014-0646-4
16. Hutto DD, Kirchhoff M, Myin E. Extensive enactivism: why keep it all in? *Front Hum Neurosci* (2014) **8**:706. doi:10.3389/fnhum.2014.00706
17. MurphyD,SmartG.Reviewofthedisorderedmind:anintroductiontophilosophy of mind and mental illness, George Graham. *Notre Dame Philosophical Reviews.* Routledge (2010). Available from: https://ndpr.nd.edu/news/24392-the-disordered-mind-an-introduction-to-philosophy-of-mind-and-mental-illness/
18. Seager W. *Theories of Consciousness.* London: Routledge (1999).
19. Shapiro L. When is cognition embodied? In: Kriegel U, editor. *Current Controversies in Philosophy of Mind.* London: Routledge (2014). p. 73–90.
20. Hutto DD. REC: revolution effected by clarification. *Topoi* (2015). doi:10.1007/s11245-015-9358-8
21. Orlandi N. *The Innocent Eye: Why Vision Is Not a Cognitive Process.* Oxford: Oxford University Press (2014).
22. Hutto DD. Overly enactive imagination? Radically re-imagining imagining. *South J Philos* (2015) **53**(S1):68–89. doi:10.1111/sjp.12122
23. Hutto DD. *Folk Psychological Narratives: The Sociocultural Basis of Understanding Reasons.* Cambridge, MA: MIT Press (2008).
24. Goldie P. *The Mess Inside: Narrative, Emotion and the Mind.* Oxford: Oxford University Press (2012).
25. Hutto DD. Folk psychology as narrative practice. *J Conscious Stud* (2009) **16**(6–8):9–39.
26. Hutto DD. ToM rules, but it is not ok. In: Costall A, Leudar I, editors. *Against Theory of Mind.* Basingstoke: Palgrave (2009). p. 221–38.
27. Hutto DD, Kirchhoff MD. Looking beyond the brain: social neuroscience meets narrative practice. *Cogn Syst Res* (2015) **34–35**:5–17. doi:10.1016/j.cogsys.2015.07.001
28. Hutto DD. Narrative understanding. In: Carroll N, Gibson J, editors. *The Routledge Companion to Philosophy of Literature.* London: Routledge (2016). p. 291–301.

2

Unraveling Executive Functioning in Dual Diagnosis

Judith C. L. M. Duijkers[1,2], Constance Th. W. M. Vissers[2,3] and Jos I. M. Egger[2,4,5,6]*

[1] Centre of Excellence for Korsakoff and Alcohol Related Cognitive Dysfunctions/Addiction Care, Vincent van Gogh Institute for Psychiatry, Venray, Netherlands, [2] Behavioural Science Institute, Radboud University Nijmegen, Nijmegen, Netherlands, [3] Kentalis Academy, Royal Dutch Kentalis, Sint-Michielsgestel, Netherlands, [4] Centre of Excellence for Neuropsychiatry, Vincent van Gogh Institute for Psychiatry, Venray, Netherlands, [5] Donders Institute for Brain, Cognition and Behaviour, Radboud University Nijmegen, Nijmegen, Netherlands, [6] Pompe Institute for Forensic Psychiatry, Pro Persona, Nijmegen, Netherlands

Edited by:
Leandro Fernandes Malloy-Diniz, Universidade Federal de Minas Gerais, Brazil

Reviewed by:
Charles W. Mathias, University of Texas Health Science Center San Antonio, USA
Emmy Uehara, Universidade Federal Rural do Rio de Janeiro, Brazil

***Correspondence:**
Judith C. L. M. Duijkers
jduijkers@vvgi.nl;
Judithonderzoek@hotmail.com

In mental health, the term dual-diagnosis is used for the co-occurrence of Substance Use Disorder (SUD) with another mental disorder. These co-occurring disorders can have a shared cause, and can cause/intensify each other's expression. Forming a threat to health and society, dual-diagnosis is associated with relapses in addiction-related behavior and a destructive lifestyle. This is due to a persistent failure to control impulses and the maintaining of inadequate self-regulatory behavior in daily life. Thus, several aspects of executive functioning like inhibitory, shifting and updating processes seem impaired in dual-diagnosis. Executive (dys-)function is currently even seen as a shared underlying key component of most mental disorders. However, the number of studies on diverse aspects of executive functioning in dual-diagnosis is limited. In the present review, a systematic overview of various aspects of executive functioning in dual-diagnosis is presented, striving for a prototypical profile of patients with dual-diagnosis. Looking at empirical results, inhibitory and shifting processes appear to be impaired for SUD combined with schizophrenia, bipolar disorder or cluster B personality disorders. Studies involving updating process tasks for dual-diagnosis were limited. More research that zooms in to the full diversity of these executive functions is needed in order to strengthen these findings. Detailed insight in the profile of strengths and weaknesses that underlies one's behavior and is related to diagnostic classifications, can lead to tailor-made assessment and indications for treatment, pointing out which aspects need attention and/or training in one's self-regulative abilities.

Keywords: executive functioning, dual-diagnosis, comorbidity, substance use disorder, alcohol use disorder, addiction, schizophrenia, bipolar

INTRODUCTION

In dual-diagnosis, a Substance Use Disorder (SUD) co-occurs with another psychiatric condition such as psychotic disorder, mood disorder, anxiety disorder or personality disorder (Ziedonis and Brady, 2005). The Epidemiologic Catchment Area study, a comprehensive study of comorbidity, showed that the lifetime SUDs-rate in the general population was 17%, compared to 48% for persons with schizophrenia and 56% for persons with bipolar disorder (Regier et al., 1990). SUD is described in respectively 27 and 24% of patients with a depressive disorder or an anxiety disorder (Mueser et al., 2011; Dom et al., 2013). Studying a dual-diagnosis population is relevant, because of the threat that SUD and dual-diagnosis form to health, society, and the presence of relapses in addiction-related behavior and destructive lifestyles (De Jong et al., 2006; World Health Organisation [WHO], 2011). In clinical practice dual-diagnosis frequently occurs whereas ideally distinguishable single disorder groups are rare. Disorders in dual-diagnosis can have a shared cause, or can cause/intensify each other's expression (Mueser et al., 1998). It is not always easy or possible to distinguish in which way the disorders causally interact or influence each other.

In most SUDs and other mental disorders self-regulatory behavior to manage daily life situations (involving work and relationships) falls short. Coping strategies are impaired, resulting in affective breakdowns (American Psychiatric Association, 2013). These frequently observed symptoms of psychiatric disorders point directly to deficits in executive functioning (EF) (among others: Barkley, 2001; Egger et al., 2007; Fernandez-Serrano et al., 2010; Wiers et al., 2012; Janssen, 2013; Luijten et al., 2013; Thoma and Daum, 2013; Goschke, 2014; Smith et al., 2014; Snyder et al., 2015). Executive (dis)-functioning is currently even seen as a shared underlying key component of most mental disorders (Egger et al., 2007; Janssen, 2013; Goschke, 2014; Snyder et al., 2015).

Executive functioning can be defined as all cognitive processes that regulate behavior in such a manner that it can be efficient and goal-orientated (Miyake et al., 2000; Barkley, 2001; Friedman et al., 2008; Miyake and Friedman, 2012; Snyder et al., 2015). Barkley (2001) describes EF as serving to "shift the control of behavior from the immediate context, social others, and the temporal now to self-regulation by internal representations regarding the hypothetical social future". Miyake et al. (2000) introduced a model of EF in which three key EF aspects were presented. Firstly, *Shifting* concerns the switch of attention between tasks/operations and/or mental sets. Translated into daily life, it involves mental flexibility to repeatedly let go of irrelevant and/or inappropriate behaviors (for example, drug use or attention bias to alcohol related cues) and switch to more adequate/relevant behaviors (like sporting or switch of television-channel). Secondly, *Updating* involves the process of actively manipulating and monitoring relevant information in working memory, in order to keep track of information that is old and needs actualization (Miyake et al., 2000). For SUD, it can involve craving. When longing for drugs, a patient may usually tend to call the drug dealer. But, in a recent relapse prevention session he or she learned about putting the numbers of supporting friends in their phone. As this is the first moment of intense craving after the session and intrusive substance-use thoughts already come to mind, the patient has to monitor his or her own behavior and promptly update these thoughts by thinking of the newly learned information and healthier thoughts. He or she needs to replace the old information about the drug dealer with the new information regarding their supportive friend's phone number. *Inhibition* is also needed in this scenario, and it is defined as the ability to inhibit dominant, automatic responses when necessary (Miyake et al., 2000; Barkley, 2001). *Inhibition is*, for instance, the suppression of approaching alcohol/drugs and/or calling the drug dealer. *Shifting, updating* and *inhibition* are all needed to some extent when making daily life decisions. For instance, when one wants to succeed in arriving at work on time tomorrow, thereby stopping destructive-avoidant behavior that was linked to one's SUD lifestyle: (i) *shifting* is needed to get up earlier than before and to repeatedly let go of attention biases triggering late night out fantasies, (ii) *inhibition* is needed to prevent this late night 'going out' with friends by stopping yourself from drinking/using and going home, (iii) *updating* is involved in checking an alternative work-route, thereby avoiding and replacing the old, coffee-shop route that would trigger craving. The interplay between EF aspects can influence self-regulation in daily life by reducing problem-behavior and raising more goal-directed behavior. In addition, EF can facilitate one's controlled coping with negative feelings and externalizing problem behaviors like substance-abuse/aggressive outbursts. On the contrary part, executive *dys*function can cause/aggravate negative feelings/behavioral outbursts by the perceived lack of control (Goschke, 2014).

The both unified and diverse aspects of EF can be placed in a model (Snyder et al., 2015, p. 13). EF can be assessed by global or more specific neurocognitive tasks (**Figure 1** for specific tasks). If severe executive dysfunctioning is expected, the use of both global and specific EF tasks is recommended by Snyder et al. (2015). *Inhibition* can be measured by Go–NoGo, Stop Signal, Approach Avoidance Tasks, the Stroop, Anti-saccade, Event Related Potential components like P300, self-report/rating measures such as the Frontal Systems Behavioral Scale, BIS-BAS scales (Behavioral Inhibition System-Behavioral Approach System) and by the MMPI-2 Impulse-Control index[1] (Stroop, 1935; Hallett, 1978; Butcher et al., 1989; Carver and White, 1994; Robbins et al., 1994; Roberts et al., 1994; Rogers and Monsell, 1995; Mayr and Kliegl, 2000; Grace and Malloy, 2001; Miyake et al., 2004; Handy, 2005; Franken et al., 2006; Friedman et al., 2008; Wiers et al., 2009; Wiers et al., 2010). *Shifting* can be measured by the Trail Making Test (Reitan, 1958), the Wisconsin Card Sorting Test (Berg, 1948), and other Category Switching Tasks. *Updating* can be measured by the letter memory task (Morris and Jones, 1990), keep track task (Yntema, 1963) or spatial n-back task.[1] *Updating* tasks involve monitoring of incoming information to check task-relevance, and replacement, update, of old non-relevant information by new information[1] (Snyder et al., 2015).

Impairments in EF aspects can trigger the appearance of mental disorders by several mechanisms such as (i) a failure to maintain goals when confronted with interfering desires that are difficult to *inhibit* and/or complicate *shifting* to more healthy goals, (ii) *inhibitory* impairment of impulsive responses, (iii) sticking attention to disorder-linked cues like substances that interfere with adequate *shifting*, (iv) impaired cognitive control (*inhibition*) and distorted anticipational planning, (v) reduced (emotional) stress regulation, and (vi) cognitive *in*flexibility (Goschke, 2014). These mechanisms negatively interfere with adequate impulse control and decision making, consequently also thwarting proper self-regulatory behavior in daily life.

Executive functioning impairments were described in several mental conditions like schizophrenia, bipolar-, anxiety-,

[1] Most of the tasks are described and categorized in a review by Snyder et al. (2015).

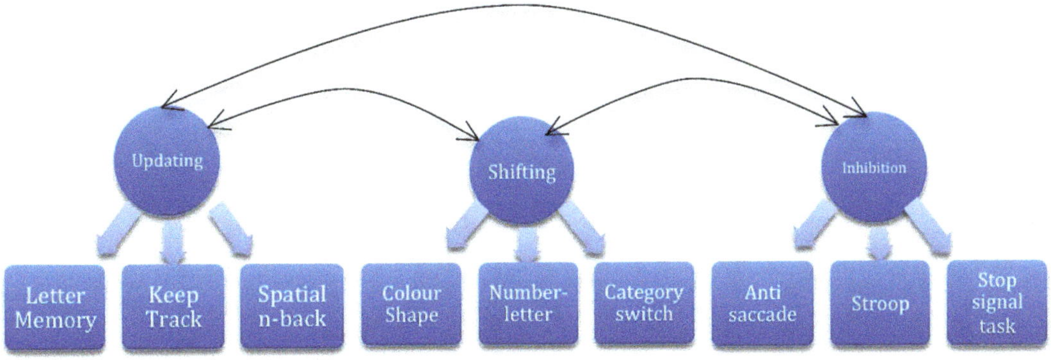

FIGURE 1 | Unified and diverse aspects of executive functioning (Snyder et al., 2015.)

personality-, developmental disorder, and SUD. For the separate disorders, a high number of studies have been undertaken and multiple reviews are present (see, among others, Verdejo-Garcia et al., 2006; Egger et al., 2007; Fernandez-Serrano et al., 2010; Wiers et al., 2012; Luijten et al., 2013; Thoma and Daum, 2013; Goschke, 2014; Smith et al., 2014; Snyder et al., 2015). Elaborating on this, one can expect that in dual-diagnosis EF will also be impaired. The majority of SUD-patients and half of schizophrenia/bipolar disorder patients are dually diagnosed. That makes insight into EF profiles for dual-diagnosis highly relevant, striving to unravel strengths and pitfalls for daily life behavior. For instance, the indications for treatment differ if one's pitfall primarily is the *inhibition* of undesired responses, or a flexible *shift* from one behavioral strategy to another. Recommendations for treatment can be formed when one oversees the differentiated profile of strengths and weaknesses, particularly in EF.

This article presents an overview of EF studies in dual-diagnosis.

MATERIALS AND METHODS

The inclusion criteria for studies were as follows: (i) A Method section that contains information concerning: (a) gender, age, test-materials and pre-assessment abstinence period of patients, and (b) diagnostic procedures that were used to determine if a dual-diagnosis was present or not; (ii) Comparisons by use of a healthy control group and/or a group without dual-diagnosis; and (iii) An abstinence period involving less risk for interfering influence of (sub-) acute substance effects, in order to only measure residual effects. The substance of study should not be traceable anymore. Studies with an abstinence period of at least one week were included. For cannabis, a period of four weeks was adhered to (for substance detection times see Verstraete, 2004; for interfering effects see Walvoort et al., 2013). Guidelines for PRISMA analysis were used to select papers (Moher et al., 2009). PRISMA analysis for Web of Science and PubMed resulted in 155 papers including the primary search terms of Executive Functioning AND dual-diagnosis. Four additional papers were found using other search term-combinations, and two additional papers were found by other sources such as on topic reviews (Rabin et al., 2011; Benaiges et al., 2010; Balanza-Martinez et al., 2015). Consequently, a total of 161 papers were screened (including duplicates). After screening, 131 papers were excluded for the following reasons: 121 papers involved the use of search terms in off-topic contexts: for instance, "dual" in "dual-task". Five studies concerned theoretical/qualitative research/reviews and five papers involved medical/different use of the dual-diagnosis term. 30 articles were assessed for eligibility. Of these, 19 were excluded after analysis, for the following reasons: 12 papers did not mention abstinence periods, two papers' method-sections did not contain gender/age/test materials, one paper was not found in full-text despite contacting authors and four papers were duplicates between searches. Finally, a total of 11 studies were selected based on the criteria (**Table 1**). Search terms were Executive Functioning, dual-diagnosis, Substance Use Disorder, alcohol use disorder, inhibition, updating, shifting, comorbidity, schizophrenia, bipolar disorder, personality disorder, anxiety disorder, mood disorder, developmental disorder, and addiction. The independent variable was the dual-diagnosis; the dependent variable was the level of functioning on EF tasks.

RESULTS

Findings are presented for 11 studies that involve the dual-diagnoses of SUD-Schizophrenia (six), SUD-Bipolar disorder (two), SUD-Personality disorders (two) and SUD-Conduct disorder (one). For SUD-Anxiety and SUD-Developmental disorder no studies were found. Results are organized by disorder, tasks and EF aspect. Significance levels and effect sizes are described if present (**Table 1**).

SUD-Schizophrenia

Rodriguez-Jiminez et al. (2010) performed the largest schizophrenia-SUD dual-diagnosis study, involving 82 patients with dual-diagnosis (Sch+) and 121 patients with Schizophrenia without SUD (Sch−). Results mostly showed comparable *Shifting* and EF general abilities for Sch+ and Sch−. The Sch+ group only functioned less at *Inhibitory* control as compared to the Sch− group. In two more studies, patients

TABLE 1 | Findings.

Dual-diagnosis	Authors	Tasks	*N*	Abstinence	Significant results
Schizophrenia and SUD	Benaiges et al., 2013	Trail Making Test (*Shifting*), Tower of Hanoi (*EF general*), Wisconsin Card Sorting Test (*Shifting, EF general*), Backwards digit subtest (*Working memory*), Iowa Gambling Task (*Decision Making*), Vocabulary (Other: premorbid verbal IQ)	30 DD 30 Schizophrenia without SUD 35 SUD	4 months	DD and SUD > Schizophrenia without SUD on: **Shifting* ($P < 0.05$, Effect Size 0.08) **Number of errors* ($P < 0.01$, Effect Size 0.13) *Speed ($P < 0.01$, Effect Size 0.10) SUD > Schizophrenia without SUD on: **Decision making* ($P < 0.05$, Effect Size 0.07)
Schizophrenia and SUD	Jockers-Scherübl et al., 2007	Trail Making Test (*Shifting*), Wisconsin Card Sorting Test (*Shifting, EF general*), Continuous Performance Test (Other); Wechsler Memory Scale (Other), WAIS-R subtests (Other)	19 DD 20 Schizophrenia without SUD 21 HC 18 SUD	28 days	#Premorbid IQ difference and education level (DD < SUD) (IQ $F = 7.88$, $P = 0.00$) #No Effect Sizes reported DD = Schizophrenia without SUD on: all measures (*Shifting, EF General*, Other) DD = SUD on: **Shifting* (Wisconsin Card Sorting Test) DD < SUD on: **Shifting* (Trail Making Test) ($F = 6.15$, $P = 0.02$) *WAIS Comprehension ($F = 18.71$, $P = 0.00$) Picture arrangement ($F = 4.45$, $P = 0.04$) Digit Symbol ($F = 4.66$, $P = 0.04$) *Verbal Memory($F = 11.29$, $P = 0.00$) *Attention (Symbols $F = 5.49$, $P = 0.03$; Digits $F = 6.80$, $P = 0.01$)

Schizophrenia and SUD	Rodriguez-Jiminez et al., 2010	Wisconsin Card Sorting Test (*Shifting, EF general*), Trail Making Test (*Shifting*), Stroop (*Inhibition*)	82 DD 121 Schizophrenia without SUD	1 month	#DD patients significantly younger age, more males and more psychotic episodes
					#No Effect Size reported #Age difference groups is factor of influence
					DD = Schizophrenia without SUD on: most executive measures (*Shifting, EF General*) DD < Schizophrenia without SUD on *Inhibition* task $P = 0.015$

Schizophrenia and SUD	Rodriguez-Jimenez et al., 2008	Wisconsin Card Sorting Test (*Shifting, EF general*)	65 DD 48 Schizophrenia without SUD	30 days	DD = Schizophrenia without SUD on: **Shifting* ($F = 0.382$, $P = 0.538$) **Perseverative Errors* ($F = 0.396$, $P = 0.530$)
Schizophrenia and SUD	Schnell et al., 2009	Trail Making test (*Shifting*), Verbal Fluency (*EF general*), Dual-Tasking (*EF*), Letter Number Span (*Working Memory*), Digit Symbol Test (Other), Auditory Verbal Learning and Memory Test (Other)	35 DD 34 Schizophrenia without SUD	3 weeks	DD > Schizophrenia without SUD on **Executive Function* **Working Memory* (Sum tasks $T = 2.923$, $P = 0.005$) (Max. span $T = 2.349$, $P = 0.022$) **Shifting* ($T = -2.590$, $P = 0.012$) *Verbal memory (Delayed recall $T = 2.263$, $P = 0.027$) (Recognition $T = 2.246$, $P = 0.028$) DD < Schizophrenia without SUD on academic achievement and vocabulary #Level of education in DD is lower than in Schizophrenia without SUD group #No Effect Sizes reported

(Continued)

TABLE 1 | Continued

Dual-diagnosis	Authors	Tasks	*N*	Abstinence	Significant results
Schizophrenia and SUD	Sevy et al., 2007	Trail Making Test (*Shifting*), Iowa Gambling Task (*Decision Making*), Controlled oral word association test (*EF*), CPT Identical Pairs test, Digit span subtest Wechsler Adult Intelligence Scale, California Verbal Learning test (all Other)	14 DD, 20 HC 13 Schizophrenia without SUD	1 week	#DD less education than Schizophrenia without SUD and HC group Schizophrenia (DD AND Schizophrenia without SUD) < HC on: **Shifting* ability *Other measured neurocognitive functions (NB: Not study topic!) DD and Schizophrenia without SUD = HC on: **Emotion-based decision-making* DD > Schizophrenia without SUD on: Digit span ($P < 0.048$)
Bipolar disorder and SUD	Marshall et al., 2012	Wisconsin Card Sorting Test (*Shifting, EF general*), Stroop (*Inhibition*), Parametric Go/No-Go task (*Inhibition*), FAS verbal fluency test (*EF*), Rey Complex Figure Test (*planning and other*), California verbal learning test-II, Purdue Pegboard test, Emotion Perception Test, Facial Emotion Perception Test, Digit Symbol Coding (all Other)	158 DD 97 HC 98 Bipolar without SUD	6 months	#Less education DD #No Effect Sizes reported DD < HC on: **Conceptual Reasoning and set-Shifting* (*Shifting*) ($F = 9.68$, $P = 0.001$) *Processing Speed and interference resolution (*Inhibition*) ($F = 15.88$, $P < 0.001$) **Inhibitory control* ($F = 5.50$, $P = 0.007$) *Visual Memory ($F = 8.84$, $P = 0.001$) *Fine Motor skill ($F = 10.32$, $P < 0.001$, DD < Bipolar without SUD on: **Shifting* ($P < 0.01$) *Visual memory ($P < 0.01$) *Conceptual reasoning ($P < 0.01$)
Bipolar disorder and SUD	Van Gorp et al., 1998	Wisconsin Card Sorting Test (*Shifting, EF general*), Stroop (*Inhibition*), Trail Making Test (*Shifting*), FAS verbal fluency test (*EF*), Rey Complex Figure Test (*Planning and other*) California verbal learning test (Other), National Adult Reading Test (Other)	12 DD 22 HC 13 Bipolar without SUD	6 months	#No Effect Sizes reported DD < HC on: **Shifting* (less finished categories on Wisconsin Card Sorting Test; $F = 4.2469$, $P = 0.02$) **Errors* Wisconsin Card Sorting Test ($F = 3.627$, $P = 0.04$) *Verbal memory ($F = 6.0427$, $P = 0.005$) Bipolar without SUD < HC on: *Verbal memory ($F = 6.0427$, $P = 0.005$) **Errors* Wisconsin Card Sorting Test ($F = 3.627$, $P = 0.04$)
Personality disorder and SUD	Albein-Urios et al., 2014	Letter-number sequencing (*Updating*), 2-back task (*Updating*), Delis-Kaplan Executive Function System Color Word Interference Test (*Inhibition and Shifting*), Category test (*Shifting*), D2 (Other)	37 DD 36 SUD 34 HC	>15 days	DD Cluster B PD < HC on: **Attention/Inhibition* ($F = 5.832$, $P < 0.001$, Effect Size 1.0) ($F = 2.866$, $P < 0.05$, Effect Size 0.7) ($F = 3.643$, $P < 0.05$, Effect Size 0.7) *Concentration ($F = 6.735$, $P < 0.001$, Effect Size 1.1) DD Cluster C PD < HC on: **Working memory* ($F = 5.591$, $P < 0.001$, Effect Size 1.1) **Updating* ($F = 4.021$, $P < 0.01$, Effect Size 1.1) *Concentration (no significance digit Effect Size 1.0) *Efficiency ($F = 5.433$, $P < 0.01$, Effect Size 1.0) SUD < HC on: **Shifting* ($F = 3.818$, $P < 0.05$, Effect Size 0.7) **Working memory* (no significance digit Effect Size 1.0) *Concentration (no significance digit Effect Size 0.9) *Efficiency (no significance digit Effect Size 0.8)

(Continued)

TABLE 1 | Continued

Dual-diagnosis	Authors	Tasks	*N*	Abstinence	Significant results
Personality disorder and SUD	Albein-Urios et al., 2013	Letter-number sequencing (*Updating*), 2-back task (*Updating*), Stroop (*Inhibition*), Category test (*Shifting*), D2 (Other)	32 DD 44 SUD 34 HC	>15 days	DD < HC on: **Shifting* ($F = 6.59$, $P = 0.002$, Effect Size 0.85) **Updating* ($F = 5.10$, $P = 0.008$, Effect Size 0.76) **Inhibition* ($F = 5.98$, $P = 0.003$, Effect Size 0.79) *Attention Total D2 score ($F = 10.85$, $P = 0.000$, Effect Size 1.01) Concentration D2 ($F = 14.60$, $P = 0.000$, Effect Size 1.24) Fluctuation D2 ($F = 12.27$, $P = 0.000$, Effect Size 1.05) DD < SUD on: *Attention (Effect Size 0.79, no significance digit) **Inhibition* (Effect Size 0.50, no significance digit)
Conduct disorder and SUD	Giancola and Mezzich, 2000	Porteus Maze Test (*Planning*), Vigilance Test (*Inhibition*), Motor restraint test (*Inhibition*), Stroop (*Inhibition*), Test Language Competence (Other), Peabody Individual Achievement Test-Revised (Other), WISC/WAIS-R (Other)	239 DD 63 SUD (+other disorders) 58 Conduct dis. without SUD 110 HC	2 weeks	#SUD and Conduct Disorder groups also have other psychiatric disorders, so not "only" disorders DD < HC on: **Inhibition* ($F = 5.48$, $P < 0.01$; $F = 4.55$, $P < 0.01$) **Planning* ($F = 4.41$, $P < 0.01$) *Intelligence, *Language *Academic Achievement

DD, Dual -diagnosis; HC, healthy controls; <functioning: worse level of functioning; >functioning: better functioning; SUD, Substance Use Disorder.

with Sch+ and patients with Sch− had similar results for several *shifting* tasks (Jockers-Scherübl et al., 2007; Rodriguez-Jimenez et al., 2008). Contradictory to those findings, two studies showed better functioning for patients with Sch+ as compared to Sch− on *shifting* abilities (Schnell et al., 2009; Benaiges et al., 2013). Furthermore, in one study, patients with Sch+ functioned less adequate at *shifting* (Trail Making Test) and *inhibition* tasks than patients with Sch− (Jockers-Scherübl et al., 2007). Lastly, Sevy et al., 2007; including a healthy control group) showed worse *shifting* abilities for Sch+ patients (schizophrenia-cannabis) as compared to healthy controls.

SUD-Bipolar Mood Disorder

Patients with SUD-bipolar disorder showed poorer functioning on mental *shifting* ability as compared to healthy controls, measured by the Wisconsin Card Sorting Test. That is, dual-diagnosis patients completed fewer categories than controls (Van Gorp et al., 1998). Marshall et al. (2012) described that patients with SUD-bipolar disorder had more executive (*inhibitory control, set-shifting,* and *interference resolution*) dysfunctions than controls and patients with bipolar disorder without SUD.

SUD-Personality Disorders

In 2013 and 2014, cocaine abusing patients with cluster B (borderline, narcissistic, histrionic, and anti-social) and cluster C (avoidant, dependent, and obsessive compulsive) personality disorders were studied at diverse EF. Patients with SUD-cluster B personality disorders, that is, more impulsive personality types, showed impairments in nearly all EF aspects as compared to controls and most specifically in *inhibitory control.* Patients with SUD-cluster C personality disorders, that is, more inhibited and obsessive personality types, showed more problems in *working memory* and *updating* ability. Patients with SUD as compared to the dual-diagnosis group had a better *inhibitory control.* However, compared to healthy controls, the SUD group also showed impairments in *shifting* and *working memory.* Patients with dual-diagnosis SUD-Personality disorders as a group consistently functioned less on *shifting, updating* and *inhibitory* abilities as compared to healthy controls (Albein-Urios et al., 2013; Albein-Urios et al., 2014).

SUD-Conduct Disorder

One study compared 239 females with dual-diagnosis to healthy controls. Impairments were shown for the dual-diagnosis group on *inhibition* and *planning* ability as compared to healthy controls (Giancola and Mezzich, 2000).

SUD-Anxiety Disorders, Developmental Disorders

Despite frequent co-occurrence of SUD-anxiety or SUD-developmental disorders (for prevalence numbers see Dom et al., 2013), we found no studies on EF for these groups.

DISCUSSION

Aim and Model

Aim and Model Gaining a prototypical profile of EF for dual-diagnosis. This is expected to contribute to tailor-made directions for treatment.

Findings

Findings Shifting and *inhibitory control* mostly are compromised in patients with dual-diagnosis as compared to healthy controls. If one were to think of dual-diagnosis and its overt behavioral symptoms, it is quite conceivable that dual-diagnosis implicates a high amount of (affective) turbulence and sensory sensitivity, since both substances and psychotic/bipolar/other symptoms have an interfering influence on the balance of several brain processes. Elaborating on this, maintaining a realistic view of daily life situations with flexible participation and properly timed inhibition when needed, is likely to be impaired. As compared to Sch−, patients with Sch+ show less *inhibitory control*. One possible explanation for this difference may be that patients with a SUD-combination show relatively more impulsivity, partly because the use of substances may negatively influence their dopaminergic *inhibitory* brain processes. Thereby, they seem to be less capable of inhibiting desires than patients without SUD. Furthermore, with a view to negative symptomatology, the schizophrenia patient-group is possibly more avoidant/*inhibited* than approaching in behavior manner. In terms of impulsivity, this hypothetical explanation also applies to the finding that patients with cluster B (impulsive type) personality disorder and SUD perform *inhibitory control* tasks less adequately than patients with only SUD. Whereas impulsive behavior has shown to negatively interfere with *inhibitory control*, it can also be influenced vice versa: common impulsive behavior in dual-diagnoses such as SUD-Bipolar disorder, SUD-cluster B Personality disorder and SUD-Conduct disorder (American Psychiatric Association, 2013) may be maintained or even urged by executive impairments. Impulsivity however seems to have a positive counterpart as well: the finding that Sch+ patients function slightly better on *shifting* abilities than Sch− patients may be linked to a higher tendency for impulsiveness and search for novelty in patients with SUD-combinations. This means that a flexible switch from familiar pathways to other routes may be easier for persons that are more impulsive and less rigid in behavior than for more avoidant persons that may seek and/or persevere in familiar styles of behavior.

Limitations Concerning Dual-Diagnosis Research

Some conflicting findings reduce the certainty with which conclusions can be stated. These contradictions may be partly caused by factors that influenced several studies, and that may have restricted the validity and reliability of the observed empirical findings in those studies. For instance, the study of Jockers-Scherübl et al. (2007), that of Schnell et al. (2009) and that of Sevy et al. (2007) involved differences in education levels between the Sch+ (lower education level) and Sch− group. Furthermore, in one study the Sch+ group included younger patients and involved more males than the Sch− group. The differences in age actually showed to be a factor in differences found between the groups; so the observed weakened inhibitory control may be affected by the younger age of the dual-diagnosis group (study of Rodriguez-Jiminez et al., 2010). Complications in dual-diagnosis research are possibly due to several reasons. Sample sizes are mostly modest because it is difficult to recruit patients that (i) are in a mild psychiatric state needed for sufficient testability, (ii) are motivated to cooperate and stop using substances, and (iii) have achieved substance-abstinence for a reasonable time prior to assessment, ideally confirmed by tests. A pre-assessment abstinence period of at least six weeks is best, in case of alcohol, but probably for other substances as well, due to the recovery that the body undergoes in this period of time (Weeda et al., 2006; Walvoort et al., 2013). The length of substance abstinence and methods are not always clearly documented, which reduces the validity and reliability of conclusions. Furthermore, when testing patients with dual-diagnosis, it is not clear which disorder and/or substance contributes to which specific empirical finding (Balanza-Martinez et al., 2015). Partly for that reason, disorders and substances are usually studied "separately". But procedures for dual-diagnosis presence are not always described. This makes it ambiguous whether separate disorders or dual-diagnosis is studied. For example, Giancola and Mezzich (2000) described a "SUD without dual-diagnosis" group in which no Conduct Disorder was present (2000); however, other psychiatric diagnoses were present in this "SUD" group, making it still a "dual-diagnosis" group.

Future Research

Findings lead to the following future research recommendations. Firstly, studying dual-diagnosis has value, when methods are described in a valid manner. Secondly, sufficiently long abstinence periods before assessment, preferably approximately 6 weeks, should be attained to prevent findings from being influenced by acute or sub-acute substance use effects (Weeda et al., 2006; Walvoort et al., 2013). Thirdly, the use of healthy control groups is highly recommended to enable valid comparisons. Fourthly, studies need to be performed in patient groups that also exist in clinical practice, such as dual-diagnosis involving anxiety and developmental disorders. Fifthly, research on all diverse aspects of EF is recommended, also involving Updating processes/working memory. Impairments in flexible shifting abilities, updating processes, or impairments in inhibitory control over undesired responses will most probably lead to different indications for treatment. Finally, findings as described should get more strength through follow up research, including the test of the stated impulsivity hypothesis. Elaborating on these recommendations, there are promising results regarding EF treatment interventions, for instance with Dys-executive Syndrome Treatment Programs and Approach-Avoidance/Inhibitory Intervention Training (among others, Boelen et al., 2012; Rinck et al., 2013; Sharbanee et al., 2014). Hence, unraveling EF in dual-diagnosis has great value for coaching and treatment of patients, and it illustrates how the gap between neuroscience and psychotherapy can be bridged.

AUTHOR CONTRIBUTIONS

JD was first and corresponding author. She performed the literature search for this mini-review and wrote several concepts of the manuscript. She consulted CV on a regular basis as second author to revise concept manuscript versions and sharpen the described theoretical and empirical issues. CV revised concept versions and JE as last author was available for consultation during the project and revised the final concept version of the manuscript. In the end, the final manuscript and cover letter to be submitted was carefully revised by all three authors en JD eventually submitted the manuscript as first author.

ACKNOWLEDGMENTS

The authors express their thanks to Mr. Remco. J. Somers, Mrs. Ingeborg L. Kiers, MSc, and Mrs. Anja J. C. M. Haaze-Schoof for english language evaluation of the manuscript.

REFERENCES

Albein-Urios, N., Martinez-Gonzalez, J. M., Lozano, O., Moreno-Lopez, L., Soriano-Mas, C., and Verdejo-Garcia, A. (2013). Negative urgency, disinhibition and reduced temporal pole gray matter characterize the comorbidity of cocaine dependence and personality disorders. *Drug. Alcohol Depend.* 132, 131–137. doi: 10.1016/j.drugalcdep2013.02.008

Albein-Urios, N., Martinez-Gonzalez, J. M., Lozano-Royas, O., and Verdejo-Garcia, A. (2014). Executive functions in cocaine-dependent patients with cluster B and cluster C personality disorders. *Neuropsychology* 28, 84–90. doi: 10.1037/neu0000007

American Psychiatric Association (2013). *Diagnostic and Statistical Manual of Mental Disorders, DSM-5*, 5th Edn. Arlington: American Psychiatric Association.

Balanza-Martinez, V., Crespo-Facorro, B., Gonzalez-Pinto, A., and Vieta, E. (2015). Bipolar disorder comorbid with alcohol use disorder: focus on neurocognitive correlates. *Front. Physiol.* 6:108. doi: 10.3389/fphys.2015.00108

Barkley, R. A. (2001). The executive functions and self-regulation: an evolutionary neuropsychological perspective. *Neuropsychol. Rev.* 11, 1–29. doi: 10.1023/A:1009085417776

Benaiges, I., Prat, G., and Adan, A. (2010). Neuropsychological aspects of dual diagnosis. *Curr. Drug Abuse Rev.* 3, 175–188. doi: 10.2174/1874473711003030175

Benaiges, I., Serra-Grabulosa, J. M., Prat, G., and Adan, A. (2013). Executive functioning in individuals with schizophrenia and/or cocaine dependence. *Hum. Psychopharmacol.* 28, 29–39. doi: 10.1002/hup.2279

Berg, E. A. (1948). A simple objective technique for measuring flexibility in thinking. *J. Gen. Psychol.* 39, 15–22. doi: 10.1080/00221309.1948.9918159

Boelen, D., Spikman, J. M., Lamberts, K., Brouwer, W. H., and Fasotti, L. (2012). *Behandeling Van het Ddysexecutief Syndroom.* Amsterdam: Boom.

Butcher, J. N., Dahlstrom, W. G., Graham, J. R., Tellegen, A., and Kaemmer, B. (1989). *The Minnesota Multiphasic Personality Inventory-2 (MMPI-2): Manual for administration and scoring.* Minneapolis, MN: University of Minnesota Press.

Carver, C. S., and White, T. L. (1994). Behavioural inhibition, behavioural activation, and affective responses to impending reward and punishment: the BIS/BAS scales. *J. Pers. Soc. Psychol.* 62, 319–333. doi: 10.1037/0022-3514.67.2.319

De Jong, C. A. J., Schellekens, A. F. A., Ellenbroek, B., Franke, B., and Verkes, R.-J. (2006). *The Course of Addiction: Neurobiological Predictors of Chronicity.* Cambridge, MA: Academic publications.

Dom, G., Dijkhuizen, A., van der Hoorn, B., Kroon, H., Muusse, C., van Rooijen, S., et al. (2013). *Handboek Dubbele Diagnose.* Utrecht: de Tijdstroom.

Egger, J. I. M., De Mey, H. R. A., and Janssen, G. T. L. (2007). Assessment of executive functioning in psychiatric disorders: functional diagnosis as the ouverture of treatment. *Clin. Neuropsychiatry* 4, 111–116.

Fernandez-Serrano, M. J., Perez-Garcia, M., Schmidt Rio-Valle, J., and Verdejo-Garcia, A. (2010). Neuropsychological consequences of alcohol and drug abuse on different components of executive functions. *J. Psychopharmacol.* 24, 1317–1332. doi: 10.1177/0269881109349841

Franken, I. H. A., Muris, P., and Georgieva, I. (2006). Gray's model of personality and addiction. *Addict. Behav.* 31, 399–403. doi: 10.1016/j.addbeh.2005.05.022

Friedman, N. P., Miyake, A., Young, S. E., Defries, J. C., Corley, R. P., and Hewitt, J. K. (2008). Individual differences in executive functions are almost entirely genetic in origin. *Gen. J. Exp. Psychol.* 137, 201–225. doi: 10.1037/0096-3445.137.2.201

Giancola, P. R., and Mezzich, A. C. (2000). Neuropsychological deficits in female adolescents with a substance use disorder: better accounted for by conduct disorder? *J. Stud. Alcohol* 61, 809–817. doi: 10.15288/jsa.2000.61.809

Goschke, T. (2014). Dysfunctions of decision-making and cognitive control as transdiagnostic mechanisms of mental disorders: advances, gaps and needs in current research. *Int. J. Methods Psychiatr. Res.* 23, 41–57. doi: 10.1002/mpr.1410

Grace, J., and Malloy, P. F. (2001). *Frontal Systems Behavioral Scale (FrSBe): Professional Manual.* Lutz, FL: Psychological Assessment Resources.

Hallett, P. E. (1978). Primary and secondary saccades to goals defined by instructions. *Vision Res.* 18, 1279–1296. doi: 10.1016/0042-6989(78)90218-3

Handy, T. C. (2005). *Event-Related Potentials.* Cambridge, MA: The MIT Press.

Janssen, G. T. L. (2013). *Diagnostic Assessment of Psychiatric Patients: A Contextual Perspective on Executive Functioning.* Nijmegen: Donders Series.

Jockers-Scherübl, M. C., Wolf, T., Radzei, N., Schlattmann, P., Rentzsch, J., Gomez-Carrillo de Castro, A., et al. (2007). Cannabis induces different cognitive changes in schizophrenic patients and in healthy controls. *Prog. Neuropsychopharmacol. Biol. Psychiatry* 31, 1054–1063. doi: 10.1016/j.pnpbp.2007.03.006

Luijten, M., Machielsen, M. W. J., Veltman, D. J., Hester, R., de Haan, L., and Franken, I. H. A. (2013). Systematic review of ERP and fMRI studies investigating inhibitory control and error processing in people with substance dependence and behavioural addictions. *J. Psychiatry Neurosci.* 39, 149–169. doi: 10.1503/jpn.130052

Marshall, D. F., Walker, S. J., Ryan, K. A., Kamali, M., Saunders, E. F. H., Weldon, A. L., et al. (2012). Greater executive and visual memory dysfunction in comorbid bipolar disorder and substance use disorder. *Psychiatry Res.* 200, 252–257. doi: 10.1016/j.psychres.2012.06.013

Mayr, U., and Kliegl, R. (2000). Task-set switching and long-term memory retrieval. *J. Exp. Psychol. Learn. Mem. Cogn.* 26, 1124–1140. doi: 10.1037//0278-7393.26.5.1124

Miyake, A., Emerson, M. J., Padilla, F., and Ahn, J. C. (2004). Inner speech as a retrieval aid for task goals: the effects of cue type and articulatory suppression in the random task cuing paradigm. *Acta Psychol.* 115, 123–142. doi: 10.1016/j.actpsy.2003.12.004

Miyake, A., and Friedman, N. P. (2012). The nature and organization of individual differences in executive functions: four general conclusions. *Curr. Dir. Psychol. Sci.* 21, 8–14. doi: 10.1177/0963721411429458

Miyake, A., Friedman, N. P., Emerson, M. J., Witzki, A. H., and Howerter, A. (2000). The unity and diversity of executive functions and their contributions to complex "frontal lobe" tasks: a latent variable analysis. *Cogn. Psychol.* 41, 49–100. doi: 10.1006/cogp.1999.0734

Moher, D., Liberati, A., Tetzlaff, J., Altman, D. G., and The Prisma Group (2009). Preferred reporting items for systematic reviews and meta analyses: the PRISMA statement. *PLoS Med.* 6:e1000097. doi: 10.1371/journal.pmed1000097

Morris, N., and Jones, D. M. (1990). Memory updating in working memory: the role of the central executive. *Br. J. Psychol.* 81, 111–121. doi: 10.1111/j.2044-8295.1990.tb02349.x

Mueser, K. T., Drake, R. E., and Wallach, M. A. (1998). Dual diagnosis: a review of etiological theories. *Addict. Behav.* 23, 717–734. doi: 10.1016/S0306-4603(98)00073-2

Mueser, K. T., Noordsy, D. L., Drake, R. E., and Fox, L. (2011). *Geïntegreerde Behandeling Van Dubbele Diagnose. Een Richtlijn Voor Effectieve Behandeling.* Utrecht: de Tijdstroom.

Rabin, R. A., Zakzanis, K. K., and George, T. P. (2011). The effects of cannabis use on neurocognition in schizophrenia: a meta-analysis. *Schizophr. Res.* 128, 111–116. doi: 10.1016/j.schres.2011.02.017

Regier, D. A., Farmer, M. E., Rae, D. S., Locke, B. Z., Keith, S. J., Judd, L. L., et al. (1990). Comorbidity of mental disorders with alcohol and other drug abuse. Results from the Epidemiologic Catchment Area study. *JAMA* 264, 2511–2518. doi: 10.1001/jama.264.19.2511

Reitan, R. M. (1958). Validity of the trail making test as an indicator of organic brain damage. *Percept. Motor Skills* 8, 271–276. doi: 10.1080/13803395.2015.1052732

Rinck, M., Telli, S., Kampmann, I. L., Woud, M. L., Kerstholt, M., Velthuis te, S., et al. (2013). Training approach-avoidance of smiling faces affects emotional vulnerability in socially anxious individuals. *Front. Hum. Neurosci.* 7:481. doi: 10.3389/fnhum.2013.00481

Robbins, T. W., James, M., Owen, A. M., Sahakian, B. J., Mc Innes, L., and Rabbitt, P. (1994). Cambridge neuropsychological test automated battery (CANTAB): a factor analytic study of a large sample of normal elderly volunteers. *Dementia* 5, 266–281. doi: 10.1159/000106735

Roberts, R. J., Hager, L. D., and Heron, C. (1994). Prefrontal cognitive processes: working memory and inhibition in the antisaccade task. *Gen. J. Exp. Psychol.* 123, 374–393. doi: 10.1037/0096-3445.123.4.374

Rodriguez-Jimenez, R., Aragües, M., Jiminez-Arriero, M. A., Ponce, G., Martinez, I., Hoenicka, J., et al. (2008). Psychopathology and Wisconsin card sorting test performance in male schizophrenic patients: influence of Dual Diagnosis. *Psychopathology* 41, 58–64. doi: 10.1159/000110627

Rodriguez-Jiminez, R., Bagney, A., Martinez-Gras, I., Ponce, G., Sanchez-Morla, E. M., Aragües, M., et al. (2010). Executive function in schizophrenia: influence of substance use disorder history. *Schizophr. Res.* 118, 34–40. doi: 10.1016/j.schres.2009.09.0259

Rogers, R. D., and Monsell, S. (1995). Costs of a predictable switch between simple cognitive tasks. *Gen. J. Exp. Psychol.* 124, 207–231. doi: 10.1037/0096-3445.124.2.207

Schnell, T., Koethe, D., Daumann, J., and Gouzoulis-Mayfrank, E. (2009). The role of cannabis in cognitive functioning of patients with schizophrenia. *Psychopharmacology* 205, 45–52. doi: 10.1007/s00213-009-1512-9

Sevy, S., Burdick, K. E., Visweswaraiah, H., Abdelmessih, S., Lukin, M., Yechiam, E., et al. (2007). Iowa gambling task in schizophrenia and co-occurring cannabis use disorders. *Schizophr. Res.* 92, 74–84. doi: 10.1016/j.schres.2007.01.005

Sharbanee, J. M., Hu, L., Stritzke, W. G., Wiers, R. W., Rinck, M., and MacLeod, C. (2014). The effect of approach/avoidance training on alcohol consumption is mediated by change in alcohol action tendency. *PLoS ONE* 9:e85855. doi: 10.1371/journal.pone.0085855

Smith, J. L., Mattick, R. P., Jamadar, S. D., and Iredale, J. M. (2014). Deficits in behavioural inhibition in substance abuse and addiction: a meta-analysis. *Drug Alcohol Depend.* 145, 1–33. doi: 10.1016/j.drugalcdep.2014.08.009

Snyder, H. R., Miyake, A., and Hankin, B. L. (2015). Advancing understanding of executive function impairments and psychopathology: bridging the gab between clinical and cognitive approaches. *Front. Psychol.* 6:328. doi: 10.3389/fpsyg.2015.00328

Stroop, J. R. (1935). Studies of interference in serial verbal reactions. *J. Exp. Psychol.* 18, 643–662. doi: 10.1037/0096-3445.121.1.15

Thoma, P., and Daum, I. (2013). Comorbid substance use disorder in schizophrenia: a selective overview of neurobiological and cognitive underpinnings. *Psychiatry Clin. Neurosci.* 67, 367–383. doi: 10.1111/pcn.12072

Van Gorp, W., Altshuler, L., Theberge, D. C., Wilkins, J., and Dixon, W. (1998). Cognitive impairment in euthymic bipolar patients with and without prior alcohol dependence: a preliminary study. *Arch. Gen. Psychiatry* 55, 41–66. doi: 10.1001/archpsyc.55.1.41

Verdejo-Garcia, A., Bechara, A., Recknor, E. C., and Perez-Garcia, M. (2006). Executive dysfunction in substance dependent individuals during drug use and abstinence: an examination of the behavioral, cognitive and emotional correlates of addiction. *J. Int. Neuropsychol. Soc.* 12, 405–415. doi: 10.1017/S1355617706060486

Verstraete, A. G. (2004). Detection times of drugs of abuse in blood, urine, and oral fluid. *Ther. Drug Monit.* 26, 200–205. doi: 10.1097/00007691-200404000-00020

Walvoort, S., Wester, A. J., and Egger, J. I. M. (2013). Neuropsychologische diagnostiek en cognitieve functies bij alcoholabstinentie. *Tijdschr. Voor Psychiatr.* 55, 101–111.

Weeda, M. R., Peters, B. D., De Haan, L., and Linszen, D. H. (2006). Blijvende neuropsychologische stoornissen en structurele en functionele hersenafwijkingen na langdurig cannabisgebruik. *Tijdschr. Voor Psychiatr.* 48, 185–193.

Wiers, R. W., Cousijn, J., Mors-Schulte, M., den Uijl, T., Goudriaan, A., Schilt, T., et al. (2012). *State of the Art Neurocognitieve Effecten van Verslaving.* Den Haag: ZonMW.

Wiers, R. W., Rinck, M., Dictus, M., and van den Wildenberg, E. (2009). Relatively strong automatic appetitive action-tendencies in male carriers of the OPRM1G-allele. *Genes Brain Behav.* 8, 101–106. doi: 10.1111/j.1601-183X.2008.00454.x

Wiers, R. W., Rinck, M., Kordts, R., Houben, K., and Strack, F. (2010). Retraining automatic action-tendencies to approach alcohol in hazardous drinkers. *Addiction* 105, 279–287. doi: 10.1111/j.1360-0443.2009.02775.x

World Health Organisation [WHO] (2011). *Global Status Report on Alcohol and Health.* Geneva: WHO Press.

Yntema, D. B. (1963). Keeping track of several things at once. *Hum. Fact.* 5, 7–17. doi: 10.1177/001872086300500102

Ziedonis, D., and Brady, K. (2005). Dual diagnosis in primary care: detecting and treating both the addiction and mental illness. *Med. Clin. N. A.* 81, 1017–1036. doi: 10.1016/S0025-7125(05)705617

3

Circadian Rhythms and Mood Disorders: Are the Phenomena and Mechanisms Causally Related?

William Bechtel

Department of Philosophy and Center for Circadian Biology, University of California San Diego, San Diego, CA, USA

Edited by:
Leon De Bruin,
VU University Amsterdam,
Netherlands

Reviewed by:
Oksana Sorokina,
The University of Edinburgh, UK
Kyle B. Gustafson,
École Polytechnique Fédérale de Lausanne, Switzerland
Victor Gijsbers,
Universiteit Leiden, Netherlands

Correspondence:
William Bechtel,
Department of Philosophy, University of California San Diego, 9500 Gilman Drive, San Diego, CA 92093-0119, USA
bechtel@ucsd.edu

This paper reviews some of the compelling evidence of disrupted circadian rhythms in individuals with mood disorders (major depressive disorder, seasonal affective disorder, and bipolar disorder) and that treatments such as bright light, designed to alter circadian rhythms, are effective in treating these disorders. Neurotransmitters in brain regions implicated in mood regulation exhibit circadian rhythms. A mouse model originally employed to identify a circadian gene has proven a potent model for mania. While this evidence is suggestive of an etiological role for altered circadian rhythms in mood disorders, it is compatible with other explanations, including that disrupted circadian rhythms and mood disorders are effects of a common cause and that genes and proteins implicated in both simply have pleiotropic effects. In light of this, the paper advances a proposal as to what evidence would be needed to establish a direct causal link between disruption of circadian rhythms and mood disorders.

Keywords: mood disorders, circadian rhythms, mechanistic explanations, causal relations between mechanisms

Introduction

Much biological research over the past 200 years has proceeded by delineating individual phenomena and explaining each distinct phenomenon by characterizing the responsible mechanism (1). Discovering mechanisms involves localizing the phenomenon in a responsible system that is taken to be the mechanism and then decomposing that system structurally to discover its component parts and functionally to discover the operations those parts perform (2–4). To show that the parts and operations suffice for the phenomenon requires recomposing the mechanism by mentally rehearsing the operations or employing computational models. When the organization is non-sequential, and the operations, non-linear, computational modeling is often necessary to establish that the mechanism could generate the phenomenon (5). Overall, this has been a highly productive strategy. Much has been learnt about the mechanisms for various biological phenomena, but it has also succeeded in revealing the limitations of the approach. One important limitation is that the supposedly independent phenomena and mechanisms are not nearly as independent as initially thought.

Understanding the ways mechanisms are connected is turning out to be an important challenge in twenty-first century biology and medicine, in part because such connections afford useful ways of intervening on systems to control particular phenomena (e.g., to treat specific diseases). This paper explores the challenges in establishing that the mechanism advanced to explain the fact that one phenomenon is causally affected by that put forward to explain another. As in the project of advancing a philosophical analysis of mechanistic explanation, my aim is to ground an account of what is involved in establishing causal relations between mechanisms in the practice of scientific researchers. To do this, I focus on two biological phenomena in which important progress has been made in identifying mechanisms – circadian rhythms and moods – and engage in a detailed review of the research and the causal claims that have been advanced as to how the mechanisms relate to each other[1].

As much of the research on mood has focused not on the moods of healthy individuals, but mood disorders such as major depressive disorder (MDD) and bipolar disorder (BD), and these have been related to disruptions of normal circadian rhythms, I will generally treat the related phenomena as mood disorders and disruptions of circadian rhythms. While making for a somewhat complex discussion, this does not pose a substantive problem since disrupted phenomena often serve to guide development of the understanding of the mechanism underlying the normally occurring phenomenon (6).

Progress in characterizing and understanding circadian rhythms and moods has largely stemmed from treating the two independently. But research in the later decades of the twentieth century also revealed connections between the two phenomena by showing that mood disorders are accompanied by disruptions of circadian rhythms. During the last two decades research on both circadian rhythms and mood disorders has increasingly focused on the molecular components of the two mechanisms. This research has revealed that molecular components of the circadian clock mechanism also play a role in mood disorders. This has raised the possibility of causal links between the mechanisms so that either disruptions in the circadian mechanism might be viewed as a cause of mood disorders, or mood disorders might be the cause of altered circadian rhythms. Of course the causality could also go in both directions, but my focus is on another alternative – that despite involving shared components, the two mechanisms are really independent and that what researchers are observing are effects of a common cause or pleotropic effects of common components.

My goal in this paper is not to argue for a particular stance on whether circadian rhythm disorders cause mood disorders; rather I will show how research has raised and addressed the question of possible connections between the two phenomena in the Section "Establishing a Relation between Circadian Rhythms and Mood Disorders" and between the two mechanisms in the Section "Research Implicating Molecular Components of the Circadian Clock in Mood Disorders." I then explore whether a causal connection is supported by the evidence in the Section "How are the Mechanisms Related?" In particular, I am concerned with what it would take to establish a causal connection between these mechanisms. Focusing only on the relation between phenomena, the standard measure of independence is that each can be dissociated from the other. There is evidence that some features of mood disorders and circadian disruptions are independent, but the same is true of different features that are treated as aspects of just one phenomenon. The separateness or relatedness of the mechanisms is what ultimately will determine whether researchers judge the phenomena to be causally linked. Mechanisms comprise parts performing operations, which explains the focus on determining whether parts of the circadian mechanism are also implicated in mood phenomena. However, just knowing that two mechanisms employ the same type of part, even if it performs the same operation in each, does not causally link the two mechanisms. Two car engines may employ pistons, but that does not causally connect them. What is required is that the same individual part is a component of both mechanisms and that the parts of the first mechanism affect the second mechanism differently as the first mechanism is in different states. Only then can researchers relate activities in one mechanism to activities in another mechanism. In the case of circadian and mood mechanisms, one needs to show that a protein, for example, affects mood differently as a consequence of its role in different circadian states. This is a demanding standard that has not yet been realized. But before raising these skeptical worries about how circadian disruptions and mood disorders relate, I turn first to the evidence that has been invoked in relating them. As noted above, my objective is to show that the question of how to understand the relation between the generation of circadian rhythm disorders and mood disorders is a real concern for science, not purely an abstract philosophical concern. Subsequent sections, thus, provide a review of how claims about the relation between circadian rhythms and mood developed and the current state of attempts to evaluate whether a causal claim can be substantiated.

Establishing a Relation between Circadian Rhythms and Mood Disorders

Reports of daily cycles of leaf folding in plants stem from ancient times and were first shown experimentally not to be a response to light when De Mairan (7) placed plants in a dark cupboard and observed that they continued to fold. Other examples of daily rhythms followed, such as, Wunderlich's (8) demonstration that body temperature in humans oscillates by over 1°C/day. Although a variety of researchers tried to maintain that these were responses to external cues, by the time of the International Symposium on Biological Clocks in 1960, the recognition that these oscillations continue but with periods of only approximately 24 h (thus, *circa* + *dies*) when light, temperature, and other environmental cues are removed had established that these rhythms were generated endogenously. That fact, plus the ability of these oscillations to be entrained by light or other cues (referred to as *Zeitgebers*) and the determination that they were maintained with the same period at different temperatures, has come to characterize the phenomenon of circadian rhythmicity. Although many researchers sought clues as to the nature of the mechanism, little progress was made until the 1990s. Instead, during the period 1960–1990, much circadian research focused on developing more detailed accounts of circadian phenomena, such as, how the phase of circadian oscillations is affected by light pulses of different strengths and durations.

Whereas the focus on circadian rhythms was largely motivated by trying to understand the phenomenon as it is normally manifested (disruptions of circadian rhythms were largely used to

[1] The relation between circadian rhythms and mood disorders is just one example of relations between circadian and other phenomena/mechanisms that have been the focus of intense research in recent years. Two other major examples are the relations between circadian rhythms and basic metabolism and circadian rhythms and cognition. See Venkataraman et al. (47) for a review of recent research addressing all three of these linkages between circadian rhythms and other phenomena.

identify the responsible mechanism), mood, like other psychiatric phenomena, is typically characterized in terms of disorders. The identification of *melancholia* stems from ancient times, with the term *depression* acquiring general currency by the end of the nineteenth century. DSM-I, in 1952, included the category of *depressive reaction*, and DSM-II (1968) included *depressive neurosis*. Mania, and the shifting from manic to depressive states, was also recognized in the DSM-II as manic-depressive psychosis. The former was subsequently labeled *unipolar* and the later *bipolar*. The terms *major depressive disorder* (MDD) and *bipolar disorder* (BD) were introduced in the 1970s and incorporated into DSM-III in 1980.

Suggestions of a link between mood disorders and circadian rhythms developed about the same time as the endogenous nature of circadian rhythms was established. Many of these focused on sleep disruptions in patients with mood disorders, for which there were case reports but no systematic studies until Hinton (9) performed a detailed study of currently depressed and recovered patients. He showed less sleep during each hour of the night as well as greater motility in those currently depressed. Sleep, however, is only partially under circadian control and Hinton's, as well as a number of other studies in the 1960s and 1970s, such as, Taub and Berger's (10) examination of the effects of altered sleep patterns on mood in healthy individuals, faced the problem of how to differentiate the effects of disrupted sleep and disrupted circadian rhythms. By employing a forced desynchrony protocol using a light–dark period longer than the circadian system could adapt to, Boivin et al. (11) were able to establish that although subjective happiness declined over each daily awake period, it clearly also oscillated in accord with underlying circadian rhythms (as measured, for example, by core body temperature).

A number of researchers in the 1970s and 1980s demonstrated correlations between measures of mood and measures of circadian rhythms. For example, Kripke et al. (12) found altered circadian periods in the manic-depressive patients they studied and determined that only those with shortened rhythms responded to lithium treatment. In another example, Souetre et al. (13) measured body temperature, plasma cortisol, norepinephrine, thyrotropin, and melatonin concentrations in depressed, recovered, and controls with no diagnosis of depression and demonstrated that the phase remained normal but the amplitude was significantly diminished in depressed participants but returned to normal after recovery.

A different strategy for establishing the linkage between mood disorders and circadian rhythms focused on various therapies found to be effective for mood disorders. Perhaps the best known is light therapy for seasonal affective disorders (SADs). After establishing that sunlight and bright artificial light (2000 lux) can suppress melatonin levels in humans, Lewy et al. (14) employed bright light therapy during 3 h after awakening on a seasonally manic-depressive patient during winter when his depression was greatest. This considerably reduced his depressive symptoms. Based on studies with additional patients, Rosenthal et al. (15) introduced the category SAD and presented further evidence of temporary reduction in depression with bright light therapy (the effects usually ceased when light treatment was stopped). The researchers went beyond the correlation to propose the *phase shift hypothesis*, which holds that depression results from the delayed phase of circadian rhythms (or, in a few cases, from an advanced phase) and that the therapeutic effect of light on depression resulted from shifting the phase of circadian rhythms earlier (or later in phase advanced patients). They supported this with evidence of advance (or delay) in the phase of melatonin expression in treated patients [(16, 17); for a more recent review, see Ref. (18)].

The evidence reviewed in this section demonstrated a connection between the phenomena of mood disorders and circadian rhythms. Mood changes according to circadian time and correlates with a number of other measures of circadian rhythmicity. Therapies that treat mood disorders, such as bright light at dawn, serve to alter the phase of circadian rhythms. The success of light therapy alleviating depression suggested a causal account, whereby circadian rhythms when altered are a causal factor in depression. Light therapy, on this account, restores normal rhythmicity and relieves depression. This idea was picked up in other theoretical proposals, such as, the *social Zeitgeber theory* (19), which proposed that in individuals vulnerable to depression, social stress events can disrupt circadian rhythms and that this in turn leads to depression. But to show that there is a direct causal connection between the phenomena requires more than evidence that they are correlated or even that the same treatments affect both. Information about the mechanism is required. Otherwise, one cannot discount the possibility that neither phenomenon directly affects the other but both phenomena are the product of other factors that are correlated or causally related.

Research Implicating Molecular Components of the Circadian Clock in Mood Disorders

The initial clues to the mechanism responsible for circadian rhythms in animals were developed in the early 1970s when circadian researchers both linked the central clock mechanism in mammals to a structure in the hypothalamus known as the suprachiasmatic nucleus (SCN) (20, 21) and, in fruit flies, identified a gene, *Period* (*Per*)[2], in which mutations caused short or long period oscillations or rendered the organisms arrhythmic (22). However, little progress was made until it was possible to clone *Per* and measure concentrations of its mRNA and protein at different times of day. This revealed that both *Per* mRNA the PER protein oscillated, with the protein peaking several hours after the mRNA. Hardin et al. (23) proposed on this basis a delayed negative feedback mechanism in which the protein PER would feedback on its own gene, temporarily inhibiting its own synthesis until concentrations decayed, at which point the inhibition would cease and new PER could be synthesized (**Figure 1**).

In the 15 years after 1990, many more clock genes were identified, including many homologs between the genes found in fruit

[2]Conventions for naming genes differ between insects and mammals. For this paper, I will adopt the mammalian convention of italics and capitalizing the first letter in the case of genes and upper case Roman for proteins regardless of species.

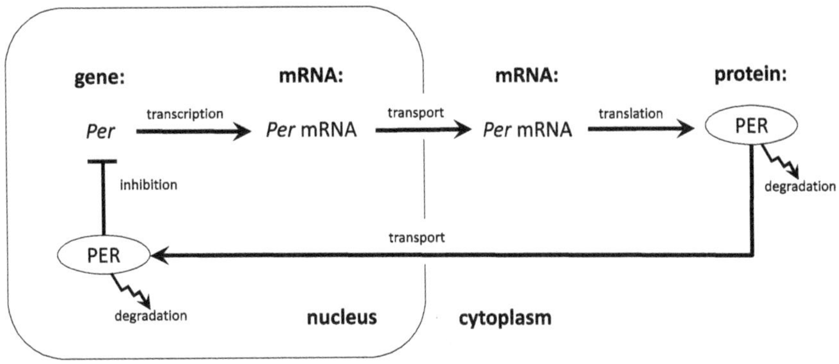

FIGURE 1 | The transcription–translation feedback loop proposed by Hardin et al. (23) to explain circadian rhythms. Transcription of the gene *Per* and translation into protein, PER is followed by the transport of PER back to the nucleus where it inhibits the transcription of its own gene.

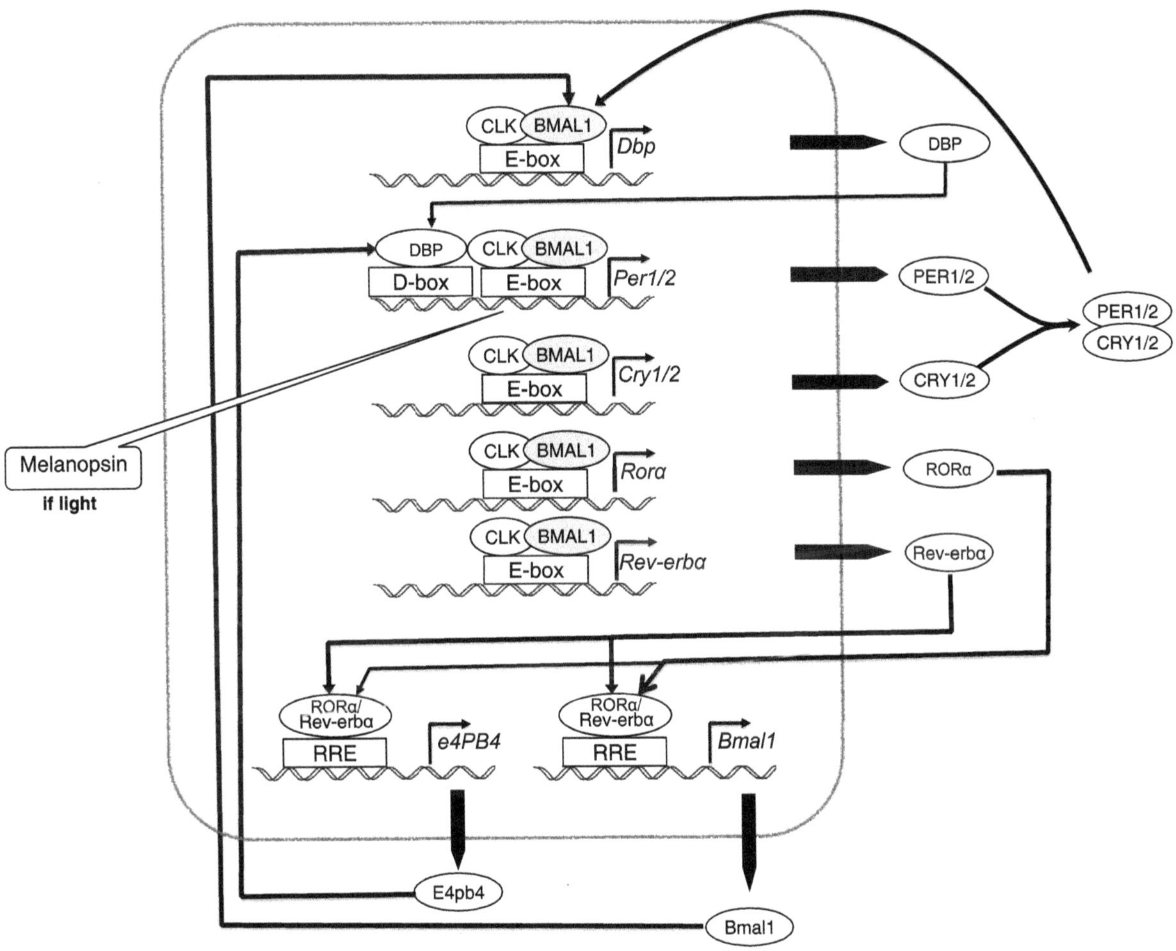

FIGURE 2 | The parts, operations, and organization of the mammalian circadian clock, as understood circa 2005.

flies and mice. Of particular, relevance for the relations between circadian rhythms and mood was the discovery of *Clock* in mice (24), which was shown to bind to the *Per* promoter and to be the target of inhibitory activity by PER. **Figure 2** shows the conception of the circadian mechanism in mammalian cells that had been generated by 2005. Two variant proteins, PER1 and PER2, were now recognized as forming dimers with CRY1 and CRY2, respectively. The inhibition is directed at a dimer between CLOCK (CLK) and BMAL1, which otherwise would bind to the promoter on *Per* and several other genes, activating their transcription. In addition, there is a negative feedback loop involving *E4pb4* and a positive feedback loop involving *Bmal1*.

Much of the research on the mechanisms underlying depression has focused on several monoamine neurotransmitters, especially serotonin, but also norepinephrine and dopamine. These were identified primarily through the fact that many antidepressant drugs increase levels of these monoamines (25). Caspi et al. (26) targeted serotonin as playing a mediating role between stressful life events and depression since individuals with short alleles of serotonin transporter were more prone to experience depression after such events. The different monoamines are associated with particular brain regions that figure centrally in research on depression. The dorsal raphe nuclei are the only source of serotonin in the brain. Dopamine, which is synthesized in decreased amounts in depression, functions in projections from the ventral tegmental area (VTA) to the nucleus accumbens. Norepinephrine is expressed in the locus coeruleus.

One clue to the linkage between circadian rhythms and these neurotransmitters that are altered in depression is that serotonin, norepinephrine, and dopamine all exhibit circadian oscillations in their concentrations (27). Moreover, the connection between the circadian mechanism and synthesis of these monoamines is quite direct: *monoamine oxidase A*, *Maoa*, is a transcriptional target of clock genes *Bmal1* and *Per2* and the protein MAOA serves to terminate dopamine signaling. On the other side, several clock genes have been linked to mood disorders. *Clock*, *Bmal1*, and *Per3* have been implicated in bipolar disease. SNPs of *Per2*, *Npas2*, and *Bmal1* are linked to increased risk for SAD, while there is suggestive evidence of a link between *Cry2* and depression (28). There is also evidence suggestive of a role of mood disorders in affecting circadian rhythms. The SCN has among the densest serotonergic innervation in the brain (all five 5-HT receptor types are employed) and the innervated region of the SCN significantly overlaps areas that receive retinal input and figure in entrainment. This suggests that mood may modulate the ability of the circadian clock to be entrained to local environments, a hypothesis supported by the fact that lesioning the raphe nucleus, thereby eliminating serotonergic innervation of the SCN, alters entrainment. Moreover, applying an agonist of 5-HT receptor generates phase advances (29).

Even stronger evidence indicative of a connection between parts of the circadian mechanism and mood is found in the affects of mutant forms of clock genes on mood. Vitaterna et al.'s discovery that *Clock* is a circadian gene resulted from the generation of a mutant (*ClockΔ19*) that exhibited a long period (27 h) and arrhythmia after several days in darkness. This same mutant has provided a mouse model for mania (30). Both the mutant mice and humans with mania exhibit (1) disrupted circadian rhythms, (2) hyperactivity, and (3) decreased sleep. In addition, the mice exhibit other traits closely resembling those of mania in humans: (4) humans describe feelings of extreme euphoria, while the mice exhibit hyperhedonia and less helplessness, (5) humans engage in increased risk taking, while the mice exhibit reduced anxiety, and (6) while humans exhibit a propensity to drug abuse, the mice show increased preference for cocaine. The mutant mice exhibit increased dopamine in the VTA, rendering neurons there more excitable. As in humans, lithium normalizes manic behavior, and since one effect of lithium is to increase dopamine levels in the VTA, the link appears to be causal.

McClung and her colleagues have investigated *ClockΔ19* mice to acquire clues into the mechanism underlying human mania. They have found deficits involving the entrainment of low gamma (30–50 Hz) oscillations to delta (1–4 Hz) oscillations in the nucleus accumbens in these mutant mice. In wild-type mice, such entrainment is negatively correlated with amount of exploration in a novel environment. This entrainment is seriously impaired in ClockΔ19 mice, which also exhibit hyperactivity in response to novelty. When treated with lithium, the coupling is restored and the hyperactivity stops (31). Knockdown of *Clock* in the VTA alone results in a manic-like state of less anxiety and hyperactivity but also depressive behavior (32), which seems to fit the fact that manic patients typically also exhibit depressive episodes. Lithium has been shown to lengthen circadian period, likely by inhibiting GSK3β, which phosphorylates PER2 and REV–ERBα, and to produce phase delays as well as affecting the amplitude and period of circadian oscillations (33). It, thus, has the opposite effects on the clock as light treatment, appropriate since it affects mania, not depression.

In an extremely ambitious study, Li et al. (34) provided yet additional evidence pointing to a causal link between circadian genes and mood disorders. They examined gene expression in six brain areas in cadavers of 55 normal controls and 34 patients with MDD post-mortem, analyzing them by circadian time of death. By plotting concentrations of mRNA by the patient's circadian time of death, they generated pseudo-time series data for each gene across the subject pool. In the controls, they identified several hundred genes exhibiting cyclic expression in the dorsolateral prefrontal cortex, amygdala, cerebellum, nucleus accumbens, anterior cingulate cortex, and hippocampus. Many core clock genes were among the genes with the strongest cyclic patterns. These are labeled in yellow on the left in **Figure 3**, in which the p-values for those genes with the highest overall significance levels on a measure of oscillation are shown. Red indicates genes whose oscillation is significant ($p < 0.05$) in a given tissue. On the right are the comparable data for the patients with MDD. Comparing the two plots reveals that oscillation reaches statistical significance for many fewer genes in many fewer tissues among the patients. Especially noteworthy is the decrease of rhythmicity in ARNTL (BMAL1) and PER2, two central clock genes, in most brain tissues.

As a measure of the power of the post-mortem gene expression data, Li et al. used the data from 60 randomly selected subjects (both normal controls and patients) to construct an algorithm designed to predict time of death from the pattern of gene expression at death. **Figure 4** shows, for all subjects, the actual time of death in the outer circle and the predicted time of death in the inner circle. Lines connect the corresponding data points and it is clear that the predictions for normal controls align better than for those for patients with MDD. This indicates substantial disruption in the circadian pattern of gene expression in the depressed patients.

Another type of evidence suggestive of a causal connection between the circadian mechanism and that involved in mood disorders is that several of the interventions designed to affect either mood or circadian rhythms also affect the other. One of the most popular drugs used to treat depression, the serotonin reuptake inhibitor (SSRI) fluoxetine, also induces phase advance in the SCN in slices of rat brain in culture. Other SSRIs shorten

A

Symbol	DLPFC	AnCg	HC	AMY	NAcc	CB
ARNTL*	0.0005	0.0005	0.001	0.001	0.0005	0.0005
PER2*	0.001	0.0005	0.0005	0.005	0.008	0.0005
PER3*	0.0005	0.0005	0.0005	0.094	0.0005	0.001
NR1D1*	0.0005	0.0005	0.0005	0.102	0.0005	0.008
DBP*	0.0005	0.0005	0.003	0.066	0.002	0.001
SFPQ	0.0005	0.152	0.013	0.134	0.001	0.029
ITIH5	0.0005	0.021	0.009	0.577	0.007	0.027
LDLR	0.001	0.002	0.004	0.014	0.561	0.204
PER1*	0.0005	0.005	0.008	0.559	0.044	0.071
INSIG1	0.007	0.003	0.001	0.025	0.727	0.183
SLC39A14	0.007	0.0005	0.029	0.067	0.077	0.262
NFIL3*	0.011	0.0005	0.104	0.181	0.03	0.198
SNTB2	0.023	0.038	0.17	0.001	0.013	0.368
PDZRN3	0.002	0.001	0.037	0.333	0.207	0.195
BHLHE40*	0.0005	0.014	0.147	0.42	0.02	0.127
BHLHE41	0.005	0.003	0.997	0.751	0.051	0.003

Color scale: 1, 0.8, 0.6, 0.4, 0.2, 0

B **MDD:**

	DLPFC	ACG	HC	AMY	NACC	CB
ARNTL	0.121	0.072	0.732	0.084	0.005	0.141
PER2	0.015	0.083	0.213	0.342	0.075	0.582
PER3	0.42	0.652	0.432	0.999	0.29	0.531
NR1D1	0.04	0.029	0.285	0.097	0.003	0.111
DBP	0.102	0.236	0.025	0.79	0.121	0.118
SFPQ	0.135	0.124	0.165	0.265	0.047	0.089
ITIH5	0.936	0.47	0.117	0.603	0.15	0.832
LDLR	0.012	0.385	0.315	0.307	0.005	0.028
PER1	0.006	0.21	0.137	0.619	0.124	0.061
INSIG1	0.056	0.534	0.668	0.869	0.318	0.88
SLC39A14	0.641	0.21	0.301	0.393	0.157	0.354
NFIL3*	0.565	0.326	0.633	0.478	0.179	0.617
SNTB2	0.928	0.194	0.123	0.765	0.365	0.293
PDZRN3	0.13	0.003	0.503	0.229	0.075	0.139
BHLHE40	0.19	0.897	0.433	0.963	0.14	0.009
BHLHE41	0.497	0.781	0.754	0.433	0.875	0.246

Color scale: 1, 0.8, 0.6, 0.4, 0.2, 0

FIGURE 3 | (A) Top oscillating genes in six brain tissues in normal controls in a cadaver study in which time of death was known. Shown in yellow are genes known to figure in the circadian clock. The numbers indicate significance levels on a measure of oscillation and color coding, with color coding differentiating five groups. **(B)** Data for patients with major depressive disorder analyzed in the same manner, making it clear that these genes achieved much lower significance levels in almost all tissues. Reproduced from Li et al. (34), Figures 2 and 4A. Copyright (2013) National Academy of Sciences, USA.

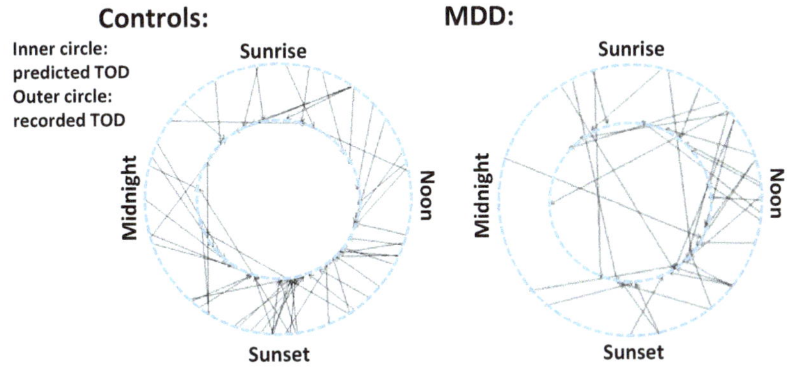

FIGURE 4 | In normal controls, as shown on the left, the pattern of gene expression at death, shown on the inner circle, was a good predictor of time of death, shown on the outer circle. Most of the lines connect nearby points on the two circles. In depressed patients (shown on the right), however, gene expression at death provided a must less reliable predictor of time of death. Reproduced from Li et al. (34), Figure 4C. Copyright (2013) National Academy of Sciences, USA.

the circadian period. Agomelatine, a relatively recent drug that advances the phase in melatonin expression, has proven effective in treating depression (it also, though, functions as an agonist to serotonin 2C receptors so the effects might not just be through altering circadian phase).

In this section, I have discussed the development of mechanistic accounts of both circadian rhythms and mood disorders. What the research has revealed is a host of possible connections between these mechanisms and many have found these highly suggestive that circadian disruption might cause mood disorders, or vice versa. But is such evidence sufficient to establish that the mechanisms are causally linked? I turn to that question in the next section.

How are the Mechanisms Related?

The evidence discussed in the previous sections, claiming both phenomenal and mechanistic connections between circadian rhythms and mood, invites a causal interpretation: disrupted circadian rhythms cause mood disorders (or vice versa). In fact, though, there are four different possibilities to consider:

1. Circadian disruptions cause mood disorders.
2. Mood disorders cause circadian disorders.
3. Causation goes in both directions.
4. Both circadian disruptions and mood disorders are common effects of something else or pleiotropic effects of common components.

Most interpretations adopt the first possibility. Yet, if there is a connection in that direction, there is likely also to be feedback from mood disorders to circadian disorders. However, my concern in this section is with the fourth possibility, which rejects a direct causal connection between circadian rhythms and mood disorders. I will argue that the evidence to date does not allow one to reject possibility.

One way some researchers have tried to support a causal connection is to identify intervening pathways between the two mechanisms. McClung (35) identifies several pathways by which circadian rhythms might regulate mood, of which I discuss three.

There are no direct projections from locus of the central circadian clock, the SCN, to the main loci of mood mechanisms, the dorsal raphe nucleus, the VTA, or the locus coereleus. But McClung shows that there are indirect pathways through a number of hypothalamic nuclei (e.g., the SCN projects to the dorsomedial hypothalamus which then projects to all three areas). These pathways appear to enable circadian oscillations in the SCN to regulate monoamine synthesis in these tissues. These pathways would explain how monoamine levels are altered in mutant mice in which clock genes are mutated or knocked down. McClung identifies a second pathway through the immune system. Alternations to circadian rhythms have effects on the immune system, leading to increased levels of proinflammatory cytokines. Increased levels of proinflammatory cytokines have previously been implicated in depression (36) as well as reduced neurogenesis, neural plasticity, and long-term potentiation. Moreover, the reduction in neurogenesis as well as depressive behaviors can be blocked in environments otherwise inducing stress by applying an inhibitor of nuclear factor-κB (NF-κB). This points to the NF-κB pathway as figuring in generating depression in animals with altered circadian rhythms. The determination that CLOCK itself interacts with NF-κB to activate transcription at NF-κB responsive promoters (37) further supports this as a candidate pathway for linking circadian mechanisms and mood disorders. A third pathway McClung proposed involves glucocorticoids. Concentrations of glucocorticoids increase in stress situations, a condition correlated with mood disorders. A neuronal and hormonal excitatory pathway from the SCN through the paraventricular nucleus (PVN) and the pituitary to the adrenal gland results in the rhythmic synthesis and release of glucocorticoids that then feed back onto the PVN and adrenal glands to maintain stable levels. Two clock proteins figure in regulating glucocorticoid levels. CRY proteins repress glucocorticoid receptors on the PVN and adrenal glands, thereby generating oscillation in the response to glucocorticoids. The receptors are also acetylated by CLOCK, which also decreases their sensitivity to glucocorticoids in the morning and increases it in the evening when acetylation is reversed (38).

Together with the evidence that components of the circadian clock are involved in mood, the evidence of pathways through which the circadian clock could regulate moods makes the case that the circadian clock plays a role in regulating seem plausible. But such evidence alone does not address the question as to whether the mechanisms themselves are actually linked. They may share components, but the roles these components play in each mechanism may be impendent of the role they play in the other. If that were the case, then, even if there are pathways that could connect the two mechanisms, the two mechanisms are not affecting each other – the generation of circadian rhythms is not affecting moods. Each mechanism operates on its own. Establishing that the circadian mechanism is what is affecting moods requires demonstrating that when common components contribute to one phenomenon, they do so in a way that is responsive to their role in the mechanism responsible for the other phenomenon.

Invoking the phenomenon of pleiotropy – the same gene having multiple functions – Landgraf et al. (39) make the case that the mechanisms responsible for circadian rhythms and moods may operate independently while sharing components:

> it is important to point out that, although commonly called 'clock genes', the molecular components of the circadian clock have pleiotropic functions, including many functions that have nothing to do with the clock: manipulating clock genes affects more than just circadian rhythms.

Landgraf et al. marshal their argument by considering several of the kinds of evidence for a causal link from circadian phenomena or mechanisms to mood such as I have presented in previous sections. In response to each, they argue that the evidence is compatible with the circadian and mood mechanisms operating independently while using common components. In fact, given differences in the way the two mechanisms operate, Landgraf et al. suggest there is reason to distinguish, not integrate, the two mechanisms. I will briefly present four of their examples.

One phenomenal linkage between circadian rhythms and mood involves the use of sleep deprivation as a means of transiently ameliorating symptoms of depression in both MDD and BD patients (40, 41). Sleep deprivation has also been found to induce mania in mice (42), which could then be successfully treated with lithium or tamoxifen. Sleep deprivation has been shown as well to have effects on circadian rhythms in mice, hamsters, and humans. A possible explanation for the dual affects of sleep deprivation on both mood and circadian rhythms is that they are the product of one integrated mechanism. But Landgraf et al. note there are also important differences between the phenomena. For example, a brief nap the following day can result in a relapse of depression, but does not have any effect on the circadian system. Sleep is only partially a circadian phenomenon, and it is possible that the effects on depression depend on a non-circadian pathway, perhaps involving cytokines, cortisol, or brain-derived neurotrophic factor.

A second example involves one of the possible pathways that might link circadian disruptions and mood disorders I discussed above: the NF-κB signal transduction pathway. Monje et al. (43) have provided intriguing evidence that the immune system, specifically the NF-κB signal transduction pathway, may be a common cause of circadian disruption and mood disorders, not an intermediary. They appeal to the effects of constant darkness, a known strategy for inducing depression-like behavior in rats. It is known that total darkness results in apoptosis of noradrenergic neurons in the locus coeruleus, serotinergic neurons in the dorsal raphe, and dopaminergic neurons in the VTA. Citing evidence of the role of the immune system in depression, they show that constant darkness results in increased levels of proinflammatory cytokine IL-6 in the hippocampus, leading to increased ERK activation. Manipulation of NF-κB inhibitors indicates that NF-κB played a causal role in mood disorders. The authors also demonstrated a causal effect of NF-κB in decreasing PER2 and increasing BMAL1 levels in the hippocampus. Rather than the effect of constant darkness on mood being mediated by an effect on the circadian system, the two may be independent consequences mediated by a common immunological pathway.

I turn now to claim about two common components of the circadian and mood mechanisms: *Clock* and *Per2*. Without challenging that the appearance of manic symptoms in the *Clock*Δ19 mouse are a result of higher dopamine levels in the VTA, which are themselves the result of the *Clock* gene mutation, Landgraf et al. note that there is little evidence of endogenous circadian rhythms in the VTA (when projections from the SCN are cut, the VTA exhibits no sustained PER2:LUC rhythms). Rather, when rhythms are found in the VTA, they may be driven by the SCN. In the VTA, where *Clock* has an effect on mood, it may not be performing a circadian function at all. It might instead be an independent contribution of the same genes.

PER2 is one of the proteins most clearly oscillating in brain tissues of normal controls. As we saw in discussing Li et al.'s study, its oscillation is greatly reduced in patients with MDD. Mouse studies have shown that stress, which leads to depression-like behaviors, results in lower amplitude oscillations in PER2 (44). But the effects can be dissociated. PER2 rhythms are restored more rapidly than recovery from depression-like behaviors. The link between PER2 and mood is thought to involve MAOA, which, as discussed above, serves to terminate dopamine signaling. MAOA contains an E-box through which its transcription is made rhythmic by fluctuating PER2 and BMAL1 concentrations (45). However, one *Per2* mutant, $Per2^{Brdm1-/-}$, despite no longer generating rhythmic expression of *Maoa*, still exhibits oscillation in dopamine levels in the VTA and its overall dopamine levels are higher than in the wild type. It exhibits much less depression-like behavior in response to a stressful activity like forced swim. Landgraf et al. suggest that the behavioral changes may be due to decrease in constitutive expression of dopamine, not its oscillation.

These and other examples that Landgraf et al. present illustrate a variety of ways to discount the suggestive links between the phenomena of circadian disruption and mood disorders and between the mechanisms for each. The two phenomena may be independent effects of a common cause[3] and the responses to therapeutic intervention, while similar, may show differences to yet other manipulations. The two mechanisms may involve the same parts without the parts figuring in a common mechanism. The roles in the different mechanisms may be pleiotropic. Moreover, the mood mechanism may not be responsive to the oscillation in dopamine but to how much is expressed. Altogether these results raise doubts about whether the correlations discussed earlier between circadian disruptions and mood disorders are due to a causal linkage between the mechanisms responsible for the two phenomena.

Raising doubts about whether two phenomena or their respective mechanisms are causally connected is very different from showing that they are not. Given the variety of correlations between mood disorders and circadian disruptions, it seems highly plausible that they are causally connected. What the challenges by Landgraf et al. indicate is that different evidence is required to establish a causal link than has been provided by most of the research to date. What would seem to be required is a demonstration that perturbations that alter one phenomenon affect the other in virtue of the way they altered the first phenomenon. This might be most clearly shown in by focusing on common parts of the circadian mechanism and the mood mechanism and the way they function in each mechanism. If the effect the part has on mood depends on how it behaves in the circadian mechanism that would indicate a causal link between the mechanisms. Experimental perturbations would provide the most compelling evidence: if perturbing how a part functions within the circadian clock thereby perturbs how it behaves in the mood mechanism, then one would have strong evidence that the two mechanisms are causally integrated. Procuring such evidence will be experimentally challenging and the evidence available to date does not support such direct causal connections.

Conclusion

Research on both circadian rhythms and mood disorders has been pursued in the quest for mechanistic explanations of each. This requires delineating the respective phenomena, linking the phenomena with a particular mechanism, and decomposing that mechanism into its parts and operations. I have reviewed several major studies that provide evidence that the phenomena of altered circadian rhythms and mood disorders are correlated and of common components in that the respective mechanisms share components. This research strongly suggests that altered circadian rhythms are a causal factor in the generation of mood disorders. Drawing on arguments advanced by Landgraf et al., however, I have argued that the evidence advanced so far does not yet justify such a claim. The phenomena may be due to common causes and the components of the mechanisms may function independently in each one. My goal, however, is not simply to make the point that correlation does not establish causation but rather to point to what would provide stronger support for the claim that circadian disruptions cause mood disorders. What is required is to show that it is as a contributor to the circadian mechanism that a component affects moods. One way this can be done is to establish that as its state in the circadian mechanism changes, the contribution of the component to the generation of moods and mood disorders changes.

The general issue of how mechanisms hypothesized to explain different phenomena are connected to one another is becoming increasingly important in biology and medicine. The investigation of proteins or the genes that code for them has often revealed components that figure in two or more cellular functions, sometimes in the same tissue. The question, as I have tried to argue here, is then whether the common component actually provides a causal linkage between the mechanisms. One factor accelerating the need to address this question is that researchers are moving beyond classical techniques that typically only identify a handful of very important components to a mechanism, such as *Per*, *Cry*, *Clock*, and *Bmal1*, in the case of circadian rhythms. Newer techniques reveal a plethora of components. For example, using small interfering RNAs to screen the whole

[3]If one opens the investigation into common causes, one finds many possible candidates. In footnote 1, I alluded to the growing evidence of multiple points of connection between circadian mechanisms and metabolic processes. Metabolic processes are one for common causes between the circadian mechanisms and mood mechanisms.

genome, Zhang et al. (46) identified an additional 200 genes beyond those thought to constitute the core clock which have affects on the amplitude or period of circadian rhythms. Many of these genes were previously characterized in terms of their roles in other cellular functions and it becomes relevant to know whether they are operating within their role in these other cellular functions in affecting circadian rhythms. If they do, then manipulating these other phenomena may be a viable strategy for altering circadian rhythms, or vice versa.

My concern has been to present issues of this sort as arising within ongoing science. Accordingly, I have examined in detail how the issue has arisen in the case of circadian rhythm research and mood. But the issue is a general one. Finding relations between phenomena and common parts within the mechanisms proposed to explain them can be very suggestive of a causal relation. Yet, until one has shown that a component has its effect on one mechanism in virtue of its role in the other, one has not established a causal connection between the phenomena.

References

1. Bechtel W, Richardson RC. *Discovering Complexity: Decomposition and Localization as Strategies in Scientific Research.* 1993 ed. Cambridge, MA: MIT Press, Princeton University Press (1993/2010).
2. Bechtel W, Abrahamsen A. Explanation: a mechanist alternative. *Stud Hist Philos Biol Biomed Sci* (2005) **36**:421–41. doi:10.1016/j.shpsc.2005.03.010
3. Craver CF, Darden L. *In Search of Mechanisms: Discoveries Across the Life Sciences.* Chicago, IL: University of Chicago Press (2013).
4. Machamer P, Darden L, Craver CF. Thinking about mechanisms. *Philos Sci* (2000) **67**:1–25. doi:10.1086/392759
5. Bechtel W, Abrahamsen A. Dynamic mechanistic explanation: computational modeling of circadian rhythms as an exemplar for cognitive science. *Stud Hist Philos Sci* (2010) **41**:321–33. doi:10.1016/j.shpsa.2010.07.003
6. Simon HA. *The Sciences of the Artificial.* 2nd ed. Cambridge, MA: MIT Press (1980).
7. De Mairan J. Observation botanique. *Histoire de l'Académie royale des sciences* (1729). p. 35.
8. Wunderlich KRA. *Das Verhalten der Eigenwärme in Krankheiten.* Leipzig: Otto Wigard (1868).
9. Hinton JM. Patterns of insomnia in depressive states. *J Neurol Neurosurg Psychiatry* (1963) **26**:184–9. doi:10.1136/jnnp.26.2.184
10. Taub JM, Berger RJ. Performance and mood following variations in the length and timing of sleep. *Psychophysiology* (1973) **10**:559–70. doi:10.1111/j.1469-8986.1973.tb00805.x
11. Boivin DB, Czeisler CA, Dijk DJ, Duffy JF, Folkard S, Minors DS, et al. Complex interaction of the sleep-wake cycle and circadian phase modulates mood in healthy subjects. *Arch Gen Psychiatry* (1997) **54**:145–52. doi:10.1001/archpsyc.1997.01830140055010
12. Kripke DF, Mullaney DJ, Atkinson M, Wolf S. Circadian rhythm disorders in manic-depressives. *Biol Psychiatry* (1978) **13**:335–51.
13. Souetre E, Salvati E, Belugou JL, Pringuey D, Candito M, Krebs B, et al. Circadian rhythms in depression and recovery: evidence for blunted amplitude as the main chronobiological abnormality. *Psychiatry Res* (1989) **28**:263–78. doi:10.1016/0165-1781(89)90207-2
14. Lewy AJ, Kern HA, Rosenthal NE, Wehr TA. Bright artificial light treatment of a manic-depressive patient with a seasonal mood cycle. *Am J Psychiatry* (1982) **139**:1496–8. doi:10.1176/ajp.139.11.1496
15. Rosenthal NE, Sack DA, Gillin JC, Lewy AJ, Goodwin FK, Davenport Y, et al. Seasonal affective disorder. A description of the syndrome and preliminary findings with light therapy. *Arch Gen Psychiatry* (1984) **41**:72–80. doi:10.1001/archpsyc.1984.01790120076010
16. Lewy AJ, Sack RL, Singer CM, White DM. The phase shift hypothesis for bright light's therapeutic mechanism of action: theoretical considerations and experimental evidence. *Psychopharmacol Bull* (1987) **23**:349–53.
17. Lewy AJ, Sack RL, Singer CM, White DM, Hoban TM. Winter depression and the phase-shift hypothesis for bright light's therapeutic effects: history, theory, and experimental evidence. *J Biol Rhythms* (1988) **3**:121–34. doi:10.1177/074873048800300203
18. Lewy AJ, Emens JS, Songer JB, Sims N, Laurie AL, Fiala SC, et al. Winter depression: integrating mood, circadian rhythms, and the sleep/wake and light/dark cycles into a bio-psycho-social-environmental model. *Sleep Med Clin* (2009) **4**:285–99. doi:10.1016/j.jsmc.2009.02.003
19. Ehlers CL, Frank E, Kupfer DJ. Social zeitgebers and biological rhythms: a unified approach to understanding the etiology of depression. *Arch Gen Psychiatry* (1988) **45**:948–52. doi:10.1001/archpsyc.1988.01800340076012
20. Moore RY. Retinohypothalamic projection in mammals: a comparative study. *Brain Res* (1973) **49**:403–9. doi:10.1016/0006-8993(73)90431-9
21. Moore RY, Eichler VB. Loss of a circadian adrenal corticosterone rhythm following suprachiasmatic lesions in the rat. *Brain Res* (1972) **42**:201–6. doi:10.1016/0006-8993(72)90054-6
22. Konopka RJ, Benzer S. Clock mutants of *Drosophila melanogaster*. *Proc Natl Acad Sci U S A* (1971) **89**:2112–6. doi:10.1073/pnas.68.9.2112
23. Hardin PE, Hall JC, Rosbash M. Feedback of the *Drosophila period* gene product on circadian cycling of its messenger RNA levels. *Nature* (1990) **343**:536–40. doi:10.1038/343536a0
24. Vitaterna MH, King DP, Chang A-M, Kornhauser JM, Lowrey PL, McDonald JD, et al. Mutagenesis and mapping of a mouse gene, *Clock*, essential for circadian behavior. *Science* (1994) **264**:719–25. doi:10.1126/science.8171325
25. Nutt DJ. Relationship of neurotransmitters to the symptoms of major depressive disorder. *J Clin Psychiatry* (2008) **69**(Suppl E1):4–7.
26. Caspi A, Sugden K, Moffitt TE, Taylor A, Craig IW, Harrington H, et al. Influence of life stress on depression: moderation by a polymorphism in the 5-HTT gene. *Science* (2003) **301**:386–9. doi:10.1126/science.1083968
27. Hampp G, Ripperger JA, Houben T, Schmutz I, Blex C, Perreau-Lenz S, et al. Regulation of monoamine oxidase A by circadian-clock components implies clock influence on mood. *Curr Biol* (2008) **18**:678–83. doi:10.1016/j.cub.2008.04.012
28. Albrecht U. Circadian clocks and mood-related behaviors. In: Kramer A, Merrow M, editors. *Circadian Clocks.* (Vol. 217), Berlin: Springer (2013). p. 227–39.
29. Sollars PJ, Pickard GE, Sprouse JS. Serotonin and the regulation of mammalian circadian rhythms. In: Squire LR, editor. *Encyclopedia of Neuroscience.* Oxford: Academic Press (2009). p. 723–30.
30. Roybal K, Theobold D, Graham A, DiNieri JA, Russo SJ, Krishnan V, et al. Mania-like behavior induced by disruption of CLOCK. *Proc Natil Acad Sci U S A* (2007) **104**:6406–11. doi:10.1073/pnas.0609625104
31. McClung CA. Circadian rhythms and mood regulation: insights from preclinical models. *Eur Neuropsychopharmacol* (2011) **21**(Suppl 4):S683–93. doi:10.1016/j.euroneuro.2011.07.008
32. Mukherjee S, Coque L, Cao J-L, Kumar J, Chakravarty S, Asaithamby A, et al. Knockdown of *Clock* in the ventral tegmental area through RNA interference results in a mixed state of mania and depression-like behavior. *Biol Psychiatry* (2010) **68**:503–11. doi:10.1016/j.biopsych.2010.04.031
33. Li JZ, Lu WQ, Beesley S, Loudon AS, Meng QJ. Lithium impacts on the amplitude and period of the molecular circadian clockwork. *PLoS One* (2012) **7**:e33292. doi:10.1371/journal.pone.0033292
34. Li JZ, Bunney BG, Meng F, Hagenauer MH, Walsh DM, Vawter MP, et al. Circadian patterns of gene expression in the human brain and disruption in major depressive disorder. *Proc Natl Acad Sci U S A* (2013) **110**:9950–5. doi:10.1073/pnas.1305814110
35. McClung CA. How might circadian rhythms control mood? Let me count the ways. *Biol Psychiatry* (2013) **74**:242–9. doi:10.1016/j.biopsych.2013.02.019
36. Miller AH, Maletic V, Raison CL. Inflammation and its discontents: the role of cytokines in the pathophysiology of major depression. *Biol Psychiatry* (2009) **65**:732–41. doi:10.1016/j.biopsych.2008.11.029
37. Spengler ML, Kuropatwinski KK, Comas M, Gasparian AV, Fedtsova N, Gleiberman AS, et al. Core circadian protein CLOCK is a positive regulator of NF-κB-mediated transcription. *Proc Natil Acad Sci U S A* (2012) **109**:E2457–65. doi:10.1073/pnas.1206274109
38. Charmandari E, Chrousos GP, Lambrou GI, Pavlaki A, Koide H, Ng SSM, et al. Peripheral CLOCK regulates target-tissue glucocorticoid receptor transcriptional activity in a circadian fashion in man. *PLoS One* (2011) **6**:e25612. doi:10.1371/journal.pone.0025612

39. Landgraf D, McCarthy MJ, Welsh DK. The role of the circadian clock in animal models of mood disorders. *Behav Neurosci* (2014) **128**:344–59. doi:10.1037/a0036029

40. Giedke H, Schwarzler F. Therapeutic use of sleep deprivation in depression. *Sleep Med Rev* (2002) **6**:361–77. doi:10.1016/S1087-0792(02)90235-2

41. Selvi Y, Gulec M, Agargun MY, Besiroglu L. Mood changes after sleep deprivation in morningness-eveningness chronotypes in healthy individuals. *J Sleep Res* (2007) **16**:241–4. doi:10.1111/j.1365-2869.2007.00596.x

42. Armani F, Andersen ML, Andreatini R, Frussa R, Tufik S, Galduroz JCF. Successful combined therapy with tamoxifen and lithium in a paradoxical sleep deprivation-induced mania model. *CNS Neurosci Ther* (2012) **18**:119–25. doi:10.1111/j.1755-5949.2010.00224.x

43. Monje FJ, Cabatic M, Divisch I, Kim E-J, Herkner KR, Binder BR, et al. Constant darkness induces IL-6-dependent depression-like behavior through the NF-κB signaling pathway. *J Neurosci* (2011) **31**:9075–83. doi:10.1523/JNEUROSCI.1537-11.2011

44. Jiang WG, Li SX, Zhou SJ, Sun Y, Shi J, Lu L. Chronic unpredictable stress induces a reversible change of PER2 rhythm in the suprachiasmatic nucleus. *Brain Res* (2011) **1399**:25–32. doi:10.1016/j.brainres.2011.05.001

45. Hampp G, Albrecht U. The circadian clock and mood-related behavior. *Commun Integr Biol* (2008) **1**:1–3. doi:10.4161/cib.1.1.6286

46. Zhang EE, Liu AC, Hirota T, Miraglia LJ, Welch G, Pongsawakul PY, et al. A genome-wide RNAi screen for modifiers of the circadian clock in human cells. *Cell* (2009) **139**:199–210. doi:10.1016/j.cell.2009.08.031

47. Venkataraman A, Ballance H, Hogenesch JB. The role of the circadian system in homeostasis. In: Walhout AJM, Vidal M, Dekker J, editors. *Handbook of Systems Biology: Concepts and Insights*. Amsterdam: Elsevier (2013). p. 407–26.

4

Factor Analysis of the Brazilian Version of UPPS Impulsive Behavior Scale

*Cristina Y. N. Sediyama[1], Ricardo Moura[2], Marina S. Garcia[3], Antonio G. da Silva[4], Carolina Soraggi[5], Fernando S. Neves[3], Maicon R. Albuquerque[6], Setephen P. Whiteside[7] and Leandro F. Malloy-Diniz[3,8]**

[1] *Faculty of Medicine, Federal University of Minas Gerais, Belo Horizonte, Brazil,* [2] *Department of Basic Psychological Processes, Institute of Psychology, University of Brasília, Brasília, Brazil,* [3] *Molecular Medicine Department at Federal University of Minas Gerais – INCT, Federal University of Minas Gerais, Belo Horizonte, Brazil,* [4] *Latin American Psychiatry Society, Porto University, Porto, Portugal,* [5] *Department of Psychology, Federal University of Minas Gerais, Belo Horizonte, Brazil,* [6] *Department of Sports, Federal University of Minas Gerais, Belo Horizonte, Brazil,* [7] *Mayo Clinic, Rochester, MN, USA,* [8] *Brazilian Society of Dual Pathology, Ilumina Neurosciences and Mental Health, Belo Horizonte, Brazil*

Edited by:
Jasmin Vassileva, Virginia Commonwealth University, USA

Reviewed by:
Bruno Kluwe Schiavon, Universität Zürich – Psychiatrische Universitätsklinik Zürich, Switzerland
Danilo Assis Pereira, Brazilian Institute of Neuropsychology and Cognitive Sciences, Brazil

****Correspondence:***
Leandro F. Malloy-Diniz
malloy.diniz@iluminaneurociencias.com.br

Objective: To examine the internal consistency and factor structure of the Brazilian adaptation of the UPPS Impulsive Behavior Scale.

Methods: UPPS is a self-report scale composed by 40 items assessing four factors of impulsivity: (a) urgency, (b) lack of premeditation; (c) lack of perseverance; (d) sensation seeking. In the present study 384 participants (278 women and 106 men), who were recruited from schools, universities, leisure centers and workplaces fulfilled the UPPS scale. An exploratory factor analysis was performed by using Varimax factor rotation and Kaiser Normalization, and we also conducted two confirmatory analyses to test the independency of the UPPS components found in previous analysis.

Results: Results showed a decrease in mean UPPS total scores with age and this analysis showed that the youngest participants (below 30 years) scored significantly higher than the other groups over 30 years. No difference in gender was found. Cronbach's alpha, results indicated satisfactory values for all subscales, with similar high values for the subscales and confirmatory factor analysis indexes also indicated a poor model fit. The results of two exploratory factor analysis were satisfactory.

Conclusion: Our results showed that the Portuguese version has the same four-factor structure of the original and previous translations of the UPPS.

Keywords: impulsivity, UPPS Impulsive Behavior Scale, psychometric, UPPS (urgency, lack of premeditation, lack of perseverance, sensation seeking), executive function

INTRODUCTION

Impulsivity is an important aspect of personality and is a central role in many forms of psychopathology. In general, impulsivity has been broadly defined as quick unplanned actions that lead to thoughtless behaviors and a tendency to act with a lower level of planning compared to individuals of similar intellectual level (Moeller et al., 2001). The lack of consensus regarding the definition of impulsivity is probably one of the main reasons for the great variation of results among studies that assess impulsivity (Malloy-Diniz et al., 2009). Such inconsistencies hamper efforts to understand the role of impulsivity in many forms of psychopathology, such as, substance abuse (Verdejo-García et al., 2007) and bipolar disorder (Malloy-Diniz et al., 2011).

Impulsivity is present in several psychiatric conditions and predictor of severity of medical, employment, alcohol, drug, family/social, legal and psychiatric problems in individuals with substance dependence (Verdejo-García et al., 2007). For example, in patients with bipolar disorder, the manifestation of impulsivity has been linked to suicidal behavior, as well as activities with high output of negative consequences and low quality of life (Malloy-Diniz et al., 2009; Kim et al., 2013).

To validate the main existing models of impulsivity Whiteside and Lynam (2001) analyzed the responses of 437 undergraduates in 17 widely used measures of impulsivity. The study resulted in the four factors UPPS Impulsive Behavior Scale. The first factor is lack of premeditation, which is characterized by the inability to think about the consequences of a decision. The second factor relates to sensation seeking, which is the tendency of an individual to engage in exciting activities and the urge to live new experiences that may or may not be dangerous. The third factor is urgency that represents a tendency to act impulsively in the presence of negative emotions at the expense of long-term gains. The last factor is lack of perseveration, and is characterized by the difficulty of maintaining focus on a particular task.

The UPPS Impulsive Behavior Scale has been translated into many languages and has been found to have strong psychometric properties in French and German (i.e., internal consistency coefficients scale between 0.77 and 0.85) as well as exploratory and confirmatory factor analysis (CFA) replicating the original four factors (Van der Linden et al., 2006; Schmidt et al., 2008). The validation and structuring of the UPPS for the Brazilian student sample, will contribute for future analysis of researches of other cultures, and in the future it will assist in clinical profiling in Brazil.

For the reasons presented above, the current authors translated the UPPS to Portuguese (Sediyama et al., 2013). However, before the UPPS can be used in researches or clinical work in Brazil, the psychometric properties of the Portuguese UPPS have to be established. Therefore, the aim of the present study was to examine in a student sample the internal consistency and factor structure of Brazilian adaptation of the UPPS Impulsive Behavior Scale.

TABLE 1 | Cronbach's alpha coefficient, mean, and standard deviation.

Scale	Mean score (*SD*)	Range	α ($IC_{95\%}$)
Lack of premeditation	20.32 (5.72)	11–44	0.87 (0.86–0.89)
Urgency	28.75 (7.40)	12–47	0.85 (0.83–0.87)
Sensation seeking	28.98 (8.47)	11–48	0.84 (0.82–0.87)
Lack of perseverance	19.20 (4.56)	10–32	0.75 (0.72–0.79)

MATERIALS AND METHODS

Participants

The study analyzed 384 participants (278 women and 106 men) that were convenient sample recruited from schools, universities, leisure centers, and workplaces. The mean age for female participants was 31-years-old ($SD = 11.94$) while male participants had a mean age of 34 years of age ($SD = 13.89$). Participants did not meet criteria for any psychiatric disorder relating to the MINI-Plus v5.0 (Amorim, 2000). Criterion analyses excluded participants younger than 18 or older than 62 years, with illiteracy, and with reported neurological disorders (such as cerebrovascular accident and epilepsy).

The participants were approached to in class, and asked to participate in the research by filling in the UPPS scale, socio-demographic scale, and MINI-Plus 5.0 (Amorim, 2000). Each candidate took an average of 60 min to finish.

The data from this study have all been drawn and have received ethical approval from the local research ethics committee of the Federal University of Minas Gerais, number ETIC 553/08. All participants provided written consent agreeing to the conditions before taking part of the experiment.

Instruments

Portuguese Impulsive Behavior Scale (UPPS)

The original version (Whiteside and Lynam, 2001) was adapted to Portuguese by Sediyama (Sediyama et al., 2013). It is a self-report scale which consists of 45 items that address the four personality factors associated to impulsive behavior in a Likert-type format ranging from 1 to 4: (1) strongly agree, (2) partially agree; (3) partially disagree and (4) strongly disagree. Besides the total scores of impulsivity, the UPPS also provides the subscale scores of each subtype of impulsivity: lack of premeditation, urgency, sensation seeking and lack of perseverance.

Mini International Neuropsychiatric Interview (MINI Plus v.5)

The MINI Plus is a structured diagnostic interview compatible with DSM-III-R/IV and ICD-10. This instrument was developed for clinical practice and research in psychiatric and primary care settings. The MINI Plus is a more detailed version that mainly helps diagnose psychotic and mood disorders in DSM-IV (Amorim, 2000).

Statistical Analysis

Descriptive statistics were calculated by mean and standard deviation. Normality of data distribution was verified by the Kolmogorov–Smirnov test. The internal consistency of the scale

TABLE 2 | Fit indices for confirmatory factor analysis models.

	Number of items	Excluded items	χ^2	gl	χ^2/gl	CFI	TLI	RMSEA	Interpretation
AFE1	45	0	12820.84*	990	12.95	0.94	0.93	0.048 (0.044–0.052)	Not suitable
AFE2	42	20, 30, 43	1341.29*	699	1.92	0.94	0.93	0.050 (0.046–0.054)	Suitable

*$p < 0.05$.

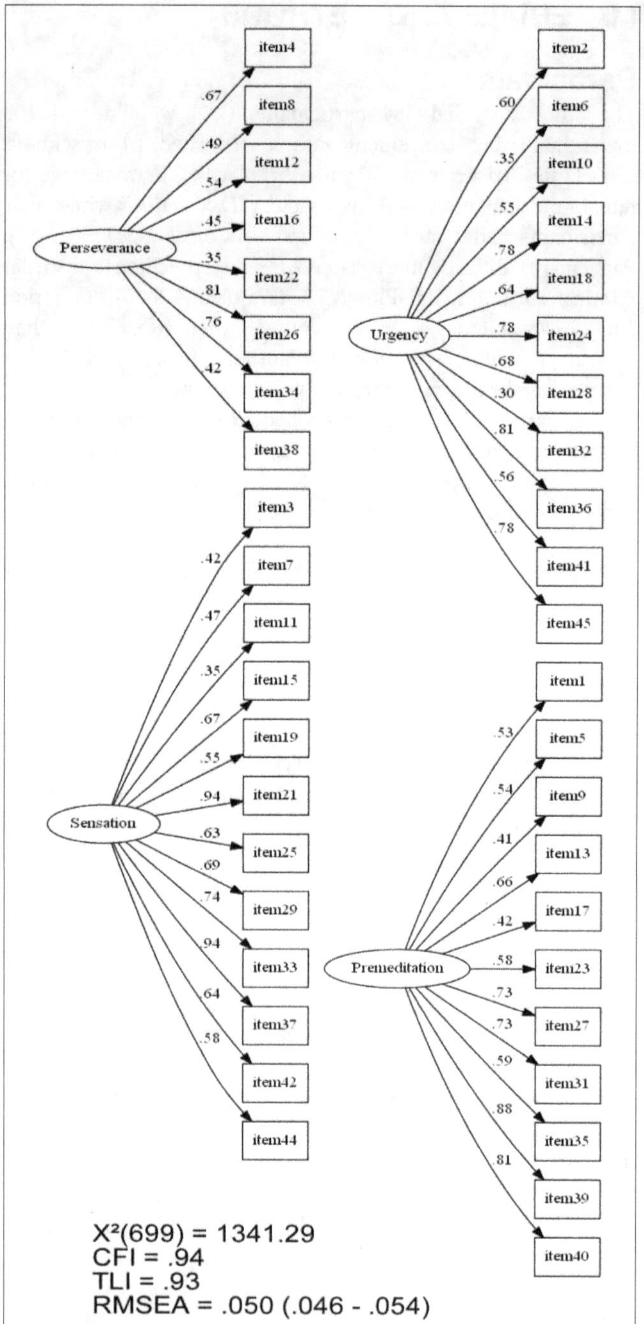

FIGURE 1 | Model fit indices for the final model by second exploratory factor analysis with factor loadings.

was calculated using the McDonald's omega and Cronbach's alpha. The One-way ANOVA with Tukey *post hoc* test were used to compare age groups. Kaiser-Meyer-Olkin (KMO) and Bartlett's test of sphericity were used for the evaluation of model sufficiency (Field, 2009). High values of KMO (more than 0.70) and values lower than 0.05 of significance of Bartlett's test probability indicate a satisfactory factor analysis (Field, 2009).

The analysis of the construct validity was done in two steps. First, a CFA was conducted to test the four-component structure of UPPS, with uncorrelated factors, found in previous studies (Magid and Colder, 2007). Second, an exploratory factor analysis (EFA) was performed. Weighted least squares method (WLSMV) estimator, once this estimator is recommended as a good alternative for items answered in an ordinal categorical scale (Chen et al., 2015). Geomin oblique rotation was used in EFA, and a range of indices were used to estimate how well the data fits the proposed model. These indexes included the chi-square and its corresponding *p*-value, the relative chi-square statistic, the root mean square error of approximation (RMSEA), the comparative fit index (CFI), and the Tucker-Lewis Index (TLI). Here we used widely adopted guidelines to interpret the adequacy of model fit, considering χ^2/df index less than 2, and RMSEA of 0.08 or lower, and both CFI and TLI with a value of 0.90 (Brown, 2006; Kline, 2011).

RESULTS

Descriptive Statistics and Internal Consistency

A Kolmogorov–Smirnov test on the UPPS total scores indicated normal distribution of the data, $D = 0.03$, $p > 0.05$. In order to analyze the effect of age in UPPS scores the sample was divided in four age-groups: below 30, between 30 and 39, between 40 and 49, and above 50 years of live. Results showed a decrease in mean UPPS total scores with age, $F = 7.37$, $p < 0.001$. *Post hoc* analysis corrected for multiple comparisons showed that the youngest participants (below 30 years) scored significantly higher than the other groups (all *p*'s < 0.05), and all other comparisons did not reveal significant differences (all *p*'s > 0.05). Moreover, UPPS scores were also similar across gender, $t(244) = 1.09$, $p > 0.05$.

Answers to items 2, 3, 6, 7, 8, 10, 11, 14, 15, 18, 19, 21, 24, 25, 28, 29, 32, 33, 36, 37, 38, 21, 42, 44 and 45 (2 through 45), were reversed in order to keep the value of 1 corresponding to the lowest level of impulsivity, and the value of 4 to the highest level of impulsivity. Scores in the UPPS scale ranged from 49 to 139 points, with an average of 94.93 points (standard deviation = 15.39). **Table 1** shows means and standard deviation for each subscale of the UPPS.

Internal consistency of UPPS was assessed using McDonald's omega and Cronbach's alpha coefficient to measure scale reliability. For a structure with four factors, using maximum likelihood as the extraction method, the omega hierarchical

TABLE 3 | Factor correlation.

Factor	Lack of premeditation	Urgency	Sensation seeking	Lack of perseverance
Lack of premeditation	1			
Urgency	0.36	1		
Sensation seeking	0.11	0.09	1	
Lack of perseverance	0.48	0.17	0.08	1

(ω_h) was 0.40, suggesting that around 40% of test variance is attributable to a general factor common to all items. The omega total (ω_t), in turn, reached an index of 0.91, thus indicating that a large part of overall test variance (91%) is due to a general but also to the other four specific factors. Omega total (ω_t) for the individual factors were also high (ω_t factor 1 = 0.91; ω_t factor 2 = 0.88; ω_t factor 3 = 0.83; ω_t factor 4 = 0.74). Additionally, the Cronbach's alpha, results indicated satisfactory values for all subscales, with similar high values for the subscales; Lack of premeditation (0.87), Urgency (0.85), Sensation seeking (0.84), and a smaller value for the subscale Lack of perseverance (0.75). Item-total correlation (dropping corresponding items from total scores in order to avoid overestimated correlations) also corroborated these findings, as the coefficients were generally high (0.61 on average), and no item exhibited a coefficient less than 0.37 (**Table 1**).

Construct Validity

The Kaiser-Meyer-Olkin (KMO) coefficient showed a sufficient magnitude (0.86), and the sphericity Bartlett's test was significant ($p < 0.001$). First, we conducted a CFA on all items of the Brazilian version of UPPS. CFA evaluated the adequacy of fit of the orthogonal model four-factor solution. Results revealed a significant Chi-square statistic, $\chi^2 = 2424.15, p < 0.05, df = 939$, $\chi^2/df = 2/58$. Other CFA indexes also indicated a poor model fit, CFI = 0.87, TLI = 0.87, and RMSEA = 0.065 ($IC_{95\%}$ = 0.062–0.068).

As CFA suggested that orthogonal model four-factor solution of the Brazilian version of UPPS was not suitable, the EFA was used to investigate the UPPS factorial structure.

As shown in **Table 2**, the initial EFA suggested that four-factor solution of the Brazilian version of UPPS was not suitable (see EFA1). Based on the Factor Loading, three items (20, 30, and 43) were excluded in the next analysis (EFA2) because showed large loading values in different factor than in the original theoretical structure.

The final version of four-factor solution of the Brazilian version of UPPS presented suitable (**Figure 1**) [$\chi^2_{(699)} = 1341.29$; $p < 0.001$; CFI = 0.94; TLI = 0.93; RMSEA = 0.050, with Geomin Rotated factor loadings greater or equal than 0.30 for all items].

Correlation between all four factors is present in **Table 3**. All latent variables but Sensation seeking correlated with at least one other variable. Similar findings were reported in previous studies (Van der Linden et al., 2006; Schmidt et al., 2008).

DISCUSSION

The present study showed that results supported the four factors of the Portuguese version, applied in a student sample, and it was consistent with previous research, that found the same factors in UPPS Impulsive Behavior Scale (Whiteside and Lynam, 2001; Magid and Colder, 2007). In addition, the consistency of UPPS demonstrated in omega score, poor homogeneity in the scale and the Cronbach's alpha, exploratory and CFA were satisfactory. These results are consistent with other translations that found internal consistency ranging from 0.75 to 0.87 (Van der Linden et al., 2006; Schmidt et al., 2008). Therefore, we can assume the four-dimensional structure and the distinct facets of Lack of premeditation, Urgency, Sensation seeking and Lack of perseverance as operationalized by the UPPS appear applicable to the Brazilian student population.

The adaptation of UPPS will provide an important tool for both clinical and research use. Since there's no scale in Brazilian context to assess this factors of impulsive behavior. In addition, the identification of these four facets corroborates the literature that impulsivity is a heterogeneous category that includes several different features. However, more studies should be conducted to assess the psychometric properties of the scale.

Like previous research that demonstrate lifespan changes in impulsivity, this study found differences in UPPS according to age, (Steinberg et al., 2008; Burnett et al., 2012). In relation to sex differences, we did not observe this in our sample, but it should be emphasized that in a prior study reported such differences, using a different version of the UPPS, the UPPS-P (Cyders et al., 2007). This study reported that male participants differed from female ones in relation to positive urgency and sensation seeking (Cyders, 2013). Our hypothesis is that study sample was larger (n = 1,372 undergraduates), and probably favored a robust statistical analysis in relation to the sex difference. However, it should be noted that our study undergoes limitations, such as the vast majority of female samples, a problem also observed in the original study (Whiteside and Lynam, 2001) and others (Van der Linden et al., 2006; Schmidt et al., 2008).

The range application in other contexts, such as psychiatric Brazilian samples is necessary to show evidence of effectiveness studies which include the UPPS, and for example, whether these factors differ according to the psychiatric diagnosis or can be predictive of some disorder. In summary, our study showed that the Portuguese version of the UPPS has adequate psychometric properties, similar to those reported in different cultures.

AUTHOR CONTRIBUTIONS

All authors listed, have made substantial, direct and intellectual contribution to the work, and approved it for publication.

ACKNOWLEDGMENT

The study is funded by Grant INCT-MM (FAPEMIG: CBB-APQ-00075-09/CNPq 573646/2008-2), grants from the Sociedade Interdisciplinar de Neurociências Aplicadas à Saúde e Educação (SINApSE).

REFERENCES

Amorim, P. (2000). Mini International Neuropsychiatric Interview (MINI): validation of a short structured diagnostic psychiatric interview. *Rev. Bras. Psiquiatr.* 22, 106–115. doi: 10.1590/S1516-44462000000300003

Brown, T. A. (2006). *Confirmatory Factor Analysis for Applied Research*. New York, NY: Guilford Press.

Burnett, H. S., Adam, R. J., Urner, M., van, L. L., Bahrami, B., Bays, P. M., et al. (2012). Impulsivity and rapid decision-making for reward. *Front. Psychol.* 3:153. doi: 10.3389/fpsyg.2012.00153

Chen, P. Y., Yang, C. M., and Morin, C. M. (2015). Validating the cross-cultural factor structure and invariance property of the insomnia severity index: evidence based on ordinal EFA and CFA. *Sleep Med.* 16, 598–603. doi: 10.1016/j.sleep.2014.11.016

Cyders, M. A. (2013). Impulsivity and the sexes: measurement and structural invariance of the UPPS-P impulsive behavior scale. *Assessment* 20, 86–97. doi: 10.1177/1073191111428762

Cyders, M. A., Smith, G. T., Spillane, N. S., Fischer, S., Annus, A. M., and Peterson, C. (2007). Integration of impulsivity and positive mood to predict risky behavior: development and validation of a measure of positive urgency. *Psychol. Assess.* 19, 107–118. doi: 10.1037/1040-3590.19.1.107

Field, A. P. (2009). *Discovering Statistics Using SPSS*. London: SAGE.

Kim, Y. S., Cha, B., Lee, D., Kim, S. M., Moon, E., Park, C. S., et al. (2013). The relationship between impulsivity and quality of life in euthymic patients with bipolar disorder. *Psychiatry Investig.* 10:246. doi: 10.4306/pi.2013.10.3.246

Kline, R. B. (2011). *Principles and Practice of Structural Equation Modelling*. London: The Guilford Press.

Magid, V., and Colder, C. R. (2007). The UPPS impulsive behavior scale: factor structure and associations with college drinking. *Pers. Individ. Dif.* 43, 1927–1937. doi: 10.1016/j.paid.2007.06.013

Malloy-Diniz, L. F., Neves, F. S., Abrantes, S. S. C., Fuentes, D., and Corrêa, H. (2009). Suicide behavior and neuropsychological assessment of type I bipolar patients. *J. Affect. Disord.* 112, 231–236. doi: 10.1016/j.jad.2008.03.019

Malloy-Diniz, L. F., Neves, F. S., de Moraes, P. H. P., De Marco, L. A., Romano-Silva, M. A., Krebs, M. O., et al. (2011). The 5-HTTLPR polymorphism, impulsivity and suicide behavior in euthymic bipolar patients. *J. Affect. Disord.* 133, 221–226. doi: 10.1016/j.jad.2011.03.051

Moeller, F. G., Barratt, E. S., Dougherty, D. M., Schmitz, J. M., and Swann, A. C. (2001). Psychiatric aspects of impulsivity. *Am. J. Psychiatry* 158, 1783–1793. doi: 10.1176/appi.ajp.158.11.1783

Schmidt, R. E., Gay, P., d' Acremont, M., and Van der Linden, M. A. (2008). German adaptation of the UPPS impulsive behavior scale: psychometric properties and factor structure. *Swiss J. Psychol.* 67, 107–112. doi: 10.1024/1421-0185.67.2.107

Sediyama, C. Y. N., Carvalho, A. M., Gauer, G., Tavares, N., Santos, R. M. M., Ginani, G., et al. (2013). Translation and adaptation of impulsive behavior scale (UPPS) to the Brazilian population. *Clin. Neuropsychiatry* 10, 79–85.

Steinberg, L., Albert, D., Cauffman, E., Banich, M., Graham, S., and Woolard, J. (2008). Age differences in sensation seeking and impulsivity as indexed by behavior and self-report: evidence for a dual systems model. *Dev. Psychol.* 44, 1764–1778. doi: 10.1037/a0012955

Van der Linden, M., d'Acremont, M., Zermatten, A., Jermann, F., Laroi, F., Willems, S., et al. (2006). A french adaptation of the UPPS impulsive behavior scale. *Eur. J. Psychol. Assess.* 22, 38–42. doi: 10.1027/1015-5759.22.1.38

Verdejo-García, A., Bechara, A., Recknor, E. C., and Pérez-García, M. (2007). Negative emotion-driven impulsivity predicts substance dependence problems. *Drug Alcohol Depend.* 91, 213–219. doi: 10.1016/j.drugalcdep.2007.05.025

Whiteside, S. P., and Lynam, D. R. (2001). The five factor model and impulsivity: using a structural model of personality to understand impulsivity. *Pers. Individ. Dif.* 30, 669–689. doi: 10.1016/S0191-8869(00)00064-7

5

Beyond Scientism and Skepticism: An Integrative Approach to Global Mental Health

Dan J. Stein[1] and Judy Illes[2]*

[1] MRC Unit on Anxiety and Stress Disorders, Department of Psychiatry, Groote Schuur Hospital, University of Cape Town, Cape Town, South Africa, [2] National Core for Neuroethics, Division of Neurology, Department of Medicine, University of British Columbia, Vancouver, BC, Canada

Edited by:
Annemarie Kalis, Utrecht University, Netherlands

Reviewed by:
Oksana Sorokina, The University of Edinburgh, UK
Eleftheria Pervolaraki, University of Leeds, UK

***Correspondence:**
Dan J. Stein
dan.stein@uct.ac.za

The global burden of disorders has shifted from infectious disease to non-communicable diseases, including neuropsychiatric disorders. Whereas infectious disease can sometimes be combated by targeting single causal mechanisms, such as prevention of contact-spread illness by handwashing, in the case of mental disorders multiple causal mechanisms are typically relevant. The emergent field of global mental health has emphasized the magnitude of the treatment gap, particularly in the low- and middle-income world and has paid particular attention to upstream causal factors, for example, poverty, inequality, and gender discrimination in the pathogenesis of mental disorders. However, this field has also been criticized for relying erroneously on Western paradigms of mental illness, which may not be relevant or appropriate to the low- and middle-income context. Here, it is important to steer a path between scientism and skepticism. Scientism regards mental disorders as essential categories, and takes a covering law approach to causality; skepticism regards mental disorders as merely social constructions and emphasizes the role of political power in causal relations. We propose an integrative model that emphasizes the contribution of a broad range of causal mechanisms operating at biological and societal levels to mental disorders and the consequent importance of broad spectrum and multipronged approaches to intervention.

Keywords: neuroethics, global mental health, scientism, skepticism, causal mechanisms

INTRODUCTION

In recent decades, there has been a shift from infectious disease to non-communicable diseases throughout the world. Mental, neurological, and substance use disorders are already the largest contributor to the burden of disease; these prevalent, chronic, and costly disorders now account for 22% of disablilty adjusted life years (DALYs) from all medical causes in those aged 15–49 (1). Furthermore, forecasts indicate that in the foreseeable future they will become even more central to global public health, with the World Economic Forum predicting that neuropsychiatric disorders will comprise the largest costs of chronic, non-communicable diseases globally in the next two decades (2).

Increased recognition of the burden of neuropsychiatric disorders has given impetus to the emergence of the discipline of global mental health (3). Additional key considerations are that interventions for mental disorders impact positively on individual well-being and country development and are highly cost-efficient, but that neuropsychiatric disorders are often underdiagnosed and undertreated, with the treatment gap particularly large in low- and middle-income countries. Furthermore, this treatment gap is a human rights issue; levels of stigmatization of people living with mental illness are too high, and levels of mental health literacy are too low in communities, clinicians, and policy makers (4, 5).

Clinical and research work on neuropsychiatric disorders raises a number of conceptual and ethical questions, many of which are relevant to the field of global mental health (6). In considering some of these conceptual and ethical questions, we have argued that clinicians and researchers should steer a course between a scientism that regards mental disorders as natural kinds, and a skepticism that views all mental disorders as mere sociocultural constructions (7–9). Integrative approaches are needed to address fully the complex reality of mental disorders. In this commentary, we discuss this view in relation to global mental health, considering in turn issues of diagnosis, pathogenesis, and intervention (**Table 1**).

GLOBAL MENTAL HEALTH AND DIAGNOSIS

Global mental health has emphasized that mental disorders are prevalent and associated with significant suffering, impairment, and socioeconomic costs. Thus, for example, data from the World Mental Health Surveys have emphasized that mental disorders are more impairing than physical disorders, but are less likely to be diagnosed and treated (10). While such conclusions are pertinent around the globe, in low- and middle-income countries, a lack of resources is particularly likely to exacerbate the treatment gap. These sorts of data provide an important foundation for the rallying cry of global mental health that there is no health without mental health (11).

Nevertheless, global mental health has also come under fire for its emphasis on these sorts of data. In particular, critics have argued that the field relies erroneously on Western paradigms of mental illness, which may not be relevant or appropriate to the low- and middle-income context (12). Such constructs run the risk of ignoring how symptoms vary from time to time and from place to place, and of downplaying the complex ways in which illnesses are expressed and experienced differently in different sociocultural contexts (13). Indeed, Jacob and Patel have emphasized that global mental health needs new diagnostic approaches, a view that is perhaps partially consistent with attempts in clinical neuroscience to reformulate approaches to evaluation of neuropsychiatric disorders (14, 15).

At the same time, international classification systems have significant clinical advantages, and there are currently no viable alternatives in practice. We would, therefore, argue that although it is clearly important to recognize the limitations of current psychiatry nosology and biopsychosocial models (16, 17), we ought to be wary of unrealistic expectations of such approaches (18). For example, medicine does not require that its diagnostic systems are essentialist in nature; rather medical syndromes provide clinicians with a practical set of tools for assessing patients. Rather than insisting that assessment systems will ultimately be supported solely by data on endophenotypes – intermediate phenotypes with high heritability – we can also ask that more work is also needed on exophenotypes, such as societal, structural, and other upstream contributors to disease and illness (19), and their intersections.

GLOBAL MENTAL HEALTH AND PATHOGENESIS

Although infectious diseases may involve a range of biological and psychosocial factors, it is sometimes possible to combat these conditions by targeting single causal mechanisms. Locating the geographic source of a cholera epidemic, employing handwashing to decrease bacterial transmission, developing vaccines to prevent polio and smallpox, and using mosquito nets to prevent malaria have been seminal exemplars of success for public health. In contrast, global mental health has had to contend with multiple upstream factors that impact mental disorders: poverty, inequality, gender discrimination, and more.

At the same time, any emphasis of global mental health on only one set of causal factors can potentially be problematic.

TABLE 1 | Moving beyond scientism and skepticism in global mental health: integrative approaches to diagnosis, pathogenesis, and intervention.

	Scientism	Skepticism	Integrative
Diagnosis	Diagnostic systems rely on essentialist categories or natural kinds. Assessment systems will be ultimately be supported by data on endophenotypes	Mental illness is expressed and experienced differently in different sociocultural contexts. Symptoms vary from time to time and place to place	Mental illness is a complex reality. Nosologies are theory bound and value laden, but may improve as the relevant science and debate advance
Pathogenesis	May approach causality in terms of covering laws. May focus on a single set of associations, such as those which characterize the health care system	May emphasize the role of sociocultural values and powers in explanations. May focus on differences in conceptualization of disorders across history and geography	Emphasizes that a broad range of factors are involved in the pathogenesis of mental disorders, with causal mechanisms operating at multiple interacting levels
Intervention	May take a single-bullet approach, looking for focused interventions, whether biological or community focused that will target the essence of the disorder	May emphasize that interventions reflect local values and powers. Both biological and community-focused interventions reinforce existing societal structures	Incorporates a range of insights about the nature of mental disorders, and targets a broad range of factors involved in their pathogenesis, including biological and social ones

Some research priority setting exercises have indicated that global mental health should focus primarily on health systems research, for example, and should pay less attention to the biological causes of mental disorders (20). This is consistent with a criticism of global mental health which emphasizes that it is ironic that a field that purports to be concerned with a broad range of socioeconomic factors relies on neuroessentialist DSM-5 categories. After all, key considerations for Western-based typologies of illness are that they have diagnostic validity, that disorders demonstrate high heritability, or that they predict response to interventions such as pharmacotherapy.

Our own view is that there are important opportunities at the intersection of global mental health and clinical neuroscience in addressing the pathogenesis of mental disorders (21). There has been significant progress on understanding how nature and nurture intersect to create vulnerabilities for mental disorder, and indeed in recognizing how multiple levels of causal factors contribute to these conditions (7, 22). We have previously noted, for example, that while basic neuroscience has shed a great deal of insight into addiction, a full understanding of substance use disorders requires the psychological and social levels to be included (8, 9). Only a comprehensive and integrative perspective will allow an understanding of complex phenomena, such as decreased voluntary control in addictive disorders (23).

GLOBAL MENTAL HEALTH AND INTERVENTION

Global mental health has focused on task shifting and implementation science. This is certainly important in the context of resource-limited settings, where there are simply not enough trained professionals to deliver interventions, where health systems have systemic problems, and where there is growing evidence that non-specialized community workers can make a real impact (3). Indeed, some of the concerns of global mental health mirror those of the solution-oriented bent of neuroethics; there is a focus on efforts to improve wellness, on the importance of human rights, and on an empirical approach to optimizing interventions (6).

At the same time, there are potential criticisms of the focus of global mental health on communities, task shifting, and implementation science. Sartorius and colleagues, for example, have noted that in many parts of the globe, communities have changed in significant ways and are no longer able to provide the support that those with serious mental illness need and deserve (24). Furthermore, some tasks simply cannot be shifted, and we need to focus at times rather on novel biological treatments (25) or on increasing resources; it is crucial that in attempting to strengthen resource-limited systems, we do not simply institutionalize mechanisms that can only work in impoverished systems.

Again, we would argue for an integrative approach. It is important to avoid a scientism which states that given that mental disorders are natural kinds, they will ultimately succumb to single-bullet biological interventions (26). At the same time, we do not want to fall to prey to a skepticism that indicates that interventions should be entirely focused on changing the way in which disorders are conceptualized and labeled by society, or that they should be limited to community practices. We need an integrative approach to intervention that incorporates a range of insights about the nature of mental disorders and that targets a broad range of factors involved in their pathogenesis, including psychobiological factors and community processes.

CONCLUSION

We have argued elsewhere that it is important to avoid neuroreductionism and to emphasize instead that mental and substance use disorders require an understanding of psychosocial factors. Put differently, it is important to steer a path between scientism, which regards mental disorders as essential categories and takes a covering law approach to causality, and skepticism, which regards mental disorders merely as social constructions and reduces causality to considerations of political power. Here, we have applied these arguments to the newly emergent field of global mental health, considering issues relevant to diagnosis, pathogenesis, and treatment (**Table 1**), and emphasizing that a broad range of causal mechanisms operating at biological, psychological, and societal levels, and at the interactions between these levels, contribute to mental disorders, and that clinical interventions and research practices must match this complexity.

FUNDING

DS is supported by the Medical Research Council of South Africa. JI is Canada Research Chair in Neuroethics.

REFERENCES

1. Murray CJ, Vos T, Lozano R, Naghavi M, Flaxman AD, Michaud C, et al. Disability-adjusted life years (DALYs) for 291 diseases and injuries in 21 regions, 1990-2010: a systematic analysis for the Global Burden of Disease Study 2010. *Lancet* (2012) **380**(9859):2197–223. doi:10.1016/S0140-6736(12)61689-4
2. Bloom DEC, et al. *The Global Economic Burden of Non-Communicable Diseases*. Geneva: World Economic Forum (2011).
3. Patel V. Global mental health: from science to action. *Harv Rev Psychiatry* (2012) **20**(1):6–12. doi:10.3109/10673229.2012.649108
4. Ganasen KA, Parker S, Hugo CJ, Stein DJ, Emsley RA, Seedat S. Mental health literacy: focus on developing countries. *Afr J Psychiatry (Johannesbg)* (2008) **11**(1):23–8.
5. Semrau M, Evans-Lacko S, Koschorke M, Ashenafi L, Thornicroft G. Stigma and discrimination related to mental illness in low- and middle-income countries. *Epidemiol Psychiatr Sci* (2015) **24**(5):382–94. doi:10.1017/S2045796015000359
6. Stein DJ, Giordano J. Global mental health and neuroethics. *BMC Med* (2015) **13**(1):274. doi:10.1186/s12916-015-0509-y
7. Stein DJ. *Philosophy of Psychopharmacology*. Cambridge: Cambridge University Press (2008).
8. Buchman DZ, Skinner W, Illes J. Negotiating the relationship between addiction, ethics, and brain science. *AJOB Neurosci* (2010) **1**(1):36–45. doi:10.1080/21507740.2010.490168
9. Di Pietro N, Illes J, Canadian Working Group on Antipsychotic Medications and Children. Rising antipsychotic prescriptions for children and youth:

cross-sectoral solutions for a multimodal problem. *CMAJ* (2014) **186**(9):653–4. doi:10.1503/cmaj.131604
10. Wang PS, Angermeyer M, Borges G, Bruffaerts R, Tat Chiu W, De Girolamo G, et al. Delay and failure in treatment seeking after first onset of mental disorders in the World Health Organization's World Mental Health Survey Initiative. *World Psychiatry* (2007) **6**(3):177–85.
11. Prince M, Patel V, Saxena S, Maj M, Maselko J, Phillips MR, et al. No health without mental health. *Lancet* (2007) **370**(9590):859–77. doi:10.1016/S0140-6736(07)61238-0
12. Summerfield D. Afterword: against 'global mental health'. *Transcult Psychiatry* (2012) **49**(3–4):519–30. doi:10.1177/1363461512454701
13. Stein DJ. Cross-cultural psychiatry and the DSM-IV. *Compr Psychiatry* (1993) **34**(5):322–9. doi:10.1016/0010-440X(93)90018-Y
14. Cuthbert BN, Insel TR. Toward the future of psychiatric diagnosis: the seven pillars of RDoC. *BMC Med* (2013) **11**:126. doi:10.1186/1741-7015-11-126
15. Jacob KS, Patel V. Classification of mental disorders: a global mental health perspective. *Lancet* (2014) **383**(9926):1433–5. doi:10.1016/S0140-6736(13)62382-X
16. McLaren N. A critical review of the biopsychosocial model. *Aust N Z J Psychiatry* (1998) **32**(1):86–92;discussion93–86. doi:10.3109/00048679809062712
17. Ghaemi SN. The rise and fall of the biopsychosocial model. *Br J Psychiatry* (2009) **195**(1):3–4. doi:10.1192/bjp.bp.109.063859
18. Nesse RM, Stein DJ. Towards a genuinely medical model for psychiatric nosology. *BMC Med* (2012) **10**:5. doi:10.1186/1741-7015-10-5
19. Stein DJ, Lund C, Nesse RM. Classification systems in psychiatry: diagnosis and global mental health in the era of DSM-5 and ICD-11. *Curr Opin Psychiatry* (2013) **26**(5):493–7. doi:10.1097/YCO.0b013e3283642dfd
20. Tomlinson M, Rudan I, Saxena S, Swartz L, Tsai AC, Patel V. Setting priorities for global mental health research. *Bull World Health Organ* (2009) **87**(6):438–46. doi:10.2471/BLT.08.054353
21. Stein DJ, He Y, Phillips A, Sahakian BJ, Williams J, Patel V. Global mental health and neuroscience: potential synergies. *Lancet Psychiatry* (2015) **2**:178–85. doi:10.1016/S2215-0366(15)00014-0
22. Kendler KS. The dappled nature of causes of psychiatric illness: replacing the organic-functional/hardware-software dichotomy with empirically based pluralism. *Mol Psychiatry* (2012) **17**(4):377–88. doi:10.1038/mp.2011.153
23. Stein DJ. Philosophy of psychopharmacology. *Perspect Biol Med* (1998) **41**(2):200–11. doi:10.1353/pbm.1998.0037
24. Volpe U, Mihai A, Jordanova V, Sartorius N. The pathways to mental healthcare worldwide: a systematic review. *Curr Opin Psychiatry* (2015) **28**(4):299–306. doi:10.1097/YCO.0000000000000164
25. Collins PY, Patel V, Joestl SS, March D, Insel TR, Daar AS, et al. Grand challenges in global mental health. *Nature* (2011) **475**(7354):27–30. doi:10.1038/475027a
26. Stein DJ. Psychopharmacology and natural kinds: a conceptual framework. In: Kincaid H, Sullivan JA, editors. *Classifying Psychopathology: Mental Kinds and Natural Kinds*. Cambridge, MA: MIT Press (2014). p. 65–74.

6

Causality in Psychiatry: A Hybrid Symptom Network Construct Model

*Gerald Young**

York University, Toronto, ON, Canada

Edited by:
Annemarie Kalis,
Utrecht University, Netherlands

Reviewed by:
Stijn Vanheule,
Ghent University, Belgium
Riet Van Bork,
University of Amsterdam, Netherlands

***Correspondence:**
Gerald Young
gyoung@glendon.yorku.ca

Causality or etiology in psychiatry is marked by standard biomedical, reductionistic models (symptoms reflect the construct involved) that inform approaches to nosology, or classification, such as in the DSM-5 [Diagnostic and Statistical Manual of Mental Disorders, Fifth Edition; (1)]. However, network approaches to symptom interaction [i.e., symptoms are formative of the construct; e.g., (2), for posttraumatic stress disorder (PTSD)] are being developed that speak to bottom-up processes in mental disorder, in contrast to the typical top-down psychological construct approach. The present article presents a hybrid top-down, bottom-up model of the relationship between symptoms and mental disorder, viewing symptom expression and their causal complex as a reciprocally dynamic system with multiple levels, from lower-order symptoms in interaction to higher-order constructs affecting them. The hybrid model hinges on good understanding of systems theory in which it is embedded, so that the article reviews in depth non-linear dynamical systems theory (NLDST). The article applies the concept of emergent circular causality (3) to symptom development, as well. Conclusions consider that symptoms vary over several dimensions, including: subjectivity; objectivity; conscious motivation effort; and unconscious influences, and the degree to which individual (e.g., meaning) and universal (e.g., causal) processes are involved. The opposition between science and skepticism is a complex one that the article addresses in final comments.

Keywords: causality, symptom, mental disorder, construct, network

CAUSALITY IN PSYCHIATRY: A HYBRID SYMPTOM NETWORK CONSTRUCT MODEL

The article tackles fundamental issues in psychiatry while proposing novel solutions. In particular, it considers the relationship between symptoms and disorder by examining extant models and current research. It attempts to disambiguate some of the confusions related to understanding and researching the models, preparing the way for presentation of a genuinely hybrid one based on systems theory thinking. Moreover, it presents other novel concepts related to emergent causality, and the relationship of meaning and causality in symptoms (hermeneutic insight and causal explanation; Verstehen, Erklären, respectively). The article presents a complex view of the relationship between meaning and causality involving three dimensions.

INTRODUCTION

Opposing Models

The article reflects on two types of models, a latent variable model (or construct model), which is seen as a top-down approach to understanding the relationship between symptoms and disorders, and a symptom interaction model (or network model), which is seen as a bottom-up approach to understanding the relationship between symptoms and disorders. In latent variable modeling, an underlying construct (e.g., depression) is considered causal of the relationship of the items or behaviors (e.g., symptoms) that are subsumed by the variable. In an item or behavior interaction or networked model (e.g., symptoms), relatively few direct relations are considered causal of the item/behavior/symptom relationships, which are deemed to lie among the latter themselves.

In the first model of the two involved, which is the traditional approach, symptoms (items) reflect a common underlying psychological construct and, therefore, this type of model is considered "reflective" (4). In this construct model, the cause of the mental symptom/disorder derives from the central construct, whether a disorder or a cluster, downward to the symptoms. In the symptom-interactive model, symptoms (items) mutually affect each other, and can be represented by a composite variable, but the direction of the causality is from the symptom interactions to the composite. The model is referred to as "formative" (4).

In this network model, which is the second of the two involved, causality springs from the symptoms (or clusters) interacting among themselves, a process that acts to change the symptoms/clusters (or initiate them). The composite variable is involved only as representation.

Before describing the hybrid model in depth, some of the challenges in doing so are described. This leads to presentation of a literature review preparatory to it.

Systems

The article will consider the following crucial questions. First, what do we miss when we represent disorders solely with top-down models such as the construct model? What do we miss when we represent disorders solely with bottom-up models such as a network model? In order to answer these questions, the hybrid model that has been created is framed in Non-Linear Dynamical Systems Theory (NLDST), which can be viewed both as a model that is an umbrella one or superordinate one to the construct and network ones. Therefore, the article presents a novel hybrid model, which combines these two types of models (top-down, bottom-up) into a framework that both respects them yet adds to them without detracting from them.

In this work, researchers might obtain a covariance matrix related to the multiple symptoms in a study (referring to the covariance among scores of participants with respect to the symptoms that were measured). Once the matrix is established, the covariance obtained could be explained from either a common construct perspective or from that of symptom network interactions (i.e., common cause vs. direct causal relations). In this regard, the researcher evaluates either (a) the shared variance of all measured variables of a putative construct, e.g., estimating factor loadings, and the causal pattern is from the construct to the variables; or (b) the parameters for the direct relations between symptoms. Furthermore, in one type of hybrid approach, the variance that is not explained by the common construct might be explained residually through direct relations between networked symptoms.

That being said, the present hybrid model is not built on statistical synergies but conceptual ones. It presents a theoretically plausible causal model and the statistical task, then becomes to fit extant statistical approaches to the model or expand them for this purpose. The conceptual hybrid model is built on NLDST, and the multilevel hierarchical structure that it includes allows for upper levels of the system to work with lower levels in establishing the system whole. That is, if we equate psychological constructs with emergent higher-order system levels that might derive from lower-order levels and their bottom-up interactions, such as in networks, then the stage is set for having higher-order levels reciprocally influence in turn in a top-down fashion the networks involved. For example, depression might not only be constructed by its symptoms but also it might exist as a subjective mental content or disorder and influence the configuration of its symptoms (in context, and for the individual in her/his uniqueness).

If one excludes psychological constructs from consideration as a higher-order level in a systems model, the hybrid model as presented will be dismissed. However, if one allows for its inclusion in a systems framework, as described, the framework can readily be conceived as one that has emergent higher-order levels (or constructs, e.g., mental content and disorder) that can interact top-down and reciprocally with symptom networks in their bottom-up influence on the system.

Clusters

Another complication in developing a hybrid model involving construct and network approaches to symptom–disorder relationships involves clusters, which stand intermediate between symptoms and disorders. In network modeling, subsets (clusters) of items, behaviors, or symptoms (variables) might be found, but they are not considered as independent sources of causation relative to the direct relationships among the variables. Rather, variables within any one cluster might causally influence each other in their network. Inter-variable correlations will result, but they would not reflect the causal influence of a common underpinning construct. The article will deal with this issue as it proceeds in creating a genuine hybrid model.

On the one hand, the DSM-5 [Diagnostic and Statistical Manual of Mental Disorders, Fifth Edition; (1)] includes many disorders that, through its polythetic approach to symptom identification, involve symptom clusters. However, the research on how many clusters are needed in the DSM's disorders stands as an ongoing enterprise. For example, in posttraumatic stress disorder (PTSD), the empirical findings on how to group its symptoms keeps finding an increasing amount of clusters. The number of factors or dimensions involved in research on PTSD has moved it from the DSM-5's four-dimensional model to ones with even seven and eight dimensions (see below). On the other hand, in systems modeling, there is no reason why intermediate levels cannot constitute both top-down causal levels working on lower ones and levels that can be influenced by those lower ones, while having levels superordinate to them influence them, while they form networks among themselves that can influence their superordinate levels. Therefore, systems modeling can accommodate the concept of clusters in symptoms.

The final prefatory note about the present hybrid model of symptom–mental disorder relations (with its mutual bottom-up and top-down influences) is that its hybrid nature is not synonymous with an attempt to explain everything related to the question to the point that its inclusivity can really explain nothing. In this regard, there are many multifactorial models in causal explanation that are acceptable; there are many systems models in this regard; and there are many advancing conceptual and statistical notions that are hybrid and explanatory without being obtuse and untestable [e.g., Ref. (5, 6)].

ISSUES

In the following, the first substantive section of the article considers relevant concepts and terms. This lays the foundation for the literature review, model building, and applications.

Concepts

Psychiatry has been criticized at multiple levels, including its difficulties with its diagnostic manuals and their assumptions. It embraces mostly the medical model of disorder and diagnosis, the biocentric model of the causality of disorder, or etiology, and the psychopharmacological model of disorder treatment and management (6–9). Even the basic concept of what constitutes a mental disorder has been disputed. In the following, I review aspects of these issues, preparing the way for presentation of my own work in the area. The section ends with an integrated view of what is mental disorder.

The RDoC project [Research Domain of Criteria; (10, 11)] contends that it offers a broad approach to causation in psychiatry, but its critics maintain that it is especially biomedical, neurocentric, and reductionistic [e.g., Ref. (6, 12, 13)]. Similarly, the DSM-5 is a psychiatric classificatory system that aims to include reliable and valid categories of mental disorder with clear causes (etiology), an aspiration that, if realized, would facilitate effective treatment; however, its critics maintain that it fails to achieve its objective [e.g., Ref. (6–9)]. Also, in terms of causal explanations, they maintain that it is still steeped in the biocentric model.

Multifactorial causal models in psychiatry have been formulated, such as the biopsychosocial model [e.g., Ref. (5, 6)]. Moreover, newer modeling efforts are specifying the mechanisms in the interactions among causal influences on behavior and its disturbance, such as work on networks [e.g., Ref. (2, 14)] and attractor dynamics [e.g., Ref. (15)].

To highlight in more depth the main argument of the article, bottom-up causality in psychiatry refers to the interaction and mutual influence of symptoms in mental illness, while top-down ones refer to the influence of underlying latent variables or constructs on symptom expression. A genuinely interactive bottom-up, top-down model would acknowledge both the reality of an underlying latent variable or construct in influencing symptomatology and also networked symptom connections as influencing the underlying construct.

This approach might be antithetical to those who hold either a network or construct view of system–disorder relations, but there are advantages to the model. Moreover, it fits the overarching model of systems theory. In this regard, the next section of the article explains in depth the concept of systems, which includes different levels, self-organization, emergence, and attractors.

Non-Linear Dynamical Systems Theory

This section of the article reviews some critical concepts in NLDST. Detailed presentation of systems theory is beyond the scope of the present work; the reader should consult Thelen and Smith (16); Young (3), and also Bielczyk et al. (15).

NLDST is distinguished by its emphasis on self-organized emergence in system component interactions within and across levels. In particular, higher-order levels of systems might emerge through bottom-up interactive processes. For example, Vallacher et al. (17) referred to the emergence of "global properties" or "coherent higher-order" states through the adjustment to each other of the individual system elements involved in a bottom to top (bottom-up, instead of top-down) self-organizational process. Typically, self-organization does not reach the new system end-state instantaneously. Rather, there are many ongoing mutual system element adjustments that take place.

Through its concepts of emergence and self-organization, NLDST allows for explanation of how higher-order patterns in behavior, from the simplest limb movements to the most profound thoughts, are part of the species' repertoire. New systems states that emerge in a system function to constrain behavior emanating from the system. New state system input transforms toward state characteristics even if they are discrepant with them. That is, systems maintain stability once formed, even if perturbed, until further mutual element and input interactions lead to critical state transition points.

System states might change over time, but when they consistently return to the same state after perturbation, the state involved is considered an attractor. Attractors reside in landscapes with basins; and the wider are the basins, the more likely a range of states in the system will converge on one attractor, which metaphorically could be considered to reside at the bottom of the basin involved. In this model, the "deeper" is the basin, the greater is the attractor's resistance to perturbation.

When a system has two or more states, it is considered multistable. The attractors could involve negative or undesirable states, such as having in the same person antagonism in conjunction with antagonism avoidance. Or, the two members of a couple could be living antagonistic regimes [e.g., Ref. (18)]. Beyond attractors on which system dynamics converge, an attractive force could be like a "repellor," or one that scrupulously avoids regions in its state space rather than returning to it. Metaphorically, instead of in a basin, a repellor resides on top of a hill in the system's landscape.

Systems might have no attractors, and therefore be more susceptible to external influences. Or, systems might have one attractor, sustain a perturbation that is critical (19), and produce self (re)organization through the effect on set points in control parameters in the system.

Finally for Vallacher et al. (17), dynamic properties can be found at "different levels of psychological reality," and dynamic transformations can take place at different time scales (seconds, years). Also, network concepts fall under the rubric of dynamic ones. That is, network nodes represent elements in systems. This notion is important for present purposes in that it justifies considering network models as part of larger ones in NLDST that includes higher-order levels that can be represented as constructs.

Samuelson et al. (20) emphasized the relevance of emergence in NLDST. Emergence takes place through systems components that interact and mutually influence each other in a soft-assembly process, or from the ground, rather than from pre-specified central, top-down (deterministic) explicit coding or organization. It takes place over multiple time scales; can happen on the moment; and is conditioned by context and the history of the organism, so that the outcome is unique and variable. Systems might also have subsystems, which are strongly coupled or integrated components that are only weakly coupled at best to other components. The authors give the example of seeking hidden objects in a first location even after viewing its hiding in a second one. Research shows that, in infants, the error involved (A-not-B) is a product of cognitive and motor components in interaction, with temporal and neural dynamics at work, too.

Hayes et al. (21) noted that dynamic systems concern pattern formation and change. The principles in dynamic systems science cut across biology, ecology, political science, and other disciplines, including physics and chemistry. Systems are adaptive when they maintain a dynamic tension between stability and variability. Although resilience to perturbation can be beneficial, it should not be overly rigid. For example, from a network perspective, in depression, negative emotions exhibit stronger temporal connections (22). Psychotherapy can help in shifting maladaptive connections to adaptive ones, as demonstrated in the research of Hayes and colleagues and Schiepek et al. (23).

NLDST is a mathematical model that is conducive to psychological theorizing. For example, attractors can be represented by mathematical formalisms, and state spaces or trajectories in a system can be represented by graphical representation of differential equations (24). In this regard, modeling could include approaches such as dynamic factor analysis and application of ergodic theory (25). Butner et al. (24) explained that, mathematically, Lyapunov exponents represent the strength of system topological features, for example, the rate a system changes toward or away from a particular state (the basin steepness). They can be calculated locally (e.g., at a set point) or globally (for the whole system).

Rabinovich et al. (26) described dynamic transformation as allowing cognition and mind to emerge from brain and computation. Cognition is not reflected in any one brain center or even in the entire brain, but is a product of interconnected cooperativity over many elements. The spatiotemporal patterns in brain dynamics that are highly coherent could be called modes, and they reflect the play of extinction and stabilizing inhibition. Brain center clusters that form in tasks represent dynamical modes and correspond to transient system states. Superordinate levels in systems can be conceived as hierarchically arranged chunking networks, e.g., from sentences to paragraphs to chapters in texts.

Wichers et al. (27) indicated how moment-to-moment affect dynamics can be viewed from NLDST. They referred to research showing that symptom networks in (severe) psychopathology are more strongly interconnected than those of people with less severe psychopathology [e.g., Ref. (14)]. The networks exhibit vicious circles because their nodes reinforce each other. In dynamical terms, a system could be "very" stable and therefore even "strong" perturbations might not create variability, let alone a small one allowing for "critical transition" to another state at a "tipping point." However, in psychopathology, if there is high, mutually reinforcing connectivity with networks, such that vicious circles develop in the background without being noticed, the mood system could become fragile and vulnerable to transition, even when one node (affective state) is triggered for the reason that others are also activated in the network. A cascade effect results that continues to resonate in the network such that the "little" perturbation of the one node involved leads to a disproportionate mood change or critical transition (as in the well-known butterfly effect).

Mental Disorder and Symptoms

Before continuing in the article with the literature review and detailed modeling, the concept of a symptom needs clarification. This is undertaken toward better understanding mental disorder, which is also discussed in this section.

Symptom

A symptom is defied as a physical or mental feature that is a departure from a typical state or feeling and that might be indicative of a disease, disturbance, disorder, unusual state, or condition (and which might be noticed by the patient). Symptoms might be subjectively experienced and phenomenologically reported or objectively obtained (signs, e.g., in laboratory tests). Symptoms include the contents of mental states that might recursively influence other symptoms, such as through the vicious circles that take place after catastrophic thinking and fears. Beliefs are powerful engines driving symptomatology, as are moods, affect, emotions, drives, desires, and motivation.

Much of the work in psychotherapy relates to these mental contents, the narratives people tell about themselves and to others, and the meanings ascribed to events, as well as one's past experiences, and one's place in the present and future, in addition to other people's actions and reactions to the person and their relationships with the person. In this sense, the person is as much, if not more, a seat of the causality of symptomatology experienced as are biological (nature) and environmental (nurture) factors (as per the biopsychosocial/biopersonalsocial models mentioned previously). That being said, not all symptoms can be taken at face value or are even genuine. This is especially true because of the influence of unconscious processes on symptom expression, as well as even conscious ones, such as those related to feigning or malingering for monetary gain, as might happen with PTSD, the exemplar chosen in the article. This difference between patient presentation and actual symptomatology constitutes the quandary confronting clinicians, as well as the challenge that they and their patients must work through.

Mental Disorder

As for defining mental disorder, there is no one accepted definition. The approach of the DSM-5 involves a clinically significant disturbance reflecting dysfunction usually associated with distress or disability in activity. In contrast, for the DSM, normally neither an expected, culturally approved loss to a common stressor/loss nor individual-society conflicts, involving socially deviant behavior, are representative of mental disorder.

The DSM-5's definition of mental disorder includes an error in reasoning (8). It indicates tautologically that a mental disorder is caused by a disturbance in mental functioning, which simply uses the same words on both sides of the definitional equation. The World Health Organization (28) definition of mental disorder does not help resolve the matter. It refers to a disorder as a combination of thoughts, perceptions, emotions, behavior, and relationships that are "abnormal."

Closer inspection of the DSM-5 definition of mental disorder indicates that it is constituted by different levels. The DSM-5 definition has implicit in it several levels. They include mental function atop the hierarchy, then mental disorder as one branch. The collection of signs (objective) and symptoms (subjective) happen behaviorally, emotionally (in regulation) and cognitively, and together constitute a syndrome. Furthermore, the ensemble of signs and symptoms are associated with a "clinically" significant disturbance and usually a "significant distress, or disability." Finally, at another level implicating causality, there are "dysfunctions" in psychological, biological, or developmental "processes." Aside from these levels, often, mental disorder in the DSM-5 includes clusters of symptoms intermediate between the disorder and symptom list.

Both the DSM-5 definition of mental disorder and the WHO's definition do not include directly environment, support or its lack, or context. A relational and systemic approach to mental disorder might better arrive at its acceptable and inclusive definition [e.g., Ref. (8)].

Young (6) developed a more elaborative definition of mental disorder. According to him, it involves "a behavioral syndrome (or pattern or network of symptoms) in context that is characterized as a clinically significant disturbance, distress, or dysfunction potentially evaluated as harmful to the individual, to others, or to both." To establish clinical significance, well-informed (and trained) individuals should rely on reliable and relevant evidence. The mental disorder can be expressed in cognition, mood, relations, interactions, self-regulation, and other behavior and its organization. Biological, social, and personal (i.e., psychological), as well as developmental processes, might be factors. Social, occupational, or other important functional activities might be involved in impairment, and they might meet disability thresholds. The definition of mental disorder that I have provided is based on the DSM's approach, but broadens it, for example, by mentioning symptom networks, which is important in the present context.

Diagnostic and Statistical Manual of Mental Disorders, Fifth Edition

According to Vanheule (9), a diagnostic category needs to be both reliable and valid. For reliability, he noted that the range of kappa results in reliability studies of DSM categories has shifted in the qualitative attribute given to the best results, the next best, and so on. In particular, Clarke et al. (29) used a shift in describing kappa results that seemingly allowed for acceptable reliability for quite a few DSM-5 categories in the DSM-5 field trials, when use of the kappa ranges used in research on prior versions of the DSM would have shown questionable reliability for those DSM-5 results had the prior adjectives in summarizing kappa results had been applied without change. That being said, I note that the best results were obtained for PTSD (along with a few others; PTSD reliability results for the DSM-5 were considered at least fair or very good, depending on the criteria).

As for validity, Vanheule (9) queried whether the DSM-5 accounts well for context and whether its categories apply well to individual cases. He concluded that, rather than symptoms being signs or indices, they should be conceived as personal constructions.

The next section of the article examines recent literature related to topics in mental disorder. They include work on network models and the construct approach at issue in the article, preparing the way for the hybrid model developed over the two approaches. In brief, the articles cited have helped lead to the present top-down (construct)/bottom-up (symptom network) causal model relating symptom and mental disorder. In addition, the review provides comments that prepare elaboration of the present model.

LITERATURE REVIEW

The literature review concentrates on the disorders of posttraumatic stress and depression, in particular. It especially analyzes the research by McNally et al. (2) for the former, and Wigman et al. (14) for the latter.

Posttraumatic Stress Disorder

Dimensions

In a literature review and conceptual analysis, Rosen and Lilienfeld (30) evaluated the core assumptions of PTSD. They found that research findings provided no compelling or consistent support for its core assumptions. They queried whether it is a diagnostic category that should be kept in the DSM. In a later publication, Rosen and colleagues called for a process of active questioning to determine its validity (31). That being said, the literature has consistently engaged in scientific investigation of PTSD and its validity. Previously, I noted that the DSM-5 field trials found it to be reliable. In the following, I examine one aspect of its validity – concerning its symptom structure. The review will show that, rather than the current four-cluster model for PTSD in the DSM-5, models with more factors better fit the 20-symptom symptom list for PTSD as found in the DSM-5. In particular, a seven-factor model has been found to be the most powerful and, moreover, it has been found to have associations indicative of its clinical and theoretical value (32, 33).

Table 1 indicates the basic symptoms of PTSD both in the psychiatric diagnostic (nosological) manual, the DSM-IV [Diagnostic and Statistical Manual of Mental Disorders, Fourth Edition; (34)] and the DSM-5, and how the symptoms of PTSD

TABLE 1 | DSM-5 PTSD symptom cluster model (seven) and the dissociative subtype (one), with hypothesized core/non-core symptoms specified.

Number	Symptom	Cluster	Non-core	Core
PTSD				
1	Memories (intrusive)	Re-experiencing	–	✓
2	Nightmares (recurrent)	Re-experiencing	✓	–
3	Dissociative reactions/ flashbacks	Re-experiencing	✓	–
4	Emotional reactivity (heightened; to signals)	Re-experiencing	✓	–
5	Physiological reactivity to reminders (marked)	Re-experiencing	✓	–
6	Avoid thoughts/feelings/ memories (reminders)	Avoidance	✓	–
7	Avoid external reminders	Avoidance	–	✓
8	Amnesia: inability to recall important aspects	Negative affect	✓	–
9	Negative beliefs (persistent, heightened)	Negative affect	✓	–
10	Self/other blame (persistent)	Negative affect	✓	–
11	Negative emotional state (persistent)	Negative affect	–	✓
12	Loss of interest (marked)	Anhedonia	✓	–
13	Detachment	Anhedonia	–	✓
14	Restricted positive affect	Anhedonia	✓	–
15	Irritability/anger	Externalizing behavior	–	✓
16	Reckless/ self-destructive	Externalizing behavior	✓	–
17	Hypervigilance	Alterations in arousal and reactivity	✓	–
18	Startle (exaggerated)	Alterations in arousal and reactivity	–	✓
19	Difficulty concentrating	Dysphoric arousal	✓	–
20	Sleep disturbance	Dysphoric arousal	–	✓
Dissociative subtype				
1	Depersonalization	Dissociation	–	✓
2	Derealization	Dissociation	✓	–

The table indicates the 20 symptoms in the DSM-5 [Diagnostic and Statistical Manual of Mental Disorders, Fifth Edition; (1)], and the 17 in the DSM-IV [Diagnostic and Statistical Manual of Mental Disorders, Fourth Edition; (34)]. There have been changes in wording for some of the symptoms from one version to the next, and the abbreviated versions in the table refer to the DSM-5 symptom list. One of the symptoms in the table (sense of foreshortened future) applies only to the DSM-IV. The table also gives the arrangement of the symptoms into clusters in the DSM-5 and in the DSM-IV. There are four clusters for the former and three for the latter. The DSM-5 clusters essentially involve splitting the DSM-IV avoidance/numbing cluster, consistent with the factor analytic model on the DSM-IV factor structure (37). There are other competing models. Moreover, other research (38) points to a separate cluster related to the DSM's dissociative subtype. The table indicates which of the symptoms for each of the eight clusters in the table appear to be predominant, essential, or core (39).
Adapted from Young (36).

are organized into clusters in these manuals. Moreover, the factor analytic research on how the symptoms cluster have not supported the way the DSMs have parsed the PTSD symptoms into clusters. In this regard, as mentioned, the most recent research of PTSD symptom clustering has indicated that a seven-factor model fits best how the 20 symptoms of PTSD in the DSM-5 organize into clusters [Ref. (32); and replicated by Wang et al. (35); as summarized in Ref. (36)]. Furthermore, the research supports a dissociative PTSD subtype. In this regard, I have argued that there are really eight dimensions to consider in PTSD as described in the DSM-5 (36). Finally, the tables show my approach to which are core symptoms rather than non-core ones among the PTSD symptoms in each of the eight clusters involved in PTSD and the dissociative subtype in the DSM-5 (36).

The factor analytic research on PTSD uses confirmatory factor analysis (CFA), which is based on *a priori* models that are tested. Until recently, only four-factor models had been supported, but the work of Elhai et al. (40) had shown that there might be five factors involved in PTSD, and more recently two six-factor models were tested and supported (32, 41) before they were combined in the seven-factor model. Therefore, the understanding of PTSD is becoming more refined and each cluster found represents some psychological construct related to it (e.g., re-experiencing, avoidance, hyperarousal/reactivity). This research is valuable for differentiating models of PTSD at the level of the higher-order constructs that comprise it, because working with 17 to 20 symptoms or so is quite difficult clinically. This is one reason why I tried to isolate the core symptoms in each of the clusters involved.

Zelazny and Simms (42) conducted CFA in a study of psychiatric outpatients assessed using DSM-5 symptom criteria of PTSD. For both samples studied (those meeting either criteria in interview or a subthreshold stressor), the best fit of the data involved the above-mentioned seven-factor model. However, a new six-factor model also fit well the data (named alternate dysphoria, in which difficult concentrating and sleep problems are removed from the dysphoric arousal factor in these models and placed in the dysphoria factor).

Clearly, the research continues on the factor structure of PTSD. That being said, the lack of final response to the question cannot be taken to invalidate PTSD.

Networks

Partly in reaction to the complexity of working with long lists of symptoms, researchers using the symptom network approach to PTSD are attempting to discern how symptoms coordinate into nodes and their relations, referred to as edges. Also, they seek the centrality of symptoms in networks, such as in measures of betweenness. The approach statistically is quite different than that of CFA, which focuses on underlying constructs. In network approaches, the nodes and edges are the foci, and symptom themselves in their networking create and influence each other outside of any putative underlying construct.

In the network approach, symptoms covary, or couple variably, and affect each other through feedback loops, homeostatic relations, and so on, allowing sensitivity to individual differences in symptom expression and their causality. For example, an episode of PTSD would follow a course related to symptom nodes in the network "turning on" and "transmitting their activation" to nodes connected to them.

McNally et al. (2) presented a network approach to the symptoms of PTSD. They conducted a questionnaire study of survivors of a 2008 Chinese earthquake, with over 360 respondents. They used a translated version of the PCL [Posttraumatic Checklist - Civilian; (43); Mandarin Chinese version; (44)]. The questionnaire is keyed to the DSM-IV. According to the questionnaire, 38% met the criteria for probable PTSD (5 years after the earthquake when the data were gathered).

The data showed that with exclusion of results at $r \leq 0.30$, strong associations become more evident, for example, for hypervigilance and startle and also avoidance of thoughts and activities (about the trauma and associated with it, respectively). Numbing and dissociation symptoms were strongly linked (loss of interest in enjoyable activities; feeling distance from others, respectively). Finally, nightmares, flashbacks, and intrusive memories related to the trauma were tightly linked. The authors noted that these various symptom linkages appear related to the three DSM-IV symptom clusters of hyperarousal, avoidance/numbing, and re-experiencing, respectively. However, other symptom linkages did not conform to these DSM clusters - those of startle-concentration problems, and anger-concentration problems.

Other results included that concentration networking indicated that two re-experiencing symptoms were not connected to the others (physiological reactivity, feeling upset at reminders), but quite connected to each other. Centrality calculations showed that a highly central symptom concerns perceiving the future as foreshortened. Overall, the authors concluded that hypervigilance, future foreshortening, and sleep appear predominant symptoms in PTSD symptom network analysis, with multiple symptom linkages involved, including some not previously considered.

To conclude this section of the paper, I note that in Young et al. (45), I attempted to show how a network model of PTSD symptoms could distinguish primary (core), secondary, and tertiary ones. That work indicates that network thinking can be applied to mental disorder in multiple ways.

Depression and Other Disorders

Bielczyk et al. (15) adopted a similar model for major depressive disorder. According to them, causal relations in network dynamics are the cause of clinical constructs such as depression.

Bielczyk et al. (15) added a role in depression of attractor dynamics and also for the regulation of excitation–inhibition balance across brain circuits. These latter concepts are quite consistent with my own (6), in that I argue that NLDST can help explain shifts to health and illness attractors and that activation/inhibition coordination is an important mechanism at all levels in brain–behavior relations.

Conway and Kovacs (46) have shown how the field of human intelligence is moving away from the traditional latent psychological construct model (*g*, general factor of intelligence) in which *g* is considered a causal general ability, to new models that interpret *g* as an emergent property reflecting the positive correlations found among test scores. This research shows how the concept that underlying constructs need to be complemented if not replaced by other models is gaining traction in areas other than psychopathology.

These newer models are "formative" ones, and not the traditional "reflective," essentialist, or "entity realism" ones. In formative models, there still are psychological constructs, but as causal effects or consequences rather than causal initiators.

Conway and Kovacs (46) concluded that hybrid models of intelligence exist, and they are partly reflective in nature and partly formative, too, such as found in their own "process overlap" theory. As has been emphasized, for the topic of psychopathology, the present work also is proposing a hybrid reflective (top-down) and formative (bottom-up) causal model of the relationship between symptom and illness. The model that I have created derives from the seminal work of McNally et al. (2) and also that of Wigman et al. (14), presented next.

Wigman et al. (14) examined data gathered by experience sampling methodology (ESM) in a pooled sample ($N = 599$) of three groups (depression in past; current status mild; psychotic symptoms, with disorder diagnosed; controls). Participants were given wristwatches that beeped quasi-randomly 10 times per day over a period of 5 to 6 days (depending on the particular sample). The signal required them to fill in a self-assessment diary. The focus of their study was to analyze the relations of participants' responses, as given on a 7-point Likert scale, for five items, which were - at this moment, I feel: cheerful; content; insecure; down; suspicious.

Wigman et al. (14) reviewed the top-down psychological construct approach to mental disorder. As shown, in this approach, mental symptoms are viewed as being caused by underlying constructs. In contrast, the bottom-up approach that they reviewed maintains that psychopathology involves a complex interacting network of components. At the symptom level, this approach views mental states as nodes that, when activated, might trigger other mental states (47). Symptom networks might be non-linear in their mutual effects, reciprocal, with feedback loops, vicious circles, and increased connectivity.

Despite pointing out the major differences in the two models of how symptoms and disorder might relate, Wigman et al. (14) did not contrast in a direct fashion one model vs. the other. Rather, they compared mental state network structure over groups having the different diagnoses mentioned to healthy controls. Also, they sought clusters of network components across network data. Note that the network characteristics analyzed involved centrality indices: node strength, outward degree, inward degree, closeness, and betweenness.

Perhaps because the first type of analysis undertaken involved group comparison and the second transdiagnostic analysis, the authors referred to the cross-group network analysis as top-down even though it makes more sense to refer to network analysis as bottom-up and they referred to the principle component analysis as bottom-up even though it typically would be referred to as top-down compared to network analysis. In short, I query whether their approach by Wigman et al. (14) allows for the hybrid reflective–formative conceptualization of mental disorder and their relations to symptoms. It seems that all they did was analyze the data involved with the two types of statistics typically associated with one approach or the other, but not in the way that the statistics are typically used in this type of research. Careful analysis of their results in what follows confirms this impression.

The results in Wigman et al. (14) showed that having a diagnosis led to more strongly connected moment-to-moment mental state network structures, and more so for depression relative to psychosis. For example, in depressed patients, there were many more interconnections between negative and positive emotions, unlike the case for the group with psychosis, for which connections like this were rare. In the latter group, there appears to be two separate loops of mental state, one negative and the other positive. In terms of the connectedness measurement, it was higher in the group with depression, e.g., in terms of node strength and inward and outward degree. Depressed individuals had the highest node strength. Finally, the comparison group had the least connections going to or coming from negative mental states.

As for the principal component analysis results, seven high-order components emerged. They were based on loadings over associations such as mental state at time $t - 1$ and what follows at time t. For the first factor, all the loaded associations began with a positive emotional state at time $t - 1$. Therefore, the authors interpreted it "impact of positive mental state." The second factor seemed to reflect the negative impact of feeling down on other mental states, and so on. A primary result was that compared to the controls, the two psychiatrically disordered groups obtained higher scores on the component of "impact of insecure," suggesting that this component might be a general one in mental illness in multiple dimensions of psychopathology. The authors noted that the network paradigm appears to be a useful one in mapping transdiagnostic processes in mental state.

Wigman et al. (14) concluded that individuals with the same diagnosis might exhibit substantially different symptom patterns. Moreover, the concept itself of separate diagnoses might be problematic in that psychopathology might reflect one underlying explanatory principle – that of mental state interconnectivity underlying symptoms. These conclusions are quite accurate, but they might reflect the manner in which the analyses were conducted rather than anything like a genuinely hybrid model of reflective and formative models. In such an approach, psychological construct and network analyses would be conceptualized as equal and interacting reciprocal causality mechanisms of the relationship of symptom and psychological construct, and not be considered hybrid simply because a principal component analysis was applied to network data. In the following, I attempt to create such an integrative model of symptom–mental disorder relations. In the latter approach, only the data analysis methods are hybrid, not the conceptualization.

This penultimate section of the article follows next and outlines a genuine hybrid model of symptom–mental disorder relations from a bottom-up-top-down perspective. Once the model building is complete, the article considers further the nature of symptoms, for example, in terms of the value of perceiving them as individualized mental content and meaning.

THE HYBRID SYMPTOM–MENTAL DISORDER MODEL

Specifically for this section of the article, I re-introduce the bottom-up and top-down models of the symptom–mental disorder relationship. Then, I show how the two models can reciprocally interrelate.

Modeling

In models of symptoms and mental disorder relations, one set of models concerns higher-order (latent variable) constructs (e.g., PTSD) that cause or influence in a top-down manner the lower-order manifest symptoms and their clusters (which in turn might be an intermediate level of influence on symptoms). In contrast, according to network models, cluster/symptom interactions cause their pattern of expressions and the term associated with mental disorder (e.g., PTSD) is a representation of the symptoms and their interactions rather than being a causal influence on their manifestation.

One way of accommodating the different views on psychopathology of what constitutes bottom-up and top-down processes is to consider a systems model with different levels (see **Figure 1**). Systems thinking is best exemplified by NLDST [e.g., Ref. (3, 16)], in which different levels of a system might interact and even be created in the interaction, just as different elements in any one level of the system (or of the system as a whole) might interact and even create new elements. Moreover, changes in system state might take place because of minor perturbations when the system is at far-from-equilibrium, while living systems generally might be poised at this state preparatory to change because of its adaptive value.

Figure 1 illustrates the difference between a hybrid conceptualization of symptom–mental state relations and a hybrid statistical analysis of the relations. There is no reason why it cannot be the case that with each of the classic top-down, psychological construct approach and the bottom-up, symptom-driven approach, there are both network and cluster statistics that could be used.

Although powerful, the network approach to symptom causality and connection is more descriptive than mechanistic. It might indicate that symptoms connect and even in unique ways compared to conjectures and findings based on other approaches. However, the causes of the connectivities involved are not specified except by indicating that the symptom interactions are the cause. This might represent tautology, although I am sympathetic to the lower-order, grounded, and micromoment dynamics producing the connectivities. We need to know which symptoms emerge as predominant in any one moment of time, and the work of Wigman et al. (14) provides methods for tackling this issue. Moreover, they also refer to dynamic temporal processes in network expression.

Nevertheless, at another level, systems theory could tell us more about emerging connectivities over symptoms and their relations to mental state. In this regard, the work of Bielczyk et al. (15) indicates that mechanisms that might cohere symptoms (or repel them) might act through dynamical system processes [including activation/inhibition balancing, which is a concept central in my work: (3, 6)]. Symptom system dynamics can be measured in different ways in dynamical systems approaches compared to network ones, for example, in terms of control and order parameters and of exponents related to bifurcation points in which systems split into new attractor regimes or chaotic–antichaotic adaptive systems, fractal patterns, and so on.

That being said, the micromoment approach to symptom connectivity at times $t - 1$, t, $t + 1$, etc., could inform these analyses in complementary ways. For example, patients might

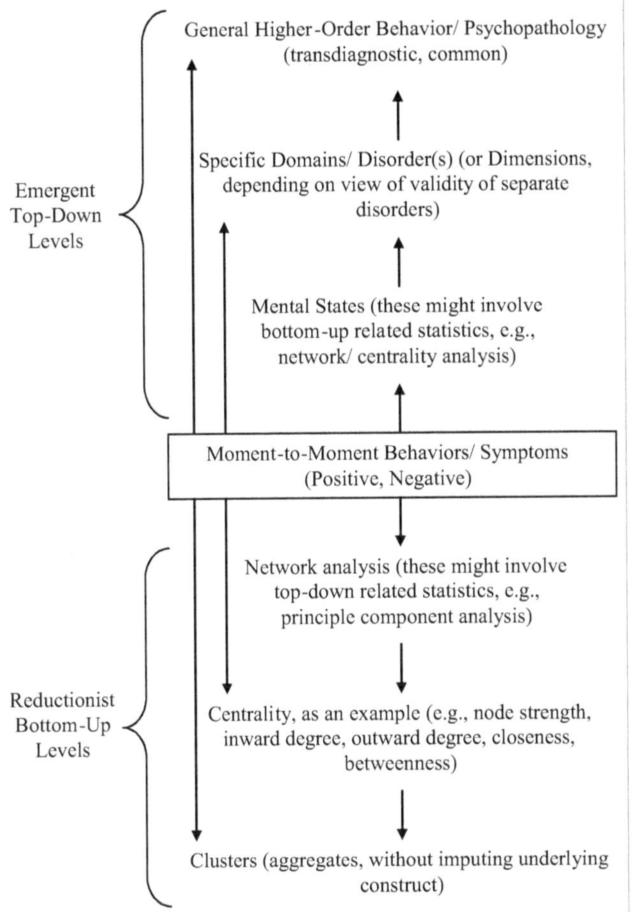

FIGURE 1 | Top-down and bottom-up levels in behavior/symptom normality/psychopathology. The figure illustrates the complementarity of top-down and bottom-up models of the causal relationship between symptoms and mental disorder. In systems, different levels might exist with higher-order levels emergent or distinct in characteristics from lower-order ones on which they are built. In terms of the constituents of the levels, they might be single elements, patterns, or networks, or even superordinate structures. Statistical techniques, such as network analysis or principle component analysis, can be applied to both emergent, higher-order levels and more basic ones. In terms of psychological constructs, at the higher-order emergent levels, in psychopathology, they might be specific disorders, dimensions, or overarching constructs (e.g., internalizing/ externalizing disorders).

have a more powerful symptom at any one time among their suite of symptoms, or one symptom might lead the way at any one moment in bringing a subthreshold one to disorder (and perhaps disability). As yet, there is no clear integrative model of how any one symptom might become primary in these senses at any one moment, although, as shown, the work of Wichers et al. (27) has made strides in these regards.

The symptom complex of the patient is crucial, as are symptom linkages over individualized patterns, or the network of nodes/ edges (relations) expressed by the patient over time. Based on this approach, the clinician might develop individual mappings of the dynamic evolution of symptoms over sessions and apply individualized approaches to intervention and treatment.

To conclude this portion of the article, hybrid conceptualizations to date on the relationship of symptoms and disorder have much to offer, but there might be conceptual limitations in the work that bar further progress. In this regard, current hybrid models [e.g., Ref. (14)], as argued above, might not allow for genuine reciprocity between the causal effects of the higher-order construct and the lower-order symptoms. Only by avoiding to equate any statistical modeling with conceptual ones and also by finding a common conceptual umbrella for both types of models can a genuine hybrid one over them be constructed. The next section presents a systems model-informed hybrid model of symptom–mental disorder relations based on these premises.

The Model

Figures 2 and **3** present core material of the present model of how symptoms and mental disorder interrelate in a hybrid fashion. The second of these two figures specifies how the concept of emergent circular causality (3) can be applied equally to the bottom-up and top-down approaches to causality. Specifically, **Figures 2** and **3** depict the difference between the latent variable/psychological construct model of the relationship between PTSD and its clusters/symptoms and the symptom-interactive or network model.

In considering development of a genuine hybrid model over the construct and symptom network approaches to how symptoms and mental disorder relates such that construct and symptoms causally interact, primacy should not be given to either component. Moreover, the statistical models that one might choose to work within each paradigm constrain the model building involved.

The next section of the article specifically demonstrates how a more integrative model of the reflective construct and formative network models could be constructed for the question of symptom–mental disorder relationship. It avoids some of the pitfalls of prior attempts to do the same. Nevertheless, it is an initial conceptualization that itself has limitations, such as not yet being mathematically grounded nor empirically tested.

Figures 4 and **5** present a genuine hybrid reflective and formative model of causality over mental symptom and disorder. For any one construct or cluster, there is not only influence/creation downward to symptoms but also feedback upward from symptom interactions to construct/cluster. Moreover, these top-down and bottom-up models function at multiple intermediary levels (intermediate, superordinate) and the interactions can take place not only horizontally (among symptoms; among levels/sublevels; and their configurations/patterns) but also vertically (downward or upward over (sub) levels).

Therefore, causality does not reside in one nexus node, level, element, element (sub)set, construct, or multiple aspects of these constituents of the symptom and disorder but in all the rich dynamical systemic interactions and reciprocal influences among them. Symptoms have causal effects on each other but constructs have causal effects on them. Constructs, such as mental disorder, are not ephemeral, reducible entities to symptoms, but emergent, irreducible entities that can affect and even initiate the symptoms. They reflect dynamical system characteristics, and can take on a life of their own at higher-order levels of a system. Perhaps they are not directly observable, but their role

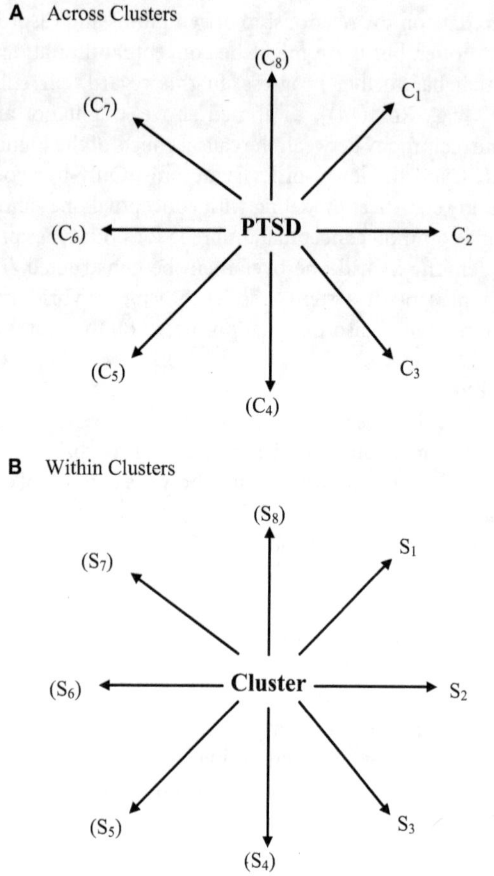

FIGURE 2 | A latent variable construct (top-down) causal model of PTSD symptoms (S) and clusters (C). (A) Across clusters, **(B)** within clusters. In latent variable or construct models of psychological phenomena, an "essential" underlying psychological entity, trait, characteristic, or superordinate attribute is considered as a valid higher-order behavioral reality that is not caused by or conditioned by the lower-order behaviors/symptoms associated with it but, to the contrary, conditions or causes in a top-down manner how they are manifested (in context, over time/development). Mental disorders might have several clusters and each can be characterized as a quasi-dependent sub-disorder that conditions/causes its associated symptoms. In this model, individual differences derive from the overarching construct involved and not from the manifested symptoms themselves, which merely reflect, in their patterns, the higher-order individual differences involved.

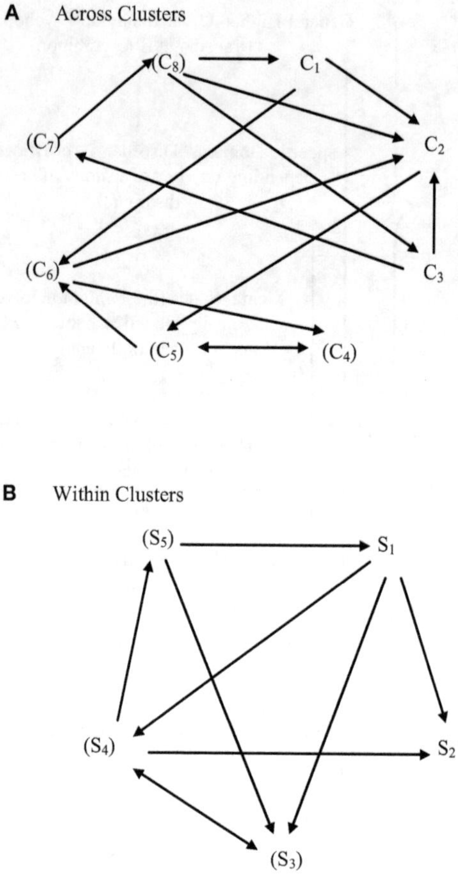

FIGURE 3 | A symptom-interactive (bottom-up) causal model of PTSD symptoms (S) and clusters (C). (A) Across clusters, **(B)** within clusters. In "non-essentialist" system-interactive or behavior/symptom network, connective models, behaviors/symptoms interact amongst themselves and constitute the cause of the pattern of behaviors/symptoms expressed. For example, if sleep is poor, other symptoms might be exacerbated. Individual differences in behavior/symptom expression derive from the behavior/symptom interactions in context (and over time/development). There is no higher-order "essential" (latent) psychological variable, construct, entity, trait, characteristic, or attribute that influences the behavior/symptom interactions. If terms relating to these levels of behavior are used in this model, it is only to represent the interactions and not as a factor that causes or influences them. In this regard, behaviors/symptoms in interaction do so at a level that is bottom-up rather than top-down.

can be inferred and the mechanisms that being them about are increasingly understood.

In short, emergence is a common construct in systems theory, but in my approach to it, circular causality constitutes an important driving mechanism in emergence (48). That is, as system levels interact with one another, new ones can emerge at higher orders, and they can become overarching and overriding drivers of behavior and symptom expression (3, 6). Specifically, I had written in Young (3) that in "circular emergence" different levels of systems can form and integrate, with higher-order ones gaining degrees of freedom through their flexibility even as their degrees of freedom are constrained through the intercoordinations involved. Also, I noted that activation/inhibition coordination can serve as the critical mechanism in stabilizing systems, in keeping them at the cusp of change, and in recreating equilibrium after they change.

CONCLUSION

First, the article has provided background information, such as relevant definitions and issues related to nosology, causality, and network and construct models of symptom–disorder relations. Then, it reviewed the relevant literature in the field, tackling alternative models and trying to disambiguate them. Next, it gave a genuinely hybrid model for the relationship of symptom network and psychological constructs in mental disorder.

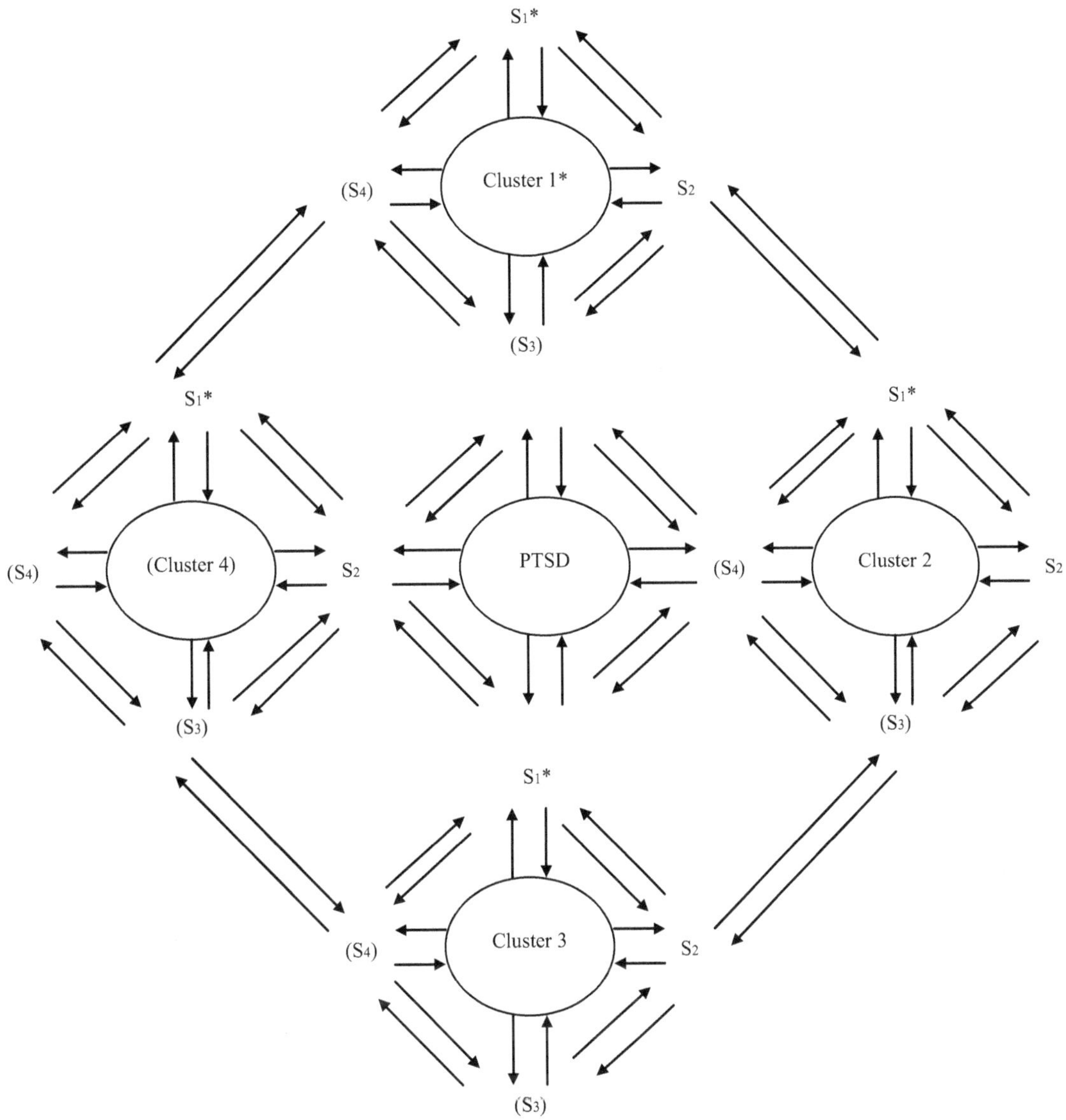

FIGURE 4 | Integrative causal symptom-construct model in mental disorder. The figure depicts the relationship between symptoms and mental disorder (or a symptom cluster of one) as dynamically reciprocal in causation. The mental disorder constitutes an underlying, higher-order level in the patient's mental state symptoms, while the symptoms interact at lower levels of the system, with both the top-down and bottom-up influences dynamically influencing each other in context and over time. Note: the parentheses indicate that PTSD might have only three clusters (as in the DSM-IV), and a cluster might have only two symptoms. Of course, depending on the disorder involved either might have more items (i.e., clusters or symptoms, respectively). Of the clusters in any mental disorder, for their symptoms, it would be beneficial to specify which ones are core/primary. For the model presented in the figure, these could be the first clusters or symptoms that are specified by the asterisks.

To conclude the article, in the next section, I return to considering the nature of symptoms by querying their unconscious, subjective, descriptive, and meaning side compared to their conscious, objective, and reductionist universal causal side. I present a novel model that addresses the question in an integrated manner.

One could ask even whether overarching illness entities could impact symptoms, and that mental disorders could be reducible to symptoms sets, as in the DSM-5. One answer to this conundrum would be to abandon the DSM-5 because of its multiple critics [see Ref. (7, 49)]. For them, the DSM-5 has theoretical, epistemological, and social weaknesses; was the result of a chaotic revision process; does not consider sufficiently the causality related to the listed mental disorders; they are artificial; and so on. However, continued research and revision of its categories could be improving its clinical usage.

Psychiatry needs to address critical questions on the nature of symptoms and mental disorder but, at the same time, balance scienticism and skepticism, or create hybrid models that integrate them and go beyond them. We need pause for thought

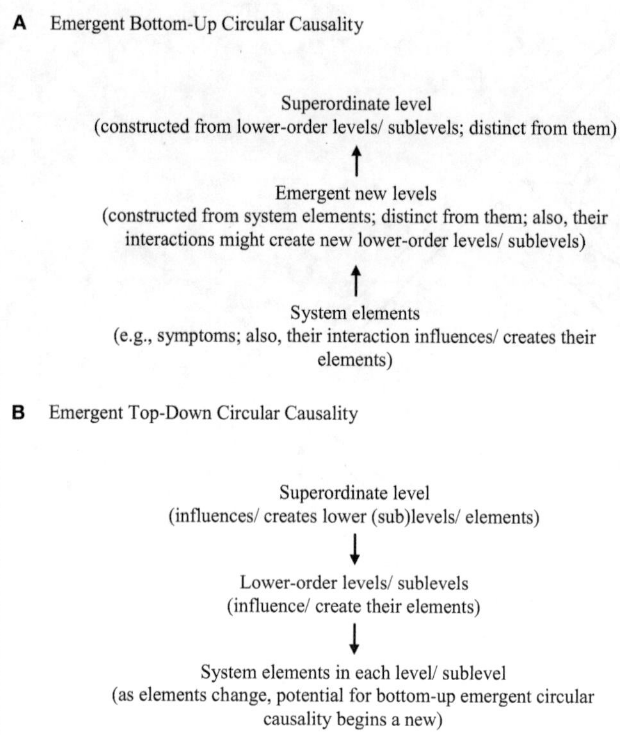

FIGURE 5 | The interaction of top-down and bottom-up emergent circular causality. **(A)** Emergent bottom-up circular causality, **(B)** emergent top-down circular causality.
Note: (1) Configuration/pattern changes possible, too, within and between (sub)levels. (2) Bottom-up and top-down causal processes work together reciprocally in system causality.
The figure illustrates the dynamic interaction of bottom-up and top-down processes both within and across levels in a system, including the possibility of emergence of new symptoms, levels, and sublevels. It also indicates the change of patterning or configuration possible within and between levels in the system dynamics involved. Briefly, as system elements (e.g., symptoms) or levels/sublevels interact, they might influence/create their configuration/patterning, expression, or even de novo emergence. This process may occur both through movement from lower to higher levels in the level hierarchy involved (bottom-up), or from higher to lower levels (top-down), or reciprocally in both ways. In essence, the figure clarifies that, in system function, bottom-up processes work both within and between levels, as do top-down processes.

in evaluating the relative roles of hermeneutic insight and causal explanation in psychiatry (Verstehen, Erklären, respectively). Whether we accept that symptom meaning/content, or phenomenology can be influenced by hermeneutic insight, "Verstehen" has important consequences. Are symptoms and their meaning/content only what can be observed, and therefore, reduced to what is measurable, or are there other levels to consider? In this regard, symptom meaning or content might be a higher-order level in the symptom/disorder complex, whether the symptoms are observed or self-reported. Moreover, observed and self-reported symptoms could be tapping different patient realities, and what might these differences mean for symptom meaning/content? For cause, are reductionist, biological views used to explain symptoms/disorders rather than higher-order mental content or constructs? Can the latter causally influence lower-order (and more easily observed/self-reported) symptoms (Erklären)?

Figure 6 presents a model of symptom expressions that illustrates the difficulty in addressing these types of questions, while proposing a nuanced solution. On the one hand, symptom meaning and causality do not necessarily stand in opposition. For example, at the level of individualization and universalization, symptoms could be unique to the person's history and current mental content, as well as unique in the coalition of forces that had created them. As well, symptoms could reflect universal themes and concerns, and also reflect standard common causal mechanisms.

Ultimately, both individual and universal mental content and symptoms might not be what they appear, either to the person expressing them phenomenologically and subjectively or to the observer using empirical methods, e.g., in observations, interviews, self-report questionnaires, in discerning them. Both subjective and objective understanding of symptoms might approach their reality.

Certainly, a complicating factor in all these regards relates to the play of unconscious processes in symptom creation and expression. This could apply in the sense of (a) classic Freudian repression, (b) automaticity in thought without deliberative reflection or insight, or (c) a lack of awareness of the overall system in which the symptoms are embedded.

Specifically for the area of PTSD and some other related conditions/disorders that are subject to legal dispute (e.g., chronic pain/somatic symptom disorder), the answers to these types of questions are complicated by court considerations. One needs to veer toward the more objective side as much as possible in order to vet possible confounds, such as malingering and unconscious influences on clinical presentation and self-report. **Figure 6** illustrates that intention is very difficult to evaluate and can never be evaluated uniquely by test results or clinical interview. Young (13, 36, 39, 50, 51) has presented work relevant to the question, calling for a scientifically-informed comprehensive impartial approach to assessment in these types of cases.

Ultimately, the network approach to symptom and mental disorder relationship addresses some of the issues raised about individual insight vs. universal explanation in symptomatology because, in this view, how symptoms interact becomes the seat of causal explanation and understanding. Nevertheless, in my hybrid model, one needs to consider top-down psychological construct influences on symptoms as much as their bottom-up interactions, so that their meaning and causation lay in not only symptom networking processes but also in higher-order levels in the symptom structure and the causes associated with them.

Often issues in our field are presented as a dichotomy, or in black and white. For example, for the causes of behavior, too often they are phrased as Nature vs. Nurture. Yet, behavioral causation reflects an interaction of biological, personal (e.g., self, free will belief), and environmental factors (6). Similarly, for the issue of scientism vs. skepticism and how it relates to considering symptoms in terms of individualized meanings or universal (read reductionist) causal mechanisms (Verstehen, Erklären, respectively), the opposition is presented too simply. The question of whether the nature of symptoms are either more unconscious, subjective/phenomenological, and meaningful in content or more conscious, observable, objective, and expressions of universal

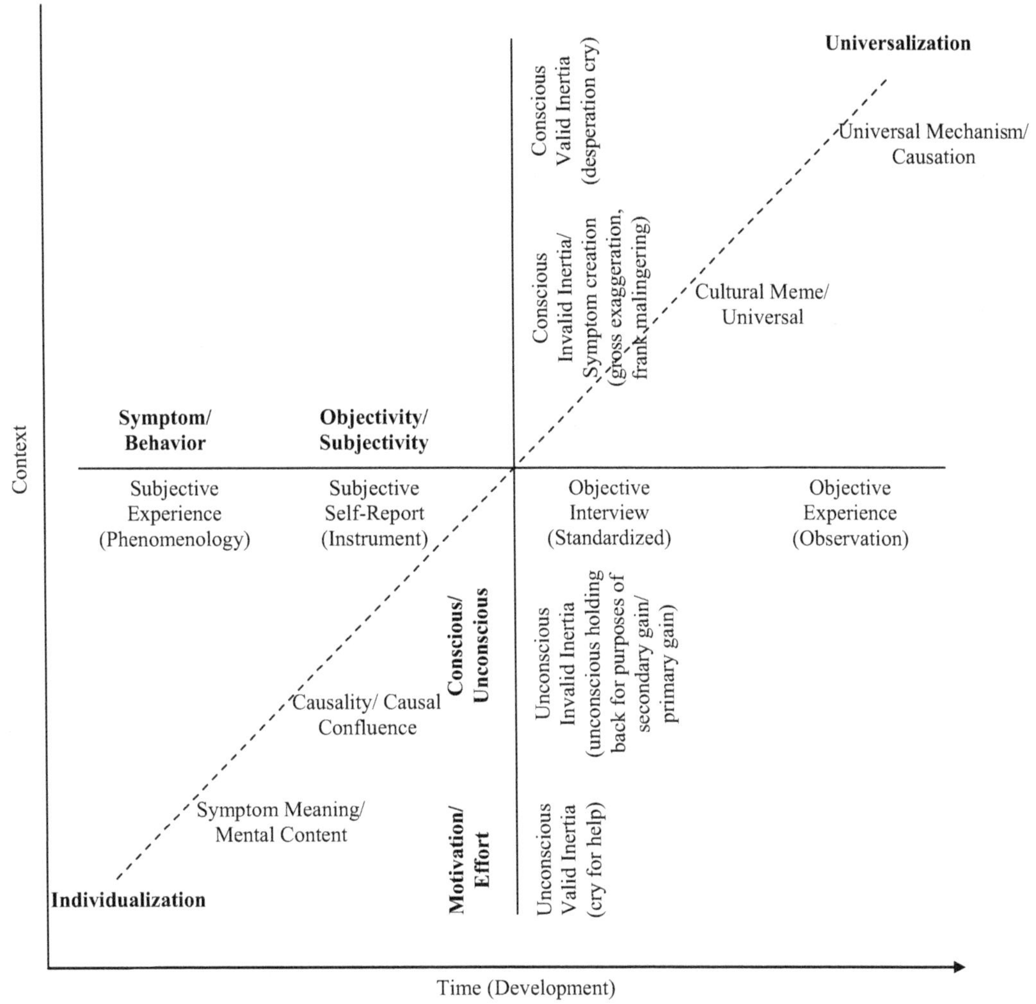

FIGURE 6 | The dimensions of symptom expression in psychiatry. The figure places symptoms along three dimensions that concern: motivation/effort (are symptoms valid?); subjectivity/objectivity (e.g., phenomenological, empirical); and individuality/universality. (a) Symptoms might not be valid, or they could be ones that should not be taken at face value. For example, about the former, there might be conscious malingering for secondary gain that is taking place. About the latter, there might be unconscious influences at work; for example, an unconscious cry for help could take place or a conscious desperation cry. (b) Also, symptoms vary in terms of they are ascertained subjectively or objectively. For example, they might derive from the person's self-report, in particular, or from the evaluator's more controlled efforts to observe/discern them. (c) Finally, symptoms vary in their individuality/universality. At one extreme, each symptom has a personal meaning or value for the patient/client that is unique to her/his history/narrative/experience. Or the causes of the symptoms constitute a unique constellation. On the other hand, they might indicate some cultural universal or meme/mythic narrative. In addition, they might reflect a universal causal or mechanism in behavior to which we are all subject and in constant, invariant ways.

causality might be one that masks a greater underlying complexity in understanding them, such as in the three-dimensional model presented in the figure.

In the article, I have presented an integrated top-down (psychological construct)/bottom-up (symptom network interaction) model of the relationship between symptom and disorder. The same model can be applied to understanding the relationship between mental content and their causes. Because of the multiple levels in systems of behavior, emergent contents can develop at higher-order levels that are not totally reflective of, reducible to, or transcribable from the lower levels, including of the causes involved. Mental contents, such as beliefs, emotions, and desires, can emerge and influence symptoms that might be closer to the lower-order biological or physical substrate, including neurobehaviorally, because of the process of circular emergence and the creation of higher-order levels in behavioral systems that the process allows.

In this regard, one example of higher-order mental state influences on lower-order symptoms is found in the how catastrophic and hopeless thought and related cognitive and emotional processes could cause downward spirals in helplessness and amotivation, and then in the specific symptoms of disorders, such as depression or PTSD. In another example, the personally-exaggerated appraisal of stress that then leads to stress-induced headaches is all too real for many of our patients.

Symptoms and mental disorder co-exist in a system in which all relevant levels need to be recognized and researched. There should be no room for exclusive reductionist or constructionist approaches in understanding them, as both are needed. Reductionism and the search for cause in the most basic biological processes should not be equated with scientism. Nor should seeking emergent phenomena that could influence behavior be treated with skepticism. Behavioral, symptom, and mental content states exist coactively with their causes, and science should examine the relations among all these levels with the clarity that patients deserve.

The present article has presented, hopefully, refined thinking in the area of mental disorder. Further effort along these lines might examine a possible systems model of the definition of mental disorder, one that includes levels for – symptoms, clusters, higher-order mental content, mental disorder, and related concepts such as disability. Similarly, treatment can be conceived systemically, e.g., in terms of cascades that might result from effective treatment shifting the patient into the region of health attractors [e.g., Ref. (27)]. Network concepts can be embedded in systems models and, therefore, the two types of models conceptualized together, and even hybridly, can provide a powerful language for grasping the nature of symptoms, mental disorder, causality, and cure (or treatment).

ACKNOWLEDGMENTS

The reviewers made excellent points and recommendations that greatly improved the manuscript. Many thanks. Grants have been involved in supporting this article.

REFERENCES

1. American Psychiatric Association. *Diagnostic and Statistical Manual of Mental Disorders: DSM-5*. 5th ed. Washington, DC: American Psychiatric Association (2013).
2. McNally RJ, Robinaugh DJ, Wu GWY, Wang L, Deserno MK, Borsboom D. Mental disorders as causal systems: a network approach to posttraumatic stress disorder. *Clin Psychol Sci* (2014):1–14. doi:10.1177/2167702614553230
3. Young G. *Development and Causality: Neo-Piagetian Perspectives*. New York, NY: Springer Science + Business Media (2011).
4. Markus KA, Borsboom D. Reflective measurement models, behavior domains, and common causes. *New Ideas Psychol* (2013) **31**:54–64. doi:10.1016/j.newideapsych.2011.02.008
5. Melchert TP. *Biopsychosocial Practice: A Science-Based Framework for Behavioral Health Care*. Washington, DC: American Psychological Association (2015).
6. Young G. *Unifying Causality and Psychology: Being, Brain, and Behavior*. New York, NY: Springer Science + Business Media (2016; in press).
7. Frances A. *Essentials of Psychiatric Diagnosis: Responding to the Challenge of DSM-5*. New York, NY: Guilford Press (2013).
8. Thyer BA. The DSM-5 definition of mental disorder: critique and alternatives. In: Probst B, editor. *Essential Clinical Social Work Series: Critical Thinking in Clinical Assessment and Diagnosis*. Cham: Springer (2015). p. 45–68.
9. Vanheule S. *Diagnosis and the DSM: A Critical Review*. Hampshire: Palgrave MacMillan (2014).
10. Insel TR, Cuthbert BN, Garvey MA, Heinssen RK, Pine DS, Quinn KJ, et al. Research domain criteria (RDoC): toward a new classification framework for research on mental disorders. *Am J Psychiatry* (2010) **167**:748–51. doi:10.1176/appi.ajp.2010.09091379
11. Insel TR, Lieberman JA. *DSM-5 and RDoC: Shared Interests*. The National Institute of Mental Health (2013). Available from: http://www.nimh.nih.gov/news/science-news/2013/dsm-5-and-rdoc-shared-interests.shtml
12. Blumenthal-Barby JS. Psychiatry's new manual (DSM-5): ethical and conceptual dimensions. *J Med Ethics* (2014) **40**:531–6. doi:10.1136/medethics-2013-101468
13. Young G. *Malingering, Feigning, and Response Bias in Psychiatric/Psychological Injury: Implications for Practice and Court*. Dordrecht: Springer Science + Business Media (2014).
14. Wigman JTW, van Os J, Borsboom D, Wardenaar KJ, Epskamp S, Klippel A, et al. Exploring the underlying structure of mental disorders: cross-diagnostic differences and similarities from network perspective using both a top-down and a bottom-up approach. *Psychol Med* (2015) **45**:2375–87. doi:10.1017/S0033291715000331
15. Bielczyk NZ, Buitelaar JK, Glennon JC, Tiesinga PHE. Circuit to construct mapping: a mathematical tool for assisting the diagnosis and treatment in major depressive disorder. *Front Psychiatry* (2015) **6**:29. doi:10.3389/fpsyt.2015.00029
16. Thelen E, Smith LB. Dynamic systems theories. 6th ed. In: Damon W, Lerner RM, editors. *Handbook of Child Psychology: Vol. 1. Theoretical Models of Human Development*. Hoboken, NJ: Wiley (2006). p. 258–312.
17. Vallacher RR, Van Geert P, Nowak A. The intrinsic dynamics of psychological process. *Curr Dir Psychol Sci* (2015) **24**:58–64. doi:10.1177/0963721414551571
18. Gottman J, Swanson C, Swanson K. A general systems theory of marriage: nonlinear difference equation modeling of marital interaction. *Pers Soc Psychol Rev* (2002) **6**:326–40. doi:10.1207/S15327957PSPR0604_07
19. Bak P. *How Nature Works: The Science of Self-Organized Criticality*. New York, NY: Springer-Verlag (1996).
20. Samuelson LK, Jenkins GW, Spencer JP. Grounding cognitive-level processes in behavior: the view from dynamic systems theory. *Top Cogn Sci* (2015) **7**:191–205. doi:10.1111/tops.12129
21. Hayes AM, Yasinski C, Barnes JB, Bockting CLH. Network destabilization and transition in depression: new methods for studying the dynamics of therapeutic change. *Clin Psychol Rev* (2015) **41**:27–39. doi:10.1016/j.cpr.2015.06.007
22. Pe ML, Kircanski K, Thompson RJ, Bringmann LF, Tuerlinckx F, Mestdagh M, et al. Emotion-network density in major depressive disorder. *Clin Psychol Sci* (2015) **3**:292–300. doi:10.1177/2167702614540645
23. Schiepek G, Eckert H, Aas B, Wallot S, Wallot A. *Integrative Psychotherapy: A Feedback-Driven Dynamic Systems Approach*. Göttingen: Hogrefe Publishing (2015).
24. Butner JE, Gagnon KT, Geuss MN, Lessard DA, Story TN. Utilizing topology to generate and test theories of change. *Psychol Methods* (2015) **20**:1–25. doi:10.1037/a0037802
25. Molenaar PCM, Nesselroade JR. 7th ed. In: Overton WF, Molenaar PC, editors. *Handbook of Child Psychology and Developmental Science, Vol. 1. Theory and Method*. Hoboken, NJ: Wiley (2015). p. 652–82.
26. Rabinovich MI, Simmons AN, Varona P. Dynamical bridge between brain and mind. *Trends Cogn Sci* (2015) **19**:453–61. doi:10.1016/j.tics.2015.06.005
27. Wichers M, Wigman JTW, Myin-Germeys I. Micro-level affect dynamics in psychopathology viewed from complex dynamical system theory. *Emot Rev* (2015) **7**:362–7. doi:10.1177/1754073915590623
28. World Health Organization. *Mental Disorders* (2015). Available at: http://www.who.int/mediacentre/factsheets/fs396/en/
29. Clarke DE, Narrow WE, Regier DA, Kuramoto SJ, Kupfer DJ, Kuhl EA, et al. DSM-5 field trials in the United States and Canada, part I: study design, sampling strategy, implementation, and analytic approaches. *Am J Psychiatry* (2013) **170**:43–58. doi:10.1176/appi.ajp.2012.12070998
30. Rosen GM, Lilienfeld SO. Posttraumatic stress disorder: an empirical evaluation of core assumptions. *Clin Psychol Rev* (2008) **28**:837–68. doi:10.1016/j.cpr.2007.12.002
31. Rosen GM, Frueh BC, Elhai JD, Grubaugh AL, Ford JD. Posttraumatic stress disorder and general stress disorder. In: Rosen GM, Frueh BC, editors. *Clinician's Guide to Posttraumatic Stress Disorder*. Hoboken, NJ: John Wiley & Sons (2010). p. 3–31.

32. Armour C, Tsai J, Durham TA, Charak R, Biehn TL, Elhai JD, et al. Dimensional structure of DSM-5 posttraumatic stress symptoms: support for a hybrid anhedonia and externalizing behaviors model. *J Psychiatr Res* (2015) **61**:106–13. doi:10.1016/j.jpsychires.2014.10.012
33. Pietrzak RH, Tsai J, Armour C, Mota N, Harpaz-Rotem I, Southwick SM. Functional significance of a novel 7-factor model of the DSM-5 PTSD symptoms: results from the national health of resilience in veterans study. *J Affect Disord* (2015) **174**:522–6. doi:10.1016/j.jad.2014.12.007
34. American Psychiatric Association. *Diagnostic and Statistical Manual of Mental Disorders*. 4th ed. Washington, DC: American Psychiatric Association (1994).
35. Wang L, Zhang L, Armour C, Cao C, Qing Y, Zhang J, et al. Assessing the underlying dimensionality of DSM-5 PTSD symptoms in Chinese adolescents surviving the 2008 Wenchuan earthquake. *J Anxiety Disord* (2015) **31**:90–7. doi:10.1016/j.janxdis.2015.02.006
36. Young G. Dimensions and dissociation in PTSD in the DSM-5: towards eight core symptoms. *Psychol Inj Law* (2015) **8**:219–32. doi:10.1007/s12207-015-9231-5
37. King D, Leskin G, King L, Weathers F. Confirmatory factor analysis of the Clinician-Administered PTSD scale: evidence for the dimensionality of posttraumatic stress disorder. *Psychol Assess* (1998) **10**:90–6. doi:10.1037/1040-3590.10.2.90
38. Armour C, Hansen M. Assessing DSM-5 latent subtypes of acute stress disorder dissociative or intrusive? *Psychiatr Res* (2015) **225**:476–83. doi:10.1016/j.psychres.2014.11.063
39. Young G, Wang JXT. PTSD-SUDs comorbidities in the context of psychological injury and law. *Psychol Inj Law* (2015) **8**:233–51. doi:10.1007/s12207-015-9229-z
40. Elhai JD, Biehn TL, Armour C, Klopper JJ, Frueh BC, Palmieri PA. Evidence of a unique PTSD construct represented by PTSD's D1-D3 symptoms. *J Anxiety Disord* (2011) **25**:340–5. doi:10.1016/j.janxdis.2010.10.007
41. Tsai J, Armour C, Southwick SM, Pietrzak RH. Dissociative subtype of DSM-5 posttraumatic stress disorder in U.S. veterans. *J Psychiatr Res* (2015) **66-67**:67–74. doi:10.1016/j.jpsychires.2015.04.017
42. Zelazny K, Simms LJ. Confirmatory factor analyses of DSM-5 posttraumatic stress disorder symptoms in psychiatric samples differing in criteria A status. *J Anxiety Disord* (2015) **34**:15–23. doi:10.1016/j.janxdis.2015.05.009
43. Weathers FW, Litz BT, Herman DS, Huska JA, Keane TM. The PTSD checklist (PCL): reliability, validity, and diagnostic utility. *Paper Presented at the Meeting of the International Society for Traumatic Stress Studies*. San Antonio, TX (1993).
44. Li H, Wang L, Shi Z, Zhang Y, Wu K, Liu P. Diagnostic utility of the PTSD Checklist in detecting PTSD in Chinese earthquake victims. *Psychol Rep* (2010) **107**:733–9. doi:10.2466/03.15.20.PR0.107.6.733-739
45. Young G, Lareau C, Pierre B. One quintillion ways to have PTSD comorbidity: recommendations for the disordered DSM-5. *Psychol Inj Law* (2014) **7**:61–74. doi:10.1007/s12207-014-9186-y
46. Conway ARA, Kovacs K. New and emerging models of human intelligence. *WIREs Cogn Sci* (2015) **6**:419–26. doi:10.1002/wcs.1356
47. Borsboom D, Cramer AOJ. Network analysis: an integrative approach to the structure of psychopathology. *Annu Rev Clin Psychol* (2013) **9**:91–121. doi:10.1146/annurev-clinpsy-050212-185608
48. Lewis MD. Bridging emotion theory and neurobiology through dynamic systems modeling. *Behav Brain Sci* (2005) **28**:169–245. doi:10.1017/S0140525X0500004X
49. Demazeux S, Singy P. *The DSM-5 in Perspective: Philosophical Reflections on the Psychiatric Babel*. Dordrecht, Netherlands: Springer Science + Business Media (2015).
50. Young G. Resource material for ethical psychological assessment of symptom and performance validity, including malingering. *Psychol Inj Law* (2014) **7**:206–35. doi:10.1007/s12207-014-9202-2
51. Young G, Drogin E. Psychological injury and law I: causality, malingering, and PTSD. *Mental Health Law Policy J* (2014) **3**:373–416.

7

What is Constructionism in Psychiatry? From Social Causes to Psychiatric Classification

Raphael van Riel[1,2*]

[1] *Philosophy, Philipps-University Marburg, Marburg, Germany,* [2] *Philosophy, University Duisburg-Essen, Essen, Germany*

Edited by:
Leon De Bruin, VU University Amsterdam, Netherlands

Reviewed by:
Anna Welpinghus, Technical University Dortmund, Germany
Lieke Asma, VU University Amsterdam, Netherlands

***Correspondence:**
Raphael van Riel
raphael.vanriel@uni-due.de

It is common to note that social environment and cultural formation shape mental disorders. The details of this claim are, however, not well understood. The paper takes a look at the claim that culture has an impact on psychiatry from the perspective of metaphysics and the philosophy of science. Its aim is to offer, in a general fashion, partial explications of some significant versions of the thesis that culture and social environment shape mental disorders and to highlight some of the consequences social constructionism about psychiatry has for psychiatric explanation. In particular, it will be argued that the alleged dependence of facts about particular mental disorders and about the second order property of being a mental disorder on social facts amounts to a robust form of constructivism, whereas the view that clinician–patient interaction is influenced by cultural facts is perfectly compatible with an anti-constructivist stance.

Keywords: philosophy of science, explanation in psychology, metaphysics, social construction, psychiatric classification

INTRODUCTION

It is common to note that social environment and cultural formation shape mental disorders. For instance, the Surgeon General David Satcher states in the preface to *Mental Health: Culture, Race, and Ethnicity* (Supplement) that

> [t]he cultures from which people hail affect all aspects of mental health and illness, including the types of stresses they confront, whether they seek help, what types of help they seek, what symptoms and concerns they bring to clinical attention, and what types of coping styles and social supports they possess. Likewise, the cultures of clinicians and service systems influence the nature of mental health services. [(1): preface]

The details of the claim that social or cultural facts or events have a significant or systematic impact on mental disorders are, however, not well understood. Some construe it as a purely epistemological claim (2), on other occasions it is mentioned without any further explication. For instance, in the supplement *Mental Health: Culture, Race, and Ethnicity* just quoted, it is stated that

> [c]ultural differences in the expression and reporting of distress are well established among American Indians and Alaska Natives. These often compromise the ability of assessment tools to capture the key signs and symptoms of mental illness [...] Words such as "depressed" and "anxious" are absent from some American Indian and Alaska Native languages [...]. Other research has demonstrated that certain DSM diagnoses, such as major depressive disorder, do not correspond directly to the categories of illness recognized by some American Indians. Thus, evaluating the need for mental health care among American Indians and Alaska Natives requires careful clinical inquiry that attends closely to culture. [(1): chapter 4.]

We will turn to similar examples below. Typically, such claims are regarded as articulating versions of *social constructivism*, as opposed to objectivism; authors quickly move from the idea that sociocultural environment has an impact on mental disorders to constructivist rhetoric. The paper takes a look at the claim that culture has an impact on psychiatry from the perspective of metaphysics and the philosophy of science. Its aim is to offer, in a general fashion, partial explications of versions of social constructivism about mental disorders and to show which claims regarding a sociocultural influence on mental disorders amount to social constructivism, and which claims do not. In particular, I will discuss constructivist claims about mental disorders themselves, such as posttraumatic stress disorder (PTSD), about the subjective experience, the phenomenology, and symptoms that are indicative of a disorder, about the second order property of being a mental disorder, instantiated by, for instance, PTSD or autism, and about constructivism about aspects of the clinician–patient interaction. It will turn out that social constructivist rhetoric, in many cases, does not amount to social constructivism, properly construed.[1]

Social constructivism in psychiatry can be tentatively characterized by contrasting it with what one may want to call *radical objectivism* (a view I will use for illustrative purposes only).[2] According to radical objectivism about psychiatry, types of mental disorders, and the type *mental disorder* itself, are just like the types the natural sciences deal with, in that they are in some sense *explanatorily independent* of social facts or events.[3] Neither do facts about mental disorders have to be explained in terms of underlying social facts nor should the occurrence of mental disorders be explained by reference to social causes, in a sense to be specified.[4] This is what the dispute between objectivism and constructivism is about. Compare events of evaporation of water and what they, as such, depend on with events of elections and what elections, as such, depend on. Neither do explanations of events of *evaporation of water* in physics or chemistry cite social causes nor is the evaporation of water, in these sciences, explained in terms of underlying social facts. Although the evaporation of water in the ocean may depend on social facts, namely, the social causes of global warming, in an explanation of what evaporation of water *is*, we should not cite the social causes of actual evaporation of water. By contrast, it seems reasonable to assume that *elections* are to be explained in terms of social causes, such as joint decisions to vote, or decisions to hold an election by individuals or groups who have a certain social status within a society. Moreover, unlike facts about the evaporation of water, the fact that the election takes place, facts about how it develops, etc., explanatorily depend on other social facts – facts about actions of individuals that count, in the relevant context, as votings. Social constructivism about psychiatry assumes that facts about mental disorders are, with respect to what they, as such, explanatorily depend on, a bit-like facts about elections. Radical objectivism assumes that facts about mental disorders are, in this respect, more like facts about the evaporation of water. They may sometimes be caused by social facts, but this is irrelevant when it comes to understanding what they are.

Social constructivism is widespread; in some circles, it may even be regarded as trivially true. So, why bother? The aim of this paper is not to *defend* or *argue against* social constructivism; it aims at a clarification of what social constructivism about mental disorder consists in, or *may* consist in. It will turn out that in the literature, one can find different versions of social constructivism. As these forms of social constructivism are often only implicit, part of the work will consist in uncovering some hidden constructivist commitments.

The paper proceeds as follows. The first section introduces some basic elements of social constructivism, including an elaboration on the difference between causal and non-causal, or, as I will also sometimes say, *metaphysical* explanation or explanatory dependence.[5] The section "Versions of Social Constructivism about Psychiatry" sketches, in an abstract way, the various versions of social constructivism about psychiatry, and introduces the different targets of constructivist claims, such as mental disorders, their symptoms, and the property of being a mental disorder. Each of the remaining Sections ["Social Constructivism about Mental Disorders", "Social Context, Experience, Phenomenology, and Symptoms", and "Mental Disorder and Social Norms"] deals with a particular version of social constructivism about psychiatry. Some consequences for psychiatric explanation and, thus, for psychiatry as a science are highlighted in the conclusion. Note that the conclusions drawn in this paper are somewhat preliminary, in three respects. First, the way I will present the different explications of social constructivism is non-committal as to the metaphysical details of social constructivism. From the perspective of metaphysics, this may appear dissatisfying. But in order to pave the way for a more thorough theory of social constructivism in psychiatry, we should remain neutral on some of the metaphysical details. Second, the conclusions drawn below are preliminary in that the distinctions discussed here may not exhaust the field. I have focused on versions of social constructivism that appear to surface within prominent areas in philosophy and psychiatry. And although the taxonomy offered here is inspired by systematic

---

[1]Throughout this paper, I will ignore the possible cultural impact on experiments in psychiatric research, for two reasons. First, I doubt that it requires special treatment, if constructivism about experiments in psychiatry poses a problem at all. If social environment significantly shapes experimentation in psychiatry, it will do so in other sciences as well, and for similar reasons. By contrast, the targets of social constructivism discussed in this paper are, prima facie, *special*. Second, I am not aware of any form of constructivist rhetoric about experimentation in psychiatry that is relevantly distinct from constructivist rhetoric that shows in descriptions of patient–clinician interaction.

[2]Social facts, whatever these are, are no less *objective*, in the sense of "*real*," than non-social ones, on the view endorsed here. It is a distinction inside naturalism. Social facts are part of nature in that they depend on natural facts about individual brains. This is an articulation of my conviction – most of the points made in the paper are compatible with more liberal views.

[3]I use the term "types," in line with the literature, to designate what is signified by predicates, not to designate predicates or concepts expressed by predicates.

[4]Some such view can be ascribed to Kendell (3) and Boorse (4), at least about the second order property of being a mental disorder, a similar view is defended by Kendler et al. (5), who admit that social aspects may have an impact on disorders, but who assume that mental disorders can be individuated in a way similar to types in the natural sciences.

[5]There is a vast literature on the metaphysics of these forms of dependence; for introductory texts, see Ref. (6); for recent work on metaphysical dependence and explanation, see, for instance, the papers published in Ref. (7).

considerations about candidate versions of social constructivism, I will not offer an argument to the effect that the versions of social constructivism discussed below exhaust the field. Finally, each of the versions discussed below deserves further attention. The paper offers partial explications of versions of social constructivism. Some aspects will be left out.

Basic Tenets of Social Constructivism

Social constructivism about psychiatry is opposed to radical objectivism. Both claims concern the subject matter of psychiatry, the types of objects and the connections psychiatry deals with. The present section introduces the conceptual tools of social constructivism.

A quick look at social constructivism in other areas of philosophy will offer a more thorough idea of what social constructivism about some subject matter consists in. A prominent example that has been extensively discussed in the past years (8–11) is social constructivism about institutions or institutional facts. Social constructivism about institutions holds that institutions (or institutional facts) depend on specific intentional states of individuals. For instance, on this view, the fact that some sea-shell, dollar-bill, or coin is money depends on the fact that people collectively accept it as money [famously argued by Searle (8, 9)]. This form of social constructivism is characterized by its *target* (facts about social institutions, such as money), the relevant facts upon which its target is supposed to depend, or the target's *social grounds* (in this case: facts about collective acceptance), and the *relation* that is supposed to hold between the two – in this case: some form of *metaphysical dependence*.

Here is the second example. Feminist philosophers have suggested that in some sense, gender is socially constructed (12, 13). On one version of this thesis, the idea is that women and men *become women* and *men* (in at least one significant sense of these terms) not due to their hard-wired biological make-up, but rather due to social causes, such as among other things, shared expectations on the side of caregivers, discursive practices (repeatedly marking the distinction between boys and girls/men and women), and esthetic practices within a society. Again, this form of social constructivism can be characterized in terms of its target (the occurrence of gender identities in individuals), the alleged grounds of this target (causal influences, such as expectations and discursive practices), and the connection between the two – here, *causation*.

Versions of social constructivism about psychiatry can be characterized in a similar format – in terms of their *target*, the alleged *grounds* of the target (I use "ground" for both, causal and non-causal grounds), and the *relation* that is supposed to hold between the two. We need to distinguish between two types of dependence relations – causal and non-causal dependence. As the reader might not be familiar with this distinction, let me illustrate the difference by way of some examples. An avalanche that occurs due to an earthquake is *caused* by the latter – and the avalanche can be causally explained by reference to the earthquake. When a rock hits a window so that the window shatters, the fact that the window shatters can be causally explained by reference to the fact that to rock hit the window. And when the heating of water leads to a transition from liquid to vapor, then the vaporization of water can be causally explained in terms of the heating of water. Causal explanations involve a temporal component – causes precede their effects. By contrast, the objects involved in *non-causal* explanations do not necessarily stand in a temporal successor relation. The existence of a forest depends on the existence of trees, and that there is a forest can be explained by reference to the presence of trees. But the existence of the trees does not cause the forest to exist, and the existence of the trees need not precede the existence of the forest. The hole in the Swiss cheese depends on the cheese; and the existence of the hole can be explained by reference to features of the cheese. But it need not be the case that there was, first, the cheese and then the hole. On naturalistic accounts of the mind, the processing of visual information depends on particular physiological processes. These processes underlie the processing of visual information, and the latter can be explained in terms of the former. But the physiological processes do not cause the processing of visual information and need not precede it.

"Because"-statements typically express explanations. Some explanations are causal, others are not. When speaking of dependence in what follows I mean *explanatory* dependence. An intuitive understanding of the difference between causal and non-causal explanation along these lines, in terms of examples and based on the observation that causal explanation essentially involves a temporal component non-causal explanation does not require, is sufficient for our present purposes. In the present context, non-causal dependence will sometimes be referred to as "constitution."

As already indicated, versions of social constructivism may, in general, differ with respect to the relation they postulate between the social grounds of their targets and these targets. Versions of social constructivism fall into two categories – those that credit social facts with a relevant causal role for the etiology of the given target and those according to which the target non-causally depends on social facts. These categories mirror, to some extent, the following distinction drawn by Sally Haslanger:

> *Causal Construction*: Something is causally constructed iff social factors play a causal role in bringing it into existence or, to some substantial extent, in its being the way it is.
>
> *Constitutive Construction*: Something is constitutively constructed iff in defining it we must make reference to social factors (13, p. 98).[6]

This distinction applies in the context of theorizing about psychiatry. Consider the claim that some mental disorders depend on social norms (we will turn back to this view below, Section

[6]It is worth noting that the claim about causal construction should be interpreted as a claim about types, rather than tokens. To return to our example from the introduction: the actual evaporation of water in the ocean is caused by social factors, and the way it proceeds also hinges on these social causes; but evaporation as such is independent of social factors; its being actually caused by social factors is irrelevant when it comes to understanding what it consists in, namely, some form of phase state transition. By contrast, to understand what gender categories consists in, social factors that played a role in the causal development of gender identities are in fact relevant. Why this is so is a question that transcends the boundaries of the present paper; it is a general question regarding classification in the social sciences.

"Mental Disorder and Social Norms") – that reference to social norms is relevant in an explanation for why a patient suffers from a mental disorder. Social norms may have a causal impact on the development of disorders, and facts about social norms may ground, in the non-causal sense, facts about disorders.

To illustrate, consider Stier's [(2), p. 28] interpretation of Wakefield's critique of current diagnostic practices in the case of anxiety disorders. Wakefield explains the fact that "current criteria allow diagnosis when someone is, say, intensely anxious about public speaking in front of strangers" by reference to "American society's high need for people who can engage in occupations that require communicating to large groups" [(14), p. 154]. Stier appears to suggest that considerations like these reveal that there is a "[normative] impact of society on the concept of mental disorder" [(2), 28f.]. Although I doubt that Wakefield's considerations concerning anxiety disorders support any such view,[7] let us assume that the diagnostic practices, based on a given cultural background, in fact, ground facts about anxiety disorders. In this spirit, one may come up with an explanation of the following type:

> [1] She suffers from anxiety disorder because her behavior violates a specific social norm, or shared expectation concerning the ability to speak publicly in front of strangers.

Taken in isolation, this explanation has *two* interpretations, corresponding to the two versions of social constructivism, a causal and a non-causal one. On the former, norm-violation plays a causal role in the occurrence of the anxiety disorder; and it may, in this respect, be similar to the case of evaporation of water and the human causes of global warming. On the latter, a behavioral pattern *counts* as an instance of anxiety disorder (in part), *because* it is an instance of a norm-violation.

Consider the *causal* reading first. Assume that, for some reason, a subject develops a minor anxiety concerning a particular type of social situation, say, to deliver a speech in front of strangers, in a social context where this form of anxiety, and the behavioral patterns that go together with it, are conceived of as socially awkward, or at least as not fulfilling a shared expectation. Showing the relevant behavior (say, some form of avoidance behavior, or specific behavior while delivering a speech) constitutes a norm violation; people react to the norm violation, thereby enforcing the anxiety in the subject – to a degree that it becomes pathological. In this case, actual social feedback in response to norm violation may trigger a feeling of shame, which, in turn, may cause the person to experience distress, which, in turn, may cause further deviations from socially expected behavior up to a degree that makes the condition pathological. Here, violation of social norms plays a causal role for the etiology of the disorder. This can easily be seen once we note the temporal component involved in the underlying process: *first*, there was norm violation which caused a certain behavior in the audience. The behavior in the audience *then* caused further distress, which, *after some time* and repeated stressful experiences, resulted in the development of an anxiety disorder.

On the other interpretation, the explanation does not commit one to there being a *development from* norm-violation *to* mental disorder. This is the interpretation (Stier's) Wakefield appears to have in mind, when claiming that there is a normative impact of society on the concept of a mental disorder (on my interpretation: that the social norms sometimes determine, in a conceptual or metaphysical sense, what is a disorder and what is not). On this interpretation, *norm-violation* (or *being disposed to violate certain norms*) and *suffering from anxiety disorder* occur synchronically. The former partly grounds the latter, or, put differently, the latter can be metaphysically explained in terms of the former. There are several ways in which one can cash out talk of metaphysical explanation. For instance, one may suggest that the truth of a proposition that a person has a mental disorder is explained by a truth about the violation of social norms. Or, alternatively, one may want to claim that the instantiation of the property of having a mental disorder metaphysically depends on the occurrence of norm-violations. We need not go into the details here. For our present purposes, suffice it to note that there are at least two interpretations of the explanation that a person suffers from a mental disorder due to some social facts, a causal and a non-causal one, and that whatever the correct explication of the non-causal interpretation is, it will render the explanation true without any implications concerning a possible causal (and, thus, temporal) connection between norm-violation and having a mental disorder. An understanding of the distinction between causal and metaphysical dependence along these lines is sufficiently precise for the goals of the present paper. Social constructivism may involve both, a causal and a non-causal claim concerning the relation between mental disorders and social facts. Although this is probably true of most scientific explanation, it is worth pointing out that these explanations are, of course, only *partial* explanations; the presence of the explanans phenomenon is not fully explained in terms of its social causes or some underlying social facts. Versions of constructivism we will be dealing with in what follows are claims about the *partial* social construction of mental disorders. Purely physiological, behavioral, or experiential aspects that are not themselves socially constructed may be required to offer a full explanation of the relevant phenomena of mental disorders.

Before we turn to the specific versions of social constructivism about psychiatry – shouldn't we say bit more about what makes social constructivism about psychiatry *social*? Intuitively, what depends on shared attitudes (like money), what varies with cultural context (like the social status of, say, a widow), or what itself essentially depends on a social object (like the property of playing in the NBL), is, in a sense, itself a social object. As a social object, it requires, at some stage, a sort of construction. There are straightforward examples of socially constructed objects; but this does not mean that there is a straightforward characterization of what social constructivism consists in. Any (at least partly

[7] Stier is, as it seems, not quite right when suggesting that Wakefield *thereby* supports the claim that "the cultural setup [...] tends to dictate the boundary between the normal and the deviant on the basis of the expected values and virtues of its members" [(2), p. 28]. Rather, Wakefield's observation supports the epistemic claim that the perceived boundaries between the normal and the deviant are dictated (or maybe better: partly influenced) by the cultural setup. Wakefield stresses that there is a difference between false diagnostic practices and "social phobia [which is] a real disorder in which people can sometimes not engage in the most routine social interaction" [(14), p. 154].

successful) attempt to deliver a general answer to the question of what social constructivism is would transcend the boundaries of the present paper; but a general answer is not required – the theses we will be concerned with here are committed to the social dimension of their targets (such as particular mental disorders) in a *straightforward* sense; and we will be able to relate, in passing, these cases to intuitive formulations of social constructivism. Short reflection on two versions, one might, at first sight, want to classify as versions of social constructivism will help to get a better understanding of what makes social constructivism about psychiatry a version of *social* constructivism, and it will reveal that not all constructivist rhetoric amounts to constructivism as opposed to objectivism.

Versions of Social Constructivism about Psychiatry

Social constructivism about psychiatry, as introduced above in contrast with radical objectivism, is heavily underdetermined. It is underdetermined with respect to its *target*, it is underdetermined with respect to the target's *grounds*, and it is underdetermined with respect to the *relation* allegedly holding between the target and the target's grounds. In this section, I will introduce five candidate targets for social constructivism about mental disorder: mental disorders themselves, the system of symptoms, phenomenology, and experience associated with a mental disorder, the second order property of being a mental disorder, and articulation of experiences and interpretation of utterances in patient–clinician interaction. The latter two can be dismissed immediately – they invite constructivist rhetoric at best. The candidate targets will have an impact on the candidate grounds and the relevant relation supposedly holding between the two.

Consider a person who has been diagnosed with PTSD and is, based on this diagnosis, classified as suffering from a mental disorder. This will, on the side of the patient, involve (a) PTSD itself, with its specific history, including the etiology or the trigger of PTSD, (b) a specific subjective experience and, possibly, a specific phenomenology, and a set of symptoms that are indicative of PTSD. Note that depending on the view one adopts regarding the nature of mental disorders, these may ultimately collapse into one single target, if the phenomenology, the subjective experience and particular symptoms enter the individuating criteria for the disorder itself;[8] but even if this were the case, talk about symptoms, phenomenology, experience, and the disorder would still be acceptable. Drawing the terminological distinction appears to be innocent.

Furthermore, the classification of PTSD as a mental disorder will involve (c) a specific aspect of PTSD in virtue of which it counts as a mental disorder (rather than, say, a stressful episode of minor importance) and becomes clinically relevant. Finally, being diagnosed with and treated for PTSD typically requires that the patient interact with a clinician. She will (d) express her experiences and inner perspective as well as report symptoms in a particular way. On the side of the clinician, (e) an interpretation of the observed and reported (verbal and non-verbal) behavior of the patient is required.

For each of these targets, one can subscribe to the view that it is shaped by social facts. We have thus identified five candidate targets for social constructivism, all of which may give rise to a form of social constructivism about psychiatry, or at least may go together with some constructivist rhetoric. And indeed, all of these can be found in the literature. Before we turn to the more promising candidates for serious versions of social constructivism, let me briefly comment on the last two alleged targets, and corresponding claims concerning the impact of culture and social environment. Little reflection will reveal that cultural influence on patient–clinician interaction is irrelevant in the context of social constructivism about psychiatry, properly construed.

The DSM 5 contains a section "Cultural Formulation," a revised version of what had already been presented in the previous manual. Its goal is somewhat difficult to identify. It contains information on mental disorder in relation to, well, *anything culture*, so to speak, beautifully illustrated by the suggested "Overall cultural assessment":

> Summarize the implications of the components of the cultural formulation identified in earlier sections of the Outline for diagnosis and other clinically relevant issues or problems as well as appropriate management and treatment intervention. (DSM 5, 750)

Information gathered about cultural background – including religious background and, possibly, gender identity – should inform diagnosis, clinician–patient interaction, and intervention. One particular reason for an assessment of cultural background is that differences in cultural background may cause confusion and misunderstandings. So, the manual includes questions that aim, in particular, at a clarification of *cultural concepts* and *idioms of distress* (DSM 5, 758 ff.), *some* of which concern the way the individual or members of the group the individual belongs to verbalize a given experience. One contention is, in this context, that knowledge of sociocultural background may facilitate access to underlying conditions; the idea does not seem to be that cultural expression of a disorder forms an integral part of the disorder itself (we will turn back to this below, in Section "Social Context, Experience, Phenomenology, and Symptoms").

Does the claim that clinicians should be sensitive the culture-specific articulations of the underlying disorder constitute a version of social constructivism, in any interesting sense? This does not seem to be the case. To use an idiom from the natural science: some of the *data* we gather may be difficult to interpret. In psychiatry, the data may be difficult to interpret because they, first, involve verbal reports, whose real or intended meaning may escape the interpreter; and, second, the interpreter may exhibit something like a cultural bias, which makes interpretation of data

[8] Let me give just two examples of views according to which symptoms may enter the individuating criteria for psychiatric types. If you assume, with Wakefield (15), that disorders are harmful dysfunctions, and that whether or not a certain psychological condition is harmful or a dysfunction may depend on the symptoms it produces, then symptoms may enter the individuating criteria for psychiatric taxonomies. You will end up with a similar result if you subscribe to what Murphy calls the "neo-Krapelinian picture" according to which "mental illnesses are regularly co-occurring clusters of signs and symptoms that doubtless depend on physical processes but are not defined or classified in terms of those physical processes" (16).

difficult, too. But once properly interpreted, the content of the knowledge we acquire need not be knowledge involving cultural facts, just because access to such knowledge required reflection on cultural background. Let me illustrate the point by way of a (fictional) example, building on what one may want to call an informed stereotype: assume you enter a shop in Berlin, run by locals, say, a bakery. You buy a roll and a cake, adding up to € 2.45. You offer a € 20 bill. It may very well happen that the clerk looks at you like you've insulted him, refuses to take the bill, rolls his eyes and says: "Damn, I don't have any change left!" Interestingly, this really does not mean that he does not have any change left. It appears to be some form of culturally determined expression of what elsewhere would probably have been expressed by something like: "Excuse me, do you have small change?" To properly interpret the utterance, knowledge of the cultural background is required. But of course, this does not mean that the fact (that there is only little change left) is constituted by these social facts knowledge of which is required to interpret the data. Claiming that in order to properly interpret the utterance in this context you have to take cultural considerations into account, does not imply that the content of the knowledge you end up with (if you're successful) is knowledge about social facts.

Analogously, the claim that cultural considerations should play a role in clinician-patient interaction has no impact on the subject matter of psychiatry. It does have an impact on the practice of psychiatry. Data may be culturally determined. But data are not what psychiatry is ultimately about. We are mainly interested in the commitments of current psychiatry (and parts of philosophy of psychiatry) with respect to the relation between psychiatry and the natural sciences. The key question is not whether cultural differences may pose difficulties in the *assessment* of whether or not an individual suffers from a particular mental disorder. The question is, rather, whether the subject matter of psychiatry involves social explanations in terms of social facts or causes.

A similar point could be made about the recent trend to take cultural considerations into account in the context of health management [also present in the "Cultural Formulation" in DSM 5, see, for instance, questions regarding "expectations for services" that may depend on the individual's cultural background (p. 752)]. The Supplement *Mental Health: Culture, Race, and Ethnicity*, edited by he U.S. Department of Health and Human Services, calls attention to the fact that cultural or racial background may have a significant impact on access conditions to mental health institutions. Thus, reflection on cultural aspects is of utmost importance in the context of psychiatric practice. But this does not amount to social constructivism about psychiatry.

The following three sections will introduce explications of the thesis that social context and culture shape mental disorder, which amount to forms of social constructivism about psychiatry in a more demanding sense.

Social Constructivism about Mental Disorders

As noted above, one may subscribe to social constructivism concerning mental disorders themselves, such as schizophrenia, PTSD, or dissociative identity disorder. Social constructivism about mental disorders comes in two radically different forms. According to one view, which appears to be a minority view (at best), facts about mental disorders are like facts about Searlean institutions – whether or not someone is, say, an alcoholic depends, in a non-causal sense, on attitudes of other people according to which that person is an alcoholic. Being regarded as an alcoholic makes one an alcoholic. According to the other view, at least some mental disorders are individuated by their social causes, so that their instantiation non-causally depends on their etiology. This makes these disorders social in nature, although it remains to be seen whether it amounts to social constructivism, properly construed. Let me briefly comment on the first view, and then turn, in more detail, to the second.

Constructivist claims in metaphysics often take the following form:

> [2] F's are F's because they are considered/regarded to be/experienced as F's.

A famous instance of this schema is Searle's claim that "[m]oney is money because the actual participants in the institution regard it as money" [(9), p. 17]. Some formulations in statements about the nature of mental disorders allow for a similar reading. Pickering, for instance, suggests that:

> The relevant features of alcoholism do not, contrary to what it demands, exist independently of the category into which alcoholism is placed [viz. illness, *RvR*]. [(17), p. 27].

One can interpret this claim as follows: some features of alcoholism depend on specific attitudes toward alcoholism within a social context – namely, that it is regarded as alcoholism [rather than a mere moral weakness (Pickering) or, alternatively, as "manly" behavior].[9] In their critical discussion of social constructivism about mental disorders, Kendler et al. [(5), p. 1145] appear to interpret social constructivism in a similar way, associating it with Haack's characterization of a kind that is not real, i.e., not "independent of how we believe it to be" [(18), 132]. I am not entirely sure whether anyone ever held some such belief; but it appears that self-declared objectivists often tend to credit constructivists with some such view (so that the opponent of Kendler et al. would turn out to be a straw-man). One may suspect that Foucault accepted this form of constructivism (19), although Foucault, in later years, explicitly subscribed to a form of causal constructivism that is based on causal effects of discursive practices.[10] Be that as it may – on this version of social constructivism, the *targets* are categories of mental disorder, the *grounds* of the targets are attitudes or discursive practices that

[9] Pickering distances himself from a social constructivist interpretation of this view – he regards the sort of construction involved in the classification of a condition as a mental illness as non-social. On his conception of social construction, social constructivists are wedded to the idea that what is socially constructed "exists only in certain cultural or social frames of reference" [(17), p. 98].

[10] The relevant power relations involve, according to Foucault, not only attributive practices but also causal feedback, for instance, in what he called biopolitics (20).

involve the psychiatric category itself and attribute it to certain people, and the relation is that of non-causal dependence.[11]

This version of constructivism is not the only form of social constructivism regarding mental disorders. Some mental disorders seem to be *typically* caused by particular social events. PTSD is *typically* caused by experiences such as incarceration as a prisoner of war, or traumatic experiences that often have a social dimension, such as interpersonal violence or sexual assault.

Being typically brought about by social causes alone does, of course, not amount to social constructivism. To see that, consider the question of whether it contradicts radical objectivism about psychiatry. The radical objectivist may hold that mental disorders can be caused by social events, as long as we need not cite the social dimension among the relevant causes in an appropriate explanation that enables us to fully understand the mental disorder we are dealing with. The evaporation of water may often be caused by social events. A large part of the evaporation of water is currently caused by global warming (or so let us assume for the sake of the example). Global warming, in turn, is caused by our joint actions. And if global warming has a significant impact on the natural evaporation of water on earth, then, currently, the evaporation of water on earth is *typically* caused by social facts. However, this does not amount to social constructivism about the current evaporation of water – the question of whether or not evaporation of water is brought about by social causes is irrelevant to our understanding of what evaporation of water consists in. Put differently: *evaporation of water due to global warming caused by social events* is not an interesting type in physics or chemistry (though it may be an interesting type in the context of politics). The radical objectivist about mental disorders will maintain that similarly, questions regarding the causes of a disorder are, or should be, irrelevant in psychiatry.

However, trauma- and stressor-related disorders are partly *characterized* in terms of their etiology. Consider the general characterization of these types of disorder, taken from the DSM 5:

> Trauma and stressor-related disorders include disorders in which exposure to a traumatic or stressful event is listed explicitly as a diagnostic criterion. (DSM 5, 265)

If the diagnostic criteria enter the taxonomy of mental disorders, then there are mental disorders that are partly individuated by their etiology. The motivation for this relational characterization is straightforward. Different experiences cause different subtypes of trauma- or stressor-related disorders, and knowledge of the cause may bear on clinical decisions. Often, the traumatic or stressful event involves a *social* dimension. Typical examples include experience of war, torture, incarceration as a prisoner of war, or sexual abuse. DSM 5 states explicitly that "[t]he disorder may be especially severe or long-lasting when the stressor is interpersonal and intentional" (DSM 5, 275). Interpersonal and intentional stressors involve a social dimension – not because any intentional action is social, bur rather because any intentional action directed at another person – here: the patient – is social. Witnessing a death by accident of a close relative and experiencing a catastrophe such as an anaphylactic shock form the *only* exceptions in the list included in DSM 5, waking during surgery forms a borderline case (in this case, it is not clear whether the fact that surgeons appear to interfere intentionally with the patient's body plays a relevant explanatory role).

So, the family of trauma- and stressor-related disorders involves types of disorders that are, in part, defined in terms of the types of causes that actually triggered the disorder. PTSD due to traumatic experience during incarceration as a prisoner of war is different from PTSD due to traumatic experience caused by witnessing an accident involving the loss of a close relative. The difference shows at the token level, and it also shows at the level of subtypes, subtypes of the type *trauma or stressor-related disorder*, when the type of cause is referred to in a classification of the relevant disorder.

But doesn't such relational individuation of types seem odd? Upon reflection, relational classifications are common. On most accounts, *being an artwork* depends on the etiology of the artwork – namely, being intentionally produced. Similarly, being an artifact depends on the etiology of the artifact. And individual horses are, on some views, horses in part because they are descendants from horses. In the social sciences, relational types are common: someone is a president (and not merely, say, a warlord), a state (and not merely a territory), or a law (and not merely an enforced rule) only if it has a certain history.

Thus, on the view implicit in DSM 5, for some subtypes of trauma- or stressor-related disorders, if a person suffers from this subtype, she does so because of the specific etiology of the disorder. The fact that the disorder has a cause of a particular type grounds the fact that it is a disorder of the corresponding subtype (for instance, *disorder caused by an interpersonal and intentional stressor*, or *PTSD due to torture*). Expressed in terms of targets, grounds, and the alleged relation between the two: the *targets* are subtypes of trauma- and stressor-related disorders. The grounds are complex events that relevantly involve a social dimension, such as intentions directed at other persons, interpersonal actions, and social properties, such as being a war and being an incarceration, which, moreover, stand in a causal relation to the psychological condition classified as a disorder. The relation between the social grounds and the occurrences of the disorder is, thus, causal. But the relation between the disorder and the cause is not *merely* causal, it is also conceptual, or metaphysical: to instantiate one of the subtypes requires that the disorder be caused by a particular type of object. The cause not only causes the disorder, facts about the cause also ground facts about the instantiation of the disorder. This marks the difference

[11] It appears that on this view, psychiatry, conceived of as a science that deals with mental disorders, would rest on a confusion. The objects of psychiatry would turn out to be mere chimeras; psychiatry would turn out to be like a version of jurisprudence whose self-declared goal was to improve the law by empirical interventions on the minds of judges, based on the false assumption that the role judges play in the juridical system is determined by features intrinsic to judges themselves, while recognizing that typical properties relevant in the legal system are social properties. Moreover, the view appears to be at odds with the view that *suffering* correlates with the presence of conditions typically classified as disorders, or better, as (Reviewer 2) suggested, with the assumption that different types of suffering correlate with different types of disorders; so, it seems that there is more to these conditions than classification or being regarded as having a mental disorder (although this may indeed constitute part of the problem).

between the current evaporation of water, on the one hand, and the relevant types of mental disorders, on the other. Whereas, in fact, some events are evaporations of water and can be explained in terms of social events, causal explanations referring to social events are not required for an explanation of why evaporation of water is evaporation of water. Suffering from PTSD due to experience of interpersonal violence, in contrast, requires a specific causal history involving a social cause.

On this interpretation, some mental disorders are clearly *social objects* in the sense that they essentially involve a social aspect. But does this amount to social *constructivism*, in a straightforward sense? It fits Haslanger's characterization, since in defining the subtype "we must make reference to social factors" [(13), p. 98]. The classification scheme involves types that are individuated by, and whose instantiation depends on, the presence of specific social features of the causes of the disorder. In some sense, however, this does not amount to social *constructivism*: it is not the case that forms of PTSD exist in or require for their existence, as Pickering put it, "a cultural or social frame of reference" [(17), p. 98]. Not every social object, such as abusive behavior, or incarceration, is a social construction in this sense. This may speak against Haslanger's characterization or at least require elaboration on the notion of a social factor. Ultimately, this may be a verbal issue about how we want to use the term "constructivism"; what is important in the present context is that this type of classification of subtypes of disorders appears to contradict *objectivism*; in the present context, we may, then, group it with more demanding versions of social constructivism, discussed in the next sections.[12]

Social Context, Experience, Phenomenology, and Symptoms

Let us move from aspects of social construction in classification to aspects of social construction involved in experience, phenomenology, and symptoms of mental disorders. Whether constructivism about experience, phenomenology, or symptoms is compatible with robust objectivism depends on whether we take these to be constitutive of the disorder.

As we have just seen, the claim that causes of mental disorders exhibit social features alone does not amount to any interesting form of social constructivism; a claim about *metaphysical* dependence on social causes was required. This should not come as a surprise. Recall the example discussed in Section "Basic Tenets of Social Constructivism":

> [1] She suffers from anxiety disorder because her behavior violates a specific social norm, or shared expectation concerning the ability to speak publicly in front of strangers.

On its causal interpretation, according to which causal norms played a causal role in the development of the disorder, committing to [1] one does not commit to any form of social constructivism. The objectivist may maintain that disorders have social causes; and the objectivist may consistently hold that *cultural variation among disorders depends on social causes.*

As already mentioned, DSM 5 offers a guide for cultural evaluations in the "Cultural Formulation," which deals, to a significant extent, with problems in the interpretation of verbal reports; but it also deals with interpretation of experiences, calling attention to the fact that "the cultural constructs ... influence how the individual experiences [...] his or her symptoms or problems [...]" (DSM 5, 750). As long as the subject's reports are distinct from the underlying disorder, the claim that an adequate interpretation of reports requires knowledge about sociocultural background does not amount to social constructivism. The same holds for the claim that sociocultural background shapes the experience, phenomenology, and symptoms of the disorder, as long as these are not constitutive of the disorder itself, but, rather, *signs* of the disorder. On this picture, experiences, symptoms, and phenomenology may need translation just like reports. But signs of a disorder need not play an essential role in scientific classification. As long as the disorder manifests at the physiological level, and as long as types of disorders can, at least in principle, be individuated in purely physiological terms, the objectivist can happily admit that social causes have an impact on mental disorders [see, for instance, Ref. (5)]. The radical objectivist may even accept that knowledge of cultural context is epistemically relevant for clinical practice.

From the objectivist perspective, the connection between social causes and the way a disorder manifests may involve causal connections at the level of neurodevelopment. Kirmayer and Crafa (22) have, in the spirit of social or cultural neuroscience, argued that the physiological structure underlying specific conditions is shaped by social causes:

> Culture can be seen as providing essential contexts for the development and functioning of the brain on multiple timescales: through its evolutionary history, which has involved brain–culture coevolution; across individual lifespans as biographical events are inscribed in circuitry by mechanisms of epigenetics and learning; and through ongoing influences on neural functioning by specific contexts of adaptation and performance. [(22), p. 7]

[12]Although this is not the topic of the present paper, two possible objectivist responses immediately come to mind: Maybe it is not the fact that the cause has certain social features, but rather that it is *perceived as* having these features, which is relevant to the type of disorder that we are dealing with. So, if reference to social features of causes just roughly catches what really does the explanatory work – that the cause is *perceived* as being of a particular social type – social constructivism about these types of disorders appears to be mistaken. Still, it is not entirely clear how to cash out, and account for, the relevance of perceived social causes within the radical objectivist framework. Second, one could construe this form of social constructivism as a form of pragmatic constructivism. Maybe Psychiatry, in its current form, is not as good as it gets. The types current psychiatry deals with are pragmatically adequate. If, for instance, incarceration as a prisoner of war is reliably connected with showing a specific behavioral pattern and being responsive to specific treatment, then, given our current epistemic background, individuation of subtypes of PTSD with respect to the causes makes perfect sense – for purely pragmatic reasons [according to Beebee and Sabbarton-Leary (21) fulfillment of some such condition is sufficient to count as a scientific type]. On this view, the mechanism underlying the connection between particular causes and particular disorders is still missing. Once uncovered, reference to the social cause becomes idle. The view that some mental disorders should, at the present stage of development of psychiatry, be classified in terms of their social causes is, thus, compatible with versions of in-principle reductionism about mental disorders. As a consequence, one may have reservations to group pragmatic constructivism with more robust forms of constructivism.

Again, this appears to be perfectly compatible with an objectivist stance – there is no social construction involved, if Kirmayer, Crafa, and others are right. Of course, these claims raise interesting methodological issues; for instance, if sociocultural background has a significant impact on the development of the physiology underlying mental disorders, can we dispense with descriptions in terms of sociocultural background, or does it provide heuristics that, for the time being, are indispensable in clinical contexts? To repeat: epistemic questions of this sort may arise even if we adopt objectivism about mental disorders. Unless we individuate disorders with respect to sociocultural causes, as suggested in DSM 5 for PTSD, we do not end up with a form of social constructivism.

If we do, however, we would end up with a very similar form of constructivism [as (Reviewer 2) has pointed out]: one may adopt the view that experiences, symptoms, or phenomenology are constitutive of a disorder, and that experiences, some symptoms and the phenomenology that goes together with a disorder are not individuated by their underlying physiology, but, rather, require individuation in terms of their social dimension [see Ref. (23–25) for a critical perspective]. Thornton (26) has recently pointed out that Jaspers (27), in his discussion of psychiatry (for instance, in his book "Allgemeine Psychopathologie," first published in 1913), suggested that for a great number of psychological conditions that count as a mental disorder, some form of subjective understanding is required, besides observing behavior and understanding the other as rational (if possible), for an understanding of the kind of disorder the patient suffers from. Thornton tentatively agrees that an understanding of phenomenal aspects and subjective experiences may be required in understanding the nature of the disorder.

In a somewhat similar spirit, certain experiences may be regarded as forming essential parts of a disorder. Consider the following example, taken from Stier's discussion of cultural variation in psychiatry:[13]

> A [...] striking cultural difference can be found in the case of social anxiety. While in the western cultural sphere this is connected with the fear of being harmed or offended, in Japan and Korea people are in fear of harming or offending others [...]. [(2), p. 29]

Now, none of these claims makes, all by itself, for *social* constructivism; highlighting the way a disorder is presented to a subject from the first person perspective need not go together with social constructivism (although it will of course pose difficulties for forms of naturalism that typically go together with the form of objectivism we are concerned with here). However, the way a condition is presented to a subject from the first person perspective may *involve* a social dimension. Consider the case of variation across cultures in anxiety disorders: the assumption is that variation should be further explained in terms of cultural background, the role an individual is supposed to play within a community, the notion of personhood, etc. If we assume that the different forms of experience in western and Japanese and Korean culture correspond to at least two different subtypes of some disorder, subtypes any psychiatric taxonomy should be sensitive to, and if we assume that there is no unified physiological type corresponding to these experiences, we end up with a robust form of social constructivism. In Haslanger's words: the subtypes are "causally constructed" in that "social factors play a causal role in bringing [them] into existence or, to some substantial extent, in [their] being the way [they are]" [(13), p. 98]. Our objectivist would oppose a view according to which genuine social experiences that are not individuated by their physiological basis are essential to classification in psychiatry. The targets are disorders, and the grounds are experiences, phenomenology, or symptoms that are individuated only with respect to a social context. The relation is, again, non-causal; the perspective of the individual is not causally connected to the disorder; it is constitutive of it.[14]

So, does *no* thesis regarding the social cause of mental disorders, all by itself, amount to social constructivism? Is all social construction non-causal, as far as psychiatry is concerned?

Consider one particular version of the claim that some disorders have (maybe among others) social causes. It is somewhat atypical. Standard versions of social constructivism regarding causal influences of the cultural background on phenomenology, symptoms, or experiences have it that cultural background does not contain any particular "information" on the disorder itself, which would explain cultural variation. For instance, the difference between social anxiety in Europe and some parts of East Asia is explained in terms of general differences regarding the concept of a person or the expectations regarding the relation between an individual and the community it lives in. In contrast, Ian Hacking, and, from a psychiatric perspective, Piper and Merskey (28) have argued that some mental disorders evolve in response to specific theories of disorders, and the expectations that go together with specific theories. Hacking writes:

> [T]here was usually only one well-defined alter; today, sixteen alters is the norm. In France, a century or so ago, cases of doubling had the symptoms then associated with florid hysteria – partial paralyses, partial anesthesia, intestinal bleeding, restricted field of vision. English cases of double consciousness were more restrained but regularly went into a trance [...]
>
> Times change, and so do people. People in trouble are not more constant than anyone else. But there is more to the change in the lifestyle of multiples than the passage of time. We tend to behave in ways that are expected of us, especially by authority figures – doctors, for example. Some physicians had multiples among their patients in the 1840s, but their picture of the disorder was very

[13]Stier uses this example to back up an argument against biologism; it is not entirely clear to me how this example may affect even purely epistemic forms of reductionism, unless we buy, as a premise, that for biologism to be true, there must be *one physiological condition underlying both disorders*. But this does not seem to be required for some form or another of biologism to be true.

[14]There is, of course, also a relevant causal connection between the phenomenology or experience and the social environment of the subject, but this does not appear to be constitutive for the disorder.

> different because the doctors' expectations were different. That is an example of a very general phenomenon: the looping effect of human kinds. [(29), p. 21]

Hacking's view is clearly not that there is one type of disorder that can be expressed or even experienced in different ways due to the different models of the disorder offered in a given social environment (such as *first* multiple personality disorder, *then* dissociative disorder). Rather, the idea is that the discourse in psychiatry itself has a causal impact on the disorder the patient develops. The discourse causes the individual to adopt the dissociative identity disorder personality. The discourse, including expectations and specific norms, functions as an external cause of the disorder itself.

Some remarks on the details of Hacking's account are required in order to avoid misunderstandings. Basically, Hacking distinguishes between two different types of kinds, *indifferent* and *interactive kinds*. The former are kin to natural kinds; their objects are indifferent to our classification. Interactive kinds, however, involve causal feedback mechanisms, where the subjects that fall into the extension of an interactive kind respond to the classification, which, in turn, bears on the classification itself. This sort of causal looping effect is visible, according to Hacking, in psychiatric classification. But psychiatric classification is not purely interactive. According to Hacking, mental disorders have a physiological basis, which can be classified in terms of an indifferent kind. For what follows, I will be solely concerned with Hacking's characterization of the interactive aspect of psychiatric classification.

The target is, again, a particular type of disorder. The grounds are social events, involving interaction between patient and clinician or members of the social environment, with certain individual or shared expectations. The dependence relation is causal - the person is caused to adopt a certain pattern of experiences and behavioral traits, which, in turn, may have an impact on the classification. In contrast with the versions of causal constructivism about mental disorders previously discussed, Hacking assumes that the very attribution of a disorder contributes to the disorder (or the interactive aspect of the disorder). Interestingly, this renders true an explanation that looks, at its surface level, very much like Searle's constructivist claim about money:

> [3] Some people suffer from dissociative identity disorder because others regard them as suffering from dissociative identity disorder.

Unlike Searle's claim about money, however, [3] can be interpreted causally (and it is merely a partial explanation). It appears that there are causal versions of social constructivism in psychiatry. It is a form of constructivism not because of cultural variation, or because the disorder relates to attitudes like money relates to acceptance as money; it is a form of constructivism because it credits a conceptual practice, or discourse (that of multiple dissociative disorder) with the ability to literally create its own objects; and it does so in a way that masks the actual mechanisms that underlie the occurrence of multiple dissociative disorder. Of course, it is similar to cases where cultural background shapes the symptoms; discourse about multiple dissociative disorder is part of the cultural background. And if it has an impact on the development of dissociative disorders, including behavioral patterns, experiences, and symptoms, then in this case, cultural background shapes the disorder. But in this particular case, there is more: due to the tight connection between cultural background and disorder (i.e., the content of the discourse, which determines what it is to suffer from multiple dissociative disorder, and the disorder itself) the causal looping effect, if it occurs, ensures that that the current psychological condition instantiates the (first order) properties that define the interactive aspect of the disorder. Ignoring feedback mechanisms: The discourse causally contributes to the fact that the subject adopts the behavioral pattern others expect the subject to show; and showing the pattern is one mark of the disorder. If the interactive aspect of psychiatric classification were constitutive for facts about a subject falling under the relevant category,[15] then the instantiation of the property of having dissociative identity disorder would metaphysically depend on facts about adaptation to expectations (among other facts). In this case, causal construction and metaphysical dependence go together.

Now, finally, let me turn to what may be regarded as the most common, and, at the same time, the most challenging version of social constructivism regarding psychiatry: the thesis that the property of *being a mental disorder* is itself socially constructed.

Mental Disorder and Social Norms

In the tentative characterization of the notion of a mental disorder published in the introductory parts of DSM 5, the authors state that "[a]n expectable or culturally approved response to a common stressor [...] is not a mental disorder" (DSM 5, 20). It seems that thereby, the authors intend to indicate that something is a mental disorder *only if* it involves responses to stressors that are *not* expectable or culturally approved. This reading is supported by the following passage:

> The boundaries between normality and pathology vary across cultures for specific types of behaviors. Thresholds of tolerance for specific symptoms or behaviors differ across cultures, social settings, and families. Hence, the level at which an experience becomes problematic or pathological will differ. The judgment that a given behavior is abnormal and requires clinical attention depends on cultural norms that are internalized by the individual and applied by others around them, including family members and clinicians (DSM V, 14)

In contrast with the issues raised under the heading "Cultural Formulation," this is clearly more than a purely epistemological

[15]Tsou (30) has argued that if Hacking is right, then a stable classification of mental disorders in terms of the indifferent "part" of the classification should be possible. Here, we are not so much concerned with what Hacking actually claims; rather, we can, based on the work of Hacking, identify one possible version of social constructivism about mental kinds, a version of social constructivism that captures the interactive "part" of psychiatric classification.

point about access conditions. The authors suggest that whether or not a problematic experience is pathological depends in part on the social or cultural context. This idea has played a prominent role in the anti-psychiatrist movement (31), and the question of whether normative aspects involved in diagnostic procedures are social or can be cashed out in, say, descriptive or biological terminology has attracted considerable attention (3, 4, 26, 32). Being a mental disorder is a second order property, in the sense that it is supposed to be instantiated by first order properties of psychological conditions. An alcoholic exemplifies a specific psychological property, which, in turn, is supposed to exemplify the property of being a mental disorder.[16] The significance of the property of *being a mental disorder* appears to stem from the fact that it distinguishes the clinically relevant from the clinically irrelevant (just like related concepts of health and illness). Social constructivism about this second order property states that whether or not it is exemplified by a first order psychological condition depends on the social norms within a society. The boundaries between the pathological and the non-pathological determine whether or not a condition is a mental disorder, and they are themselves partly determined by social norms. Very roughly, social norms are usually regarded as a particular type of expectations about the behavior of others (33, 34); individuals are expected to follow a norm and are expected to act in a certain way when they detect norm-violation. Only if some such structure is widespread among a society, a social norm is in place. Facts about social norms are clearly social facts. Consequently, this form of social constructivism maintains that facts about the second order property *being a mental disorder* (the target of this form of social constructivism) depend on social facts, such as the presence of social norms, and that the relation between the two is non-causal dependence – the social norms do not cause a condition to be a mental disorder; they determine, in a conceptual, or logical sense whether or not some condition counts as a mental disorder.[17] Here, in a straightforward sense, instantiation of the second order property of being a mental disorder requires a certain conceptual framework; and it is shared attitudes that ground the instantiation of the property.

CONCLUSION

Let me sum up the results. Versions of social constructivism come in three different forms. Their targets are (some or all) types of mental disorders, or the second order property of being a mental disorder. Social facts and events appear among the grounds of mental disorders, and social norms or expectations shape the boundaries of the second order property of being a mental disorder. It may even be the case that sometimes, psychiatric classification itself has an impact on the occurrence of its objects, as Hacking suggests. Note that apart from versions of social constructivism about the second order property of being a mental disorder, social constructivism about psychiatry may, and probably will be limited to *some* forms of mental disorders. What is true of trauma or stressor-related disorders need not be true of schizophrenia, or, in particular, neurodevelopmental disorders.

So, what's the consequence of social constructivism for psychiatry as a science? It is difficult to give a straightforward answer. Quite a bit will hinge on general considerations about reduction, about the nature of scientific kinds, and on the nature of explanation. In order to bypass these further questions, let me begin with an observation that immediately follows from the different versions of social constructivism described above: if social constructivism about psychiatry is true, in one of the versions described above, then the conceptual apparatus psychiatry employs involves concepts of social objects, events, or facts. Moreover, it credits the so-represented events, objects, or facts with an explanatory role, in causal as well as metaphysical respects. Causal explanations in terms of social causes would turn out to be genuine and indispensable explanations within psychiatry – indispensable in the sense that the psychiatric types are partly social in nature. Although the radical objectivist may accept that some causal explanations of the occurrences of mental disorders that cite social events as causes are true, or may even play a useful heuristic role, she will deny that such explanations figure among the set of *psychiatric* explanations, properly construed. Recall: the evaporation of water from the Ocean may be caused by global warming, which, in turn, may be caused by social events. But an explanation of the evaporation of water from the Ocean based on its social causes will not count as an explanation within physics. Similarly, on the objectivist view, the explanation of mental disorders in terms of social causes will not count as a psychiatric explanation. Social constructivism, in some of its versions, is bound to deny that. Parts of psychiatry would then move toward the social sciences, as far as their explanatory practices are concerned.

Now, there is no consensus as to how we should conceive of scientific explanation, especially in the social sciences. One may take a liberal stance, suggesting that type construction and explanation mainly serve heuristic purposes, that causal generalizations merely systematize observations, and that consequently, the metaphor of the sociocultural environment *shaping* mental disorders can be given a non-committal, pragmatic, or purely epistemic interpretation. If so, the commitments of social constructivism are relatively weak; and dispute between constructivism and objectivism would be a dispute not about the nature, but rather about the pragmatically adequate or epistemically beneficial conceptualization of mental disorders. Some such considerations may have played a role in the history of DSM – the question of where to invest time and money may, by and large, be decided on pragmatic grounds.

But there is a corresponding ontic distinction that seems to better fit the nature of the dispute between constructivists and objectivists. The constructivist raises the worry that objectivism will fail for principled reasons; it just does not get the metaphysics

[16] In a derivative sense, individuals instantiate the property of having a mental disorder, namely, when they instantiate a first order property (such as alcoholism), which exemplifies the second order property of being a mental disorder.

[17] Although Wakefield departs from a biological notion of dysfunction, he arrives at a similar form of social constructivism. Wakefield characterizes the concept of a disorder in terms of a "condition [that] causes some harm or deprivation of benefit to the person as judged by the standards of the person's culture" – what he calls the "value criterion" [(15), p. 385], which complements the biologically construed dysfunction condition for the presence of a mental disorder. Wakefield assumes that disorders require biological dysfunction, but that what counts as a normal or acceptable life depends on social or cultural context.

right and, hence, looking for mechanisms or genetic profiles alone will never deliver the desired results. Rather, we should take social background, etiology, and cultural formation into account. And the objectivist maintains that at best, considerations regarding the sociocultural environment may play a heuristic role, or constitute an obstacle in the appropriate translation from behavioral observation and the subjects' reports to the language of the underlying neural mechanisms.

Social constructivism, on its metaphysical interpretation, may have ramifications that go beyond issues that pertain to the metaphysics of science in the narrow sense. Some versions of social constructivism, concerning, for instance, gender or race categories, have been proposed not as a challenging exercise in theoretical metaphysics, but rather with a critical intention. Very roughly, the critique, whatever the details, departs from the observation that what *seems* to be a distinction, or is typically regarded as a distinction grounded in natural properties, in reality is a distinction imposed on the world *by us*, to a relevant degree. If true, this may have significant political and ethical ramifications – whether a status is natural or social bears on normative considerations. Revealing the hidden social nature of an allegedly natural category may then constitute a first step in a critical enterprise [for an explication of the idea of how social constructivisms relates to the critique of current practices, cf. Ref. (35)]. Uncovering the social nature of gender categories is important not only for general metaphysical purposes but also, and primarily, for political reasons. The idea is that if what appears to be natural turns out to be social, evaluative, and political practice should change.

We cannot go into the details here; but one may expect that similar critical or ameliorative projects will be relevant in the philosophy of psychiatry whenever evaluations based on the classification of people as having a mental disorder hinge on an objectivist interpretation of the property of having a mental disorder, where, in fact, having a mental disorder depends on social facts. If social norms determine whether or not a psychological condition belongs to the category of having a mental disorder, and if being classified as having a mental disorder forms the basis of unjust treatment by others because these others mistakenly believe the property of having a mental disorder to be natural, or objective, then uncovering the social nature of the property of being a mental disorder may bear on social practice. This is precisely what Szasz intended.

Let me close with a related observation regarding the distinction between objectivists and constructivists in psychiatry. As (Reviewer 2) has stressed, variation in the occurrence of a type depending on sociocultural background (such as the occurrence of specific gender identities) is often regarded as an indication of the fact that the occurrence of this type depends on social facts; social constructivism has been the theory of choice to account for such facts. Recall Hacking's theory about the construction of dissociative identity disorders. Cultural variation is, here, clearly an indicator for the dependence of dissociative identity disorder on social facts. It is an indicator of the latter; but does cultural variation alone support some form or another of social constructivism?

Above, I have suggested that cultural variation in mental disorders is compatible with the form of objectivism discussed here. Doesn't this show that the way I use the term "objectivist," and, hence, "constructivist," is at odds with at least one important use of these terms in the general debate on social constructivism? Here, I can merely gesture at an answer. I think that there is a difference between the pair "constructivist"/"objectivist" in the context of debates about first order mental disorders and, say, in the field of gender theory. This is not an accident; it is mainly due to the fact that the type of objectivism opposed, for instance, by feminist constructivists just lacks a counterpart in the sphere of psychiatry, because gender categories differ from categories of (first order) mental disorders in one important respect. Simplifying a lot, conceptualization in terms of gender will typically go together with an implicit naturalist conception of gender properties (sometimes described as *essentialization*). Consequently, the gender-objectivist believes gender to be part of the *nature* of an individual; being a woman is supposed to be inborn, deviations from the dichotomy are regarded as, well, non-natural and, possibly, requiring intervention. These issues simply do not arise in current day psychiatry. Conceptualizing someone as suffering from a disorder does *not* suggest a conceptualization of the person as having this property by nature.

In the context of psychiatry, *naturalist* or *essentialist* objectivism typically concerns the *second order* property of being a mental disorder; objectivists claim that it is a natural or essential property of (first order) psychological conditions, whereas constructivists maintain that classification of first order psychological conditions as a mental disorder comprises an element of construction.

AUTHOR CONTRIBUTIONS

The author confirms being the sole contributor of this work and approved it for publication.

FUNDING

This work was supported by the Volkswagen Foundation as part of the generously funded project "A Study in Explanatory Power" and by the German Research Foundation within the network "Social Functions."

REFERENCES

1. US Department of Health and Human Services, editor. *Mental Health: Culture, Race, and Ethnicity – A Supplement to Mental Health: A Report of the Surgeon General*. Rockville, MD: U.S. Department of Health and Human Services; Substance Abuse and Mental Health Services Administration; Center for Mental Health Services (2001).
2. Stier M. Normative preconditions for the assessment of mental disorder. *Front Psychol* (2013) **4**:611. doi:10.3389/fpsyg.2013.00611
3. Kendell R. The concept of disease and its implications for psychiatry. *Br J Psychiatry* (1975) **127**:305–15. doi:10.1192/bjp.127.4.305
4. Boorse C. On the distinction between disease and illness. *Philos Public Aff* (1975) **5**:49–68.
5. Kendler KS, Zachar P, Craver C. What kinds of things are psychiatric disorders? *Psychol Med* (2011) **41**:1143–50. doi:10.1017/S0033291710001844
6. Hoeltje M, Schnieder B, Steinberg A, editors. *Varieties of Dependence: Ontological Dependence, Grounding, Supervenience, Response-Dependence*. Philosophia Verlag (2013).

7. Correia F, Schnieder B, editors. *Metaphysical Grounding. Understanding the Structure of Reality*. Cambridge: Cambridge University Press (2012).
8. Searle J. *The Construction of Social Reality*. London: Penguin (1995).
9. Searle J. *Making the Social World: The Structure of Human Civilization*. Oxford: Oxford University Press (2010).
10. Tuomela R. *The Philosophy of Sociality*. Oxford: Oxford University Press (2007).
11. Epstein B. *The Ant Trap. Rebuilding the Foundations of the Social Sciences*. Oxford: Oxford University Press (2015).
12. Millett K. *Sexual Politics*. London: Granada Publishing (1971).
13. Haslanger S. Ontology and social construction. *Philos Top* (1995) **23**:95–125. doi:10.5840/philtopics19952324
14. Wakefield JC. The concept of mental disorder: diagnostic implications of the harmful dysfunction analysis. *World Psychiatry* (2007) **6**:149–56.
15. Wakefield JC. The concept of mental disorder: on the boundary between biological facts and social values. *Am Psychol* (1992) **47**:373–88.
16. Murphy D. Philosophy of psychiatry. 2012 Edition. In: Zalta EN, editor. *The Stanford Encyclopedia of Philosophy*. (2010). Available from: http://plato.stanford.edu/entries/psychiatry/
17. Pickering N. *The Metaphor of Mental Illness*. Oxford: Oxford University Press (2006).
18. Haack S. *Defending Science – Within Reason: Between Scientism and Cynicism*. Amherst, NY: Prometheus Books (2003).
19. Foucault M. *Histoire de la folie à l'âge classique: Folie et déraison*. Paris: Plon (1961).
20. Foucault M. *Histoire de la Sexualité (vol. 1): La Volonté de Savoir*. Paris: Gallimard (1976).
21. Beebee H, Sabbarton-Leary N. Are psychiatric kinds 'real'? *Eur J Anal Philos* (2010) **6**:11–27.
22. Kirmayer L, Crafa D. What kind of science for psychiatry? *Front Hum Neurosci* (2014) **8**:435. doi:10.3389/fnhum.2014.00435
23. Gallagher S. Delusional realities. In: Broome M, Bortolotti L, editors. *Psychiatry as Cognitive Neuroscience: Philosophical Perspectives*. Oxford: Oxford University Press (2009). p. 245–66.
24. Ghaeme S. Feeling and time: the phenomenology of mood disorders, depressive realism, and existential psychotherapy. *Schizophr Bull* (2007) **33**:122–30. doi:10.1093/schbul/sbl061
25. Murphy D. *Psychiatry in the Scientific Image*. Cambridge: MIT Press (2006).
26. Thornton T. *Essential Philosophy of Psychiatry*. Oxford: Oxford University Press (2007).
27. Jaspers K. *Allgemeine Psychopathologie. Für Studierende, Ärzte und Psychologen* Berlin: Springer (1913).
28. Piper A, Merskey H. The persistence of folly: a critical examination of dissociative identity disorder. Part I. The excesses of an improbable concept. *Can J Psychiatry* (2004) **49**:592–600.
29. Hacking I. *Rewriting the Soul*. Princeton, NJ: Princeton University Press (1995).
30. Tsou J. Hacking on the looping effects of psychiatric classifications: what is an interactive and indifferent kind? *Int Stud Philos Sci* (2007) **21**(3):329–44. doi:10.1080/02698590701589601
31. Szasz T. *The Myth of Mental Illness*. London: Paladin (1972).
32. Fulford K. Analytic philosophy, brain science and the concept of disorder. In: Bloch S, Chodoff P, Green SA, editors. *Psychiatric Ethics*. Oxford: Oxford University Press (1999). p. 161–92.
33. Elster J. *The Cement of Society*. Cambridge: Cambridge University Press (1989).
34. Bicchieri C. *The Grammar of Society: The Nature and Dynamics of Social Norms*. New York: Cambridge University Press (2006).
35. Haslanger S. Gender and race: (what) are they? (what) do we want them to be? *Noûs* (2000) **34**:31–55.

8

Cognitive Neuroscience and Causal Inference: Implications for Psychiatry

Nadine Dijkstra[1]* *and Leon de Bruin*[2]

[1] *Donders Institute for Brain, Cognition and Behavior, Radboud University Nijmegen, Nijmegen, Netherlands,* [2] *Department of Philosophy, VU University Amsterdam, Amsterdam, Netherlands*

Edited by:
Firas H. Kobeissy, University of Florida, USA

Reviewed by:
David Papo, Technical University of Madrid, Spain
Eleftheria Pervolaraki, University of Leeds, UK
Ying Xu, University at Buffalo, USA

***Correspondence:**
Nadine Dijkstra
n.dijkstra@donders.ru.nl

In this paper, we investigate to what extent it is justified to draw conclusions about causal relations between brain states and mental states from cognitive neuroscience studies. We first explain the views of two prominent proponents of the interventionist account of causation: Woodward and Baumgartner. We then discuss the implications of their views in the context of traditional cognitive neuroscience studies in which the effect of changes in mental state on changes in brain states is investigated. After this, we turn to brain stimulation studies in which brain states are manipulated to investigate the effects on mental states. We argue that, depending on whether one sides with Woodward or Baumgartner, it is possible to draw causal conclusions from both types of studies (Woodward) or from brain stimulation studies only (Baumgartner). We show what happens to these conclusions if we adopt different views of the relation between mental states and brain states. Finally, we discuss the implications of our findings for psychiatry and the treatment of psychiatric disorders.

Keywords: interventionism, causal exclusion problem, cognitive neuroscience, psychiatry, mental causation

INTRODUCTION

Traditionally, cognitive neuroscientists have been probing the relation between brain states and mental states by manipulating the mental state of the participant through different conditions and then measuring the associated changes in neural activity, for example by means of Functional Magnetic Resonance Imaging (fMRI) or Electro-encephalogram (EEG). The results of these manipulations are usually taken to reflect a *correlation* between mental states and brain states, rather than a "genuine" *causal* relation. According to several neuroscientists, however, new brain stimulation techniques, such as Deep Brain Stimulation (DBS) and Transcranial Magnetic Stimulation (TMS), allow us to go beyond correlations and establish causal relations between mental states and brain states [for a review, see Ref. (1)]. This has important implications for other disciplines in which these techniques become increasingly popular. For example, in psychiatry, DBS has proven to be an effective treatment for patients with major depressive disorder (MDD) who do not respond to pharmacotherapy or psychotherapy (2–4).

In the current paper, we investigate whether and to what extent it is indeed justified to draw conclusions about causal relations between brain and mental states on the basis of cognitive neuroscience studies. In the next section, we start with a description of an interventionist account of causation, which is inspired by Woodward (5). We argue that this account is more or less in line with how causation is understood in scientific practice. The question is, however, whether it can be used to make causal claims about the interaction between mental states and brain states. In order to address this question, we introduce the notion of supervenience in Section "Mental States and Brain States: A Supervenience Relation." This notion aims to capture the intuition that mental states are dependent on, but not identical with, brain states. In Section "Causation in Traditional Cognitive Neuroscience Studies," we turn to Baumgartner's "causal exclusion" argument. According to this argument, the assumption of a supervenience relation violates the criteria of what counts as a good intervention. As a result, we cannot draw conclusions about the causal relation between mental states and brain states. In his reply to Baumgartner, Woodward (6) proposes to adjust these intervention criteria in order to make room for supervenience relations and to secure causal claims on the basis of traditional cognitive neuroscience studies. In Section "Causation in Brain Stimulation Studies," we discuss the consequences of both positions for causal claims on the basis of brain stimulation studies. Most importantly, we will show that Baumgartner's causal exclusion argument does not apply to these studies. That is, we can make causal claims about brain stimulation studies *even* if we assume a supervenience relation and accept Woodward's original intervention criteria. In Section "Articulating the Mind–Brain Relation," we show what happens to these conclusions if we adopt a different view of the relation between mental states and brain states. Finally, in Section "Conclusion," we briefly discuss the implications of our findings for psychiatry and the treatment of psychiatric disorders.

THE INTERVENTIONIST ACCOUNT OF CAUSATION

In most textbooks on experimental research two main requirements are described that an experiment must meet to be able to reveal a causal relation between *X* and *Y*. The first is that the levels of *X* must be systematically varied and the second is that all variables other than *X* and *Y* are to be controlled in order to eliminate other possible causes of *Y*. If these requirements are met and changes in *X* are accompanied by changes in *Y*, one is allowed to speak of a causal relation between *X* and *Y* (7, 8).

This notion of how to investigate causal relations in scientific practice is very much in line with a philosophical account of causation that has become quite popular recently: interventionism. One of the most established interventionist definitions of causation comes from Woodward (5):

> (M) A necessary and sufficient condition for *X* to be a (type-level) *direct cause* of *Y* with respect to a variable set **V** is that there be a possible intervention on *X* that will change *Y* or the probability of *Y* when one holds fixed at some value all other variables Z_i in **V**. A necessary and sufficient condition for *X* to be a (type-level) *contributing cause* of *Y* with respect to variable set **V** is that (i) there be a directed path from *X* to *Y* such that each link in this path is a direct causal relationship… and that (ii) there be some intervention on *X* that will change *Y* when all other variables in **V** that are not on this path are held fixed [Ref. (5), pp. 59].

We mainly focus on the definition of a direct cause since this comes closest to the notion of causation as it is investigated in scientific practice (i.e., it explicitly involves the two requirements mentioned above). However, for the definition to make sense, we also need a clear notion of what an appropriate intervention is. Woodward (5) defines an intervention variable as follows:

(IV) *I* is an intervention variable for *X* with respect to *Y* if:

1. *I* causes *X*;
2. *I* acts as a switch for all the other variables that cause *X*. That is, certain values of *I* are such that when *I* attains those values, *X* ceases to depend on the values of other variables that cause *X* and instead depends only on the value taken by *I*;
3. Any directed path from *I* to *Y* goes through *X*. That is, *I* does not directly cause *Y* and is not a cause of any causes of *Y* that are distinct from *X* except, of course, for those causes of *Y*, if any, that are built into the *I*–*X*–*Y* connection itself; that is, except for (a) any causes of *Y* that are effects of *X* (i.e., variables that are causally between *X* and *Y*) and (b) any causes of *Y* that are between *I* and *X* and have no effect on *Y* independently of *X*.
4. *I* is (statistically) independent of any variable *Z* that causes *Y* and that is on a directed path that does not go through *X* [(5), pp. 98].

Finally, relative to the notion of an intervention variable an (actual) *intervention* can be straightforwardly understood in terms of an intervention variable *I* for *X* with respect to *Y* taking on some value z_i such that $I = z_i$ causes *X* to take on some determinate value z_j [(5), pp. 98]. In terms of experimental design, an intervention can be seen as a manipulation that changes the variable *X*. In order for this manipulation to be able to reveal a causal relation, it has to meet the requirements in (IV).

MENTAL STATES AND BRAIN STATES: A SUPERVENIENCE RELATION

Can we use interventionism to make causal claims about the interaction between mental states and brain states? To answer this question, we will (initially) assume a very minimal relation between mental states and brain states – one that captures the intuition that mental states are dependent on brain states. In the philosophy of mind, this relation is known as "supervenience."

A schematic representation of a supervenience relation between mental states M1 and M2 and brain states P1 and P2 is depicted in **Figure 1**. Although the notion of supervenience has been much discussed, there are two features that are common in most definitions:

(S1) $\neg$(*M* causes *P*) $\wedge$ $\neg$(*P* causes *M*);
(S2) Every change in the value of M is necessarily accompanied by a change in the value of P.

This means that (i) supervenience is a non-causal relation such that neither M causes P nor vice versa[1] and (ii) any change in mental state is necessarily accompanied by a change in brain state. Furthermore, with regard to **Figure 1**, we will assume that:

(S3) P1 causes P2.

[1]Supervenience is non-causal because it represents a synchronic rather than a diachronic relation between M and P.

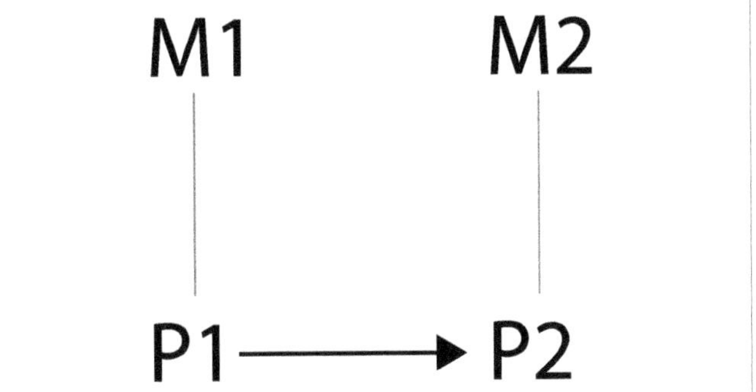

FIGURE 1 | **Schematic representation of the relation between brain states and mental states. Undirected edges indicate supervenience relations and the arrow indicates a causal relation.**

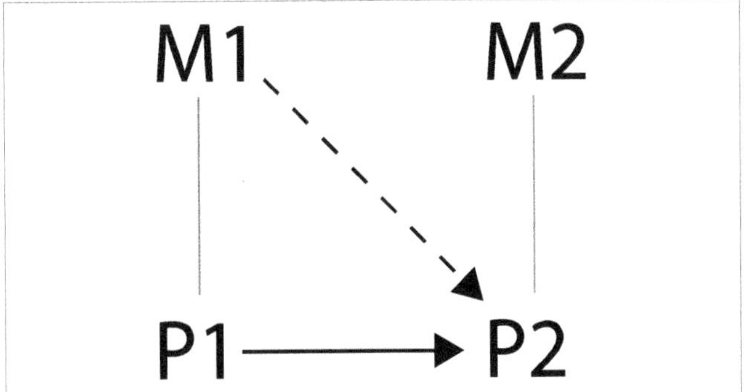

FIGURE 2 | **Schematic representation of the relation investigated in traditional cognitive neuroscience studies indicated by the dashed arrow.**

The end result is a schematic representation of two types of relations: one between *properties* (M1 and P1, M2 and P2), which is captured by a supervenience relation, and one between *events* (M1/P1 and M2/P2), which is captured by a causal relation (i.e., event 1 causes event 2).

CAUSATION IN TRADITIONAL COGNITIVE NEUROSCIENCE STUDIES

With the interventionist account of causation and the notion of supervenience in place, let us now take a closer look at traditional (non-invasive) cognitive science studies.

In most of these studies, the relation between mental states and brain states is investigated by observing the effect of changes in mental state M1 on brain state P2 (see **Figure 2**). This is done by manipulating the mental state of the subjects by letting them participate in separate conditions that differ on some stimulus characteristic or task that is meant to induce changes in M1. To investigate the effect of these manipulations on brain states, the subjects' brain activity P2 is measured in all conditions. Then, if the researcher has made sure that the conditions only differ on the manipulated mental variable (using all kinds of controls like randomization of subjects), and a (significant) difference in brain activity between the conditions is found, the researcher concludes that the manipulated mental variable M1 has had an effect on the measured brain state P2.

However, is it valid to conclude that the change in mental state M1 *caused* the change in brain state P2? According to the causal exclusion argument put forward by Baumgartner (9), it is not.

Baumgartner's Causal Exclusion Argument

In his argument, Baumgartner (9) takes together the interventionist definition of causation as described above in (M) and (IV) and the supervenience relation as described in (S1–2) to formulate the following conditional:

> (BM) If *M1* is causally relevant to *P2* with respect to the variable set **V** = {*M1, M2, P1, P2*}, then there possibly exists a variable I_1 that causes a change in the value (or the probability distribution) of *M1* and is statistically independent of any variable *Z* that causes *P2* and that is on a directed path that does not go through *M1* [(9), pp. 170].

Now we can see that no such variable I_1 can exist. Because of the supervenience relation between *M1* and *P1*, any variable I_1 that causes a change in *M1* also causes a change in *P1* (S2) and this variable *P1* is on a causal path to *P2* that does not go through *M1* (S3). In other words, every time we perform an intervention on a subjects' mental state, by manipulating some variable in separate experimental conditions, we also intervene on their brain state. This is not because the change in mental state causes the change in brain state (recall that a supervenience relation is not a causal relation; S1), but because the intervention changes both the mental state and the brain state (S2). In other words, we cannot control the effect of *P1* on *P2*. It follows that we cannot draw any conclusions about the causal effect of the intervention on the mental state. Furthermore, because the relation between *M1* and *P1* is not a causal relation, we also cannot say that *M1* is a contributing cause to *P2*. In the context of an experiment, we would say that *P1* is a confounding variable for which we cannot control, prohibiting any statement to be made about the causal effect of the independent variable on the dependent variable.

Woodward's Response

In reply to Baumgartner's argument, Woodward (6) proposes that when assessing causation in a variable set that includes supervenience relations between variables, it is not necessary to control for or hold fixed the supervenience base. Thus, it is not necessary to control for *P1* when assessing the relation between *M1* and *P2*. According to Woodward, this is because the interventionist account of causation as defined by (M) and (IV) is intended to apply to systems of causal relations in which no non-causal relations (such as supervenience relations) exist. It is not at all clear whether it is applicable to a system in which non-causal relations are present.

Woodward illustrates this by giving an example of a variable set in which non-causal relations are present that are not supervenience relations (6). His example goes along the following lines. Suppose that getting a headache (*H*) is causally influenced by the amount of alcohol consumption (*AC*), which increases the probability of getting a headache, and the amount of non-alcoholic liquid consumption (*NC*), which decreases the probability of getting a headache. We also have a variable representing the total liquid consumption (*TC*), which is the sum of *AC* and *NC*. Assume that we also think of *TC* as causally influencing *H*. We can put all these variables together to get the schematic representation in **Figure 3**.

Suppose now that we want to investigate if *AC* is causally relevant for *H*. According to Baumgartner's reading of (IV) and (M), this would mean that it has to be possible to change (intervene on) *AC* without changing any other variable in **Figure 4** that is on a directed path to *H* that does not go through *AC*. We can see that this is not possible because *TC* is defined such that if *AC* changes, *TC* also changes. It seems strange to take this finding as evidence for there not being a causal relation between *AC* and *H*. Therefore, Woodward (6) concludes, the interventionist definition as put forward in (M) and (IV) is intended to only apply to systems of causal relations in which no non-causal relations exist. In systems with non-causal relations, one needs to hold fixed only the *appropriate* variables. In the variable set described in **Figure 4**, this means that if one wants to investigate the effect of *AC* on *H*, *NC* needs to be fixed, but *TC* does not.

Similarly, Woodward (6) argues, when one wants to investigate the causal effects of supervening variables, their supervenience base does not have to be fixed. This means that *M1* can be causally relevant for *P2* or in other words, according to this interpretation of interventionist causation, investigating the relation between mental states and brain states, as done in traditional cognitive neuroscience studies, by manipulating *M1* and investigating its effect on *P2* can reveal a causal relation between *M1* and *P2*.

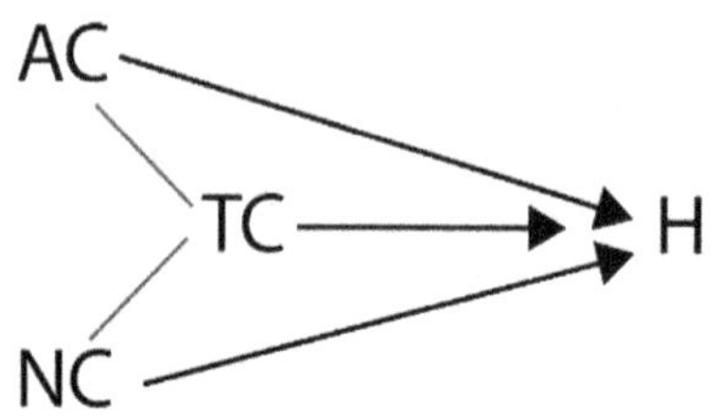

FIGURE 3 | Schematic representation of the relation between AC, WC, TC, and H.

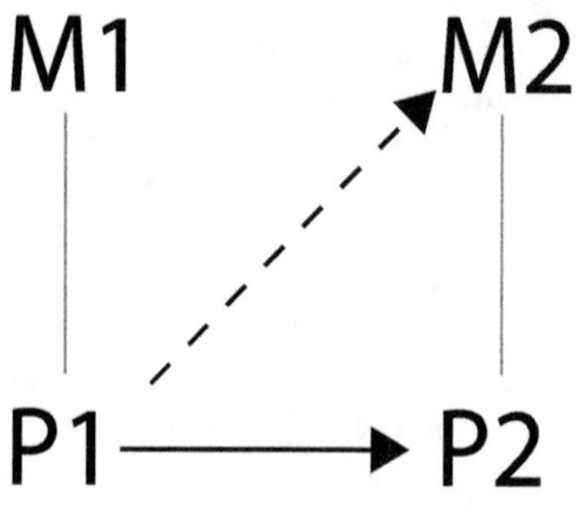

FIGURE 4 | Schematic representation of the relation investigated in brain stimulation studies as indicated by the dashed arrow.

In conclusion, according to Baumgartner (9), one cannot draw any conclusions about causal relations between mental states and brain states from traditional cognitive neuroscience studies. However, according to Woodward (6), this is perfectly valid. In the next section, we will discuss both these positions in light of brain stimulation studies in which the brain states are manipulated to investigate the effects on mental states.

CAUSATION IN BRAIN STIMULATION STUDIES

Since the introduction of brain stimulation techniques such as TMS and DBS, it has become possible for scientists to directly manipulate (intervene on) the electrical activity in the brain. Many neuroscientists have been using these techniques to draw conclusions about the causal relations between brain states and mental states. The following are quotes from TMS and DBS studies published in high-impact journals:

> "Making the causal link: frontal cortex activity and repetition priming" (10).
> "Causal implication by rhythmic TMS of alpha frequency in feature-based vs. global attention" (11).
> "DBS of the subthalamic nucleus markedly improves the motor symptom's of Parkinson's disease, but causes cognitive side effects such as impulsivity" (12).
> "Stimulation of a restricted site in the upper midbrain can cause major acute depression" (13).

Are these claims justified? In the present section, we will explore this question in light of Baumgartner's and Woodward's arguments. Before we continue, we should mention that a large part of the brain stimulation studies only focuses on the effects of changes in brain states on other brain states [e.g., Ref. (14–16)]. This is the relation between *P1* and *P2*. As described in (S3), we assume that there exists a causal relation between these variables. Therefore, in these types of brain stimulation studies, it is perfectly justified to talk about causal effects.

In the brain stimulation studies in which the relation between brain states and mental states is investigated, this seems more complicated. In these studies, the relation between *P1* and *M2* as depicted in **Figure 4** is investigated. *P1* is manipulated by stimulating a certain brain area using TMS or DBS in one condition and not stimulating it in another condition, while measuring some mental variable *M2* in both conditions. The researcher tries to make sure that the two conditions only differ on *P* and not on other variables, for example by applying sham stimulation in the control condition. If then a (significant) difference in *M2* between the two conditions is found, the researcher concludes that there was an effect of the change in brain activity on the mental state. However, is he or she justified in saying that *P1* has *caused* *M2*?

Baumgartner's Approach

To determine whether Baumgartner's argument applies to this experimental set-up, the conditional (BM) has to be redefined. If we switch the relevant terms, we get the following definition:

> (BP) If *P1* is causally relevant to *M2* with respect to the variable set **V** = {*M1, M2, P1, P2*}, then there possibly exists a variable I_1 that causes a change in the value (or the probability distribution) of *P1* and is statistically independent of any variable *Z* that causes *M2* and that is on a directed path that does not go through *P1*.

Interestingly, the causal exclusion argument used by Baumgartner (9) to conclude that *M1* is not causally relevant to *P2* does not work in this case. This is because there is no variable in **V** that causes *M2* but does not go through *P1*. It is true that, because of the supervenience relation (S2), any intervention on *P1* also changes *M1*. However, there is no causal relation between *M1* and *M2* that does not go through *P1*. Furthermore, an intervention on *P1* also changes *P2*, through the causal relation mentioned in (S3), but according to (S1), *P2* does not cause *M2*. So it seems that an intervention on *P1* is possible without intervening on another variable that causes *M2*. This suggests that we actually can make causal claims on the basis of brain stimulation studies, even if we assume a supervenience relation and accept Woodward's original intervention criteria. Let us now see whether Woodward's approach leads to a similar conclusion.

Woodward's Approach

According to Woodward, if one wants to investigate whether *P1* is causally relevant to *M2*, one needs to perform an intervention to change the value of *P*, while holding fixed all *appropriate* other variables. When investigating the relation between *P1* and *M2*, the supervenience base *P2* is not one of these appropriate variables, so even if *P2* were on a directed path to *M2* that does not include *P1*, *P2* does not have to be fixed because it is the supervenience base of *M2*.

The other possible candidate for a variable that is on a directed path to *M2* that does not include *P1*, is *M1*. Now this seems to pose a problem. According to Woodward's adjusted interpretation of interventionist causation, we can argue that *M1* causes *M2*, because *P1* and *P2* do not have to be fixed. This seems to imply that *M1* is an alternative cause for *M2* making it impossible to conclude that *P1* has caused *M2*. However, it seems that in his adaptation, Woodward (6) also argues that supervening variables do not have to stay fixed:

> (IV*) An intervention *I* on *X* with respect to *Y* will (a) fix the value of *SB(X)* in a way that respects the supervenience relationship between *X* and *SB(X)*, and (b) the requirements in the definition (IV) are understood as applying only to those variables that are causally related to *X* and *Y* or are correlated with them *but not to those variables that are related to X and Y as a result of supervenience relations* [(6), pp. 32].

This means that *M1* does not have to be fixed in order to draw a causal conclusion about the relation between *P1* and *M2* by intervening on *P1*.

Thus, according to Woodward's adjusted interpretation of interventionist causation, brain stimulation studies in which appropriate controls are applied, such as randomization of groups and application of sham stimulation in the control group, are suitable to base conclusions about the causal effect of brain states on mental states on.

In conclusion, if one follows Woodward, we can make claims about causal relations between brain states and mental states from the results of both traditional cognitive neuroscience and brain stimulation studies. However, for this to work, we do have to adjust the original interventionist criteria (5) and accept a non-causal supervenience relation. According to Baumgartner, by contrast, we cannot make claims about causation from the results of traditional cognitive neuroscience studies. However, even if we do not adjust the original criteria, we can still draw conclusions about causation from brain stimulation studies.

ARTICULATING THE MIND–BRAIN RELATION

The conclusions drawn in the previous sections rely heavily on the assumption of a supervenience relation between brain states and mental states. We believe that most neuroscientists would agree with this assumption. Quoting one of the key textbooks in cognitive neuroscience programs: "Cognitive neuroscience is an academic field concerned with the scientific study of biological substrates underlying cognition, with a specific focus on the neural substrates of mental processes" [(17), p. 12]. This definition suggests that what lies at the heart of cognitive neuroscience is a dependency relation between mental states ("cognition") and brain states (the "neural substrate").

Supervenience is not a "deep" explanatory relation; however, it only indicates the presence of a dependence relation without telling us what it is (18). A common way to further explain this dependency is by appealing to the notion of *emergence*. Central to emergentism is the idea that supervenient properties are "novel" properties over and above the properties upon, which they supervene. In the context of the mental causation debate, emergentism can be understood as the more specific claim that mental states are the emergent properties of a complex physical system, which have their own causal power and cannot be reduced to the basic physical properties of this system.[2] It is also possible to explain the dependence relation between mental and physical properties in terms of *reduction*. In contrast to emergentism, reductionism claims that supervenient properties are reducible to their base properties, and hence that mental properties are reducible to physical properties.

Thus far we have investigated whether interventionism allows us to make causal claims about the relation between mental states

[2] See, e.g., Ref. (19, 20) for specific accounts of supervenient emergentism in (cognitive) neuroscience.

and brain states, given a notion of supervenience that in principle allows mental states to be causally efficacious *qua* mental. In other words, we have assumed a dependence relation between mental states and brain states that is non-reductive, in principle compatible with the notion of emergence, and less strong than an identity relation. However, some people might not agree with this characterization of the relation between mind and brain. What happens to the conclusions drawn in this paper when one wishes to assume a reductive relation between mental states and brain states instead? In what follows we will briefly explore this option and also consider the possibility of a causal relation.

Type Identity and Functional Reduction

A radical reductive explanation of the supervenience relation is offered by the identity theory. This theory holds that mental states *are* brain states. The strongest version of the identity theory, the so-called "type-identity" theory, is reductionist in the sense that it states that specific types of mental states can be reduced to specific types of brain states (21). This theory would therefore claim that $M1 = P1$ and $M2 = P2$. Now it becomes almost trivial to show that an intervention on *P1* can show a causal effect on *M2*: since we know that an intervention on *P1* will cause a change in *P2* (S3) and since *M2* is now the same as *P2*, we can conclude that *P1* causes *M2*. Thus, assuming a type-identity relation between brain states and mental states still allows us to draw conclusions about the causal effects of brain states on mental states from brain stimulation studies. Similarly, assuming a type-identity relation also makes it possible to draw conclusions about causal relations from traditional cognitive neuroscience studies: since we know an intervention on *P1* causes a change in *P2* and $M1 = P1$, we can conclude that *M1* causes *P2*.

The identity theory faces two important problems. First of all, it does not really provide us with an explanation of *why* mental states are identical with brain states. Take the claim that water is H_2O. In this case, we can explain the properties of water in terms of the molecules that constitute it (two hydrogen atoms and a single oxygen atom) and the way they are interrelated. Stating that mental states are identical with brain states does not provide us with such an explanation. Second, there is the problem of multiple realizability (22, 23). If (at least some) mental states can be realized by different brain states, which seems plausible given what we know about the plasticity of the human brain, then they cannot be identical with specific brain states.

An alternative model of reduction, *functional reduction*, has been proposed by Kim (18, 24). According to this model, mental states can be reduced in the following way:

> *Stage 1.* Define *M* in terms of its "causal role," i.e., in terms of the causal task *C* it performs.
>
> *Stage 2.* Identify the "realizers" of *M*, i.e., the actual mechanisms that perform causal task *C*.
>
> *Stage 3.* Develop an explanatory theory that explains how the realizers of *M* perform causal task *C*.

The causal claims about brain stimulation studies and traditional cognitive neuroscience studies that can be made on the basis of functional reductionism are similar to those that can be made on the basis of the identity theory. Furthermore, functional reductionism does provide an explanation of how mental states are realized by brain states, and it is entirely consistent with the phenomenon of multiple realizability (in the sense that Stage 2 anticipates the existence of multiple lower-level realizers).

However, functional reductionism, like the identity theory, comes at a high price: it grants mental states causal power, but only in virtue of their being physical states. And this might be a hard pill to swallow, since many people believe that mental states do have causal power of their own, *qua* mental. It is precisely this intuition that is behind the debate between Baumgartner and Woodward in the first place.

A Causal Relation

The second alternative that we will consider is one that postulates a causal relation between brain states and mental states, in the sense that *P2* causes *M2*. Although most philosophers reject this possibility [with the notable exception of (25)], it might strike cognitive neuroscientists as a plausible option.

What can we conclude from brain stimulation studies if we assume that the relation between *P2* to *M2* is a causal relation (one that has been established by means of an appropriate intervention)? In particular, can we still make causal claims about the relation between *P1* and *M2*? At first glance, the problem seems to be that *P2* is now on a directed path to *M2* that does not include *P1*. However, it is precisely this relation that allows us to conclude that *P1* is a *contributing* cause according to the second part of (M):

> A necessary and sufficient condition for *X* to be a (type-level) *contributing cause* of *Y* with respect to variable set **V** is that (i) there be a directed path from *X* to *Y* such that each link in this path is a direct causal relationship… and that (ii) there be some intervention on *X* that will change *Y* when all other variables in **V** that are not on this path are held fixed [(5), pp. 59].

Note that this was not possible when we assumed a supervenience relation between *P2* and *M2* because in that case not every link on the path from *P1* to *M2* was a direct causal relation.

Unfortunately, this does not work when we want to make causal inferences from traditional cognitive neuroscience studies. *M1* cannot have a causal effect on *P2*, because it is impossible to intervene on *M1* without violating the second requirement of (IV):

> 2 *I* acts as a switch for all the other variables that cause *X*. That is, certain values of *I* are such that when *I* attains those values, *X* ceases to depend on the values of other variables that cause *X* and instead depends only on the value taken by *I*.

Criterion 2 is violated because of the assumption that *M1* is caused by *P1*. What this seems to show is that the assumption of a causal relation between brain states and mental states ultimately leads to *epiphenomenalism*, i.e., the thesis that mental states can be causally influenced by physical states, but have no causal efficacy themselves. It is probably safe to assume that most people will not really consider this an improvement over the minimal notion of mental causation provided by type identity and functional reduction.

CONCLUSION

The aim of this paper was to investigate whether we can draw conclusions about causal relations between brain states and mental states from traditional cognitive neuroscience studies and brain stimulation studies, given an interventionist account of causation. We have argued that, if one follows Woodward in embracing the notion of supervenience and revising the criteria for what counts as an intervention, both types of studies can be used to establish causal claims. If, by contrast, one follows Baumgartner and his causal exclusion argument, traditional cognitive neuroscience studies cannot be used to establish causal claims but brain stimulation studies can.

Brain stimulation is being used more and more as a form of treatment for psychiatric disorders. We have shown that from an interventionist point of view, it is valid to say that these brain stimulation treatments *cause* changes in mental states. Now this is not necessarily an argument in favor of these treatments. However, if Baumgartner is right, then it seems reasonable to conclude that brain stimulation treatments will become increasingly attractive. Unlike traditional cognitive neuroscience studies, they actually have the potential to elucidate the causal structure of certain psychiatric disorders (i.e., the underlying causal relations between mental states and brain states). It is a safe bet that this will appeal to many psychiatrists.

At the same time, this conclusion is based on a "conservative" interpretation of interventionism, and a rejection of non-causal metaphysical relations between mental states and brain states such as supervenience. In this respect, Woodward's position is much more "liberal," insofar as it proposes adjusted intervention criteria and allows for the inclusion of non-causal relations between mental states and brain states. One advantage of Woodward's position is that it allows psychiatrists to draw conclusions about the causal structure of mental disorders from traditional cognitive neuroscience (and not just brain stimulation studies). Another and perhaps even more important advantage is that it legitimates the claim that cognitive and behavioral therapy, aiming at influencing the mental state of a patient, can *cause* changes in the patient's brain state.

A note of caution is required when applying our conclusions to psychiatric practice. When defining mental states and brain states as separate targets of intervention, we assume an ideal situation in which such a separation can be easily obtained, and Woodward's intervention criteria are met. In practice, however, such a situation might be difficult to achieve. For example, in their paper on degeneracy, Price and Friston (26) have argued that different neural configurations can lead to similar mental states. This means that a disruption of one of these configurations by brain stimulation might not necessarily lead to a change in mental state. The experimenter who uses interventionism in the context of a single study would then be forced to conclude that there is no causal relation between the brain state and mental state in question. Now this scenario could be avoided by making sure that conclusions about causal relations between mental states and brain states are supported by multiple studies (controlling for both inter- and intra-individual variation). However, there might be a larger worry here, not just about the fact that the application of interventionism to single studies in practice might sometimes result in misguided causal claims, but also about the *very possibility* of applying interventionism to cognitive neuroscience studies.

For example, one might argue that various factors such as degeneracy, redundancy, path-dependency, non-linearity and complex feedback loops make it (theoretically) impossible to establish linear causal chains.[3] In the light of this, several theorists have proposed a concept of "circular causation" (27–29). Circular causation, which is taken to be typical of a self-organizing system, is realized by the cooperation of the individual parts of the system, yet it also governs or constrains the behavior of these individual parts. A good illustration of circular causation is given by McGilchrist (30) in his account of the brain as a complex system: "Events anywhere in the brain are connected to, and potentially have consequences for, other regions, which may respond to, propagate, enhance or develop that initial event, or alternatively redress it in some way, inhibit it, or strive to re-establish equilibrium. There are no bits, only networks, an almost infinite array of pathways" (2010, p. 34).

Circular causation is attractive, but also slightly misleading – at least when it is articulated in opposition to linear causation. As Von Bertalanffy (31, 32) already pointed out, to make sense of circular causation we still require a notion of linear and "unidirectional" causation. The kind of feedback regulation that is implied by circular causation is obviously not unidirectional in *spatial* terms: it moves back and forth or circles around the various components of a system (33). However, despite circling in space, feedback still proceeds forward in *linear time*, one component being separated from the next in time. Circular causation, thus understood, is compatible with the assumption of a supervenience relation between mental states and brain states. The question is whether it is also compatible with interventionism. Let us say we propose a modified version of **Figure 1** that involves feedback loops, for example one in which P1 causes P2 which in turns causes *P1* (**Figure 5A**). Now, at first glance, such a feedback loop seems to violate the second requirement of (IV), in the sense that one might think that *P1* not only depends on the value taken by *I* but also on the value of *P2*. However, the problem is that such a depiction of circular causation fails to take into account the fact

[3] We thank an anonymous reviewer for bringing this to our attention.

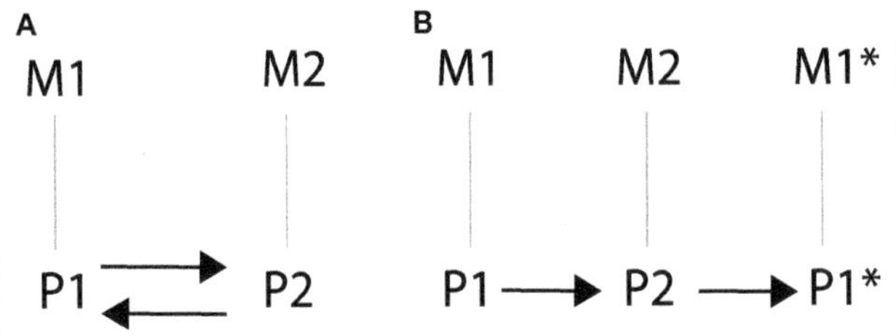

FIGURE 5 | **(A)** Incorrect depiction of circular causation that fails to take into account the temporal relation between P1 and P2, and P2 and P1. **(B)** Correct depiction of circular causation that takes into account the spatial as well as the temporal relation between P1 and P2, and P2 and P1*, and illustrates the linear nature of circular causation.

that the relations between *P1* and *P2*, and *P2* and *P1* are temporal relations between different *events,* and therefore they cannot be circular. That is, the *P1* that causes *P2* is different (not spatially, but temporally) from the *P1* that is caused by *P2* as the result of the feedback loop. The correct (linear) way to represent circular causation is shown in **Figure 5B**: *P1* causes *P2*, and *P2* causes *P1** (which is temporally different, but spatially identical with *P1*). And this seems to be compatible with interventionism, to the extent that an intervention on *P1* does not violate the second requirement of (IV).

It is important to note, at this point, that interventionism as such is relatively free of metaphysical commitments, in the sense that it does not make claims about how exactly one should spell out the relation between mental states and brain states. It only tells us what needs to be in place and which conditions need to be met for a given relation between variables to be described as "causal." Furthermore, as we have shown in Section "The Interventionist Account of Causation," one of the main attractions of interventionism is that it seems to correspond to how causal relations are investigated in scientific practice. Therefore, even if interventionism turns out to be incompatible with certain assumptions about brain functioning, such as circular causation and feedback loops, then this indicates a larger problem with mainstream scientific method and textbook accounts of experimental research. Obviously, these are issues that deserve critical attention. For the purpose of this paper, however, we have taken the mainstream scientific method as our starting point.

In the end, how psychiatrists approach these issues will probably depend on their intuitions about interventionist causation and the relation between mind and brain. However, one thing is certain. What they conclude will have important implications for the way they communicate the effect of different treatments to their patients.

AUTHOR CONTRIBUTIONS

ND wrote the core sections of this paper ("The Interventionist Account of Causation," "Mental States and Brain States: a Supervenience Relation," "Causation in Traditional Cognitive Neuroscience Studies," and "Causation in Brain Stimulation Studies") and the main argument; LB wrote the other Sections "Introduction," "Articulating the Mind–Brain Relation," and "Conclusion," revised/rewrote Sections "The Interventionist Account of Causation," "Mental States and Brain States: a Supervenience Relation," "Causation in Traditional Cognitive Neuroscience Studies," and "Causation in Brain Stimulation Studies and supervised the project."

FUNDING

LB's research was supported by a grant from the Templeton World Charity Foundation. The opinions expressed in this publication are his own and do not necessarily reflect the views of Templeton World Charity Foundation.

REFERENCES

1. Sack AT. Transcranial magnetic stimulation, causal structure-function mapping and networks of functional relevance. *Curr Opin Neurobiol* (2006) 16(5):593–9. doi:10.1016/j.conb.2006.06.016
2. Cleary DR, Ozpinar A, Raslan AM, Ko AL. Deep brain stimulation for psychiatric disorders: where we are now. *Neurosurg Focus* (2015) 38(6):E2. doi:10.3171/2015.3.focus1546
3. Holtzheimer PE, Mayberg HS. Deep brain stimulation for psychiatric disorders. *Annu Rev Neurosci* (2011) 34:289–307. doi:10.1146/annurev-neuro-061010-113638
4. Mayberg HS, Lozano AM, Voon V, McNeely HE, Seminowicz D, Hamani C, et al. Deep brain stimulation for treatment-resistant depression. *Neuron* (2005) 45(5):651–60. doi:10.1016/j.neuron.2005.02.014
5. Woodward J. *Making Things Happen: A Theory of Causal Explanation.* (Vol. 14). Oxford: Oxford University Press (2007).
6. Woodward J. Interventionism and causal exclusion. *Philos Penomenol Res* (2014). doi:10.1111/phpr.12095
7. Convenor C, Field A, Drury J. *Research Mewwthods in Psychology.* (Vol. 26). (2006). Available from: www.Sussex.ac.uk.
8. Shaughnessy JJ, Zechmeister EB, Zechmeister JS. *Research Methods in Psychology.* New York: McGraw-Hill (2012).
9. Baumgartner M. Interventionist causal exclusion and non-reductive physicalism. *Int Stud Philos Sci* (2009) 23(2):161–78. doi:10.1080/02698590903006909
10. Martin A, Gotts SJ. Making the causal link: frontal cortex activity and repetition priming. *Nat Neurosci* (2005) 8(9):1134–5. doi:10.1038/nn0905-1134
11. Romei V, Thut G, Mok RM, Schyns PG, Driver J. Causal implication by rhythmic transcranial magnetic stimulation of alpha frequency in feature-based local vs. global attention. *Eur J Neurosci* (2012) 35:968–74. doi:10.1111/j.1460-9568.2012.08020.x
12. Frank MJ, Samantha J, Moustafa AA, Sherman SJ. Hold your horses: impulsivity, and medication in parkinsonism. *Science* (2007) 318(5854): 1309–12. doi:10.1126/science.1146157
13. Bejjani B, Damier P, Arnul I, Thivard L, Bonnet A, Dormont D, et al. Transient acute depression induced by high-freuquency deep-brain stimulation. *N Engl J Med* (1999) 340:1476–80. doi:10.1056/NEJM199905133401905
14. Grossman E, Donnelly M, Price R, Pickens D, Morgan V, Neighbor G, et al. Brain areas involved in perception of biological motion. *J Cogn Neurosci* (2000) 12(5):711–20. doi:10.1162/089892900562417
15. Thut G, Miniussi C. New insights into rhythmic brain activity from TMS-EEG studies. *Trends Cogn Sci* (2009) 13(4):182–9. doi:10.1016/j.tics.2009.01.004
16. Zatorre RJ, Chen JL, Penhune VB. When the brain plays music: auditory-motor interactions in music perception and production. *Nat Rev Neurosci* (2007) 8(7):547–58. doi:10.1038/nrn2152
17. Gazzaniga MS, Irvy RB, Mangun GR. *Cognitive Neuroscience: The Biology of the Mind.* New York: W.W. Norton (2002).
18. Kim J. Supervenience, emergence, realization, reduction. In: Loux M, Zimmerman D, editors. *The Oxford Handbook of Metaphysics.* Oxford: Oxford University Press (2005). p. 556–84.
19. Haken H. *Brain Dynamics.* Berlin: Springer (2002).
20. Atmanspacher H. Identifying mental states from neural states under mental constraints. *Interface Focus* (2012) 2:74–81. doi:10.1098/rsfs.2011.0058
21. Smart J. *Philosophy and Scientific Realism.* London: Routledge (2014).
22. Putnam H. Psychological predicates. In: Capitan W, Merrill D, editors. *Art, Mind, and Religion.* Pittsburgh: University of Pittsburgh Press (1967). p. 37–48.
23. Fodor J. Special sciences: or the disunity of science as a working hypothesis. *Synthese* (1974) 28:97–115. doi:10.1007/BF00485230
24. Kim J. *Mind in a Physical World.* Cambridge, MA: MIT Press (1998).
25. Searle JR. Reductionism and the irreducibility of consciousness. In: Flanagan O, Block N, Guzeldere G, editors. *The Nature of Consciousness.* MIT Press (1997).
26. Price CJ, Friston KJ. Degeneracy and cognitive anatomy. *Trends Cogn Sci* (2002) 6:416–21. doi:10.1016/s1364-6613(02)01976-9
27. Varela F. *Principles of Biological Autonomy.* New York, NY, North Holland: Elsevier (1979).
28. Kelso JAS. *Dynamic Patterns: The Self-Organization of Brain and Behavior.* Cambridge: MIT Press (1995).

29. Freeman WF. Consciousness, intentionality, and causality. *J Conscious Stud* (1999) 6:143–72.
30. McGilchrist I. *The Master and His Emissary: The Divided Brain and the Making of the Western World.* New Haven: Yale University Press (2009).
31. Von Bertalanffy L. *General Systems Theory*. New York: George Braziller (1968).
32. Von Bertalanffy L. General theory of systems: application to psychology. In: Kristeva J, Rey-Debove J, Umiker DJ, editors. *Essays in Semiotics*. The Hague: Mouton (1971).
33. Slife BD. *Time and Psychological Explanation*. New York, NY: State University of New York Press (1993).

9

Executive Functions in Children Who Experience Bullying Situations

Wandersonia Medeiros[1], Nelson Torro-Alves[2], Leandro F. Malloy-Diniz[3] and Carla M. Minervino[4]*

[1] Laboratory of Cognitive Sciences and Perception-Laboratory of Mental Health, Education and Psychometric, Universidade Federal da Paraíba, Paraíba, Brazil, [2] Postgraduate Program in Cognitive Neuroscience and Behaviour, Laboratory of Cognitive Sciences and Perception, Universidade Federal da Paraíba, Paraíba, Brazil, [3] ILUMINA Neurosciences, LINC-INCT, Universidade Federal de Minas Gerais, Belo Horizonte, Brazil, [4] Postgraduate Program in Cognitive Neuroscience and Behaviour, Laboratory of Mental Health, Education and Psychometric, Universidade Federal da Paraíba, Paraíba, Brazil

Edited by:
Amitai Abramovitch,
Texas State University, USA

Reviewed by:
Eyal Kalanthroff,
Ben-Gurion University of the Negev, Israel
Joseph Mcguire,
Semel Institute for Neuroscience and Human Behavior, UCLA, USA

***Correspondence:**
Nelson Torro-Alves
nelsontorro@yahoo.com.br

Bullying is characterized by intentional, repetitive, and persistent aggressive behavior that causes damage to the victim. Many studies investigate the social and emotional aspects related to bullying, but few assess the cognitive aspects it involves. Studies with aggressive individuals indicate impairment in executive functioning and decision-making. The objective of this study was to assess hot and cold executive functions in children who experience bullying. A total of 60 children between 10 and 11 years of age were included in the study. They were divided into four groups: aggressors (bullies), victims, bully-victims, and control. Tests for decision-making, inhibitory control, working memory, and cognitive flexibility were used. The bully group made more unfavorable choices on the Iowa Gambling Task, which may indicate difficulties in the decision-making process. The victim group took longer to complete the Trail Making Test (Part B) than aggressors, suggesting lower cognitive flexibility in victims. The hypothesis that aggressors would have lower performance in other executive functions such as inhibitory control, working memory, and cognitive flexibility has not been confirmed. This study indicates that bullies have an impairment of hot executive functions whereas victims have a comparatively lower performance in cold executive functions. In addition to social and cultural variables, neurocognitive and emotional factors seem to influence the behavior of children in bullying situations.

Keywords: bullying, decision-making, executive function, aggressive behavior, cognitive flexibility

INTRODUCTION

The word bullying is used to characterize intentional repetitive and persistent aggressive behavior toward a victim (Olweus, 1994). There is an uneven power relationship between the aggressor and the victim in bullying due to differences in age, physique, or strength. This difference sustains the behavior of the bully even despite clear signs of discomfort and displeasure on the part of those suffering from it (Smith, 2002).

Bullying aggression can occur by direct physical contact (kicking, punching, pushing, theft, or damage to the victim's objects), psychological aggression (verbal abuse involving nicknames, insults, or mean comments about race, sexuality, religion, and physical features) or indirectly (excluding the victim from playing or group conversations) (Bullock, 2002).

In a bullying situation, children can take on different roles. Aggressing children (bullies) have the intention of causing harm or excluding others (Berger, 2007). Children that are victims suffer from the constant aggression and often fail to react or get others to stop. Children considered victims-aggressors are those that bully/offend but also suffer aggression, and they differ from aggressors because they are not as popular and usually replicate the aggression with a more fragile child (Bandeira and Hutz, 2012). Bystanders are those children who are not directly involved in the aggression but those who witness bullying. Bystander often do not know how to behave in the face of aggression and become silent for fear of becoming victims, or for not trusting the actions taken by school professionals (Lopes Neto, 2005; Miranda, 2011).

The prevalence of bullying seems to vary depending on the sociocultural context. For example, Berger (2007) reviewed the prevalence of bullying in different countries and found a range between 3 and 27% of bullies and between 9 and 32% of victims. However, methodological differences and the definition of bullying itself make it difficult to establish epidemiological comparisons. Understanding the psychological processes involved in the onset and maintenance of a bullying relationship involves clarifying the cognitive and personality factors of bullies and victims. Koh and Wong (2015) argue that the psychological traits of the aggressors reflect potential adaptive advantages related to sexual selection. However, there is evidence that cognitive deficits and certain personality traits are most frequently found in children and adolescents who bully (Medeiros et al., 2014).

Children who are bullies and bully-victims show more frequent antisocial behavior and lower levels of empathy compared to victims and children who do not experience bullying (Camodeca and Goossens, 2005; Gery et al., 2009; Viding et al., 2011). They also have lower academic performance, an increased school drop-out rate, and higher involvement with the justice system (Gini, 2006). Coolidge et al. (2004) observe that bullying behavior is associated with deficits in executive functioning, conduct disorders, oppositional-defiant disorder, attention deficit hyperactivity disorders (ADHDs), and increased use of substances such as alcohol and marijuana.

Regarding executive functions, Diamond (2013) believes that these functions involve three main centers: inhibitory control, working memory, and cognitive flexibility. According to the author, the other functions such as reasoning, planning and organization are built from these three functions.

Currently, some authors have distinguished executive functions into cold and hot. Cool executive functions are related to cognitive/rational high-order process and are used to general cognitive control. Hot executive functions, in turn, are cognitive/emotional processes related to affective decision making, motivation, and social cognition. According to Damásio (1996), decision-making processes are related to the interpretation of body states and emotional bias defined as somatic markers. The process of somatic markers interpretation is important both to risk perception and decision considering immediate and future outcomes. Antisocial behavior has been associated to impairment in somatic marker processing (Damásio et al., 1996; Séguin, 2004; Sinclair and Gansler, 2006; Tung and Chhabra, 2011). Despites the knowledge of social rules, antisocial subjects present rule-breaking behaviors due to the lack of interpretation of these emotional-somatic signals.

Verlinden et al. (2014) found that children who are not involved in bullying situations as bullies or victims have better scores on intelligence tests. Bullies, victims, and bully-victims have greater difficulty with inhibitory control according to the reports of their parents in the BRIEF Scale. This result suggests a probable deficit in executive functioning related to involvement in bullying situations. Such results, however, have certain limitations. Verlinden et al. (2014) use indirect measures of executive functioning in questionnaires that assess parents' perceptions of such cognitive processes.

Cognitive-emotional aspects of executive functions are poorly investigated in studies on bullying, however, they are particularly important in regulating behavior in social situations (Smith and Jones, 2012). Affective decision-making seems to be related to the presence of various psychopathological conditions such as ADHD; autism spectrum disorders, substance abuse such as alcohol and/or cigarettes; conduct disorders; schizophrenia, as well as behavioral problems such as high disinhibition, self-harm, and aggressive behavior (Best et al., 2002; Ernst et al., 2003, 2010; Verdejo-García et al., 2006; Suhr and Tsanadis, 2007; DeVito et al., 2008; Fairchild et al., 2009; Herrera, 2011; Mata et al., 2011; Sallum et al., 2013). Bullies often have alterations in behavior, therefore, the possibility that decision-making may also be impaired in these individuals cannot be ruled out.

In view of the likely involvement of executive functioning in different behavioral patterns related to bullying, the objective of this study was to evaluate the different components of these functions in groups of bullies, victims, bully-victims, and a control group.

As a hypothesis, we consider that bullies, victims and bully-victims child groups would achieve lower scores on the evaluation of executive functions than the group that has no direct involvement with bullying. Another hypothesis was that the group of aggressors and victims-aggressors would demonstrate lower performance on inhibitory control and decision-making in comparison to victims and controls.

MATERIALS AND METHODS

Sample

Initially, the Peer Aggression and Victimization Scale (PAVS) was applied to 225 students of the 6th grade of two public schools and a private school. After the exclusion of children who did not fit in the pre-established age group, the scales and the free informed consent form were delivered to parents. Children were recruited according to the results of the PAVS scale. Children were excluded if they were 12 years or older (as they would be at a different phase of development, in this case in adolescence), with complaints of uncorrected visual or hearing difficulties and/or those with compromising cognitive impairment. Thirty-nine children completed the individual steps, however, they were not included in data analysis because their parents did not deliver the Strengths and Difficulties Questionnaire.

The sample comprised 60 children (32 females and 28 males), with age between 10 to 11 years and attending sixth grade in middle school. A total of 34 children attended private schools and 26 attended public schools in João Pessoa.

Instruments

Strengths and Difficulties Questionnaire – SDQ (Goodman, 1997)

The instrument used to characterize the sample was the Strengths and Difficulties Questionnaire- SDQ, developed by Goodman (1997) and validated for the Brazilian context by Fleitlich et al. (2000). It is a screening questionnaire that aims to assess mental health of children and adolescents (4–16 years). It has 25 items, divided into five subscales: emotional symptoms, conduct problems, hyperactivity, relationship problems with peers and prosocial behavior. A total index of difficulty which is the sum of the subscales (except sociability) is also generated. The instrument can be used in three versions (self-reporting, a version for parents and a version for teachers). In the present study, we used the version for parents. Each item has three alternatives, false (zero), more or less true (one point) and true (two points).

Bullying Evaluation: Peer Aggression and Victimization Scale (PAVS; Cunha et al., 2009)

The PAVS is a self-reported, 18-item scale, applicable to students attending the second half of elementary school (in general, children from 10 to 15 years of age), that investigates behaviors of bullying and victimization among peers. The child selects the frequency (never, rarely, sometimes, very often, or always) with which they performed or suffered a certain behavior at school during the previous 6 months. The answers were added separately according to the following classification: direct aggression, relational aggression, indirect physical aggression, and victimization. This study did not investigate "indirect physical aggression." From the sum of the scores in each class, participants were divided into subgroups according to the cutoff points (Cunha et al., 2009). The scale was used to classify participants into groups of bullies, victims, and bully-victims, in addition to a control group, by using the following criteria:

(a) Bully group – This group comprises children with a high frequency of behavior in the direct aggression items (score $\geq$ 9) and low (score $\leq$ 12) or moderate (score $\leq$ 16) behavior in the victimization items. Children with high scores only in the relational aggression items were not included.

(b) Victim group – This group comprises children with a high frequency of victimization behavior (score $\geq$ 16) and a low level of direct physical aggression (score $\leq$ 7) and relational aggression (score $\leq$ 6).

(c) Bully-victim group – This group comprises children with a high frequency of direct aggressive behavior (score $\geq$ 9) and victimization (score $\geq$ 16). Children with a high score in victimization and high scores only in relational aggression were not included.

(d) Control group – This group comprises children with a low frequency of direct aggressive behavior (score $\leq$ 7) and victimization with a low (score $\leq$ 12) or moderate (score < 16) frequency.

Evaluation of Executive Functioning

The protocol for the analysis of cold executive functions used the model proposed by Diamond (2013). In this model, three main cores are part of executive functioning: inhibitory control, working memory, and cognitive flexibility. These three functions give rise to the other functions, such as reasoning, planning, and organization. The following instruments were used.

Digit Span Backward (DSB) Subtest (Wechsler, 2013)

A subtest of the Wechsler Intelligence Scale for Children (WISC-IV), the DSB evaluates working memory. For this task, the professional applying the test reads some numbers aloud, and the child must repeat them in descending order. The tables for 10 and 11 years of age were used to transform the raw scores into weighted scores.

Trail Making Test Part B (TMT-B)

The TMT has two parts: A and B. This study used only part B, which evaluates alternating attention and mental flexibility. The child was instructed to connect the numbers in ascending order and in alphabetical order. The execution time of the activity was considered to determine the score. When there was an error, the evaluator showed it to the participant and requested correction, which increased the execution time.

Victoria Stroop Color-Word Test

The Stroop Test was used to assess attention and inhibitory control. The Victoria version includes three cards, 1 (color), 2 (word), and 3 (color-word). The first card (color) contains colored rectangles with the colors pink, green, blue, and brown, which must be named by the child as quickly as possible. The second card (word) lists the words EACH, TODAY, NEVER, and EVERYTHING, printed in the same colors, and the child is asked to simply read the words as quickly as possible. The third card (color-word) lists the names of the four colors, printed in colors that are incompatible with the written word (e.g., the word "Blue" is printed in pink). The child is asked not to read the names but instead to name the printed colors as quickly as possible. For the assessment, the execution time for each card and the number of mistakes (errors not spontaneously corrected by the child) were taken into account (Kulaif, 2005).

For the assessment of the "hot" executive functions, the test of affective decision-making described below was used.

Iowa Gambling Task (IGT; Bechara et al., 1994)

The Brazilian version of the IGT, adapted by Malloy-Diniz et al. (2008), was used to evaluate hot executive functions as a test of emotional decision-making. In this task, participants aim to achieve the maximum gain from an initial cash loan. Individuals make 100 selections of cards, not knowing in advance how many are allowed, and they must make decisions that lead to a final positive result according to the feedback that they receive. Card decks A and B initially offer an advantage, but in the long term, they become unfavorable. Decks C and D offer an overall advantage because, although they have a lower value of rewards, the punishments are also smaller, ultimately resulting in a higher overall gain.

In this study, to increase the chances that the test evaluated hot executive functions, a reward (candy) was included, according to the following criteria:

- Gains of 25, 50, and 75 (frequent in advantageous decks): receives one piece of candy;
- Losses of 25, 50, and 75 (frequent in advantageous decks): loses one piece of candy;
- Gains ≥ 100 (frequent in disadvantageous decks): receives two pieces of candy;
- Losses ≥ 100 (frequent in disadvantageous decks): loses two pieces of candy; and
- Losses = 1500 (only in disadvantageous decks): loses all candy.

Procedures

After approval by the school and parents by means of agreement documents and free and informed consent forms, the groups were determined by applying the PAVS. For the individual step, tests for the assessment of executive functioning were applied in an isolated room arranged by the school. The professional applying the test was with the child throughout task execution to answer questions and prevent mistakes due to confusion.

The study was approved by the Research Ethics Committee of the University Hospital Lauro Wanderley (Hospital Universitário Lauro Wanderley), UFPB (CAAE process: 17883413. 5.0000.5183). All procedures were performed according to Regulation 466/96 of the National Health Council (Conselho Nacional de Saúde - CNS). Participation was voluntary, and the participants were informed in advance that they could withdraw their consent at any time during the study.

Statistical Analysis

The softwares SPSS 21.0 and Microsoft Office Excel 2007 were used for the tabulation of data and statistical analysis. The Shapiro–Wilk test and Levene's test showed that data did not present normal distribution and equality of variances (homoscedasticity), respectively. For this reason, non-parametric testing was selected. The Kruskal–Wallis test was used for comparisons between groups using a significance level of 0.05. When Kruskal–Wallis test was inferior to 0.05, we performed Mann–Whitney pairwise comparisons. In order to control the probability of Type I error, we corrected the critical value of alfa by dividing the familywise error rate (0.05) by the number of comparisons (6). Therefore, we considered as statistically significant only the probabilities values inferior to 0.0083.

In addition, we determined effect sizes estimates (Fritz et al., 2012; Field, 2013). As proposed by Cohen (1988), effect sizes were calculated using the formula:

$$r = \frac{z}{\sqrt{N}} \quad (1)$$

where r is the effect size estimate, z is the standard score of the distribution, and N is the total of the sample size.

According to Cohen's guidelines used to interpret r, a large effect is superior to 0.5, a medium effect is 0.3 and a small effect is 0.1. Large effect sizes associated to non-significant results may suggest to carry out a research with a greater power, whereas small effect sizes associated to significant results may indicate that the observed effects are not so robust (Fritz et al., 2012).

RESULTS

With regard to socio demographic characteristics, a total of 32 out of the 60 children who participated in the sample were female, and 28 were male, with 34 attending private schools and 26 attending public schools in João Pessoa, Paraíba, Brazil.

The participants were divided into four groups according to their result on the PAVS scale: bullies (n = 15; seven male), victims (n = 15; six male), bully-victims (n = 15; nine male), and control (n = 15; six male). A preliminary statistical analysis showed no differences between genders with regard to the variables investigated in the study ($p > 0.05$). **Table 1** shows the average score of the four groups in the dimensions of the PAVS scale. In **Table 2**, we present data of the four groups of participants and results of the statistical analysis.

Strengths and Difficulties Questionnaire - SDQ

We found no differences between groups with regard to the total score of difficulties ($\chi^2 = 1.088$, $p = 0.780$), emotional problems ($\chi^2 = 6.585$, $p = 0.086$), hyperactivity ($\chi^2 = 1.087$, $p = 0.780$), conduct problems ($\chi^2 = 2.517$, $p = 0.472$) and peer relationship problems ($\chi^2 = 6.920$, $p = 0.740$). In the prosocial behavior subscale, we found differences between groups ($\chi^2 = 11.347$, $p = 0.01$). Mann–Whitney tests showed that victims presented higher scores than bullies ($U = 33.00$, $z = -3.217$, $p = 0.001$, $r = -0.59$), but not in comparison to the control group ($U = 73.5$, $z = -1.703$; $p = 0.089$, $r = -0.31$) and bully-victims ($U = 54.5$, $z = -2.495$; $p = 0.013$, $r = -0.46$). Bullies, bully-victims and controls had similar scores in prosocial behavior compared one another.

Digit Span Backward (DSB) Subtest

There was no significant difference between the groups with regard to DSB ($\chi^2 = 2.587$, $p = 0.46$), indicating that they had similar patterns of performance in working memory.

Trail Making Test Part B (TMT-B)

Statistical analysis showed significant differences between groups in TMT-B ($\chi^2 = 13.839$, $p = 0.003$). Mann–Whitney tests showed that the victim group had a longer execution time in TMT-B compared to bullies ($U = 32.5$, $z = -3.322$; $p = 0.001$, $r = -0.61$), but not differed from bully-victims ($U = 65$, $z = -1.972$, $p = 0.049$, $r = -0.36$), and controls ($U = 62.5$, $z = -2.075$, $p = 0.038$, $r = -0.38$). This result indicates a lower cognitive flexibility in the victim group. The other groups did not differ one another: aggressors compared to bully-victims ($U = 66$, $z = -1.932$, $p = 0.053$, $r = -0.35$); bullies compared to controls ($U = 66$, $z = -1.93$, $p = 0.054$, $r = -0.35$); bully-victims

TABLE 1 | Means and standard deviations of age and scores in the PAVS scale dimensions in the four groups of participants.

Variable	Bully	Victim	Bully-Victim	Control
Age	10.73 (0.45)	10.87 (0.35)	10.80 (0.41)	10,73 (0.45)
Relacional aggression	8.20 (4.29)	5.93 (1.62)	8.53 (3.29)	4.87 (1.12)
Direct aggression	11.73 (2.01)	6.47 (0.91)	12.67 (1.71)	6.40 (1.18)
Victimization	13.33 (2.19)	20.73 (4.90)	23.73 (5.78)	11.07 (2.05)

TABLE 2 | Statistical analysis and scores obtained by the four groups of participants in the Strengths and Difficulties Questionnaire (SDQ), Digit Span Backward Subtest (DSB), Trail Making Test part B (TMT-B), Victoria Stroop Color-Word Test (STROOP), Iowa Gambling Task (IGT).

Instrument	Bully	Victim	Bully-Victim	Control	Kruskal–Wallis
SDQ					
Emotional symptoms	3.53 (2.26)	5.80 (3.07)	3.27 (2.86)	4.00 (2.77)	$p = 0.086$
Conduct problems	3.07 (2.65)	1.87 (1.80)	2.73 (1.43)	2.27 (1.62)	$p = 0.472$
Hyperactivity	4.60 (3.26)	3.53 (2.10)	4.33 (1.91)	3.93 (2.89)	$p = 0.780$
Peer relationship Problems	1.53 (1.72)	2.67 (1.63)	2.47 (2.56)	1.20 (1.01)	$p = 0.074$
Prosocial behavior	7.07 (2.40)	9.27 (0.96)	7.87 (1.59)	8.33 (1.54)	$p = 0.010$*
Total difficulties	12.80 (8.24)	14.07 (7.16)	12.80 (6.71)	11.40 (5.27)	$p = 0.780$
DSB	9.33 (2.52)	9.53 (2.35)	9.93 (1.94)	8.73 (2.12)	$p = 0.460$
TMT-B	40.27 (10.27)	61.40 (17.31)	48.60 (12.43)	48.20 (11.91)	$p = 0.003$*
STROOP					
Color (Time)	16.00 (0.92)	19.13 (0.89)	18.58 (1.21)	17.80 (1.03)	$p = 0.126$
Color (Errors)	0.00 (0.00)	0.07 (0.26)	0.00 (0.00)	0.13 (0.352)	$p = 0.284$
Word (Time)	11.27 (3.41)	12.40 (2.41)	12.26 (2.68)	12.67 (2.58)	$p = 0.205$
Word (Errors)	0.07 (0.26)	0.00 (0.00)	0.13 (0.51)	0.07 (0.26)	$p = 0.792$
Color-word (Time)	27.47 (1.68)	34.20 (3.25)	35.21 (2.76)	30.40 (1.84)	$p = 0.018$*
Color-word (Errors)	0.40 (0.63)	0.27 (0.59)	0.47 (1.12)	0.60 (1.24)	$p = 0.869$
IGT					
Deck A choices	25.15 (0.74)	22.60 (1.29)	20.79 (0.96)	21.07 (1.26)	$p = 0.039$*
Deck B choices	27.33 (1.55)	27.53 (1.29)	30.13 (1.60)	29.47 (1.57)	$p = 0.286$
Deck C choices	25.00 (1.17)	25.00 (0.99)	26.47 (1.04)	24.53 (0.66)	$p = 0.325$
Deck D choices	24.00 (1.82)	24.87 (1.94)	21.73 (1.37)	24.93 (1.57)	$p = 0.566$
General Trend Block 1 (1–20)	−0.93 (0.64)	−1.47 (0.74)	−1.47 (0.90)	−1.07 (0.54)	$p = 0.971$
General trend block 2 (21–40)	−1.20 (0.95)	−0.40 (1.58)	−3.07 (1.53)	−1.47 (0.71)	$p = 0.859$
General trend block 3 (41–60)	−0.27 (0.67)	1.47 (1.75)	−2.00 (1.08)	1.07 (1.40)	$p = 0.697$
General trend block 4 (61–80)	−0.13 (1.50)	−0.93 (1.24)	0.80 (1.59)	−0.67 (1.11)	$p = 0.640$
General trend block 5 (81–100)	0.53 (0.95)	1.07 (0.93)	2.13 (1.38)	1.07 (1.18)	$p = 0.995$
General trend	−2.00 (3.20)	−0.27 (3.95)	−3.60 (3.48)	−1.07 (3.03)	$p = 0.881$

Values correspond to means and standard deviations.

compared to controls ($U = 109.5$, $z = -0.125$, $p = 0.901$, $r = -0.02$; **Figure 1**).

Stroop Color-Word Test

The Kruskal–Wallis test showed significant differences between groups only for the third card (color-word; $\chi^2 = 10{,}039$, $p = 0.018$). Mann–Whitney tests showed that the bully group had a shorter execution time compared to the victim ($U = 35$, $z = -2.736$, $p = 0.006$, $r = -0.50$) and bully-victim groups ($U = 31$, $z = -2.754$, $p = 0.006$, $r = -0.50$), but not differed from control group ($U = 52$, $z = -2.109$, $p = 0.035$, $r = -0.39$; **Figure 2**). In the third card, we found no differences between victims compared to bully-victims ($U = 87$, $z = -0.195$, $p = 0.846$, $r = 0.04$); victims compared to controls ($U = 93$, $z = -0.525$, $p = 0.600$, $r = 0.10$); bully-victims compared to controls ($U = 83$, $z = -0.669$, $p = 0.503$, $r = 0.12$). For the first card (color), we found no statistically significant differences between groups ($\chi^2 = 5.718$; $p = 0.126$), but victims presented longer execution time than other groups. We find no differences between groups with regard to Stroop word (time; $\chi^2 = 4.587$, $p = 0.205$), Stroop color (errors; $\chi^2 = 3.795$, $p = 0.284$), Stroop word (errors; $\chi^2 = 1.037$, $p = 0.792$), and Stroop color-word (errors; $\chi^2 = 0.718$, $p = 0.869$) (**Figure 2**).

Iowa Gambling Task – IGT

The Kruskal–Wallis test showed significant differences between groups only for choices from Deck A ($\chi^2 = 8{,}393$, $p = 0.039$). Mann–Whitney tests showed that the bully group had the highest score considering all choices from Deck A compared to the bully-victim group ($U = 34.5$ $z = -2.755$, $p = 0.006$, $r = 0.50$), but not differed from victims ($U = 61.5$ $z = -1.666$, $p = 0.96$, $r = 0.30$) and the control group ($U = 49$, $z = -2.246$, $p = 0.025$, $r = 0.41$).

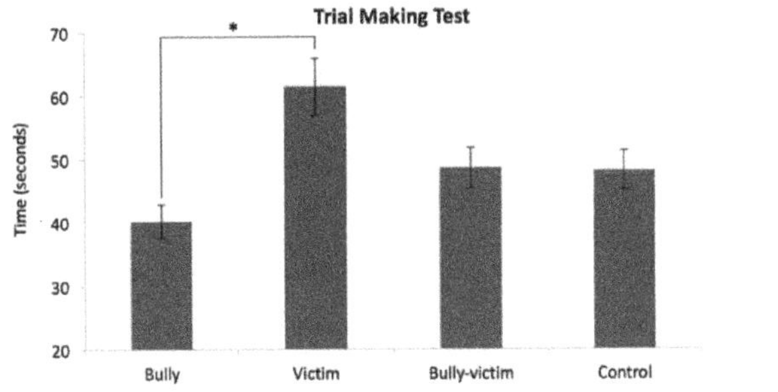

FIGURE 1 | Time, in seconds, on the Trail Making Test Part B (TMT-B). *Significant difference for the victim group compared to the bully group ($p = 0.001$).

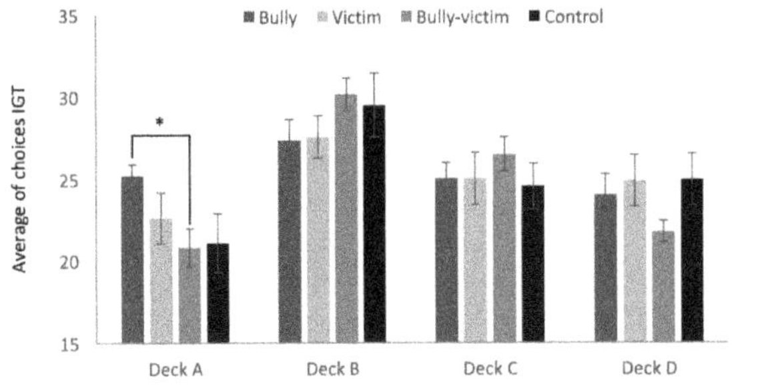

FIGURE 3 | Average of choices from decks A, B, C, and D on the Iowa Gambling Task (IGT). *Significant difference for the bully group compared to the bully-victim group in Deck A ($p = 0.006$).

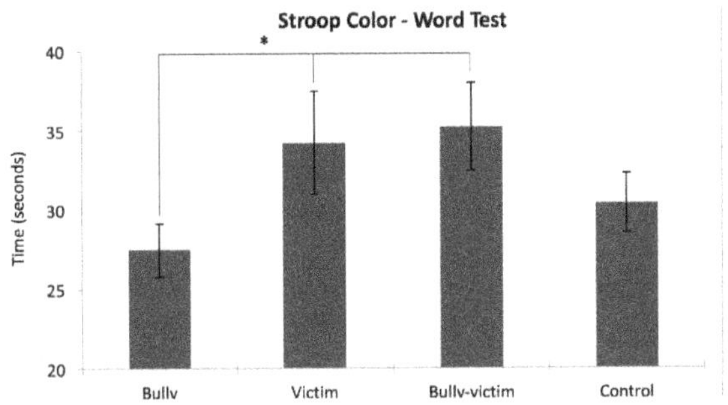

FIGURE 2 | Time, in seconds, on the Stroop Color-Word Test. *Significant difference for the bully group compared to victim ($p = 0.006$) and bully-victim ($p = 0.006$).

Other groups had a similar number of choices of cards in Deck A: victims compared to bully-victims ($U = 82$, $z = -1.006$, $p = 0.314$, $r = 0.18$); victims compared to controls ($U = 94$, $z = -0.771$, $p = 0.440$, $r = 0.14$); bully-victims compared to controls ($U = 99.50$, $z = -0.241$, $p = 0.810$, $r = 0.04$). There was no significant differences between the groups with regard to the general score trends in blocks ($\chi^2 = 0.241$, $p = 0.971$ in Block 1; $\chi^2 = 0.758$, $p = 0.859$ in Block 2; $\chi^2 = 1.435$, $p = 0.697$ in Block 3; $\chi^2 = 1.685$, $p = 0.640$ in Block 4, and $\chi^2 = 0.096$, $p = 0.995$ in Block 5) and the overall general trend ($\chi^2 = 0.668$, $p = 0.881$). There was also no difference between the total number of choices from Decks B ($\chi^2 = 3.780$, $p = 0.286$), C ($\chi^2 = 3.466$, $p = 0.325$), and D ($\chi^2 = 2.031$, $p = 0.566$) (**Figure 3**).

DISCUSSION

In this study, executive functioning (inhibitory control, working memory, and cognitive flexibility) and emotional decision-making were assessed in children who experience bullying. This study is innovative because it investigates multiple components of executive functioning and their relationship to bullying.

We used the Strengths and Difficulties Questionnaire - SDQ (parent version) to characterize chid behavior. In the SDQ, offending children (bullies) did not differ from other groups with regard to the symptoms of hyperactivity and behavior problems, contradicting the results of Coolidge et al. (2004), which found a higher prevalence of challenging behavior, conduct problems and ADHD in offending children compared to the control group. Therefore, it is clear that aggressors of this sample did not differ from controls with respect to behavior problems, probably due to this group presenting many children who also had average levels of victimization. Viding et al. (2011) claim that not all behavior problems are due to the same cause, so it is important to investigate the profile of each group.

The group of victims obtained the highest score of prosocial behavior, related to behaviors of empathy (helping others, being nice, and caring for younger children) than the group of bullies. However, there were no differences between victims compared to controls and bully-victims.

Deficits in executive functioning have been reported in several developmental and behavioral disorders (Lezak, 1982; Hamdan and Pereira, 2009). In this study, there was no significant difference between groups with regard to working memory, assessed by DSB Subtest. With regard to working memory, Best et al. (2002) found no differences between patients with aggressive and impulsive behavior compared to controls. Nevertheless, they observed that the clinical group showed impairment in the decision-making process.

Contrary to expectations, there was no deficit in inhibitory control functions and cognitive flexibility in bullies, as assessed by the Stroop test and TMT-B, respectively. The bully group had a shorter execution time on the TMT-B compared to the victims group and the third Stroop card (color-word) compared to the victims and bully-victims groups and not presented more errors. Brennan (2002) found no association between high levels of juvenile delinquency and poor performance in the executive function assessment tasks. However, our results are different from those reported by other authors who observed inhibitory control difficulties in aggressive individuals (Best et al., 2002; Ellis et al., 2009). Verlinden et al. (2014) found a relationship between low inhibitory control and involvement in bullying, whether in the bully, victim or bully-victim roles. Nevertheless, the authors used an indirect assessment with questionnaires directed to parents, which may explain the difference between the results. Compared to bullies, the victim group had a longer TMT-B execution time, indicating less efficient performance in the context of cognitive flexibility. Although not statistically significant, we found medium effect sizes to the comparisons between victims and bully-victims ($r = 0.36$) and between victims and controls ($r = 0.38$), what indicates a reduction in cognitive flexibility in victims compared to those groups. This result is consistent with those found by Dertelmann (2011), who found lower performance in cognitive flexibility tests and working memory in child victims of abuse (Dertelmann, 2011). Brennan (2002) found that children who had suffered abuse and higher delinquency levels had lower scores on the assessment of executive functioning. This result shows that the presence of victimization is a factor that may be associated with deficits in the development of cognitive impairment. Other studies also show worse performance in tasks that assess executive functioning in individuals who have suffered physical or sexual assaults (Stein et al., 2002; Coolidge et al., 2004).

The association between deficits in executive functioning and vulnerability to aggression can be explained as a consequence of exposure to violence, but it can also be understood as a factor of vulnerability to such acts. The different types of victimization investigated and the lack of longitudinal studies do not allow us to safely determine whether impairment in executive functioning is a result of aggression, whether it is associated with psychiatric disorders developed due to aggression (anxiety disorders, post-traumatic stress disorder), or whether it is part of the cognitive and personality features of these individuals, which may predispose them to suffer aggression (Stein et al., 2002). According to Teicher et al. (2003), exposure to violence or severe stress in childhood, depending on its severity and intensity, can cause neurobiological changes and affect brain development. For example, Johnson (2012) suggests that the presence of deficits in executive functioning since childhood can make individuals less efficient in problem solving and, therefore, less resilient in adverse situations.

In this study, compared with the bully-victim group, children in the bully group choose more cards from one of the disadvantageous decks (Deck A). Decks A and B are considered disadvantageous because they cause losses over the long term of task execution compared to decks C and D. Although deck B is also unfavorable, Deck A has the highest frequency of punishments but is lower in intensity (Singh, 2013). We found no statistically significant differences between bullies and controls in IGT, however, the effect size obtained in the comparison (0.41) indicates that groups might differ each other in studies involving a greater sample, with bullies choosing more disadvantageous cards.

This finding suggests that bullies are more sensitive to the intensity of punishment than they are to the frequency of punishment. The choice for one of the unfavorable decks by bullies indicates a preference for immediate gains (two pieces of candy), ignoring punishment and the future consequences of the choice. Such behavior has been designated "myopia for the future" (Bechara et al., 1994, 2002; Gomes et al., 2011).

With regard to "myopia for the future," the following analogy can be made for a situation experienced at school: a child can choose between advantageous attitudes (not attacking), which generate long-term gains (e.g., being aware of doing the right thing, building lasting and true friendships), and unfavorable behavior (aggression), which brings immediate gains (a sense of power, entertaining peers, being popular) but generate losses in the long run (complaints, punishment by parents, poor school performance, and shallow friendships). In this sense, it is possible to consider that the practice of bullying in the school context may be associated with a decrease in the decision-making process of bullies. Decision-making deficits are clearly found in children and adolescents with behavioral disorders, conduct disorders and in patients who suffered injuries to the orbitofrontal cortex (Best et al., 2002; Ernst et al., 2003; Fairchild et al., 2009).

Bully-victims present similarities and differences with regard to both groups of victims and bullies. In the IGT, bully-victims were similar to controls and victims, but choose more advantage cards as compared to bullies. In SQD, bully-victims presented scores of prosocial behavior more similar to bullies than victims. A possible explanation is that the decreasing of prosocial behavior in bully-victims may be related to the dissemination of the aggression suffered. For Bandeira and Hutz (2010), bully-victims children are more likely to present depressive symptoms, anxiety, and externalizing behaviors, and unlike children in the bullies group, they are not popular but rather rejected by their peers.

The results of this study can be analyzed by considering the dichotomy proposed by Kerr and Zelazo (2004). These authors suggest the existence of hot (more closely related to motivation and emotional control) and cold (more closely related to logical-rational aspects of cognition) executive functions. If, on one hand, victims have experienced greater difficulties in tasks that require cold executive functions, then bullies have impaired "hot" executive functions.

This study includes certain limitations, such as the sample size and the fact that some children in the bully group have shown moderate levels of victimization. Another limitation of the study is the use of a self-reported scale, which can generate interference in the division of the groups, although this problem was minimized by the application of the ICU scale in children and parents. It should also be considered that the methodology used was transversal and causal inferences about the investigated aspects cannot be made. We suggest that future studies be conducted with larger samples, longitudinal studies and different cultures.

In addition to sociocultural variables, this study shows that executive functioning, including decision-making, can also play a relevant role in bullying behavior. This type of study may lead to the development of customized intervention strategies according to the profile of students in each school because not all behavioral issues are due to the same cause and not every victim responds to aggression in the same manner (Viding et al., 2011).

AUTHOR CONTRIBUTIONS

Conceived and designed the experiments: WM, NT-A, and CM. Performed the experiments: WM. Analyzed the data: WM, NT-A, and CM. Contributed with materials and analysis tools: WM, NT-A, CM, and LM-D. Wrote the paper: WM, NT-A, CM, and LM-D.

REFERENCES

Bandeira, C. M., and Hutz, C. S. (2010). As implicações do bullying na autoestima de adolescentes. *Psicol. Esc. Educ.* 14, 131–138. doi: 10.1590/S1413-85572010000100014

Bandeira, C. D. M., and Hutz, C. S. (2012). Bullying: prevalence, implications and gender differences. *Psicol. Esc. Educ.* 16, 35–44. doi: 10.1590/S1413-85572012000100004

Bechara, A., Damásio, A. R., Damásio, H., and Anderson, S. W. (1994). Insensitivity to future consequences following damage to human prefrontal cortex. *Cognition* 50, 7–15. doi: 10.1016/0010-0277(94)90018-3

Bechara, A., Dolan, S., and Hindes, A. (2002). Decision-making and addiction (part II): myopia for the future or hypersensitivity to reward? *Neuropsychologia* 40, 1690–1705. doi: 10.1016/S0028-3932(02)00016-7

Berger, K. S. (2007). Update on bullying at school: science forgotten? *Dev. Rev.* 27, 90–126. doi: 10.1016/j.dr.2006.08.002

Best, M., Williams, J. M., and Coccaro, E. F. (2002). Evidence for a dysfunctional prefrontal circuit in patients with an impulsive aggressive disorder. *Proc. Natl. Acad. Sci. U.S.A.* 99, 8448–8453. doi: 10.1073/pnas.112604099

Brennan, S. G. C. (2002). *The Relationship between Maltreatment in Childhood and Delinquency: An Examination of IQ and Executive Functions.* Palo Alto, CA: Pacific Graduate School of Psychology.

Bullock, J. (2002). Bullying Among Children. *Child. Educ.* 78, 130–133. doi: 10.1080/00094056.2002.10522721

Camodeca, M., and Goossens, F. A. (2005). Aggression, social cognitions, anger and sadness in bullies and victims. *J. Child Psychol. Psychiatry* 46, 186–197. doi: 10.1111/j.1469-7610.2004.00347.x

Cohen, J. (1988). *Statistical Power Analysis for the Behavioral Sciences,* 2nd Edn. Hillsdale, NJ: Lawrence Earlbaum Associates.

Coolidge, F. L., DenBoer, J. W., and Segal, D. L. (2004). Personality and neuropsychological correlates of bullying behavior. *Pers. Individ. Dif.* 36, 1559–1569. doi: 10.1016/j.paid.2003.06.005

Cunha, J. M., Weber, L. N. D., and Steiner Neto, P. (2009). "Escala de vitimização e agressão entre pares (EVAP)," in *Pesquisando em Família - Instrumentos Para Coleta e Análise de Dados,* eds L. Weber and M. A. Dessen (Curitiba: Juá Editora), 108–120.

Damásio, A. (1996). *O erro de Descartes: Emoção, Razão e o Cérebro Humano.* São Paulo: Companhia das Letras.

Damásio, A. R., Everitt, B. J., and Bishop, D. (1996). The somatic marker hypothesis and the possible functions of the prefrontal cortex. *Philos. Trans. R. Soc. Lond. B Biol. Sci.* 351, 1413–1420. doi: 10.1098/rstb.1996.0125

Dertelmann, C. D. F. V. (2011). *Avaliação Neuropsicológica em Crianças Vítimas de Maus-Tratos,* Dissertação de mestrado, Pontifícia Universidade Católica do Rio Grande do Sul, Porto Alegre.

DeVito, E. E., Blackwell, A. D., Kent, L., Ersche, K. D., Clark, L., Salmond, C. H., et al. (2008). The effects of methylphenidate on decision making in attention-deficit/hyperactivity disorder. *Biol. Psychiatry* 64, 636–639. doi: 10.1016/j.biopsych.2008.04.017

Diamond, A. (2013). Executive functions. *Annu. Rev. Psychol.* 64, 135–168. doi: 10.1146/annurev-psych-113011-143750

Ellis, M. L., Weiss, B., and Lochman, J. E. (2009). Executive functions in children: associations with aggressive behavior and appraisal processing. *J. Abnorm. Child Psychol.* 37, 945–956. doi: 10.1007/s10802-009-9321-5

Ernst, M., Grant, S. J., London, E. D., Contoreggi, C. S., Kimes, A. S., and Spurgeon, L. (2003). Decision making in adolescents with behavior disorders and adults with substance abuse. *Am. J. Psychiatry* 160, 33–40. doi: 10.1176/appi.ajp.160.1.33

Ernst, M., Luckenbaugh, D. A., Moolchan, E. T., Temple, V. A., Jenness, J., Korelitz, K. E., et al. (2010). Decision-making and facial emotion recognition as predictors of substance-use initiation among adolescents. *Addict. Behav.* 35, 286–289. doi: 10.1016/j.addbeh.2009.10.014

Fairchild, G., van Goozen, S. H. M., Stollery, S. J., Aitken, M. R. F., Savage, J., Moore, S. C., et al. (2009). Decision making and executive function in male adolescents with early-onset or adolescence-onset conduct disorder and control subjects. *Biol. Psychiatry* 66, 162–168. doi: 10.1016/j.biopsych.2009.02.024

Field, A. (2013). *Discovering Statistics Using IBM SPSS Statistics.* Thousand Oaks, CA: Sage Publications.

Fleitlich, B., Cortázar, P. G., and Goodman, R. (2000). Questionário de capacidades e dificuldades (SDQ). *Infanto Rev. Neuropsiquiatria Infânc. Adolescênc.* 8, 44–50.

Fritz, C. O., Morris, P. E., and Richler, J. J. (2012). Effect size estimates: current use, calculations, and interpretation. *J. Exp. Psychol. Gen.* 141, 2–18. doi: 10.1037/a0024338

Gery, I., Miljkovitch, R., Berthoz, S., and Soussignan, R. (2009). Empathy and recognition of facial expressions of emotion in sex offenders, non-sex offenders and normal controls. *Psychiatry Res.* 165, 252–262. doi: 10.1016/j.psychres.2007.11.006

Gini, G. (2006). Social cognition and moral cognition in bullying: what's wrong? *Aggress. Behav.* 32, 528–539. doi: 10.1002/ab.20153

Gomes, F., Mata, F. S. N., Lage, G. M., Paiva de Moraes, P. H., Moraes, P., Fuentes, D., et al. (2011). Avaliação neuropsicológica do processo de tomada de decisões em crianças e adolescentes: uma revisão integrativa da literatura. *Rev. Psiquiatr. Clín.* 38, 106–115.

Goodman, R. (1997). The strengths and difficulties questionnaire: a research note. *J. Child Psychol. Psychiatry* 38, 581–586. doi: 10.1111/j.1469-7610.1997.tb01545.x

Hamdan, A. C., and Pereira, A. P. D. A. (2009).Neuropsychological assessment of executive functions: Methodological questions. *Psicol. Reflexão E Crít.* 22, 386–393. doi: 10.1590/S0102-79722009000300009

Herrera, G. M. (2011). Bulimia nervosa: emotions and making decisions. *Rev. Psiquiatr. Salud Ment.* 4, 88–95. doi: 10.1016/j.rpsm.2011.03.002

Johnson, M. H. (2012). Executive function and developmental disorders: the flip side of the coin. *Trends cogn. sci.* 16, 454–457. doi: 10.1016/j.tics.2012.07.001

Kerr, A., and Zelazo, P. D. (2004). Development of "hot" executive function: the children's gambling task. *Brain Cogn.* 55, 148–157. doi: 10.1016/S0278-2626(03)00275-6

Koh, J. B., and Wong, J. S. (2015). Survival of the fittest and the sexiest: evolutionary origins of adolescent bullying. *J. Interpers. Violence* doi: 10.1177/0886260515593546 [Epub ahead of print].

Kulaif, T. (2005). *O Teste de Cores e Palavras de Stroop Modificado Para Analfabetos,* Dissertação de mestrado, Universidade de São Paulo, São Paulo.

Lezak, M. D. (1982). The problem of assessing executive functions. *Int. J. Psychol.* 17, 281–297. doi: 10.1080/00207598208247445

Lopes Neto, A. A. (2005). Bullying: comportamento agressivo entre estudantes. *J. Pediatr.* 81, 164–172. doi: 10.1590/S0021-75572005000700006

Malloy-Diniz, L. F., Leite, W. B., Moraes, P. H. P. de Correa, H., Bechara, A., and Fuentes, D. (2008). Brazilian portuguese version of the iowa gambling task: transcultural adaptation and discriminant validity. *Rev. Bras. Psiquiatr.* 30, 144–148. doi: 10.1590/S1516-44462008005000009

Mata, F. G. D., Neves, F. S., Lage, G. M., Moraes, P. H. P. D., Mattos, P., Fuentes, D., et al. (2011). Neuropsychological assessment of the decision making process in children and adolescents: an integrative review of the literature. *Arch. Clin. Psychiatry* 38, 106–115. doi: 10.1590/S0101-60832011000300005

Medeiros, W. M. B., Moita Minervino, C. A. S., Duarte, J. S., Cavalcanti, J. D. T., and Alves, N. T. (2014). Competência emocional e bullying: uma visão da neurociência. *Pediatr. Mod.* 50, 100–110.

Miranda, R. D. S. (2011). *Bullying a Partir de Representações Sociais De Estudantes,* Dissertação de Mestrado, Universidade Federal da Paraíba, João Pessoa.

Olweus, D. (1994). *Bullying at School.* NewYork, NY: Springer.

Sallum, I., Mata, F., Miranda, D. M., and Malloy-Diniz, L. F. (2013). Staying and shifting patterns across IGT trials distinguish children with externalizing disorders from controls. *Front. Psychol.* 4:899. doi: 10.3389/fpsyg.2013.00899

Séguin, J. R. (2004). Neurocognitive elements of antisocial behavior: relevance of an órbito-frontal cortex account. *Brain Cogn.* 55, 185–197. doi: 10.1016/S0278-2626(03)00273-2

Sinclair, S., and Gansler, D. (2006). Integrating the somatic marker, and social cognition theories to explain different manifestations of antisocial personality. *New School Psychol. Bull.* 4, 25–47.

Singh, V. (2013). A potential role of reward and punishment in the facilitation of the emotion-cognition dichotomy in the iowa gambling task. *Front. Psychol.* 4:944. doi: 10.3389/fpsyg.2013.00944

Smith, P. K. (2002). "Intimidação por colegas e maneiras de evitá-la," in *Violência nas Escolas e Políticas Públicas*, eds E. Debarbieux and C. Blaya (Brasilia: Unesco), 187–205.

Smith, P. K., and Jones, A. P. (2012). The importance of developmental science for studies in bullying and victimization. *Int. J. Dev. Sci.* 6, 71–74. doi: 10.3233/DEV-2012-11093

Stein, M. B., Kennedy, C. M., and Twamley, E. W. (2002). Neuropsychological function in female victims of intimate partner violence with and without posttraumatic stress disorder. *Biol. Psychiatry* 52, 1079–1088. doi: 10.1016/S0006-3223(02)01414-2

Suhr, J. A., and Tsanadis, J. (2007). Affect and personality correlates of the iowa gambling task. *Pers. Individ. Dif.* 43, 27–36. doi: 10.1016/j.paid.2006.11.004

Teicher, M. H., Andersen, S. L., Polcari, A., Anderson, C. M., Navalta, C. P., and Kim, D. M. (2003). The neurobiological consequences of early stress and childhood maltreatment. *Neurosci. Biobehav. Rev.* 27, 33–44. doi: 10.1016/S0149-7634(03)00007-1

Tung, S., and Chhabra, N. (2011). A comparative study on the neuropsychological status of delinquent and non-delinquent boys. *Int. J. Cul. Ment. Health* 4, 121–127. doi: 10.1080/17542863.2010.530772

Verdejo-García, A., Pérez-García, M., and Bechara, A. (2006). Emotion, decision-making and substance dependence: a somatic-marker model of addiction. *Curr. Neuropharmacol.* 4, 17–31. doi: 10.2174/157015906775203057

Verlinden, M., Veenstra, R., Ghassabian, A., Jansen, P. W., Hofman, A., Jaddoe, V. W. V., et al. (2014). Executive function in gand non-verbal intelligence as predictors of bullying in early elementary school. *J. Abnorm. Child Psychol.* 42, 953–966. doi: 10.1007/s10802-013-9832-y

Viding, E., McCrory, E. J., Blakemore, S.-J., and Frederickson, N. (2011). Behavioural problems and bullying at school: can cognitive neuroscience shed new light on an old problem? *Trends Cogn. Sci* 15 289–291. doi: 10.1016/j.tics.2011.05.001

Wechsler, D. (2013). *Escala de Inteligência Wechsler para Crianças- WISC-IV: Manual de instruções para aplicação e avaliação (1a edição)*. São Paulo: Casa do Psicólogo.

10

Explanatory Pluralism and the (Dis)Unity of Science: The Argument from Incompatible Counterfactual Consequences

*Victor Gijsbers**

Institute for Philosophy, Universiteit Leiden, Leiden, Netherlands

Edited by:
Leon De Bruin,
VU University Amsterdam,
Netherlands

Reviewed by:
Markus Ilkka Eronen,
KU Leuven, Belgium
Jeroen Van Bouwel,
Ghent University, Belgium

****Correspondence:***
Victor Gijsbers
V.Gijsbers@hum.leidenuniv.nl

What is the relationship between different sciences or research approaches that deal with the same phenomena, for instance, with the phenomena of the human mind? Answers to this question range from a monist perspective according to which one of these approaches is privileged over the others, through an integrationist perspective according to which they must strive to form a unity greater than the sum of its parts, to an isolationist perspective according to which each of them has its own autonomous sphere of validity. In order to assess these perspectives in this article, I discuss the debates about the unity of science and about explanatory pluralism. The most pressing issue turns out to be the choice between the integrative and the isolationist perspective: the question is whether the integrative tendencies in science should be fully indulged in or whether they should be held in check by acknowledging that a certain amount of isolation is necessary. I argue that the issue can be further distilled into the question of whether two true explanations of the same fact can ever fail to be combinable into one single explanation. I show that this can indeed be the case, namely, when the explanations have incompatible counterfactual consequences, something that is often the case when we try to combine explanations from different sciences or research approaches. These approaches thus embody perspectives on the world that are to a certain extent autonomous. This leads to the conclusion that although interdisciplinarity may have many advantages, we should not take the project of integration too far. At the end of the day, the different research approaches with their different perspectives and insights must remain precisely that: different and somewhat disunified.

Keywords: explanatory pluralism, unity of science, disunity of science, explanation, counterfactual incompatibility, counterfactuals

INTRODUCTION

What is the relationship between the different sciences or, to use a more fine-grained term, research approaches that deal with the human mind? Faced with a variety of explanations for a psychiatric illness – for example, genetic, neurological, cognitive, psychoanalytic, and sociological explanations – a scientist could take one of three broad views. First, the view that one explanation will trump all the others, making it the only one that is needed. Second, the view that these explanations can be combined into one unified explanation that is superior to each of the individual ones. Third, the view that these explanations all add to our understanding, but cannot be combined into a single integrated account. In other words, a scientist could take a *monist*, an *integrationist*, or an *isolationist* view. Of course, combinations are also possible: one might believe that genetic and neurological explanations can be integrated, that sociological explanations are useful but will remain isolated, that explanations from cognitive psychology will be trumped by neurological ones, and that psychoanalytic explanations are simply wrong; or any other combination of options.

The distinction between these views has important practical consequences both for research and for therapy. If a monist perspective were correct, scientists and practitioners alike should learn to focus on the specific approach that provides the best explanations (which monists of today are likely to identify with neuroscience and low-level biological approaches to the human brain). But if an integrationist perspective were correct, researchers should focus on doing interdisciplinary research, and practitioners should make sure that they learn to see the interconnections between different clinical approaches and find ways to combine them. Then again, if an isolationist perspective were correct, the most fruitful approach would be one of disciplinary specialization and parallel but isolated lines of treatment.

The general heading under which these issues used to be discussed was that of the *unity of science*, but as I will make clear in Section "From Unity of Science to Explanatory Pluralism," philosophers now generally talk about the issue of *explanatory pluralism*. Those who defend explanatory pluralism – which includes almost everyone engaged in the current discussion – generally reject the monist and isolationist positions in favor of some kind of integrationism, some version of the idea that the different sciences have to work together in order to achieve results that they could not achieve separately. The arguments for this claim come in two flavors: first, arguments to the effect that interdisciplinary research is methodologically superior to monodisciplinary research, and, second, case studies that prove that scientists are actually pursuing such research and achieving their aims through it.

These methodological and empirical approaches are of course very valuable. But in the current paper, I would like to ask a more fundamental question about scientific explanation, namely, whether there is anything in the structure of explanations itself that can form a barrier to their complete integration. If two different research approaches come up with explanations of the same phenomenon, and if these are both true and not logically contradictory, is it then always possible to put them together into a single integrated perspective on the phenomenon? Or is it sometimes the case that we have no choice but to be isolationists, because the explanations themselves just do not fit together? Can true explanations be incompatible? These questions are pertinent. There may be, in our current scientific practice, a presumption in favor of interdisciplinarity and the integration of explanations; but it is far from clear that complete integration is the correct ideal to pursue. Perhaps there is a sense in which, say, a neurological and a sociological explanation of a patient's symptoms are just "too different" to be forged into a single, more complete explanation.

My task in Section "Combining Explanations" will be to analyze the conditions under which two explanations of the same phenomenon can fail to be combinable into a single explanation; in other words, I want to find out what it would mean for two explanations to be "too different." To this end, I will develop the notion of *counterfactual incompatibility*: the idea that two statements, even though they are logically consistent, can nevertheless imply different things about what would have happened under hypothetical circumstances. I then argue that explanations that are counterfactually incompatible cannot be combined into a single explanation – and far from that being a merely academic possibility, this does in fact regularly happen when we take explanations from different research approaches.

We thus find, from studying the structure of explanations themselves, that there is something in the sciences that resist integration; that, however, much we love interdisciplinarity, there is an extent to which we must remain isolationists; that different research approaches yield perspectives on the world which cannot always be fully integrated. Interdisciplinarity and the search for connections, while commendable, should be held in check by a healthy appreciation of the autonomy of each of the individual approaches scientists are using.

FROM UNITY OF SCIENCE TO EXPLANATORY PLURALISM

The 1930s saw a rising interest in the idea of the unity of science, which is perhaps nowhere more visible than in the activities of one of the fathers of logical empiricism, Otto Neurath. Neurath founded the Unity of Science Institute in 1936; organized a series of conferences between 1935 and 1941 called the International Congresses for the Unity of Science; and started the International Encyclopedia of Unified Science [see Cat (1) for historical details]. Many of the most important philosophers of the era were implicated in one or more of these enterprises, among them Philipp Frank, Charles Morris, Rudolf Carnap, Bertrand Russell, Ernest Nagel, and John Dewey.

Neurath's own overarching concern with the unity of science movement was to create an environment within which the different sciences could interact and learn from each other. As Pombo et al. (2) put it:

> Neurath's own encyclopedic conception of the unity of science is built on the notion of cooperative action in the scientific community and the accumulation of available results. [...] at the heart of the project is the goal of providing a universal medium for communicating across disciplines and languages (p. 4)

But although Neurath's own view was characterized by symmetric and non-reductionist ideas about communication, cooperation, interdisciplinarity, and interaction between different disciplines (idem, p. 6), the idea of the unity of science was soon interpreted in a much more reductive way. Thus, Oppenheim & Putnam (3) suggests that the unity of science would be achieved when all the terms and all the laws of all the sciences have been reduced to the terms and laws of a single scientific discipline. For Oppenheim and Putnam, the unity of science in this sense is an "over-arching metascientific hypothesis" (p. 6) which, even if it cannot be conclusively shown to be true, is nevertheless credible (p. 8).

It is against this background that we have to understand the position taken up in Fodor's classic anti-reductionist paper "Special Sciences, or: the Disunity of Science as a Working Hypothesis" (4), namely, the position that it is in all probability useless to search for lawful coextension of predicates from sciences at different levels. If unity of science is understood in the reductionist way that Oppenheim and Putnam understand it, then one is indeed tempted to emphasize, with Fodor, the *disunity* of science rather than its unity. Few scientists are interested in strong reductionist projects, and thus it might seem that they have no reason to seek for a unity of science.

In the philosophy of science, this attitude has been forcefully defended by Dupré (5), Cartwright (6), and Teller (7). They use metaphysical, epistemological, and methodological arguments to argue for a "disunified" and "dappled" view of science in which no overarching, all-encompassing laws can be found, and no single discipline will emerge as foundational. Dupré, in fact, insists that science is not even unified by any common sociological, methodological, or processual element.

We have no quarrel with this general view, but something seems to be missing from it. We are still, and perhaps more than ever, interested in communication, cooperation, interdisciplinarity, and interaction between the sciences; and we share with Oppenheim and Putnam, if not their views about reduction, at least their general aim of "counterbalancing specialization by promoting the integration of scientific knowledge." Insisting, as Dupré, Cartwright, and Teller do, that science cannot be unified, helps combat reductionist ideals, but does little to shed light on why integration is still seen as a worthy goal.

How can we understand the unifying tendency in science without returning to reductionism? One option is to defend non-reductive unity at a metaphysical level: examples of this are non-reductive physicalism and the idea of the "primacy of physics" defended by Ladyman and Ross (8). Such metaphysical discussions will be avoided in the current paper, in order to focus on the methodology and the products of science. Among methodologically inclined philosopher of science, there seems to be an emerging tendency to revive a Neurathian use of the term "unity of science," as some of the authors in Symons et al. (9) do. But more influential, especially among scientists themselves, has been the adoption of a new term of art for what is at bottom the same idea of unifying different research approaches: explanatory pluralism. It is this term and the debate surrounding it that we will focus on.

The term "explanatory pluralism" is not without problems, one of which is that different authors use it in sometimes quite different ways. But we can glean the core idea from some representative citations, all of them from papers which set out to defend a form of explanatory pluralism within the psychological sciences:

> Explanatory pluralism holds that simultaneously pursuing research at multiple analytical levels in science tends to aid progress at each of those levels [(10), p. 738]
>
> Explanatory pluralism hypothesizes multiple mutually informative perspectives with which to approach natural phenomena [(11), p. 436]
>
> On this view, different sciences have a degree of autonomy (they are not to be eliminated), but also interact in an effort to understand physical reality at different scales (they are not fully autonomous silos). [...] different sciences and theoretical approaches should maintain their emphasis on different proprietary scales but should also work to unify their work as much as possible, insofar as they often describe the same phenomena in different but compatible ways [(12), p. 3]

As we can see, there are two elements to the core idea: first, that science can be broken up into distinct enterprises, and, second, that it is scientifically fruitful to have interaction between these enterprises. The authors have different ideas about how to carve up science: in terms of "levels," or "perspectives," or "scales," or simply "sciences"; but in each case, we are presumably to identify them with well-known disciplines and subdisciplines, such as high-energy physics, cell biology, neuroscience, and cognitive psychology. We will ignore the question of how exactly to carve up science and assume that speaking of research approaches is clear enough.

More relevant to our current purposes is the second element of explanatory pluralism, namely, the idea that the sciences have to interact in order to achieve their full potential. As we can see, this claim is formulated in different ways by the different authors. McCauley and Bechtel frame it as a prediction about the rate of scientific progress, although one that is not, perhaps, especially clear, since it is not evident which contrast they are drawing. Kendler formulates explanatory pluralism as a methodological norm and contrasts it with reductionism. Abney et al. take explanatory pluralism to be an alternative not only to reductionism but also to an isolationist view of science that they attribute – perhaps inaccurately, since his article opposes reduction but not interaction in general – to Fodor (4). Given our interest in finding a middle ground between the unity and the disunity of science, this is an especially interesting version of the explanatory pluralism. But the formulation of Abney et al. remains vague: it exhorts us to unify the sciences "as much as possible," but it does not indicate how far that possibility extends.

Some of the most thoughtful analyses of explanatory pluralism are those of Marchionni (13), Mitchell (14), Campaner (15), and Van Bouwel (16). [Closely related, though couched in a different terminology and less focused on the technical details of explanation, is Brigandt (17) account of *explanatory integration* as an intermediate between reductionism and pluralism.] All these authors take the view that explanatory pluralism is primarily about what *explanations* the best science will end up with, and more precisely about the question whether explanations from different research approaches can all be integrated into a coherent whole.

Marchionni (13) makes a distinction between two ways in which explanations of the same phenomenon on a macro and micro level can complement each other: *weak complementarity*, which holds when the two explanations are both legitimate and autonomous, but cannot be combined; and *strong complementarity*, which holds when the two explanations can be integrated into a whole that provides a better explanation than the two explanations did separately. If weak complementarity holds, we have two research approaches that are essentially independent; this is a disunified or isolationist view of science. When strong complementarity holds, our best understanding of the world is generated when two or more research approaches interact: this is a unified or integrationist view. We thus arrive at a gliding scale ranging from the ultimate unity that is reduction/monism, to the ultimate disunity that is weak complementarity/isolationism, with strong complementarity/integrationism in between.

However, the idea of strong complementarity involves a certain instability. On the one hand, it poses different, distinct research approaches; and on the other hand, it tells us that the results of these approaches can be put together to form a single picture of the world, a picture that is more enlightening than any of the separate pictures. But if the sciences are to be integrated so tightly and do not have an autonomous domain of knowledge wherein they reign supreme, in what sense can they still be said to be distinct? Do they not reveal themselves as merely different parts of the same one-and-only scientific discipline?

This seems to be the background against which Campaner (15), in an attempt to explain how different kinds of psychiatric explanation can be combined, asks the following pertinent questions about explanatory pluralism:

> Is there any underlying idea that some sort of complete explanatory picture can be – sooner or later – elaborated, or is some more radical form of pluralism advanced here? Is pluralism suggested here as only the acknowledgement of the existence and toleration of a diversity of current explanatory theories, or also as the idea that distinctive views will persist as such in the long run? In other terms, is actual plurality treated in this context as provisional and resolvable, or is the idea that renouncing pluralism would lead to some loss of explanatory information? (pp. 98–99)

Unlike Marchionni, who comes out in favor of strong complementarity, Campaner believes that the different types of explanation in psychiatry will turn out to be impossible to integrate into a single type of explanation. She points at the very different aims and interests of different actors in the field of psychiatry, and she argues that there is little reason to suppose that the explanations constructed to advance those different interests will coincide, even in the long run. According to her, we must be "open to the possibility that, at least in principle, explanatory pluralism can be a permanent state" (idem, p. 101), where explanatory pluralism is here understood – justifiably, but somewhat confusingly when compared to Abney et al. – as the isolationist rather than the integrationist position.

Van Bouwel (16), in a commentary on Campaner and using and expanding the earlier classification of Mitchell (14), adds another level of sophistication to the analysis. Next to explanatory reductionism, Van Bouwel distinguishes no fewer than five different kinds of explanatory pluralism, ranging from the more monistic to the more pluralistic:

1. *Explanatory reductionism*: there is a single privileged research approaches, and ultimately the best understanding of the world will be achieved when all the explanations from other approaches are reduced to this privileged approach.
2. *Temporary pluralism*: it is methodologically advisable to promote a temporary plurality of competing theories, as a means of achieving, in the end, one single unified theory that gives the best explanations.
3. *Integrative pluralism*: satisfactory explanations can only be generated by integrating the findings of different research approaches. (This is equivalent to always embracing Marchionni's idea of strong complementarity.)
4. *Interactive pluralism*: research approaches often generate satisfactory explanations by themselves, but it is also often – though not invariably – the case that the integration of explanations from different sciences leads to a better explanation. (This position, which is Van Bouwel's preferred position, posits a mixture of Marchionni's two kinds of complementarity.)
5. *Isolationist pluralism*: different research approaches generate very different kinds of explanation, which are all valid but cannot be integrated. (This is equivalent to always embracing Marchionni's idea of weak complementarity.)
6. *Anything goes pluralism*: all theories and perspectives are equally valid, and the greatest understanding of the world is achieved by an unlimited proliferation of theories and perspectives.

Van Bouwel is undoubtedly right when he suggests that it would be tough to defend either the idea that isolation is always correct or the idea that integration is always correct. Interactive pluralism, which decides on a case-to-case basis whether integration will succeed or whether isolation is needed, seems to be the most rational position. But in its relaxed wait-and-see attitude, it misses out on something that is more adequately captured by the admonitions of McCauley, Bechtel, Kendler, and Abney et al. all of whom push toward integration. There is a methodological presumption in science in favor of integration: where we *can* integrate, one feels, we *should* integrate; after all, pushing toward integration has led to many great advances.[1] The scientist who insists on the splendid isolation of her discipline will come under immediate suspicion for being, perhaps, too conservative. "Interdisciplinarity" remains a word with which one can woo funding agencies. In other words, we love the unity of science, we are striving toward the unity of science, and if we fail to achieve

[1] See also Andler (18), pp. 140–141, for an appraisal of why we cannot ignore the unifying tendencies in science. Of course, there are critics of integration and interdisciplinarity too, but I venture – although I have no hard data to back this up – that most of these critics have doubts about the *possibility* of integration, rather than about the *desirability* of integration where this is possible.

it – that is, more specifically, if we fail to achieve an integrative pluralism where all the sciences work together to create one single coherent explanation of every phenomenon – than there must be some particular obstacle in the way of that integration. It is that obstacle that I wish to consider. Is the scientist who believes that her explanations stand alone and cannot fruitfully be combined with those of other sciences automatically an unintelligent conservative, or are there circumstances under which it is rational to embrace an isolationist pluralism? What, we may ask more specifically, are the circumstances under which two explanations can fail to be combinable into a single, more complete explanation?

Answering that question will be the burden of the Section "Combining Explanations" of this paper. But before I embark on that project, it will be useful to mention Van Bouwel's own approach to this question and distinguish my project from his. According to Van Bouwel et al. (19):

> [e]xplanatory pluralism consists in the claims that (i) the best form (and level) of explanation depends on the kind of question one is willing to answer by the explanation and (ii) that in order to answer all explanation-seeking questions in the best way possible we will need more than one form (and level) of explanation (p. 36)

The approach championed by these authors, which also influences Gervais' (20) account of inter-level explanations, starts not from a phenomenon, to then ask whether different research approaches should cooperate in giving a single explanation of that phenomenon, but starts from the idea that different epistemic interests lead to different explanatory questions that are best answered by explanations involving different forms and levels. This more pragmatic approach to explanation leads to a natural answer to the questions I posed above: yes, one can say, it is rational to believe that isolation is sometimes the best strategy, because under some circumstances narrow isolated explanations are more conducive to our specific epistemic goals than grand integrative stories. [In their 2011 article, Van Bouwel et al. (19) are actually concerned with showing that reductive explanations have a place in science next to high-level explanations, but I take it that they would also agree with the approach to isolation I just outlined.] Actual examples of science can then be used to prove that scientists indeed choose between integration and isolation based on pragmatic and contextual factors.

I have no quarrel with such an approach. Suppose, for a moment, that there is indeed a single best, completely integrated explanation of any phenomenon. Then, it is undoubtedly true – and I would expect even hard reductionists to agree – that there are strong pragmatic reasons against using this explanation to answer any and all questions about that phenomenon. A therapist interested in curing her patient's depression might not need to hear about the details of the patient's neurochemistry in order to prescribe the right cure, while the patient's company doctor might need to know nothing at all about the causes of the depression in order to decide whether or not to grant the patient extended sick leave. In practical contexts, the "best" explanation is often simple and idealized. And it would also be true, as the pragmatist might stress, that in practice we tend to lose important insights and information if we do not keep our practical goals in mind from the start, so that there is a more fundamental, if still practical, reason for pursuing isolated rather than integrated explanations.

So, even if it were true that there is a single best, completely integrated explanation of any phenomenon – where "best" is understood not in a pragmatic and contextual way, but in terms of an ideal state of understanding – there are still legitimate practical concerns about integration. But I want to know whether that supposition, which seems to underlie much of the theoretical defense of integration, is true. If it is, then the sciences are fundamentally one, at least as far as explanation is concerned; and we will reach the most perfect understanding of the world when we relentlessly pursue integration. If not, then the sciences are fundamentally a plurality; and we will lose some understanding if we push our quest for integration too far.

COMBINING EXPLANATIONS

Is there a single best, completely integrated explanation of any phenomenon? There are instances where one might doubt this for reasons having to do with what the explanations are *about*. For instance, one might doubt whether explanations involving the mind and explanations involving the body could ever be combined; or explanations involving facts and explanations involving values. These doubts are related to some of the thorniest metaphysical issues in all of philosophy. We will sidestep these issues – which we could not possibly do justice to here – and focus instead, not on what explanations are *about*, but on the general *form* or structure of explanations. What I want to know is what general feature of two explanations of the same phenomenon could stand in the way of their being combined into a single bigger explanation.

In order to simplify the discussion, I will make two assumptions. First, I will assume that the things that get explained by explanations – with a technical term, the *explananda* – are facts, and that these facts can be put into a contrastive form, that is, an "A rather than B" form. An explanation thus may explain why Tom is depressed rather than not being depressed; or why he is depressed rather than manic; or why he has been depressed since August rather than having been depressed for a longer or shorter time. Not much in the discussion will hinge on this assumption, but settling on one specific form of explanandum will increase both brevity and clarity. In addition, it has been made by many authors working on scientific explanation, from Van Fraassen (21) to Woodward (22).

When we start thinking about features of explanations that could stand in the way of their being combined, one rather trivial feature will come to us immediately: logical inconsistency. If I explain Tom's depression from that fact that he has been working too much and you explain it from the fact that he has been jobless, we are contradicting each other and no integration is possible. In order to avoid this, I will stipulate that in all the examples to be discussed later on, the explanations given are true; and furthermore, I assume – this is my second substantive assumption – that true statements are always logically compatible. Many will regard this assumption as a self-evident truth;

I myself do not; but I will assume its truth here in order to focus on the issues at hand.

Given this second assumption, there seems to be a strong presumption in favor of the idea that all explanations of the same explanandum will be combinable. After all, we can simply put them together; there being no logical incompatibility, nothing could stop us from doing so. This, I take it, is precisely why integrative approaches to science are so intuitively persuasive: if all our final theories are true, it surely *must* be possible to combine them. But of course, there are many ways to "combine" explanations, and it behooves us to take stock of them – and of any presuppositions they entail – before coming to a judgment about the matter.

In the following, I will identify three ways in which explanations can be combined: by presenting additive causes, by presenting different parts of a single causal tree, or by describing supervening levels. After a brief discussion of these three kinds of compatibility, I will argue that all of them share a basic presupposition that I will call *counterfactual compatibility*. This will suggest a way that even true, logically consistent explanations of the same fact can fail to be combinable: by *counterfactual incompatibility*.

As our example explanandum, let us take the fact F that patient P suffers from major depressive disorder (MDD), rather than not suffering from it. Let us postulate that P's MDD can be causally linked to a life history that has led to self-esteem and relationship issues; that the depression has been triggered by the loss of a job and the death of his best friend; that on a neural level the depressive symptoms are caused by, among other things, a disruption of neuroplasticity; and that P's self-esteem issues can be related to the exaggerated expectations his authoritarian father had of his only son. Given this situation, both of the following are acceptable explanations of F:

(1) P suffers from MDD because he lost his job.
(2) P suffers from MDD because his best friend died. These explanations both present causal factors that increased the likelihood of a depression and were in fact causally linked to it. Irrespective of whether either of them was sufficient for the occurrence of MDD, or whether both together were needed to trigger it, these causes can be added to each other in a single, more encompassing explanation:
(3) P suffers from MDD because he lost his job and his best friend died. This is what I call the *presentation of additive causes*: when two or more explanations present different causal factors that are independent but both increase the probability of the explanandum, we can simply combine them into a single conjunctive causal factor that is more informative than either of the factors alone. Of course, it is also possible that a set of explanations presents causal factors that are not independent, but that depend on each other because they are causally linked. Take, for instance, the following:
(4) P suffers from MDD because he lost his job and has been unable to find a new one.
(5) P suffers from MDD because he has self-esteem issues, which made him ineffective in his last job and caused him to lose it. The loss of his job triggered MDD.
(6) P suffers from MDD because the economy is in a slump and that has made him unable to find a new job. If he had found a new job soon after losing his last one, MDD would not have been triggered.

The relationship between these explanations is that each of them traces out a different part of a single causal *tree*, where a causal tree is the structure that is generated by providing the direct causes of one event, and then continuing to provide causes for any event in the tree whose causes have not been given yet. In this case, (4) explains F by giving two of its causes: the loss of the job and the inability to find a new one. (5) explains F by giving only one of those causes – the loss of the job – but by also explaining what caused that cause, thus moving up a level in the explanatory tree. Explanation (6) gives another of the causes of F – the inability to find a new job – and gives the causes of that cause. It is of course possible to combine (4–6) into a single, more complete description of the explanatory tree:

(7) P suffers from MDD because he has self-esteem issues and because the economy is in a slump. The self-esteem issues caused him to be ineffective at his last job, which in turn caused him to be fired. Because of the economic slump, he has been unable to find a new job. The prolonged joblessness was one of the things that triggered P's current episode of MDD.

This is what I call the *presentation of different parts of a causal tree*. Of course, the addition of causes and the presentation of different parts of a causal tree can be combined more or less *ad infinitum* in order to trace out the entire causal history of the event in the explanandum. Each of the explanations gives a different part of the tree, gives us a different set of events and causal links between them, and as this proceeds, we know about a larger part of the tree and understand the explanandum better.

These two ways of combining explanations are straightforward and important in practice, but they pose few theoretical problems. Things become more interesting when we move to two explanations like these:

(8) P suffers from MDD because he has a high stress level and stress causes the symptoms known as depression.
(9) P suffers from MDD because he has abnormal levels of cortisol, serotonin, and norepinephrine. These abnormal levels reduce the neuroplasticity of P's brain, which in turn causes the symptoms known as depression.[2]

We cannot understand (8) and (9) as tracing out different parts of a causal tree, for the simple reason that – at least on standard theories of the mental – they trace out the *same* part, but described at different levels or in different vocabularies. Where (8) speaks about stress, (9) speaks about the abnormal levels of

[2] For the potential relation between stress hormones, neuroplasticity, and depression, see Maletic et al. (23) and Pittenger and Duman (24).

certain hormones, but these are two descriptions of the same state. It is both possible and enlightening to combine (8) and (9):

(10) P suffers from MDD because he has a high stress level, which involves him having abnormal levels of cortisol, serotonin, and norepinephrine. These abnormal levels reduce the neuroplasticity of P's brain, which in turn causes the symptoms known as depression.

Philosophical questions about this situation remain, especially about the status of the word "involves" in (10). Is having stress *identical* to having certain hormonal levels, or does having stress instead *supervene*[3] on hormone levels? If it supervenes, could there be a reduction of theories about stress to theories about hormones, or are reductions impossible? Might it even be the case that this description of the situation is wrong, and that stress and certain hormone levels are merely accidentally cooccurring? Such questions are familiar from the philosophy of mind and will not be resolved any time soon. But for our current discussion, it turns out, perhaps surprisingly, that the answers to these questions make no difference. On any of the options in the debate, either (8) and (9) can be combined into (10) or at least one of them is false:

- On a reductionist theory, the two explanations are simply saying the same things in different vocabularies; once this is seen, the combination is trivial, because it turns out that there is nothing to combine.
- On a non-reductionist theory which sees psychological notions like "stress" as supervening on neurochemical states, the two explanations can both be given, and then linked through supervenience relations to result in a more complete explanation. This is what I will call the *description of supervening levels*.
- On a non-reductionist theory that rejects the supervenience thesis and instead believes that psychological events such as stress and neurochemical events such as high hormone levels are wholly distinct but related through the relation of causation, the two explanations can be combined by giving the causal interrelations between them. In this case, combining (8) and (9) into (10) turns out to be a case of *presentation of different parts of a causal tree*.
- On a radical dualist theory which sees mental events like stress and physical events like hormone levels as wholly distinct and non-interacting, explanation (9) must be false, for hormone levels cannot cause stress. So in this case, too, we do not have two true explanations of the same phenomenon that cannot be combined; we have a true and a false explanation, and the false explanation must be rejected.

Which of these options is correct will be highly relevant to our view of the relation between psychology and neuroscience. But what anyone can seemingly agree on is that once we have found the true explanations, those explanations *can* be combined into a single story – either by identifying them, by linking them through supervenience relation, or by linking them through causal relations.

Having seen three important ways in which true explanations can be combined, and are combined in practice, we are still faced with the question of whether there are any conditions under which they cannot. To answer that question, we must think about what explanations are and how something could fail to be an explanation, even though its parts are explanations.

When we do think through the properties of explanations, we quickly find that they are not merely lists of unconnected facts. Explanations always trace links between the fact to be explained and other facts. Different theories of explanation have different ideas about what these links are like: according to Hempel's original DN-model, explanations show how the fact to be explained can be derived from other facts through laws of nature; according to unificationist theories, explanations show how the fact to be explained can be derived using unifying arguments; according to causal theories of explanation, explanations explain a fact by giving its causal antecedents [see Salmon (25) and Woodward (26) for overviews]. But what all these theories have in common, and what is indeed one of the central facts about explanation that any theory of explanation would have to do justice to, is that explanations allow us to draw *counterfactual conclusions* about the explanandum. To *know that* P suffers from MDD is to know something important; but to *understand why* P suffers from MDD is to have, in addition, a measure of insight into the conditions under which he would *not* have suffered. Explanations allow us to make claims about what *would have happened* in different circumstances. And this is indeed one of the prime reasons that we are interested in explanations at all, for by allowing us to see what would happen in different circumstances, they allows us to make an informed choice between different courses of action. [For more on the relation between explanation, causation, and counterfactuals, see Chapter 3 of Woodward (22).]

If one of the central obligations on an explanation is to allow us to draw counterfactual conclusions about the explanandum, then it is reasonable for us to require explanations to fulfill that obligation. To be precise, it is reasonable to ask of any explanation that the counterfactual consequences that follow from it are consistent: that is, that we cannot show from it both that if A had happened, C would have happened; and that if A had happened, C would not have happened. In other words, the counterfactual picture painted by any explanation should be coherent.

This in turn suggests a condition that two explanations of the same fact have to fulfill in order to be combinable into a single explanation: they should not have logically incompatible counterfactual consequences. If they do not, we will call them *counterfactually compatible*. If, on the other hand, they do have logically incompatible counterfactual consequences, we will call them *counterfactually incompatible*. The claim I am making, then, is that two true explanations of the same fact are combinable into one explanation only if they are counterfactually compatible.

[3]Supervenience is a notoriously difficult term to define adequately, but in this article, I will take it to be the relation such that (a) the values of supervening properties at time *t* are fully determined by the values at time *t* of the properties they supervene on, but (b) the supervening properties cannot be identified with the supervened-on properties. Many philosophers have defended the idea that while, say, mental states are not identical to brain states; nevertheless, our brain states fully determine our mental states. If this is so, then mental states supervene on brain states in the sense I am using the term here.

(This is a necessary condition. Perhaps it is also sufficient, but I have no argument to that effect.)

In all our previous examples, the explanations were indeed counterfactually compatible. Both (4) and (5) imply that if P had not lost his job, he would not have had MDD. In addition, (5) implies that if P had not had self-esteem issues, he would not have lost his job; this is of course compatible with the previous claim. Both (4) and (6) imply that if P had been able to find a new job soon, he would not have had MDD. In the case of (8) and (9), the counterfactual implications are different but logically compatible: (8) implies that P would not have suffered from MDD if he had not suffered from stress, whereas (9) implies that P would not have suffered from MDD if his hormone levels had been normal; and these two claims are perfectly consistent on both reductive and non-reductive theories of the mental.

We must now ask ourselves whether it is ever possible for two true explanations to be counterfactually incompatible. Let us first look at an example involving two very different explanations of the same fact, one from the perspective of textbook physics and one from the perspective of common sense teleology. Suppose that a door in my living room is open rather than closed. Why? Here are two explanations:

(11) The door is open because a force greater than F was applied to it from the inside while the handle was down.
(12) The door is open to allow fresh air to get in.

Both of these explanations can be true at the same time. But now let us ask the following question: would this door have been open if it had been a door to the cellar instead of a door to the garden? The physicist, with (11) in hand, would say that, yes, the door would still have been open. After all, cellar doors do not have physical properties that make them physically more difficult to open than garden doors. But the common sense thinker, looking at (12), would say no, the door would have been closed if it had been a cellar door. After all, cellar doors are not opened to let in fresh air. Who of the two is right? Would this door have been open if it had been a door to the cellar? Well, yes *and* no – it depends on the perspective we are taking. But this means that the explanations from the two perspectives, while both valid and true, fail the test of counterfactual compatibility and cannot be combined into a single coherent explanation.

One might object that any incompatibility here is the result of the incompatibility of a broadly causal and a broadly teleological perspective; and one might then go on to claim that teleology has no place in science. If that is true, then examples like the one above could show at most that science cannot always be integrated with common sense; but this does not disprove the integrationist claim that the sciences themselves are always capable of being integrated. Perhaps this is true; although it would already be an interesting result, since discussions about teleology are by no means dead in science. But counterfactual incompatibility can in fact also arise between two perspectives that are both purely causal.

Let us return to our poor patient P, and let us ask the following question: suppose that P had been a woman, would he still have suffered from MDD? One way to approach this question – the approach that would be favored by a neuroscientist – would be to review the differences between male and female brains. Let us supposes that there is no systematic difference between the sexes such that female brains handle abnormal levels of cortisol, serotonin, and norepinephrine differently from male brains. Then, the neuroscientist would pronounce, correctly and with ample justification, that if P had been female, (s)he would still have suffered from MDD.

But the question could also be answered by P's therapist, who has been especially interested in talking through his life history with him, with a special emphasis on traumatic events from his early childhood. According to this therapist the crucial cause of P's self-esteem issues is the way P's father treated his only son; a way that was markedly different from the way he treated his daughters. The therapist thus comes to the conclusion – just as correct and just as justified as that reached by neuroscientist – that if P had been a woman, (s)he would not have suffered from MDD.

There is nothing especially mysterious about this situation. Different scientific perspectives on P naturally lead to different ways of evaluating counterfactual claims about him. For a neuroscientist, contemplating the influence of gender means contemplating the way that gender has influenced the structure and functioning of the patient's brain. For the therapist, contemplating the influence of gender means contemplating the way that gender has influenced the patient's life history. Both of these perspectives are equally valid, and both lead to explanations that should be accepted. But these explanations cannot be accepted into one single coherent explanation; for combining them leads to a story in which P would both have suffered from MDD and not suffered from MDD if he had been a woman. So, the therapist's life-history approach and the neuroscientist's approach have to remain isolated to a certain extent. Here, we have a case of counterfactual incompatibility; and in general, counterfactual incompatibility may occur when we try to integrate explanations from different research approaches. When it does, it acts as a barrier to integrative pluralism.

This conclusion could be attacked in two ways. First, one could attack the claim that counterfactual compatibility is a requirement for two explanations to be combined. Now, admittedly, by choosing a suitable low standard for what "integration" means, one can always claim that two research approaches can be integrated. But counterfactual incompatibility is a real barrier to any substantive kind of integration, because it means that we cannot simply transfer conclusion reached in one approach to the other approach. If the neuroscientist finds that gender is irrelevant to MDD, the therapist or the sociologist cannot just accept that conclusion; for the conclusion, while true – in our example – from the neuroscientific perspective, might well be false from the other perspectives. This non-transferability of counterfactual conclusions is surely a good reason to hold that the different research approaches are to some extent isolated and autonomous.

Second, one could claim that, my examples notwithstanding, counterfactual compatibility cannot occur between true explanations. For, one could argue, it is logically impossible that "if A had happened, then B would have happened" and "if A had happened, then B would not have happened" are both true. To substantiate this conclusion, one could appeal to influential theories about the truth conditions of counterfactuals. Lewis (27), for instance, tells us that "if A had happened, then B would have happened" is true just in case that B is true in the closest possible world where A is true, where the closeness of possible worlds is defined in terms of their similarity to ours. If such a story were correct, and, crucially, *if similarity were a non-contextual affair*, something that should be evaluated in the same way across all the sciences, then either the therapist or the neuroscientist would have to be wrong. To see which, we would have to find out which world is more similar to ours, the one envisaged by the therapist or the one envisaged by the neuroscientist. And whichever of them in their imaginative flights stayed closer to home, so to speak, would be the person drawing the correct counterfactual conclusions.

Such a procedure, however, has very little to recommend itself. Theories about the truth conditions of counterfactuals should respect our everyday evaluations of counterfactuals; and it is an undeniable fact that people working from different perspectives use different scenarios to evaluate the same counterfactual claims. As Lowe (28) points out, the truth conditions of counterfactuals are highly context-dependent. Lowe then argues (pp. 54–55) that the context influences how we evaluate claims about the similarity of possible worlds, and that this context is at least partly defined by the intentions of the speaker. For our current purposes, we can slightly modify his proposal and state that the context within which counterfactuals are evaluated is at least partly defined by the research approach within which the claim appears. Counterfactual evaluation in neuroscience takes scenarios into account that are ignored in the therapeutic setting, and the other way around. The different sciences use different relevance criteria; and this does not make a difference not only for which facts they uncover but also for how they reason about counterfactual scenarios. Since explanations are tightly connected to counterfactual scenarios, these differences between research approaches translate into an incompatibility of the explanations they generate.

This concludes my argument for the claim that I set out to prove, namely, that true explanations of the same fact sometimes cannot be combined into a single bigger explanations. Counterfactual incompatibility is a barrier to such combination, and counterfactual incompatibility is real. This result nicely mirrors that of Lange (29). His point is that different research approaches take different sets of counterfactuals seriously, and that this leads to incompatible laws; my point is that different research approaches sometimes reach incompatible results when evaluating identical counterfactuals. Both points support the conclusion that research approaches can be expected to be at least partly autonomous.

Let me end this section by professing ignorance about two points. First, I am not sure whether counterfactual incompatibility can also occur within a single research approach – e.g., whether two true neurological explanations of a brain phenomenon could ever turn out to be incompatible. If this were possible, science would be even more disunified than we tend to think. Second, I do not know whether this section has covered all the ways in which explanations can be combinable or fail to be combinable. In this respect, I make no claim to having exhausted the territory.

CONCLUSION

My analysis of the debate surrounding the unity of science and explanatory pluralism revealed that the most pressing issue lies in the choice between integrative and isolationist pluralism; or rather, in finding out whether the integrative tendencies present in current science should be fully indulged in, or should be held in check by affirming that a certain amount of isolation is unavoidable. I further distilled this issue into the question of whether two true explanations of the same fact could ever fail to be combinable into one single explanation. It turns out that although many explanations are in fact combinable, this only holds when they have compatible counterfactual consequences. I then argued that true explanations from different sciences can have incompatible counterfactual consequences. This leads us to the general conclusion that a certain amount of isolation between the sciences is indeed both present and unavoidable; forcing all the sciences to use the counterfactual relevance criteria of one of them would rob us of part of the insight that the different sciences can give us and would lead to the uncritical transfer of counterfactual claims from one science into another, with potentially disastrous results (in the case of, e.g., a sociologist who rejects the possibility that gender could be related to psychological conditions because the neuroscientists tell him that there is no such relation). This does not mean that we should not strive for integration and the benefits of interdisciplinarity. But it does mean that we should not take this project too far, for, at the end of the day, there will still be the different sciences with their different perspectives and insights. The plurality of the sciences is to be cherished rather than combated.

AUTHOR CONTRIBUTIONS

The author confirms being the sole contributor of this work and approved it for publication.

REFERENCES

1. Cat J. The unity of science. Winter 2014 ed. In: Zalta EN, editor. *The Stanford Encyclopedia of Philosophy* (2014). Available from: http://plato.stanford.edu/archives/win2014/entries/scientific-unity/
2. Pombo O, Symons J, Torres JM. Neurath and the unity of science: an introduction. In: Symons J, Pombo O, Torres JM, editors. *Otto Neurath and the Unity of Science*. Dordrecht: Springer (2011). p. 1–11.
3. Oppenheim P, Putnam H. The unity of science as a working hypothesis. In: Feigl H, Scriven M, Maxwell G, editors. *Minnesota Studies in the Philosophy of Science* (Vol. **2**), Minneapolis: Minnesota University Press (1958).
4. Fodor J. Special sciences: or the disunity of science as a working hypothesis. *Synthese* (1974) **28**:97–115. doi:10.1007/BF00485230
5. Dupré J. *The Disorder of Things. Metaphysical Foundations of the Disunity of Science*. Cambridge, MA: Harvard University Press (1993).
6. Cartwright N. *The Dappled World. A Study of the Boundaries of Science*. Cambridge: Cambridge University Press (1999).
7. Teller P. Twilight of the perfect model model. *Erkenntnis* (2001) **55**:393–415. doi:10.1023/A:1013349314515
8. Ladyman J, Ross D. *Every Thing Must Go. Metaphysics Naturalized*. Oxford: Oxford University Press (2007).
9. Symons J, Pombo O, Torres JM, editors. *Otto Neurath and the Unity of Science*. Dordrecht: Springer (2011).
10. McCauley RN, Bechtel W. Explanatory pluralism and heuristic identity theory. *Theory Psychol* (2001) **11**:736–60. doi:10.1177/0959354301116002

11. Kendler KS. Toward a philosophical structure for psychiatry. *Am J Psychiatry* (2005) **162**:433–40. doi:10.1176/appi.ajp.162.3.433
12. Abney DH, Dale R, Yoshimi J, Kello CT, Tylén K, Fusaroli R. Joint perceptual decision-making: a case study in explanatory pluralism. *Front Psychol* (2014) **5**:330. doi:10.3389/fpsyg.2014.00330
13. Marchionni C. Explanatory pluralism and complementarity: from autonomy to integration. *Philos Soc Sci* (2008) **38**:314–33. doi:10.1177/0048393108319399
14. Mitchell S. *Unsimple Truths. Science, Complexity, and Policy*. Chicago: University of Chicago Press (2009).
15. Campaner R. Explanatory pluralism in psychiatry: what are we pluralists about, and why? In: Galavotti MC, et al., editors. *New Directions in the Philosophy of Science*. Cham: Springer (2014). p. 87–103.
16. Van Bouwel J. Pluralists about pluralism? Different versions of explanatory pluralism in psychiatry. In: Galavotti MC, et al., editors. *New Directions in the Philosophy of Science*. Cham: Springer (2014). p. 105–19.
17. Brigandt I. Beyond reduction and pluralism: toward an epistemology of explanatory integration in biology. *Erkenntnis*. (2010) **73**:295–311. doi:10.1007/s10670-010-9233-3
18. Andler D. Unity without myths. In: Symons J, Pombo O, Torres JM, editors. *Otto Neurath and the Unity of Science*. Dordrecht: Springer (2011). p. 129–44.
19. Van Bouwel J, Weber E, De Vreese L. Indispensability arguments in favour of reductive explanations. *J Gen Philos Sci* (2011) **42**:33–46. doi:10.1007/s10838-011-9141-5
20. Gervais R. A framework for inter-level explanations: outlines for a new explanatory pluralism. *Stud Hist Philos Sci* (2014) **48**:1–9. doi:10.1016/j.shpsa.2014.07.002
21. Van Fraassen B. *The Scientific Image*. Oxford: Oxford University Press (1980).
22. Woodward J. *Making Things Happen*. Oxford: Oxford University Press (2003).
23. Maletic V, Robinson M, Oakes T, Iyengar S, Ball SG, Russell J. Neurobiology of depression: an integrated view of key findings. *Int J Clin Pract* (2007) **61**:2030–40. doi:10.1111/j.1742-1241.2007.01602.x
24. Pittenger C, Duman RS. Stress, depression, and neuroplasticity: a convergence of mechanisms. *Neuropsychopharmacology* (2008) **33**:88–109. doi:10.1038/sj.npp.1301574
25. Salmon W. *Four Decades of Scientific Explanation*. Minneapolis: University of Minnesota Press (1989).
26. Woodward J. Scientific explanation. Winter 2014 ed. In: Zalta EN, editor. *The Stanford Encyclopedia of Philosophy* (2014). Available from: http://plato.stanford.edu/archives/win2014/entries/scientific-explanation/
27. Lewis D. *Counterfactuals*. Oxford; Cambridge, MA: Blackwell Publishers; Harvard University Press (1973).
28. Lowe EJ. The truth about counterfactuals. *Philos Q* (1995) **45**:41–59. doi:10.2307/2219847
29. Lange M. Who's afraid of *Ceteris-Paribus* laws? Or: how I learned to stop worrying and love them. *Erkenntnis* (2002) **57**:407–23. doi:10.1023/A:1021546731582

11

Predicting Medical Students' Current Attitudes Toward Psychiatry, Interest in Psychiatry, and Estimated Likelihood of Working in Psychiatry

Ingeborg Warnke[1], Alex Gamma[1], Maria Buadze[1], Roman Schleifer[1], Carlos Canela[1], Bernd Strebel[2], Tamás Tényi[3], Wulf Rössler[4,5,6], Nicolas Rüsch[7] and Michael Liebrenz[1]*

[1] Department of Forensic Psychiatry, Institute of Forensic Medicine, University of Bern, Bern, Switzerland, [2] Department of Psychosomatic Medicine, Protestant Hospital Hagen-Haspe, Hagen, Germany, [3] Department of Psychiatry and Psychotherapy, University of Pécs, Pécs, Hungary, [4] Department of Psychiatry, Psychotherapy and Psychosomatics, Psychiatric Hospital, University of Zurich, Zurich, Switzerland, [5] Laboratory of Neuroscience (LIM 27), Institute of Psychiatry, University of São Paulo, São Paulo, Brazil, [6] Department of Psychiatry and Psychotherapy, Charité University of Medicine, Berlin, Germany, [7] Department of Psychiatry II, University of Ulm and Bezirkskrankenhaus Günzburg, Ulm, Germany

Edited by:
*Adriana Mihai,
University of Medicine and
Pharmacy of Târgu
Mureş, Romania*

Reviewed by:
*Costin Roventa,
Prof. Dr. Alexandru Obregia
Psychiatry Hospital, Romania
Bulent Coskun,
Kocaeli University, Turkey
Jana Chihai,
Nicolae Testemiţanu
State University of Medicine
and Pharmacy, Moldova*

***Correspondence:**
*Ingeborg Warnke
ingeborg.warnke@fpd.unibe.ch*

Psychiatry as a medical discipline is becoming increasingly important due to the high and increasing worldwide burden associated with mental disorders. Surprisingly, however, there is a lack of young academics choosing psychiatry as a career. Previous evidence on medical students' perspectives is abundant but has methodological shortcomings. Therefore, by attempting to avoid previous shortcomings, we aimed to contribute to a better understanding of the predictors of the following three outcome variables: current medical students' attitudes toward psychiatry, interest in psychiatry, and estimated likelihood of working in psychiatry. The sample consisted of $N = 1,356$ medical students at 45 medical schools in Germany and Austria as well as regions of Switzerland and Hungary with a German language curriculum. We used snowball sampling *via* Facebook with a link to an online questionnaire as recruitment procedure. Snowball sampling is based on referrals made among people. This questionnaire included a German version of the Attitudes Toward Psychiatry Scale (ATP-30-G) and further variables related to outcomes and potential predictors in terms of sociodemography (e.g., gender) or medical training (e.g., curriculum-related experience with psychiatry). Data were analyzed by linear mixed models and further regression models. On average, students had a positive attitude to and high general interest in, but low professional preference for, psychiatry. A neutral attitude to psychiatry was partly related to the discipline itself, psychiatrists, or psychiatric patients. Female gender and previous experience with psychiatry, particularly curriculum-related and personal experience, were important predictors of all outcomes. Students in the first years of medical training were more interested in pursuing psychiatry as a career. Furthermore, the country of the medical school was related to the outcomes. However, statistical models explained only a small proportion of variance. The findings indicate that particularly curriculum-related experience is important for determining attitudes toward psychiatry, interest in the subject and self-predicted professional career choice. We therefore encourage the provision of opportunities for clinical experience by psychiatrists. However, further predictor variables need to be considered in future studies.

Keywords: attitudes toward psychiatry, interest in psychiatry, professional preference, multivariable modeling, curriculum-related experience, gender, medical school, study year

INTRODUCTION

For two decades, there has been growing worldwide concern that psychiatry as a profession, its identity, and image is in crisis (1–4). Moreover, there is an imbalance between the high numbers affected by mental disorders (5–7), the high and increasing worldwide burden attributable to mental disorders in terms of disability-adjusted life years (DALYs), years of life lost to premature mortality (YLL) and years lived with disability (YLD) (8), and the declining numbers of young academics choosing psychiatry as a career (4, 9–13). Despite its achievements, psychiatry faces challenges that might contribute to the dearth of psychiatrists and to resource shortage in the field: namely, the questionable validity of diagnostic definitions, doubts about the effectiveness of therapeutic interventions due to negative or contradictory findings, and the methodological quality of related research, opposing ideologies such as biological psychiatry vs. psychotherapy, the resulting unclear role profile of the psychiatrist, patient criticism of the formerly paternalistic discipline, overlapping responsibilities of psychiatrists and other professions (e.g., neurologists, psychologists), and, finally, its low status within medicine and society (4). Accordingly, psychiatric organizations have launched initiatives to better understand the reluctance medical students appear to feel toward psychiatry and to improve the recruitment of young academics into the field (12, 14–17).

In order to learn more about medical students' views of psychiatry, numerous studies have focused on their attitudes toward psychiatry and their intended or definite career choice in order to obtain a deeper insight into the factors which might contribute to a better standing (18–29). Most studies indicate a discrepancy between positive attitudes toward psychiatry and low willingness to work in the field (18, 21, 22). However, attitude toward psychiatry, interest in psychiatry, and intended career choice are positively interrelated (18, 20, 21). In particular, medical students acknowledge the value of psychotherapy (21), view psychiatry as intellectually challenging and personally rewarding, but are reported to entertain a certain skepticism toward factors such as scientific standing, status, prestige and financial prospects, psychiatrists, patients, and treatment (18). In previous studies, female medical students and those with previous experience with psychiatry had consistently more positive attitudes (18, 20, 21, 23, 24, 28, 29), higher general interest in psychiatry (18), or higher interest in psychiatry as a career (20, 22, 25–28). Attitudes toward psychiatry and the definite career choice might also depend on characteristics of the medical school concerned, such as selection of students by non-teachable competencies, cultural diversity among medical students or the medical school's focus on psychiatric education, and the supportiveness of the faculty (18, 20). Furthermore, how the number of study years affects attitudes (18, 24), interest, or career choice remains unclear.

However, previous research also reveals limitations. It does not indicate the most important predictors of attitudes toward psychiatry, interest in psychiatry, or intended career choice because most studies are just descriptive and did not use multivariable modeling (21–24, 26, 27, 29). In particular, it remains unclear as to which type of previous experience with psychiatry (e.g., clinical experience in the curriculum, private contact with people with mental illness or work-related experience) is mainly associated with medical students' perceptions of psychiatry. Samples are frequently small to moderately sized ($N \leq 500$) (21–26, 28, 29). Finally, there is usually no hierarchical modeling in cases of multiple catchment areas (22, 26, 27), although the generalizability of results across settings is assumed without confirmatory evidence.

Accordingly, this study aimed to contribute to a better understanding of predictors of medical students' current perceptions and attempted to avoid the limitations of previous research. Therefore, we multivariably and hierarchically analyzed sociodemographic and education-specific predictor variables such as gender and diverse types of previous experience with psychiatry (see below) for three outcomes: (1) attitudes toward psychiatry, (2) interest in psychiatry, and (3) estimated likelihood of working in psychiatry. To achieve a sufficient sample size, we used an innovative recruitment approach *via* social media. We further considered multiple medical schools with a German language curriculum: namely, in Germany, Switzerland, Austria, and Hungary. There are, of course, differences between these countries as well, which include lower thresholds in selecting prospective medical students and lower tuition fees in Hungary, the highest density of psychiatrists in Switzerland, followed by Germany and Hungary (30); no officially approved and independent mental health policy or program in Hungary (11, 31).

MATERIALS AND METHODS

Data Collection

Data were collected electronically by a secure web application called "Research Electronic Database Capture (REDCap)" for constructing and managing online surveys and databases (32, 33). The link was distributed on Facebook *via* message boards and student associations all over medical schools with a German language curriculum (or program) across Germany, Switzerland, Austria, and Hungary (34). Accordingly, we used snowball sampling based on person-to-person subject recruitment (35): "Snowball sampling yields a study sample through referrals made among people with important characteristics for the research question. It is particularly applicable when the focus of study is on a sensitive issue, and thus requires the knowledge of insiders to locate people for study."

Data collection started on November 24, 2016 and ended on January 10, 2017.

The Cantonal Ethics Committee Bern (Kantonale Ethikkommission Bern, KEK-BE), responsible for the study site, filed a letter of non-competence and stated no objection. Accordingly, approval by the KEK-BE was not required because the study type was exempt from the local legislation on research involving human beings (Human Research Act, Article 2, Section 1).

The participants declared their informed consent by participating in the study after having been fully informed about its content. They themselves decided to submit the manuscript anonymously or not. Those who gave their mailing address could participate in a lottery with the possibility to gain a smartphone by randomized selection at the end of recruitment. Data were stored and managed according to the data protection guidelines of the University of Bern (36, 37).

Online-Questionnaire

The online questionnaire was composed of a German version (21) of the original Attitudes Toward Psychiatry (ATP-30) Scale (38). The frequently used ATP-30 measures medical students' attitudes toward psychiatry (21–24, 28) and has proven validity and reliability, as assessed in a Canadian sample of medical students (38). According to the author, the split-half reliability by Spearman–Brown was $r = 0.90$ in medical and $r = 0.89$ in O.T. students. The test stability varied depending on the length and type of the test–retest period between $r = 0.51$ and $r = 0.87$, with a value of $r = 0.69/r = 0.67$ before and after psychiatry-related experience in second-, third-, and fourth-year medical students and O.T. students.

The German ATP-30-G showed high internal consistency (21). It comprises 30 Likert-scale items, with 5 = strongly disagree and 1 = strongly agree. The questionnaire includes diverse statements related to mental illness and psychiatric patients, psychiatric treatment and institutions, psychiatrists, education, knowledge, and psychiatry as a career choice. To calculate a sum score, scores of positively phrased items were subtracted from 6, resulting in higher values for a more positive attitude, and finally, item scores of positively and negatively phrased items were summed up. The sum score ranged between 30 and 150 points. A sum score of 90 would represent "the logical neutral point of the scale" (38).

We also asked participants about their general interest in the discipline of psychiatry and how likely it seemed to them that they would choose psychiatry as a career (21). Responses were given on a visual analog scale ranging from 0 to 100. Although the ATP-30 also includes specific items on interest (e.g., "Psychiatry is unappealing because it makes so little use of medical training"; "It is interesting to unravel the cause of a psychiatric illness"; "Psychiatric patients are often more interesting to work with than other patients.") or career preference (e.g., "I would like to be a psychiatrist"), we preferred the above-mentioned global and probably more robust outcome measures. However, we conducted statistical analyses for both outcome variables on the professional preference as measured by the visual analog scale and the respective ATP item.

Predictor variables included the following: age (transformed by centering on the mean of 24 years), gender (male vs. female), nationality (German, Swiss, Austrian, Hungarian/other), medical school and country of medical school (German, Swiss, Austrian, Hungarian), study year (1st- to 4th semester [first 2 years, preclinical study period], 5th- to 10th semester [third, fourth, and fifth year, clinical part], and >10 semesters [beginning of clinical rotations]), and previous experience with psychiatry and type of experience (curriculum-related, personal, work-related, other). Curriculum-related experience included practical activities such as clinical traineeship/academic assistance. Further possible free answers under "other experience" related to training or internships and teaching, usually referring to medical training and only rarely to premedical education were grouped in this category. Personal experience included experiences with psychiatry related to oneself (e.g., psychotherapy) or to one's personal environment, e.g., having friends or family members with a mental disorder. We also grouped possible free answers into this category if they were related to having mental health care professionals as parents or previous voluntary work in the social sector. Work-related experience referred to medical paid work during the course of medical studies (e.g., night shift on a ward). We also grouped information on professional work due to previous training (e.g., as a nurse or physiotherapist) into this category.

Sample Selection

The sample selection procedure is illustrated in **Figure 1**. Of 1,884 students, 1,356 (72%) students from 45 medical schools submitted the online questionnaire and gave full information on predictor variables, interest in psychiatry, and likelihood of working in psychiatry. A subsample of 1,290 students gave full information on the ATP-30-G.

Statistical Analyses

To avoid data loss, we used both samples described above ($N = 1,356$ and 1,290) for statistical analyses on outcomes.

First, we described the sample and compared sample characteristics across outcomes by t-test, ANOVA and Pearson's correlation. We further analyzed the relationship between outcomes by Pearson's correlation.

Second, we calculated linear mixed models (LMMs) (39, 40) by using the ATP-30-G sum score, interest in psychiatry, and estimated likelihood of working in psychiatry as outcome variables. LMMs are eligible for continuous outcome variables with normally distributed residuals, which may, however, not be independent or have constant variance (40). The independent variables may involve fixed effects with unknown constant parameters and random effects with levels of factors regarded as having been randomly sampled from a larger population (40). Using traditional regression models in nested data might lead to Type-I error inflation (39), whereas mixed models effectively address this issue (41). We considered the group variable "medical school" as a random variable at level 1, and other predictor variables as fixed effects. Interaction effects of the mixed-effects models were visualized by graphing marginal means.

Third, to evaluate the robustness of the mixed-model findings, we calculated complementary models by robust regression,

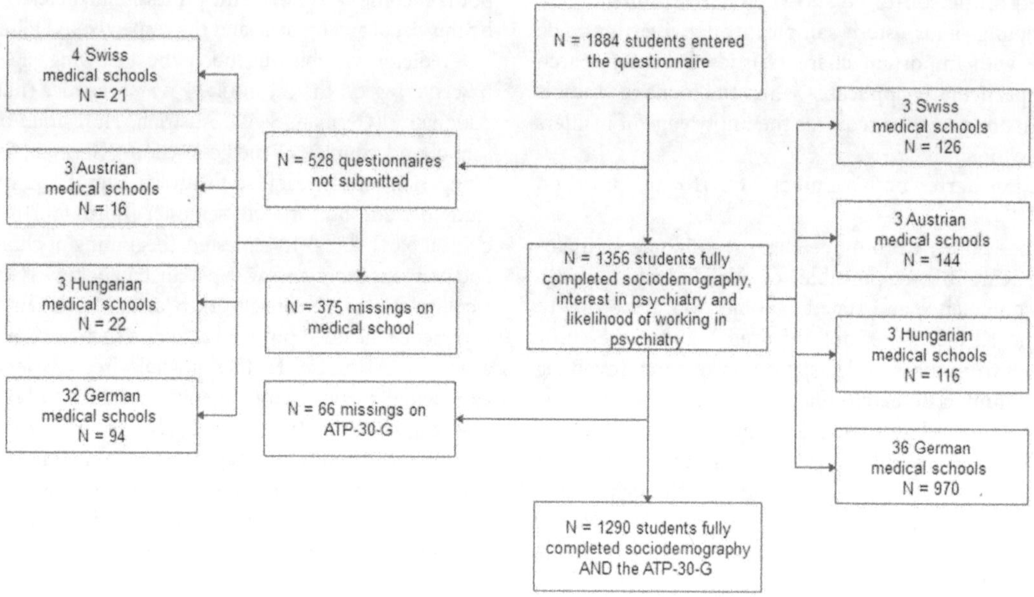

FIGURE 1 | Sample selection procedure.

using the Huber M estimation method,[1] and quantile (median) regression.[2] These methods are suitable for data contaminated with outliers and heterogeneous conditional distributions, and therefore appropriate for the outcome variables "interest in psychiatry" and "likelihood of working in psychiatry." Robust regression indicates the amount of variance explained by R^2 in order to assess the relative predictive capability of the statistical models. Results of all three regression types were illustrated by coefficient plots for each outcome.

Fourth, we considered the item "I would like to be a psychiatrist" as measured by the ATP-30-G as an outcome variable, with a higher score indicating a more positive attitude. We calculated a General Linear Model with cumulative logit function[3] and the random-effect "medical school."

Statistical models were run in SAS/STAT, Version 9.4 (42) using the procedures "proc mixed," "proc robustreg" and "proc quantreg," and "proc glimmix." The plot of margins was generated in SPSS, version 23 for Windows (43). Coefficient plots were generated by Stata, version 14.2 for Mac (44).

RESULTS

Non-Response and Sample Selection

A comparison of students who submitted the questionnaire (N = 1,356 responders) with those who did not but who

TABLE 1 | Sample characteristics.

Sample characteristics		Sample: N = 1,290[a]		Sample: N = 1,356[b]	
		N	**(%)**	***N***	**(%)**
Age (mean, SD), years		24	(3.79)	24	(3.74)
Gender					
	Female	903	(70.0)	955	(70.4)
	Male	387	(30.0)	401	(29.6)
Nationality					
	Swiss	110	(8.5)	117	(8.6)
	Austrian	102	(7.9)	111	(8.2)
	Hungarian/other	58	(4.5)	63	(4.6)
	German	1,020	(79.1)	1,065	(78.5)
Medical school, country					
	Swiss	118	(9.1)	126	(9.3)
	Austrian	135	(10.5)	144	(10.6)
	Hungarian	111	(8.6)	116	(8.6)
	German	926	(71.8)	970	(71.5)
Semesters					
	1st–4th semester	245	(19.0)	256	(18.9)
	5th–10th semester	771	(59.8)	810	(59.7)
	>10th semester	274	(21.2)	290	(21.4)
Previous experience					
	Yes	458	(35.5)	489	(36.1)
	No	832	(64.5)	867	(63.9)
Type of previous experience					
	Curriculum-related	211	(16.4)	222	(16.4)
	Personal	155	(12.0)	169	(12.5)
	Work-related	92	(7.1)	98	(7.2)
	No experience	832	(64.5)	867	(63.9)

[a]Complete information on the German version of the Attitudes Toward Psychiatry Scale.
[b]Full sample.

[1]Chen C. *Robust Regression and Outlier Detection with the ROBUSTREG Procedure [Paper 265-27].* Cary, NC: SAS Institute Inc.

[2]Chen C. *An Introduction to Quantile Regression and the QUANTREG Procedure [Paper 213-30].* Cary, NC: SAS Institute Inc.

[3]Schabenberger O. *Introducing the GLIMMIX Procedure for Generalized Linear Mixed Models [Working Paper].* Cary, NC: SAS Institute Inc.

entered sociodemographic information (N = 158 non-responders) revealed no statistically significant differences in age, gender, nationality, and number of semesters (Table S1A in Supplementary Material). The samples differed with respect to the country of the medical school, with more responders (71.5%) than non-responders (61.4%) enrolled in Germany and more responders (36.1%) than non-responders (23.2%) mentioning previous psychiatric experience. The two groups did not differ in "interest in psychiatry" (N = 11 missings in non-responders) and "likelihood of working in psychiatry" (N = 7 missings in non-responders), whereas findings on "attitudes toward psychiatry" were not interpretable (N = 145 missings in non-responders).

A comparison of the students who gave their mailing address and therefore took part in the lottery (N = 1,163) with those who did not (N = 193) showed that they differed statistically only with respect to age and gender, with women preferring to remain anonymous (Table S1B in Supplementary Material). The two groups differed neither in other sociodemographic or education-specific variables nor concerning attitude, interest or professional preference scores.

Sample Description

Tables 1 and **2** present basic sample characteristics.

The majority were females and German students enrolled at a medical school in Germany, in the clinical part of their studies (5th–10th semester) and without previous experience in psychiatry. Most previous experience was curriculum-related.

Females and those with previous experience—especially curriculum-related or personal experience—had higher scores in attitudes, interest in psychiatry, and estimated likelihood of working in psychiatry. Students from a medical school in Hungary had lower scores in all outcomes. Furthermore, a shorter length of medical study was associated with lower attitude scores (**Table 2**).

Relationship between Outcome Variables

The outcome variables were strongly and positively correlated. The ATP-30-G sum score correlated with "interest in psychiatry" by $r = 0.59$ ($p < 0.0001$) and with "likelihood of working in psychiatry" by $r = 0.54$ ($p < 0.0001$). Interest in psychiatry and likelihood of working in psychiatry correlated by $r = 0.66$

TABLE 2 | Mean outcome scores by sample characteristics.

		ATP-30-G sum score N = 1,290		Interest in psychiatry N = 1,356		Likelihood of working in psychiatry N = 1,356	
		Mean	**SD**	**Mean**	**SD**	**Mean**	**SD**
Sample characteristics							
Age (mean, SD), years							
Gender							
	Female	112.4	12.9	65.4	24.4	37.1	28.4
	Male	109.2	14.2	58.8	25.8	30.8	28.0
Nationality							
	Swiss	112.2	13.5	63.8	23.4	35.2	25.2
	Austrian	114.3	12.1	59.8	27.3	31.1	25.7
	Hungarian/other	108.7	14.6	57.9	30.8	37.0	32.1
	German	111.2	13.4	64.1	24.5	35.6	28.8
Medical school, country							
	Swiss	111.9	13.3	64.6	23.1	34.9	24.9
	Austrian	112.2	30.6	58.4	26.8	30.6	25.6
	Hungarian	106.4	13.7	57.4	24.5	28.0	27.1
	German	111.8	13.3	64.8	24.9	36.8	29.2
Semesters							
	1st–4th semester	108.8	13.4	63.6	23.7	37.1	26.8
	5th–10th semester	111.5	13.3	63.2	25.0	34.1	27.5
	>10th semester	113.5	13.3	63.9	26.1	36.7	31.9
Previous experience							
	Yes	115.7	13.1	73.0	23.0	46.2	30.6
	No	109.1	12.9	58.1	24.5	29.1	25.1
Type of previous experience							
	Curriculum-related	117.2	13.0	73.7	23.5	48.7	31.2
	Personal	115.7	12.9	75.9	20.1	46.1	29.1
	Work-related	112.2	13.2	66.2	25.5	40.6	31.4
	No experience	109.1	12.9	58.1	24.5	29.1	25.1

An ANOVA was performed in the case of more than two categories within variables; a t-test was done in the case of two categories within variables; a Pearson's correlation was done in the case of a continuous variable.

*ATP-30-G sum score: ****P < 0.0001: age, gender, semesters, previous experience, type of previous experience, **P < 0.01: medical school, country, n.s.: nationality.*

*Interest in psychiatry: ****P < 0.0001: gender, previous experience, type of previous experience, **P < 0.01: medical school, country, n.s.: age, nationality, semesters.*

*Likelihood of working in psychiatry: ****P < 0.0001: gender, previous experience, type of previous experience, **P < 0.01: medical school, country, *P < 0.05: age, n.s.: nationality, semesters.*

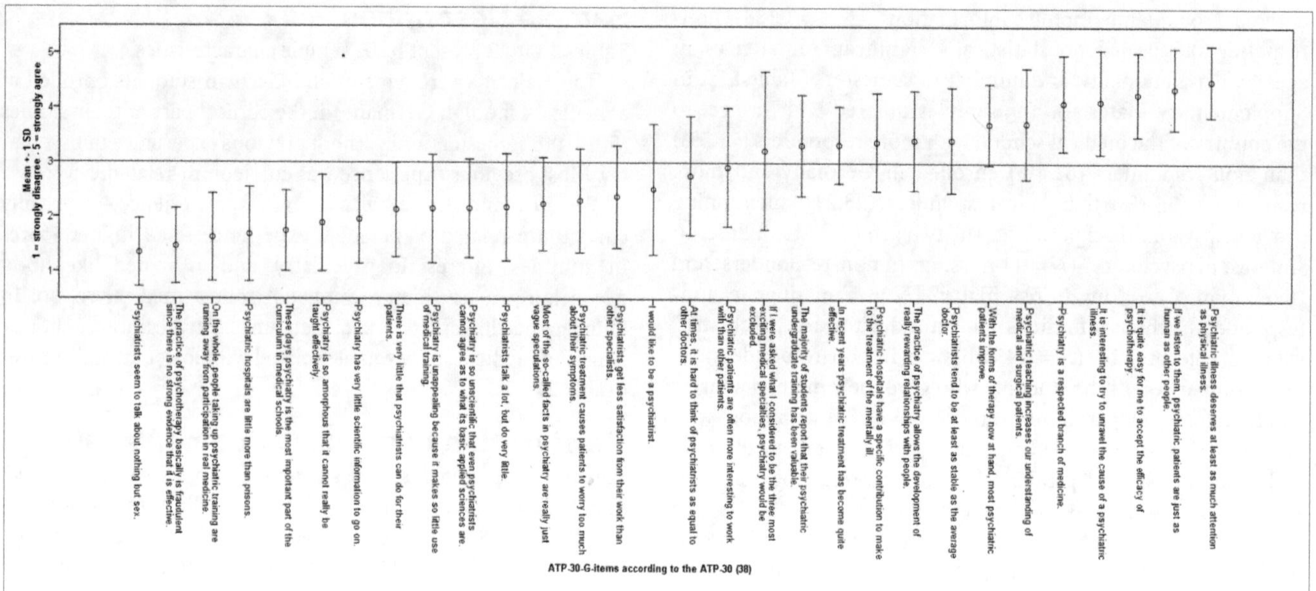

FIGURE 2 | Mean and SD of single German version of the Attitudes Toward Psychiatry Scale (ATP-30-G) items.

TABLE 3 | Mixed-effects models: German version of the Attitudes Toward Psychiatry Scale sum score (N = 1,290); interaction effect gender × type of previous experience.

Sample characteristics		Estimate	SE	df	*t*-Value/*z*-value	Pr > |*t*|
Intercept		106.85	0.92	347	116.43	<0.0001
Age (centered), years		0.18	0.11	1,290	1.69	0.091
Gender						
	Female	**3.89**	**0.96**	**1,286**	**4.03**	**<0.0001**
	Male (Ref)[a]					
Nationality						
	Swiss	4.05	4.67	1,258	0.87	0.386
	Austrian	**4.89**	**1.91**	**1,263**	**2.56**	**0.011**
	Hungarian/other	−2.01	1.78	1,289	−1.13	0.261
	German (Ref)[a]					
Medical school, country						
	Swiss	−3.37	4.61	905	−0.73	0.465
	Austrian	−1.80	1.84	60.2	−0.98	0.332
	Hungarian	**−3.60**	**1.51**	**21.9**	**−2.39**	**0.026**
	German (Ref)[a]					
Semesters						
	1st–4th semester	−1.48	1.02	636	−1.44	0.149
	>10th semester	0.73	0.95	921	0.76	0.445
	5th–10th semester (Ref)[a]					
Type of previous experience						
	Curriculum-related	**10.38**	**1.74**	**1,284**	**5.96**	**<0.0001**
	Personal	**6.69**	**2.57**	**1,267**	**2.57**	**0.009**
	Work-related	4.87	2.60	1,284	1.87	0.062
	No experience (Ref)[a]					
Gender × type of previous experience						
	Female × curriculum-related	**−4.76**	**2.10**	**1,273**	**−2.27**	**0.023**
	Female × personal	−0.93	2.86	1,272	−0.33	0.745
	Female × work-related	−3.14	3.06	1,284	−1.02	0.306
Random effects						
Residual		159.35	6.40		24.89	<0.0001
Intercept		1.30	1.64		0.80	0.213

[a]*Ref, reference category; fit statistics: AIC = 10,249.8 and BIC = 10,284.1.*
Statistically significant findings (p < 0.05) are shown in bold font.

($p < 0.0001$). Likelihood of working in psychiatry and the ATP-30-G-item "I would like to be a psychiatrist" correlated by $r = 0.79$ ($p < 0.0001$; due to missing values in the ATP item $N = 1,353$).

Outcome Scores

On average, medical students had a positive attitude toward psychiatry. The mean ATP-30-G sum score was 111.42 (SD = 13.35). The mean "interest in psychiatry score" was 63.44 (SD = 25.01), and the mean "likelihood of working in psychiatry score" was 35.22 (SD = 28.39).

Figure 2 shows means and SD for each ATP-30-G item according to the ATP-30. For readability, we inversely coded all items, with 5 indicating "strongly agree" and 1 indicating "strongly disagree." The results show that the medical students surveyed acknowledged psychiatry as a medical discipline based on scientific evidence. They believed in the efficacy of psychotherapy and, to a lesser extent, in psychiatric institutions. Attitudes toward psychiatrists were positive to ambiguous. They answered neutrally or negatively on items indicating a professional preference toward psychiatry. With respect to education, they fluctuated between a negative and a positive attitude. Overall, medical students had a neutral to positive attitude toward mental disorders and psychiatric patients.

Linear Mixed and Complementary Models

The mixed models for the three outcome variables "attitudes toward psychiatry," "interest in psychiatry," and "likelihood of working in psychiatry" and the interaction effect between gender and type of previous experience are shown in **Tables 3–5**. Mixed models including the interaction effect between gender and previous experience as a dichotomous variable are demonstrated in Tables S2–S4 in Supplementary Material. Complementary models are shown by coefficient plots (**Figures 3–5**). An additional model on the ATP item "I would like to be a psychiatrist" is shown in Table S5 in Supplementary Material.

In general, the variance between medical schools was not statistically significant in any mixed model. However, the residual variance revealed that there were individual differences among students within medical schools. The robust regression models revealed R^2 values between 8 and 11%.

Being female and having previous experience with psychiatry (compared with no experience), especially curriculum-related and personal experience, were associated with higher attitude

TABLE 4 | Mixed-effects models: interest in psychiatry (N = 1,356); interaction effect gender × type of previous experience.

Sample characteristics		Estimate	SE	df	*t*-Value/*z*-value	Pr > |*t*|
Intercept		54.64	1.62	1,356	33.66	<0.0001
Age (centered), years		0.01	0.20	1,356	0.03	0.974
Gender						
	Female	**7.05**	**1.76**	**1,356**	**4.01**	**<0.0001**
	Male (Ref)[a]					
Nationality						
	Swiss	−10.77	8.21	1,356	−1.31	0.189
	Austrian	0.73	3.36	1,356	0.22	0.827
	Hungarian/other	−5.88	3.18	1,356	−1.85	0.064
	German (Ref)[a]					
Medical school, country						
	Swiss	8.35	7.96	1,356	1.05	0.294
	Austrian	−5.29	3.03	1,356	−1.75	0.081
	Hungarian	**−4.66**	**2.36**	**1,356**	**−1.98**	**0.048**
	German (Ref)[a]					
Semesters						
	1st–4th semester	1.58	1.80	1,356	0.88	0.381
	>10th semester	−1.71	1.69	1,356	−1.01	0.311
	5th–10th semester (Ref)[a]					
Type of previous experience						
	Curriculum-related	**21.81**	**3.17**	**1,356**	**6.87**	**<0.0001**
	Personal	**20.16**	**4.62**	**1,356**	**4.36**	**<0.0001**
	Work-related	6.81	4.67	1,356	1.46	0.145
	No experience (Ref)[a]					
Gender × type of previous experience						
	Female × curriculum-related	**−7.97**	**3.81**	**1,356**	**−2.09**	**0.037**
	Female × personal	−4.83	5.13	1,356	−0.94	0.346
	Female × work-related	0.72	5.51	1,356	0.13	0.897
Random effects						
Residual		553.65	21.26		26.04	<0.0001
Intercept		–	–	–	–	–

[a]*Ref, reference category; fit statistics: AIC = 12,449.4 and BIC = 12,481.9.*
Statistically significant findings (p < 0.05) are shown in bold font.

TABLE 5 | Mixed-effects models: likelihood of working in psychiatry (N = 1,356); interaction effect gender × type of previous experience.

Sample characteristics		Estimate	SE	df	*t*-Value/*z*-value	Pr > |*t*|
Intercept		24.93	1.85	1,356	13.49	<0.0001
Age (centered), years		0.26	0.23	1,356	1.17	0.241
Gender						
	Female	**6.66**	**2.00**	**1,356**	**3.33**	**0.001**
	Male (Ref)[a]					
Nationality						
	Swiss	5.94	9.34	1,356	0.64	0.525
	Austrian	1.35	3.82	1,356	0.35	0.724
	Hungarian/other	2.04	3.62	1,356	0.56	0.573
	German (Ref)[a]					
Medical school, country						
	Swiss	−8.02	9.06	1,356	−0.88	0.377
	Austrian	−5.95	3.45	1,356	−1.72	0.085
	Hungarian	**−6.06**	**2.68**	**1,356**	**−2.26**	**0.024**
	German (Ref)[a]					
Semesters						
	1st–4th semester	**5.19**	**2.05**	**1,356**	**2.52**	**0.012**
	>10th semester	−0.92	1.92	1,356	−0.48	0.631
	5th–10th semester (Ref)[a]					
Type of previous experience						
	Curriculum-related	**25.14**	**3.61**	**1,356**	**6.96**	**<0.0001**
	Personal	**18.17**	**5.26**	**1,356**	**3.45**	**0.001**
	Work-related	**10.79**	**5.32**	**1,356**	**2.03**	**0.043**
	No experience (Ref)[a]					
Gender × type of previous experience						
	Female × curriculum-related	−7.49	4.34	1,356	−1.73	0.084
	Female × personal	−3.11	5.84	1,356	−0.53	0.595
	Female × work-related	−1.91	6.28	1,356	−0.30	0.761
Random effects						
Residual		717.79	27.57		26.04	<0.0001
Intercept		–	–	–	–	–

[a]*Ref, reference category; fit statistics: AIC = 12,801.5 and BIC = 12,834.0.*
Statistically significant findings ($p < 0.05$) are shown in bold font.

toward, interest in and likelihood of working in psychiatry scores/ATP-30-G-item score "I would like to be a psychiatrist" (**Tables 3–5**; **Figures 3–5**; Tables S2–S5 in Supplementary Material). Furthermore, there was an interaction effect between females and previous experience with psychiatry only with respect to attitudes, as shown in **Table 3**. Notably, the ATP-30-G sum score did not differ in men and women with experience (estimated mean, men = 114.63 [SE = 1.37]; estimated mean women = 115.06 [SE = 0.98]), but men without experience had lower attitude scores than did women (estimated mean, men = 106.23 [SE = 1.04]; estimated mean women = 110.10 [SE = 0.89]). In particular, curriculum-related experience was linked with comparable ATP-30-G sum scores for both genders (**Figure 6**). However, the interaction effects did not hold for robust regression (**Figure 3**).

Furthermore, the study year, nationality, and medical school were related to the outcome scores. Austrian nationality was statistically consistently linked with higher attitude scores than German nationality (**Table 3**; Table S2 in Supplementary Material; **Figure 3**).

Being enrolled at a Hungarian medical school was consistently related to lower attitude scores (**Table 3**; Table S2 in Supplementary Material; **Figure 3**), and partly to lower interest (**Table 4**; **Figure 4**) or lower likelihood of working in psychiatry (**Table 5**; Table S4 in Supplementary Material; **Figure 5**) than being enrolled at a German medical school.

Students in the preclinical part of their studies (i.e., 1st–4th semester) showed a higher estimated likelihood of working in psychiatry/higher ATP-30-G-item score "I would like to be a psychiatrist" compared with students in the clinical part (5th–10th semester) (**Table 5**; Tables S4 and S5 in Supplementary Material; **Figure 5**).

DISCUSSION

Considering the lack of young academics entering the field of psychiatry, this study aimed at analyzing medical students' perceptions of the discipline and related predictors (e.g., gender and previous experience). We also attempted to avoid certain limitations of previous research, such as mostly descriptive studies and limited sample size. We found high interest in, but low professional preference for, psychiatry and an overall positive to ambiguous attitude toward psychiatry. Multivariable analyses revealed that gender and experience with psychiatry, particularly curriculum-related and personal experience, were among the statistically significant predictors. However, the statistical models explained at most 11% of the variance.

By and large, our findings on attitudes agree with previous research (18, 21, 22). Overall, it seems that attitudes toward psychiatry have not changed over the last 20 years (21)—a time period in which new teaching models have arisen and knowledge about mental disorders has increased. Like others, we identified positive attitudes toward psychotherapy (21). According to some

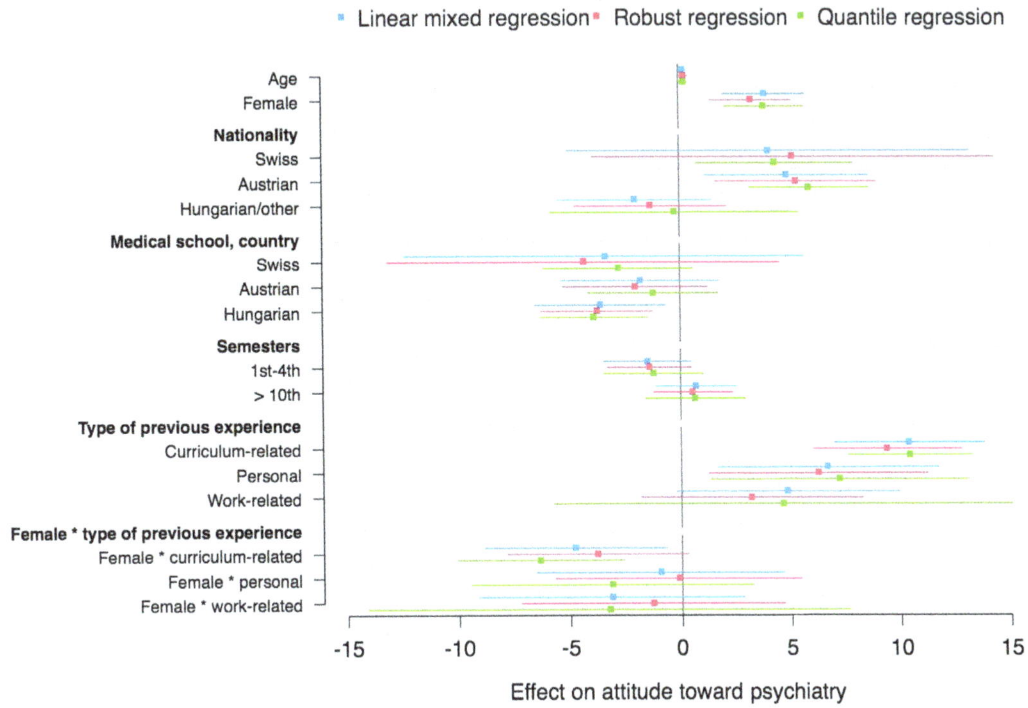

FIGURE 3 | Coefficient plot: German version of the Attitudes Toward Psychiatry Scale sum score (robust regression: $R^2 = 0.086$).

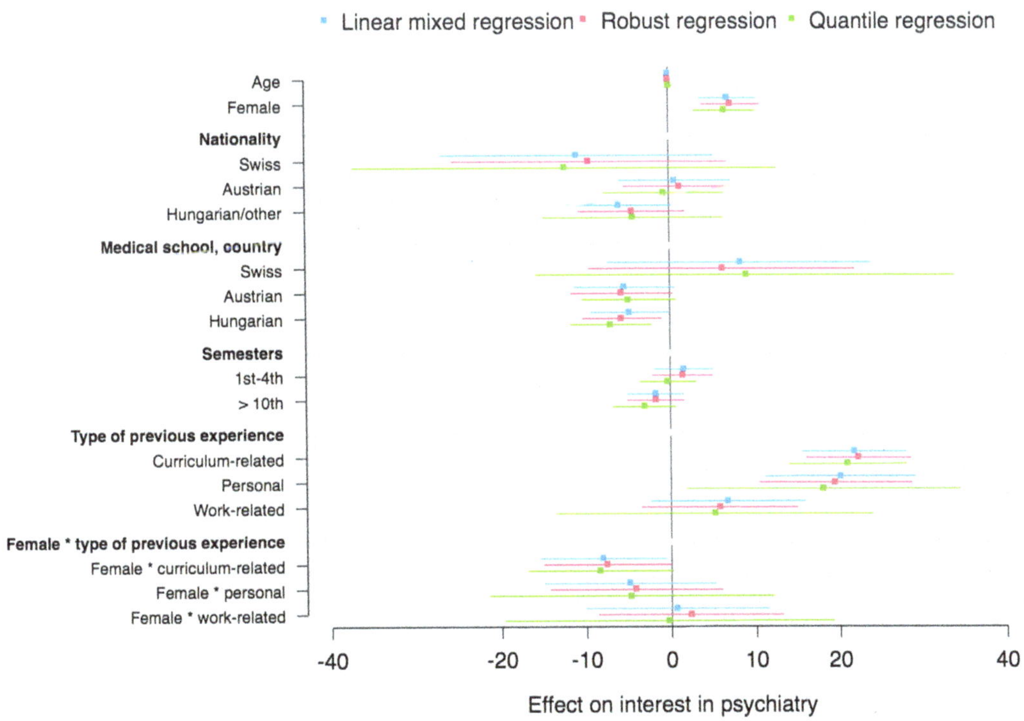

FIGURE 4 | Coefficient plot: interest in psychiatry (robust regression: $R^2 = 0.106$).

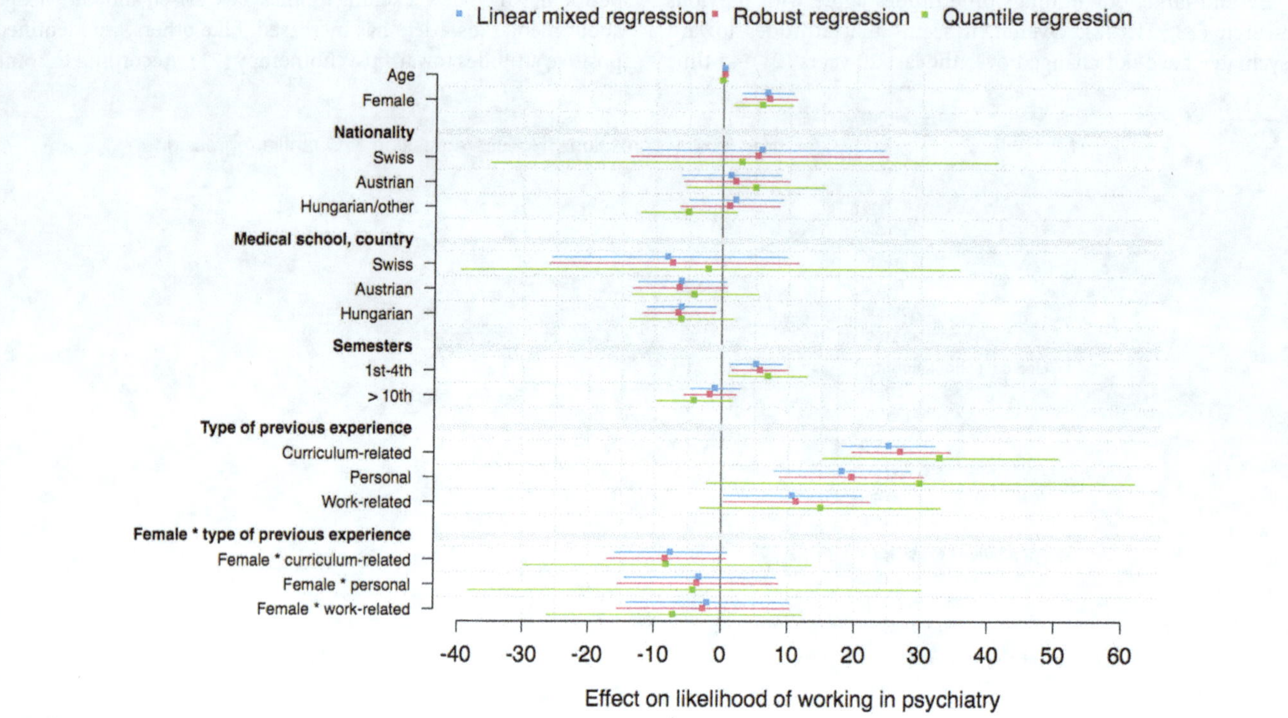

FIGURE 5 | Coefficient plot: likelihood of working in psychiatry (robust regression: $R^2 = 0.105$)

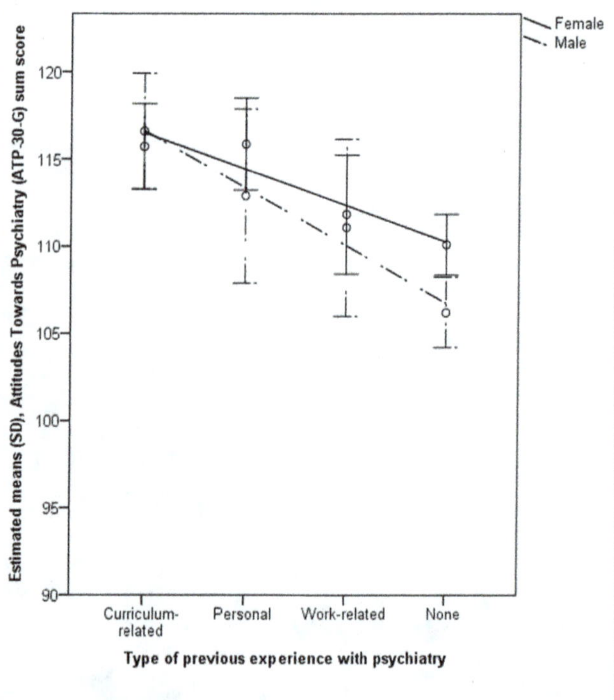

FIGURE 6 | Margins plot: gender by type of experience controlled for other predictors: German version of the Attitudes Toward Psychiatry Scale (ATP-30-G) sum score.

(21) but not all previous findings (18, 21, 45), we also found positive attitudes toward people with mental disorders. However, as previously shown, attitudes toward psychiatrists were ambiguous (18, 21) and the preference for psychiatry over other medical disciplines remained unclear (21, 25).

Women had more positive attitudes toward psychiatry, higher interest in psychiatry and a higher estimated likelihood of working in psychiatry in our study. This corresponds to most previous results (18, 20, 22–24, 28, 29) but not to all (21, 25, 27). The finding is also congruent with the fact that more women later seek a specialization in psychiatry (20), which might be linked with lifestyle aspects in terms of flexible working hours (18, 20, 25) and work-life-balance (21, 25), or with the social aspect of psychiatry rather than with medical-technical aspects (46). According to our results and previous evidence (23), attitudes toward psychiatry may improve in men after (curriculum-related) experience, whereas women's attitudes are positive irrespective of previous experience.

The positive association between previous experience with psychiatry and attitudes (18, 21, 23, 24, 47), interest in psychiatry (18), or intended career choice (20, 22, 25–27) is in line with previous evidence. Others have also identified the importance of previous personal or work-related experience with psychiatry for (early) career choice (25, 27). Due to the cross-sectional design of our study, it is impossible to make inferences about causality, but studies with repeated measures have demonstrated that attitudes toward psychiatry (28, 29, 48) or a career interest (49) can improve after curriculum-related experience.

In the meantime, widely implemented methods combining theory and practice with concepts such as problem-based learning or bedside-teaching (50, 51) or other approaches (e.g., psychiatry electives, summer institutes, exchange programs, small group teaching, simulated patients, using movies, multidisciplinary seminars, integrated teaching, attitude questionnaires, and objective structured clinical examinations, etc.) could be promising in further improving attitudes toward psychiatry (23, 52), interest in psychiatry, and/or career choice (19, 26). In particular, scenario-based learning in different settings, such as primary care or general hospitals, could prepare medical students for a potential future in psychiatry (53, 54), even if findings on the setting of clinical experience with psychiatry are contradictory (26).

As findings on attitudes toward psychiatrists were positive to ambiguous, in particular concerning a neutral attitude toward the statement that psychiatrists are not thought of as being equal to other doctors, personal contact with psychiatrists through tutorials might be helpful. The professionals themselves could contribute to overcoming stigma and to obtaining an accurate picture of psychiatry (19), given that they are aware of self-stigma (55) and stigma against their own clientele (56). Furthermore, personal experience with psychiatry might be promoted by early volunteering opportunities to come in contact with the discipline. The effectiveness of any clinical experience might rely on factors such as personal contact with patients and the development of close relationships, seeing patients recover, perceived quality of the experience or improvement in clinical skills, and understanding patients' feelings (48).

Due to our finding of a higher estimated likelihood of working in psychiatry in the first semesters, we, along with other authors (25), suggest that psychiatry as a medical discipline in a psychosocial context could be introduced earlier in the medical curriculum. However, it still remains unclear what effect an early introduction of psychiatry could have on students' general attitudes toward psychiatry. In this respect, besides timing, teaching mental disorders as being based on multiple etiologies is important. Biological explanations of mental illness (57) might increase the acceptance of medical treatment, but a holistic understanding of the etiology of mental disorders could reduce social distance (58). In any case, according to medical students themselves, psychiatry should be better integrated into the general curriculum (54), which might refer to timing and content.

Furthermore, we found differences connected with the nationality of students and the country where medical schools were located. It remains unclear why medical students from Austria had higher attitude scores than German students, as both countries have a long tradition of psychiatric medicine. Hungarian medical schools were linked with lower attitude scores. This might be related to medical faculties, education, and/or limitations in mental health politics or working conditions (11). These differences illustrate the importance of the country of the medical school for analysing medical students' attitudes toward psychiatry.

This study has strengths and limitations. We used an innovative recruitment approach in the form of snowball sampling on Facebook. Furthermore, we multivariably and hierarchically analyzed basic predictors of medical students' perceptions of psychiatry by focusing on types of previous experience with psychiatry.

However, snowball sampling does not allow for inferences about representativity in any one place. Our data include a selection bias toward German medical students from German medical schools, which might reflect different country size but also might be due to the method of recruitment. Due to the nature of online questionnaires, we could not rule out invalid data entries; for instance, diverse items on career choice showed partly inconsistent findings.

A general positive attitude toward psychiatry and psychiatric patients or choosing psychiatry as a career does not rule out negative stereotypes toward people with mental disorders (56). Accordingly, it remains moot whether some ATP-30-G statements were rated based on social desirability. Furthermore, the phrasing of certain ATP-30 items could be viewed critically (e.g., "Psychiatrists seem to talk about nothing but sex." or "If we listen to them, psychiatric patients are just as human as other people.").

Our findings have implications for future research. More specific factors need to be addressed to account for a larger proportion of the variance in statistical models. Examples of this might be: components of medical training (e.g., lectures, special psychiatric modules or clinical placement and its quality, teacher–student relationships, supportiveness, and mentoring) (18, 20, 26), personal characteristics of medical students (e.g., personality factors) (20, 23), or family history and attitudes of close social networks (25). Furthermore, future studies should include multiple medical schools and their characteristics in hierarchical models in order to better understand students' perceptions. In particular, comparable studies in other, non-German-speaking countries could help to better understand medical students' views on psychiatry and their determining factors in different educational and health systems.

In summary, in an online survey of 1,356 medical students from medical schools with German language curricula in four European countries, female gender and previous experience, particularly curriculum-related and personal experience, determined attitudes toward and interest in psychiatry, and self-predicted career choice. Opportunities for clinical experience should be promoted in medical curricula, particularly for men. Further predictor variables might contribute to a larger proportion of explained variance in statistical models.

NOMENCLATURE

ATP-30	Attitudes Toward Psychiatry Scale
ATP-30-G	German version of the Attitudes Toward Psychiatry Scale
REDCap	Research Electronic Data Capture
KEK-BE	Cantonal Ethics Committee Bern; Kantonale Ethikkomission Bern
LMMs	linear mixed models

Accordingly, approval by the KEK-BE was not required because the study type was exempt from the local legislation on research involving human beings (Human Research Act, Article 2, Section 1).

AUTHOR CONTRIBUTIONS

ML designed the study including the sample selection procedure and reviewed the manuscript. BS and his research group translated the English original version of the ATP-30 by Burra et al. (38). We further used the same predictor and "mediator variables" as described in the study of Strebel et al. (21). AG designed the statistical analysis plan and reviewed the statistical analyses as well as the manuscript. IW designed the study, conducted the statistical analyses, and wrote the manuscript. MB did the recruitment *via* Facebook and used a subset of the data for her thesis. RS, CC, BS, TT, WR, and NR reviewed the draft paper and contributed to the interpretation of the data. All authors approved the final manuscript.

ACKNOWLEDGMENTS

The authors express warm thanks to the reviewers for their advice. We thank Prof. Dr. Prakash Burra for his important work delivering the basis for our study and Dominique Rubi of the Clinical Trials Unit of the Faculty of Medicine of the University of Bern and the Inselspital, Bern University Hospital who constructed and programmed the online questionnaire by the software REDCap (32, 33). Warm thanks also to Heather Murray for language editing.

REFERENCES

1. Pincus HA. The crisis in psychiatry [correspondence]. *Lancet* (1997) 349:965. doi:10.1016/S0140-6736(05)62124-1
2. Psychiatry's identity crisis [editorial]. *Lancet* (2012) 379:1274. doi:10.1016/S0140-6736(12)60540-6
3. Barkil-Oteo A. Psychiatry's identity crisis [correspondence]. *Lancet* (2012) 379:2428. doi:10.1016/S0140-6736(12)61067-8
4. Katschnig H. Are psychiatrists an endangered species? Observations on internal and external challenges to the profession. *World Psychiatry* (2010) 9:21–8. doi:10.1002/j.2051-5545.2010.tb00257.x
5. Vigo D, Thornicroft G, Atun R. Estimating the true global burden of mental illness. *Lancet* (2016) 3:171–8. doi:10.1016/S2215-0366(15)00505-2
6. Mathers CD, Loncar D. Projections of global mortality and burden of disease from 2002 to 2030. *PLoS Med* (2006) 3:20. doi:10.1371/journal.pmed.0030442
7. WHO. editor. *The European Mental Health Action Plan*. Çeşme Izmir, Turkey Copenhagen: World Health Organization, Regional Office for Europe (2013).
8. Whiteford HA, Degenhardt L, Rehm J, Baxter AJ, Ferrari AJ, Erskine HE, et al. Global burden of disease attributable to mental and substance use disorders: findings from the Global Burden of Disease Study 2010. *Lancet* (2013) 382:1575–86. doi:10.1016/S0140-6736(13)61611-6
9. Riedel M, Czypionka T, Röhrling G, Kalmar M. *Abschätzung des zukünftigen Bedarfs an Psychiatern in Österreich. Studie im Auftrag und in Kooperation mit der Österreichischen Gesellschaft für Neuropsychopharmakologie und Biologische Psychiatrie (ÖGPB). [Estimating the future need for psychiatrists in Austria. Study on behalf of and in cooperation with the society 'Österreichischen Gesellschaft für Neuropsychopharmakologie und Biologische Psychiatrie (ÖGPB).'] [Report in German]*. Wien: Institut für Höhere Studien (IHS) [Institute for Advanced Studies] (2011).
10. Buddeberg-Fischer B, Klaghofer R, Buddeberg C. Die Motivation zur Weiterbildung in Psychiatrie und Psychotherapie: eine Untersuchung bei jungen Ärztinnen und Ärzten in der Deutschschweiz. [Young doctors' motivations for choosing psychiatry as specialty qualification in German-speaking Switzerland.] [Article in German]. *Schweiz Arch Neurol Psychiatr* (2008) 159:34–41.
11. Bitter I, Kurimay T. State of psychiatry in Hungary. *Int Rev Psychiatry* (2012) 24:307–13. doi:10.3109/09540261.2012.694856
12. WHO. *mhGAP. Mental Health Gap Action Programme. Scaling Up Care for Mental, Neurological, and Substance Use Disorders*. Geneva: World Health Organization (2008).
13. Landolt K, Giacometti-Bickel G, Bernath C, Rössler W. Möglichkeiten und Grenzen der Bedarfsschätzung in der ambulanten Psychiatrie. [Predicting the number of office-based psychiatrists needed in the future: potential and limitations.] [Article in German]. *Psychiat Prax* (2015) 42:248–54. doi:10.1055/s-0034-1369957
14. WPA. *WPA 2014-2017 Action Plan*. Chêne-Bourg, Geneva: World Psychiatric Association (2014).
15. Möller-Leimkühler AM, Möller HJ, Maier W, Gaebel W, Falkai P. EPA guidance on improving the image of psychiatry. *Eur Arch Psychiatry Clin Neurosci* (2016) 266:139–54. doi:10.1007/s00406-016-0691-8
16. RCPSych. *Recruitment Strategy 2017-2019*. London: Royal College of Psychiatrists (2017).
17. Schneider F, Falkai P, Maier W. *Psychiatrie 2020 Plus. Perspektiven, Chancen, Herausforderungen. [Psychiatry 2020 Plus. Perspectives, Prospects, Challenges.] [Report in German]*. 2nd ed. Berlin: Deutsche Gesellschaft für Psychiatrie und Psychotherapie, Psychosomatik und Nervenheilkunde [German Association for Psychiatry and Psychotherapy] (2012).
18. Lyons Z. Attitudes of medical students toward psychiatry and psychiatry as a career: a systematic review. *Acad Psychiatry* (2013) 37:150–7. doi:10.1176/appi.ap.11110204
19. Sartorius N, Gaebel W, Cleveland H-R, Stuart H, Akiyama T, Arboleda-Flórez J, et al. WPA guidance on how to combat stigmatization of psychiatry and psychiatrists. *World Psychiatry* (2010) 9:131–44. doi:10.1002/j.2051-5545.2010.tb00296.x
20. Farooq K, Lydall GJ, Bhugra D. What attracts medical students towards psychiatry? A review of factors before and during medical school. *Int Rev Psychiatry* (2013) 25:371–7. doi:10.3109/09540261.2013.823855
21. Strebel B, Obladen M, Lehmann E, Gaebel W. Einstellungen von Studierenden der Medizin zur Psychiatrie. Eine Untersuchung mit einer in das Deutsche übersetzten, erweiterten Version des ATP-30. [Attitude of medical students to psychiatry. A study with the German translated, expanded version of the ATP-30.] [Article in German]. *Nervenarzt* (2000) 71:205–12.
22. Zwerenz R, Barthel Y, Leuzinger-Bohleber M, Gieler U, Rudolf G, Schwarz R, et al. Attitudes of medical students towards psychotherapeutic treatment and training. *Z Psychosom Med Psychother* (2007) 53:258–72. doi:10.13109/zptm.2007.53.3.258
23. Kuhnigk O, Hofmann M, Böthern AM, Haufs C, Bullinger M, Harendza S. Influence of educational programs on attitudes of medical students towards psychiatry: effects of psychiatric experience, gender, and personality dimensions. *Med Teach* (2009) 31:e303–10. doi:10.1080/01421590802638048
24. Kuhnigk O, Strebel B, Schilauske J, Jueptner M. Attitudes of medical students towards psychiatry: effects of training, courses in psychiatry, psychiatric experience and gender. *Adv Health Sci Educ Theory Pract* (2007) 12:87–101. doi:10.1007/s10459-005-5045-7
25. Baller FA, Ludwig KV, Kinas-Gnadt Olivares CL, Graef-Calliess IT. Exploring the ideas and expectations of German medical students towards career choices and the speciality of psychiatry. *Int Rev Psychiatry* (2013) 25:425–30. doi:10.3109/09540261.2013.823384
26. Halder N, Hadjidemetriou C, Pearson R, Farooq K, Lydall GJ, Malik A, et al. Student career choice in psychiatry: findings from 18 UK medical schools. *Int Rev Psychiatry* (2013) 25:438–44. doi:10.3109/09540261.2013.824414
27. Aslam M, Taj T, Ali A, Badar N, Saeed F, Abbas M, et al. Psychiatry as a career: a survey of factors affecting students' interest in psychiatry as a career. *Mcgill J Med* (2009) 12:7–12.
28. Mortlock A-M, Puzzo I, Taylor S, Kumari V, Young S, Sengupta S, et al. Enrichment activities in the medical school psychiatry programme—could this be a key to engaging medical students in psychiatry? A study from a high secure forensic psychiatric hospital. *BMC Psychiatry* (2017) 17:83. doi:10.1186/s12888-017-1236-z
29. O'Connor K, Brennan D, O'Loughlin K, Wilson L, Pillay D, Clarke M, et al. Attitudes towards patients with mental illness in Irish medical students. *Ir J Med Sci* (2013) 182:679–85. doi:10.1007/s11845-013-0955-5
30. OECD. *Health Care Resources. Psychiatrists*. Paris: Organisation for Economic Co-operation and Development (2015).

31. NEFMI. *Resuscitated Health Care, Recovering Hungary—Semmelweis Plan for the Rescue of Health Care—A Professional Concept*. Budapest: Hungarian Ministry of National Resources (2011).
32. REDCap. *Research Electronic Data Capture* (2017). Available from: https://www.project-redcap.org/
33. Harris PA, Taylor R, Thielke R, Payne J, Gonzalez N, Conde JG. Research electronic data capture (REDCap)—a metadata-driven methodology and workflow process for providing translational research informatics support. *JBI* (2009) 42:377–81. doi:10.1016/j.jbi.2008.08.010
34. Buadze M. *German Medical Students Attitudes towards Psychiatry and Forensic Psychiatry as a Potential Field for Later Specialization [master's thesis]*. Bern, Pécs (CH, HU): University of Bern. University of Pécs (2017).
35. Biernacki P, Waldorf D. Snowball sampling: Problems and techniques of chain referral sampling. *SMR* (1981) 10:141–63. doi:10.1177/004912418101000205
36. Universität Bern. *Weisungen. Datenschutz im IT-Bereich der Universität Bern*. Universität Bern (2013). Available from: http://www.unibe.ch/unibe/portal/content/e152701/e322683/e325067/e323226/ul_ws_datenschutz_it_ger.pdf
37. Kanton B. *BELEX—Gesetztessammlung des Kantons Bern. BSG 152.04—Datenschutzgesetz (KDSG)*. Bern: Kanton Bern (2017).
38. Burra P, Kalin R, Leichner P, Waldron JJ, Handforth JR, Jarrett FJ, et al. The ATP 30—a scale for measuring medical students' attitudes to psychiatry. *Med Educ* (1982) 21:227–34.
39. Tabachnik BG, Fidell LS. *Using Multivariate Statistics*. 6th ed. Upper Saddle River NJ: Pearson Education (2013).
40. West BT, Welch KB, Galecki AT. *Linear Mixed Models. A Practical Guide Using Statistical Software*. Boca Raton, FL: Chapman & Hall/CRC, Taylor & Francis Group (2007).
41. Murayama K, Sakaki M, Yan VX, Smith GM. Type I error inflation in the traditional by-participant analysis to metamemory accuracy: a generalized mixed-effects model perspective. *J Exp Psychol Learn Mem Cognition* (2014) 40:1287–306. doi:10.1037/a0036914
42. SAS/STAT. *SAS® 9.4 Statements: Reference* (Cary, NC). SAS Institute Inc. (2016).
43. IBMCorp. *IBM SPSS Statistics for Windows. Release 14*. Armonk, NY: IBM Corp (2013).
44. StataCorp. *Stata Statistical Software. Release 14*. College Station, TX: StataCorp. LP (2015).
45. Rössler W, Salize HJ, Trunk V, Voges B. The attitude of medical students to psychiatric patients. *Nervenarzt* (1996) 67:757–64.
46. Tijdink JK, Soethout MB, Koerselman GF, Ten Cate TJ. The interest shown by medical students and recently qualified doctors in a career in psychiatry. *Tijdschr Psychiatr* (2008) 50:9–17.
47. Balon R. Does a clerkship in psychiatry affect medical students' attitudes toward psychiatry? *Acad Psychiatry* (2008) 32:73–5. doi:10.1176/appi.ap.32.2.73
48. Lyons Z. Impact of the psychiatry clerkship on medical student attitudes towards psychiatry and to psychiatry as a career. *Acad Psychiatry* (2014) 38:35–42. doi:10.1007/s40596-013-0017-3
49. Lyons Z, Janca A. Impact of a psychiatry clerkship on stigma, attitudes towards psychiatry, and psychiatry as a career choice. *BMC Med Educ* (2015) 15:34. doi:10.1186/s12909-015-0307-4
50. Kadmon G, Schmidt J, De Cono N, Kadmon M. Integrative vs. traditional learning from the student perspective. *GMS Z Med Ausbild* (2011) 28:Doc28. doi:10.3205/zma000740
51. Chur-Hansen A, Carr JE, Bundy C, Sanchez-Sosa JJ, Tapanya S, Wahass SH. An international perspective on behavioral science education in medical schools. *J Clin Psychol Med Settings* (2008) 15:45–53. doi:10.1007/s10880-008-9092-0
52. Nayak A. Changing medical students' attitudes to psychiatry through newer teaching techniques. *Mens Sana Monogr* (2015) 13:180. doi:10.4103/0973-1229.153338
53. Walton H. Core curriculum in psychiatry for medical students. *Med Educ* (1999) 33:204–11. doi:10.1046/j.1365-2923.1999.00390.x
54. Oakley C, Oyebode F. Medical students' views about an undergraduate curriculum in psychiatry before and after clinical placements. *BMC Med Educ* (2008) 8:26. doi:10.1186/1472-6920-8-26
55. Reich-Erkelenz D, Schmitt A, Falkai P. Psychiatrists' self-stigma, the DGPPN guideline for psychosocial interventions, and contemporary treatment strategies. *Eur Arch Psychiatry Clin Neurosci* (2015) 265:171–2. doi:10.1007/s00406-015-0586-0
56. Lauber C, Nordt C, Braunschweig C, Rössler W. Do mental health professionals stigmatize their patients? *Acta Psychiatr Scand* (2006) 113:51–9. doi:10.1111/j.1600-0447.2005.00718.x
57. Stahl S. *Stahl's Essential Psychopharmacology Online*. Cambridge, UK: Cambridge University Press (2017).
58. Schomerus G, Schwahn C, Holzinger A, Corrigan PW, Grabe HJ, Carta MG, et al. Evolution of public attitudes about mental illness: a systematic review and meta-analysis. *Acta Psychiatr Scand* (2012) 125:440–52. doi:10.1111/j.1600-0447.2012.01826.x

12

Risky Decisions in a Lottery Task are Associated with an Increase of Cocaine Use

Amrei Wittwer[1†], Lea M. Hulka[2,3†], Hans R. Heinimann[4,5], Matthias Vonmoos[2] and Boris B. Quednow[2,6]*

[1] Collegium Helveticum, University of Zurich and Swiss Federal Institute of Technology, Zurich, Switzerland, [2] Experimental and Clinical Pharmacopsychology, Department of Psychiatry, Psychotherapy, and Psychosomatics, Psychiatric Hospital, University of Zurich, Zurich, Switzerland, [3] Center for Addictive Disorders, Department of Psychiatry, Psychotherapy, and Psychosomatics, Psychiatric Hospital, University of Zurich, Zurich, Switzerland, [4] Future Resilient Systems, Singapore-ETH Centre, Singapore, Singapore, [5] Department of Environmental Systems Science, ETH Zurich, Zurich, Switzerland, [6] Neuroscience Center Zurich, University of Zurich and Swiss Federal Institute of Technology Zurich, Zurich, Switzerland

Edited by:
Rodrigo Grassi-Oliveira,
Pontifical Catholic University of Rio Grande do Sul, Brazil

Reviewed by:
Luke Clark,
University of Cambridge, UK
Joseph Kambeitz,
University of Munich, Germany

***Correspondence:**
Amrei Wittwer
awittwer@collegium.ethz.ch

† These authors have contributed equally to this work.

Cocaine use disorder is associated with maladaptive decision-making behavior, which strongly contributes to the harmful consequences of chronic drug use. Prior research has shown that cocaine users exhibit impaired neuropsychological test performances, particularly with regard to attention, learning, and memory but also in executive functions such as decision-making and impulse control. However, to what extent cocaine users show impaired decision-making under risk without feedback has not yet been investigated systematically. Therefore, to examine risk-taking behavior, 31 chronic cocaine users and 26 stimulant-naïve healthy controls who were part of the Zurich Cocaine Cognition Study, performed the Randomized Lottery Task (RALT) with winning lotteries consisting of an uncertain and a certain prospect. Results revealed that risky decisions were associated with male sex, increased cocaine use in the past year, higher cocaine concentrations in the hair, and younger age. In addition, higher levels of cocaine in the hair and cumulative lifetime consumption were associated with risky decisions, whereas potentially confounding factors including cognition and psychiatric symptoms had no significant effect. Taken together, our results indicate that cocaine users who increased their consumption over a period of 1 year show deficits in the processing of risky information accompanied with increased risk-taking. Future research should analyse whether risky decisions could potentially serve as a prognostic marker for cocaine use disorder.

Keywords: stimulants, impulsivity, gambling, addiction, risky choices, economics, reward, drug dependence

INTRODUCTION

Did cocaine use cause the financial crisis? David Nutt has been heavily criticized for his provocative statement that cocaine-using bankers with their "culture of excitement and drive and more and more and more... got us into this terrible mess" (Anderson, 2013). However, when mechanisms for dealing with uncertain information fail, as in psychiatric conditions such as cocaine use disorder, the results can really be disastrous for the individual (Bolla et al., 1998; Zack and Poulos, 2009) and result in high economic and societal costs (Olesen et al., 2012). Cocaine is the second most used illegal drug in Europe after cannabis (EMCDDA, 2014) and is considered to be the second most harmful drug after heroin (Nutt et al., 2007). Apparently, about 5–6% of cocaine users get addicted within the first year after first use, while 15–16% develop dependency in the long term (Wagner and Anthony, 2002). However, there is yet a lack of longitudinal data and, thus, it remains unclear why some individuals get addicted and others evade an addiction. Although, cocaine is an unselective monoamine reuptake inhibitor (Iversen et al., 2013), its acute rewarding effects have been primarily linked to the inhibition of dopamine transporter function and consequently, increased dopamine levels in the synaptic cleft (Ritz et al., 1987). There is mounting evidence that chronic cocaine consumption is associated with persistent structural and functional adaptive changes in brain areas involved in motivation, reward, judgment, and inhibitory control of behavior (Robinson and Kolb, 2004; Koob and Volkow, 2010). Neuropsychiatric manifestations of cocaine use disorder involve decrements in cognitive domains of attention, working memory, declarative memory, social cognition, and executive functions including decision-making and impulse control (Jovanovski et al., 2005; Nnadi et al., 2005; Verdejo-Garcia et al., 2007; Vonmoos et al., 2013a,b; Hulka et al., 2014; Preller et al., 2014). Specifically, the maladaptive decision-making strategies of cocaine users have been considered to be both: (i) similar to deficits observed in patients with lesions in the orbitofrontal and ventromedial prefrontal cortex; and (ii) an essential attribute of addictive behavior (Bechara, 2005). As effective pharmacological treatment options are currently lacking (Quednow and Herdener, 2016), an adequate characterization of maladaptive decision making as a potential core feature of cocaine addiction could be useful for the development of effective prevention and treatment strategies.

Hence, the effect of chronic drug use on decisions that involve uncertainty, or incomplete knowledge about how choices lead to outcomes, is an important field of addiction research. Indeed, in daily life we continually face trade-offs between options that promise safety and others that carry both potential for jackpot and threat. Sometimes we receive immediate feedback and are able to learn fast and, therefore, improve our decision behavior, whereas other times the outcomes of our decisions are delayed and we only learn slowly over time. In behavioral economics, uncertainty occurs in two domains with different ranges of incompleteness of information: *risk* refers to situations where the expected value of the outcomes are known (e.g., lotteries, insurance); whereas *ambiguity* indicates their likelihood is unknown and is often simply referred to as *uncertainty* (Platt and Huettel, 2008; Shafir, 2008).

Interestingly, most studies on the effect of cocaine use on decision behavior have so far focused on *ambiguous information with feedback*. They have provided evidence that chronic cocaine use is linked to deficits in the processing of reward and punishment contingencies, as measured by the Iowa Gambling Task (IGT; Bechara and Damasio, 2002; Verdejo-Garcia et al., 2007; Kjome et al., 2010). Consequently, it has been suggested that dependent cocaine users fail to incorporate ongoing feedback to guide future behaviors and instead, make impulsive decisions that are based on immediate reward availability (Bechara et al., 2002).

In this study we focussed on decisions under *risky information without feedback* in cocaine users in comparison to an age-, sex-, and verbal intelligence-matched healthy control group. Risky decisions without immediate feedback allow a derivation of solid parameters for the expected value of the outcomes, in contrast to tasks with ambiguous information, such as the IGT. We used a general linear model (GLM) approach enabling a multivariate means of establishing the predictive value of demographic (e.g., sex, age, cognitive function), task-related (e.g., probability), and cocaine- (e.g., dose) related variables concerning risky decisions. Based on a prior study demonstrating deficits in cocaine users in risky decision-making with feedback (Gorini et al., 2014), we hypothesized that cocaine users are more prone to risky decisions and that elevated risk-taking is associated with increased cocaine use.

METHODS

Participants

All individuals were tested in the 1-year follow-up measurement of the Zurich Cocaine Cognition Study (ZuCo2St; Vonmoos et al., 2013a; Hulka et al., 2014; Vonmoos et al., 2014; Hulka et al., 2015). The recruitment of participants took place at drug prevention and treatment centers, psychiatric hospitals, through advertising in local newspapers, internet platforms, and by word-of-mouth communication (for details see Vonmoos et al., 2013a). Inclusion criteria for all participants were: (1) age between 18 and 60 years, (2) proficiency in German language, (3) no use of prescription drugs affecting the CNS, (4) no current or previous Axis I DSM-IV psychiatric disorder (in cocaine users with exception of cocaine abuse/dependence and/or alcohol and nicotine abuse/dependence, attention deficit hyperactivity disorder, and a history of depression), (5) no neurological disorder or head injury, and (6) no family history of a severe DSM-IV psychiatric disorder such as schizophrenia, bipolar disorder, or obsessive-compulsive disorder. Cocaine users had to meet the DSM-IV criteria for either cocaine abuse or dependence to be included in the study.

Prior to the follow up measurements, participants were instructed to abstain from illegal drugs for $\geq$3 days and from alcohol $\geq$24 h. Additionally healthy controls were excluded if they regularly engaged in illegal drug use (>15 occasions) with the exception of occasional cannabis use. Hair samples (6 cm) from all participants were collected at baseline and follow-up and subsequently analyzed with liquid chromatography-mass spectrometry to exclude participants with opioid use and/or pronounced poly-toxic drug use patterns and to objectively characterize cocaine use over the past 6 months (for details see Vonmoos et al., 2013a). In the hair, the concentrations (pg/mg) of cocaine and its main metabolites benzoylecgonine and norcocaine were determined. The total cocaine (coc_{tot}) concentration in the hair was then calculated by the following formula according to Hoelzle et al. (2008): coc_{tot} = cocaine + benzoylecgonine + norcocaine. Additionally, the concentration of cocaethylene (coc_{eth}) was measured. Coc_{eth} is an ethyl ester of benzoylecgonine formed by the human liver metabolism when cocaine and ethanol co-occur in the blood. Thus, coc_{eth} is a reliable marker for the concomitant use of cocaine and ethanol (Pennings et al., 2002).

Of the 132 participants (79 cocaine users, 53 stimulant-naïve controls) participating in the ZuCo^{2}St follow-up, 27 (22 cocaine users, 5 controls) were excluded from the analyses, either because of illegal drug use detected in the hair and not allowed by our exclusion criteria (e.g., opioids or excessive MDMA intake), or because of newly initiated treatment with psychotropic medication (e.g., methylphenidate, antipsychotics, or antidepressants). The risk task was administered in 60 participants (34 cocaine users and 26 controls) only at the follow-up measurement. As one cocaine user had to be excluded from the analysis due to random decision-making and two cocaine users were excluded due to illegal drug use other than cocaine (see above), the final sample consisted of 31 cocaine users and 26 controls. Cocaine users were further divided into groups of (i) 10 persons with a strong increase of cocaine hair concentrations between baseline and 1-year follow-up (*increasers*), (ii) 12 persons with a strong decrease of cocaine hair concentrations (*decreasers*), and (iii) 9 users with largely unchanged cocaine use between both measurement time points (*equal users*). Criteria for increasing and decreasing cocaine use were determined by a combination of absolute and relative changes of cocaine concentration in hair samples between baseline and follow-up. The absolute criterion was based on a shift in cocaine hair concentration of at least 500 pg/mg, according to a commonly accepted cut-off value for reliable detection of cocaine use (Bush, 2008; Cooper et al., 2012). The relative criterion was based on a minimal increase of 20% or a minimal decrease of 10% in coc_{tot} (Vonmoos et al., 2014; Hulka et al., 2015).

The Ethics Committee of the Canton of Zurich approved the study. All participants provided written, informed consent and were compensated for their participation.

Clinical Interviews and Questionnaires

At the follow-up, all participants were interviewed with the Structured Clinical Interview for DSM-IV Disorders (SCID-I), which was carried out by a trained psychologist (APA, 1994). Drug use patterns were assessed by means of the Interview for Psychotropic Drug Consumption (IPDC), which has been described in detail elsewhere (Quednow et al., 2004). The brief version of the Cocaine Craving Questionnaire (CCQ) was used to assess current cocaine craving in cocaine users (Sussner et al., 2006). Current symptoms of depression were measured with the Beck Depression Inventory (BDI; Beck et al., 1961). Attention Deficit Hyperactivity Disorder (ADHD) symptoms were assessed with the ADHD Self-Rating Scale (ADHD-SR; Roesler et al., 2004).

Neuropsychological Tests

Participants underwent a broad neuropsychological and social cognitive test battery as well as psychophysiological measurements, which have been described in detail elsewhere (Preller et al., 2013, 2014; Vonmoos et al., 2013a; Hulka et al., 2014). In order to control for the influence of attention, working memory and long-term memory, four representative tests were included into the statistical model as confounding factors: The Letter Number Sequencing Task (LNST) was used to measure verbal working memory function (Wechsler, 1997), for which the dependent variable was the number of correct answers. The Spatial Working Memory task (SWM) strategy score from the Cambridge Neuropsychological Test Automated Battery (CANTAB; Strauss et al., 2006) was used to measure spatial working memory and executive function. The number of total errors tested the capability to retain spatial information and to manipulate remembered items. The Rapid Visual Processing task (RVP) from the CANTAB was administered to assess sustained attention (dependent variable: A', a signal detection measure of sensitivity that incorporates how well a person is able to detect target sequences). The German version of the Rey Auditory Verbal Learning Test (RAVLT) was administered to assess the verbal declarative memory performance (Helmstaedter et al., 2001), for which the dependent variables were learning performance (Σ trials 1–5) and delayed recall (trial 7).

Risk Task

One of the most common methods to elicit risky decisions without feedback in experimental economics involves the use of binary choice tasks that present winning lotteries in "multiple price lists" (Charness et al., 2013). Participants are presented with a set of binary lotteries where they choose from two options: (A) a lottery with an expected value; and (B) a guaranteed payoff, i.e., a cash amount that can be earned with certainty (Tversky, 1992; Schubert and Brown, 1999; Fehr-Duda, 2006). One multiple price list depicts several decisions with a fixed winning probability and decreasing guaranteed payoff, and therefore when filled out depicts the decision-maker's transition from the safe to the uncertain alternative, or their "indifference point." Anderson et al. (2007) reported three disadvantages for multiple price lists: First, they are based on internal responses only. Second, subjects often switch back and forth between the choice alternatives, resulting in inconsistent preference elicitation. Third, the multiple price list approach could be susceptible to framing effects, because subjects have a tendency to start in the middle of the table irrespective of the presented values. These disadvantages can be overcome with an experimental task with automatic data capturing that offers the single, binary lotteries in a randomized order. Here we describe such an experimental task, which simulates ecologically valid decisions under risky information with no direct feedback.

At the 1-year- follow-up, all participants performed an interactive risk task, the Randomized Lottery Task (RALT). The task presented a set of 20 binary lotteries to each subject on a computer screen, with each lottery consisting of: option A) a lottery with an expected value characterized by a randomized winning probability of 50 CHF; and option B) a guaranteed payoff that was randomly distributed between zero and the maximum outcome (50 CHF). For example, participants decided between 50 CHF with a probability of 25% *or* a guaranteed payoff of 25 CHF. Different lotteries were automatically generated for each trial: the winning probability and therefore the expected value of the lotteries as well as the guaranteed payoff were fully randomized and equally distributed in the interval between zero and one, in order to allow a comparison between trials and to avoid artifacts.

The RALT started by informing each participant that he/she will play the task for real money. Participants were informed that after completing the RALT, one of the lotteries would be randomly chosen and paid out in real money. A sequence of 20 lotteries appeared on the screen and participants had to make a choice for each of them regarding option A or B. The series of choices was recorded as a sequence consisting of 0 (guaranteed payoff rejected) and 1 (guaranteed payoff preferred) representing the choice behavior (C) in our analysis. As the task does not give any feedback, players cannot adapt their strategies over time and the monetary payoff is only revealed at the very end of the game. Therefore, each player acts independently on each decision, which is a prerequisite for the statistical analysis applied. The task additionally recorded the lotteries' so-called uncertainty premium (*up*), which is defined as the difference between the expected value of the lottery minus the value of the guaranteed payoff. Under rationality assumptions, a negative *up* of the lottery would lead to "risk-prone" behavior, whereas a positive *up* would lead to "risk-averse" behavior. The sequence of lotteries was randomized and data were recorded automatically and without immediate feedback. Both the user interface and the data-capture procedure were implemented with Visual Basic for Application (VBA) and a spreadsheet program (Microsoft EXCEL 2007).

Definition of Variables

Following Montgomery (1999), we defined four types of variables (**Table 1**), namely the response variable, covariates, factors, and nuisance covariates: risk behavior C, captured by the RALT, was our response variable that we aimed to explain with covariates (cocaine consumption, lotteries *up*, and age parameters; measured continuously on a scale), which are modified by factors (sex, cocaine user group, and cocaine craving; discrete classes) and nuisance variables (ADHD symptoms, depressive symptoms, attention, verbal, and spatial working memory, as well as verbal declarative memory). Prior findings have provided compelling evidence that dependent (Jovanovski et al., 2005; Vonmoos et al., 2013a) and to some extent also recreational cocaine users (Soar et al., 2012; Vonmoos et al., 2013a) exhibit broad neurocognitive deficits in attention, verbal, and spatial working memory, as well as verbal declarative memory. Moreover, cocaine users are more likely to suffer from depression and ADHD (Vonmoos et al., 2013a). Therefore, in order to control for potentially confounding effects of these nuisance variables on risk-taking behavior, we included them in the GLM. **Table 1** provides additional description and the acquisition method.

Statistical Analysis

The statistical analysis was based on generalized linear models (McCullagh and Nelder, 1989) using the statistical software R, aiming to identify a model that best explains the choice behavior (C) with the explanatory variables (**Table 1**). Since the response variable is binary, a logit transformation was used, assuming linearity of all the explanatory variables in the logit space (Equation 1):

$$g(n) = \mu + up + p + SEX_i + [COC_{it} + ...] + [CCQ + BZT + RAVLT_{sum}] + \varepsilon_{ij} \quad (1)$$

where η, linear predictor; $g()$, link function [logit]; μ, overall mean; *up*, lotteries uncertainty premium [CHF, risk task input]; p, probability of the uncertain alternative; SEX_j, sex [factor, i = m, f]; [coc_{lt}+...], cocaine use parameters [see **Table 1**]; [CCQ,...], nuisance due to craving and cognitive detriment [see **Table 1**]; ε_{ij}, error term, binomial distributed.

Linear and generalized linear models assume a lack of multicollinearity in the explanatory variables, which was analyzed with correlation diagnostics (R *cor* function). The model consists of three classes of explanatory variables: (1) the utility parameters (mean value μ, *up*, sex), (2) cocaine use parameters (estimated lifetime cocaine use [coc_{lt}], CCQ score, hair parameters coc_{eth} and coc_{tot},), and (3) cognitive and clinical covariates (ADHD, BDI, RVP, LNST, $RAVLT_{sum}$, $RAVLT_7$, SWM). As the number of observations in each class of sex (male, female) was unbalanced, which is typical for observational studies, a weighted squares of means analysis (Searle, 1987) was necessary.

A log transformation of the cocaine use parameters (coc_{lt}, coc_{eth}, coc_{tot}, CCQ) was calculated in order to eliminate the heavy skewness of the data distribution and increase the homogeneity of the residual variance. To identify the subset of variables with the highest explanatory power the following strategy was used: first, in order to depict the power of single effects, a type II deviance analysis was calculated, which is an analog to the variance analysis in linear models (Fox et al., 2011). A type II analysis compares the full model with all variables with (full-1) models that sequentially leave-one-out of all variables (Langsrud, 2003). Strategies for developing models and for the selection of the variables also recommend investigating the effect of first-order interactions (e.g., sex*up*). Second, an applied standard procedure was used to estimate the values and standard errors of parameters (**Tables 5, 6**), including backwards stepwise elimination based on the Akaike Information Criterion (R *stepAIC function*). Since this procedure may risk over-fitting models, we used variance inflation metrics (R *vif function*) to estimate the severity of multicollinearity and eliminate collinear explanatory variables. Third, we performed model diagnostics, such as studentized residuals, hat values and cook's distance to assess if error distributions were homogeneous and if there were influential or leveraging observations (R *influencePlot*). The outlier analysis was performed with the R *outlierTest* function.

As a risk measure derived from the choice behavior C, we calculated the indifference points, where the probabilities of choosing options A or B were both 0.5. This approach has been used widely in experimental economics. We calculated indifference points for all groups (*increasers, decreasers, equal users, control)* based on cocaine toxicological hair analyses (**Figure 1**). For each of the indifference points, confidence intervals were estimated in logit space and transformed back

TABLE 1 | Definition of variables and acquisition methods.

Variable type	Symbol	Description of variable	Acquisition method
Response	*C*	Binary variable 0 choice of the uncertain alternative 1 choice of the safe alternative	Automatically recorded by the RALT
Covariates	*up*	Uncertainty premium of the safe alternative of a lottery Expected value (x; p)–cash value (y; 1)	Automatically recorded by the RALT
	p	Probability of the uncertain alternative of a lottery	Automatically recorded by the RALT
	coc_{lt}	Lifetime amount of cocaine (g)	Drug interview
	coc_{eth}	Cocaethylene in the hair (pg/mg)	LC-MS/MS analysis of the hair
	coc_{tot}	Sum of cocaine, and its metabolites benzoylecgonine and norcocaine in the hair (pg/mg)	LC-MS/MS analysis of the hair
	age	Biological age (y)	Questionnaire
Factor	SEX	Biological aspects of femaleness/maleness	Questionnaire
	INC	Cocaine concentration measured in hair Factor 10 controls (no cocaine use) 20 increasing cocaine use 30 decreasing cocaine use 40 steady cocaine use	LC-MS/MS analysis of the hair
	CCQ	Craving for cocaine (score 0–70)	Cocaine Craving Questionnaire
Nuisance covariates	ADHD	Attention deficit hyperactivity disorder symptoms (score 0–54)	ADHD Questionnaire
	BDI	Symptoms of depression (score 0–63)	Beck Depression Inventory
	RVP	Sustained attention (score 0–1)	Rapid Visual Processing task CANTAB
	LNST	Verbal working memory (score 0–24)	Letter Number Sequencing Task
	RAVLTsum	Verbal declarative memory performance (Σtrials 1–5, score 0–75)	Rey Auditory Verbal Learning Test
	RAVLT7	Verbal declarative memory, delayed recall (score 0–15)	Rey Auditory Verbal Learning Test
	SWM	Spatial Working Memory/Executive function (score 1–37)	Spatial Working Memory task CANTAB

LC-MS/MS, liquid chromatography-tandem mass spectrometry.

to the observation space. As the indifference points depend on the *up* of the lotteries, they were depicted as a probability distribution, our additional risk metric (**Figure 2**).

RESULTS

Demographic Variables and Drug Use

Table 2 presents means, standard deviations and *t*-test statistics for demographic variables and drug use patterns. Healthy controls and cocaine users did not differ with regard to age and verbal IQ. In contrast, cocaine users had significantly fewer years of education and higher depression and ADHD scores compared to healthy controls. There was also a trend toward a greater number of males in the cocaine users than in the control group. Cocaine users had an average lifetime cocaine consumption of 744 g and hair toxicology analyses confirmed that cocaine was the primary drug of choice.

Neuropsychological Tests and Risk Task

In order to control for general neuropsychological performance with regard to preferences in the RALT risk task, verbal working memory function (LNST), spatial working memory and executive function (SWM), sustained attention (RVP'A), and verbal declarative memory performance were measured (RAVLT; **Table 2**). Healthy controls and cocaine users did not significantly differ with regard to the RVP A′, LNST, and SWM, but cocaine users performed significantly worse in both RAVLT parameters, reflecting impaired verbal declarative learning capacity and reduced delayed verbal recall. With regard to the RALT, cocaine users had significantly higher *C* values, indicating that cocaine users on average preferred the risky alternative.

Task Correlations

The correlation-matrix identifies collinearities within a data set, which is a prerequisite for proper GLM-model selection. **Table 3** depicts the correlation coefficients. In order to avoid accumulation of alpha error, the significance threshold for correlations was set at $p < 0.01$. Decision behavior *C* was significantly correlated with the *up* of the lotteries ($r = 0.46$). Moreover, coc_{lt} was negatively correlated with sustained attention (RVP), working memory (LNST), verbal learning capacity (RAVLT_sum), and verbal long-term memory (RAVLT7). Additionally, increased coc_{eth} in hair was correlated with reduced sustained attention, suggesting that the pronounced concomitant use of alcohol and cocaine is considerably worse for cognitive functioning, as shown previously (Bolla et al., 2000). These findings recapitulate the previously-reported correlations between cocaine use and cognitive impairment in this sample (Vonmoos et al., 2013a, 2014). Finally, higher age was correlated

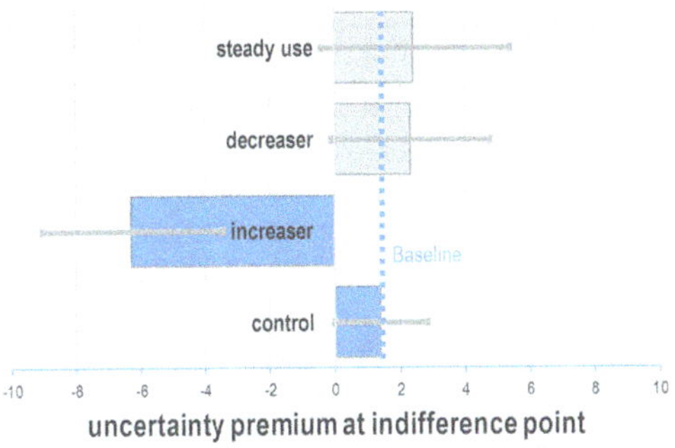

FIGURE 1 | Difference in indifference points between the controls and the groups of cocaine users. Increasers had negative indifference points indicating increased risk-taking behavior. The dotted line depicts the indifference point of the control group as the baseline condition. The estimated uncertainty premium was calculated for the four increaser classes with SEX = female; age = 30, $p = 0.5$. Bars depict estimated 95% confidence intervals.

with lower verbal working memory, while several additional cognitive parameters were intercorrelated (e.g., worse sustained attention was associated with decreased verbal declarative memory and an increased, i.e., less efficient, SWM strategy score).

The three parameters (coc_{lt}, coc_{eth}, coc_{tot}) were heavy-tailed: about 90% of the coc_{eth}, coc_{tot} data are located in the lowest 10% of the data range, whereas this amount is close to 75% for coc_{lt}. Therefore, a log-transformation of these parameters was used in further calculations to eliminate the heavy skewness of the data distribution and increase the homogeneity of the residual variance.

Analysis of Deviance

The analysis of variance likelihood ratio test of the RALT parameter *C* including all 15 explanatory variables was significant for seven variables (**Table 4**). Explanatory variables with a stronger effect on risk-taking *C* had a higher likelihood ratio, measured with the likelihood chi-square. Concerning first-order interactions, the interaction of *up* and sex was chosen in the final model, as the partial deviance of this interaction term is higher than the sum of partial deviance of the two single variables.

The interaction of the lotteries *up* and sex had the strongest effect, followed by the lotteries winning probability, increase in cocaine use, the cocaine concentration in the hair and age. A model with 15 parameters bears the risk of over-fitting and variance inflation. The variance inflation test yielded five variables with a variance inflation factor higher than 5, which indicated the presence of collinearities that were omitted in the next step.

Model Based on Changing Cocaine Use Patterns within 1 Year

The stepwise selection procedure based on the Akaike Information Criterion (AIC) resulted in a model with 5 parameters only (**Table 5**): the interaction of the lotteries *up* and sex, the lotteries winning probability, cocaine use pattern and age. Since cocaine use pattern is a factor with 4 levels, a single parameter was estimated for each level, whereas the standard

TABLE 2 | Demographic data, drug use patterns, neuropsychological and risk tasks.

	Stimulant-naïve controls ($n = 26$)	Cocaine users ($n = 31$)	*t*	*df*	*p*
DEMOGRAPHY					
Age	31.62 (9.14)	30.81 (7.87)	0.36	55	0.72
Sex (number/%)	10/16 38/62%	5/26 16/84%	3.64‡	1	0.06
Verbal IQ	109.58 (11.64)	106.32 (9.28)	1.18	55	0.25
Years of education	11.10 (1.80)	10.16 (1.49)	2.11	55	**0.04**
BDI	1.85 (2.33)	8.35 (9.50)	−3.69	55	**0.00**
ADHD-SR score	7.69 (4.92)	14.97 (8.88)	−3.90	55	**0.00**
COCAINE USE					
Lifetime (g)	–	744.04 (927.09)	–	–	–
Coc_{tot} (pg/mg)	–	14120 (37769)	–	–	–
Coc_{eth} (pg/mg)	–	818 (1750)	–	–	–
CCQ	–	18.06 (8.84)	–	–	–
NEUROPSYCHOLOGICAL TESTS					
RVP A′	0.94 (0.04)	0.92 (0.04)	1.78	55	0.08
LNST	15.19 (2.79)	14.61 (3.03)	0.75	55	0.46
RAVLT7	13.92 (1.73)	12.65 (2.51)	2.24	54	**0.03**
$RAVLT_{sum}$	66.56 (5.46)	60.65 (9.34)	2.96	54	**0.01**
SWM	30.00 (6.81)	32.48 (4.52)	−1.59	55	0.12
RISK TASK (RALT)					
C	0.39(0.49)	0.45(0.49)	−2.09	1123	**0.04**
up	−2.14(9.4)	−1.38(9.25)	−1.39	1106	0.16
p	0.49(0.26)	0.47(0.26)	1.16	1102	0.25

BDI, Beck Depression Inventory; ADHD-SR, Attention-Deficit Hyperactivity Disorder Self-Rating Scale; C, choice behavior; Coctot, cocaine + benzoylecgonine + norcocaine concentration in hair; Coceth, ethylcocaine in hair sample; CCQ, Cocaine Craving Questionnaire; p, probability of the uncertain alternative, RVP A′, Rapid Visual Processing task A′; LNST, Letter Number Sequencing Task; RAVLT sum, Rey Auditory Verbal Learning Test (Σtrials 1-5); RAVLT7, Rey Auditory Verbal Learning Test (trial 7); SWM, Spatial Working Memory; up, uncertainty premium. Significant p-values are shown in bold. Statistical tests: Independent t-tests for continuous data and ‡chi^2 for frequency data.

level equals the intercept. Only users with an increase of cocaine use (level 20) were significantly different from the controls (level 10).

Figure 1 shows that the estimated indifference points of the *increasers* were negative, indicating strong risk-taking behavior, whereas controls, steady users and *decreasers* had a positive risk premium, indicating a more risk adverse behavior. The depicted indifference points correspond to the lotteries *up* with the highest probability of choice.

Figure 2 depicts the effect of the explanatory variables on the probability distribution of the indifference point, depending on the *up* of the lotteries. Increasing cocaine use and high cocaine concentrations in the hair were associated with participants' negative *up* indicating risk-prone behavior. Male sex was associated with a smaller variability in the distribution of the indifference points.

Model Based on Cocaine Hair Concentrations

The stepwise selection procedure based on AIC resulted in a 4 parameter model (**Table 6**) consisting of the interaction of the lotteries *up* and sex, the lotteries winning probability,

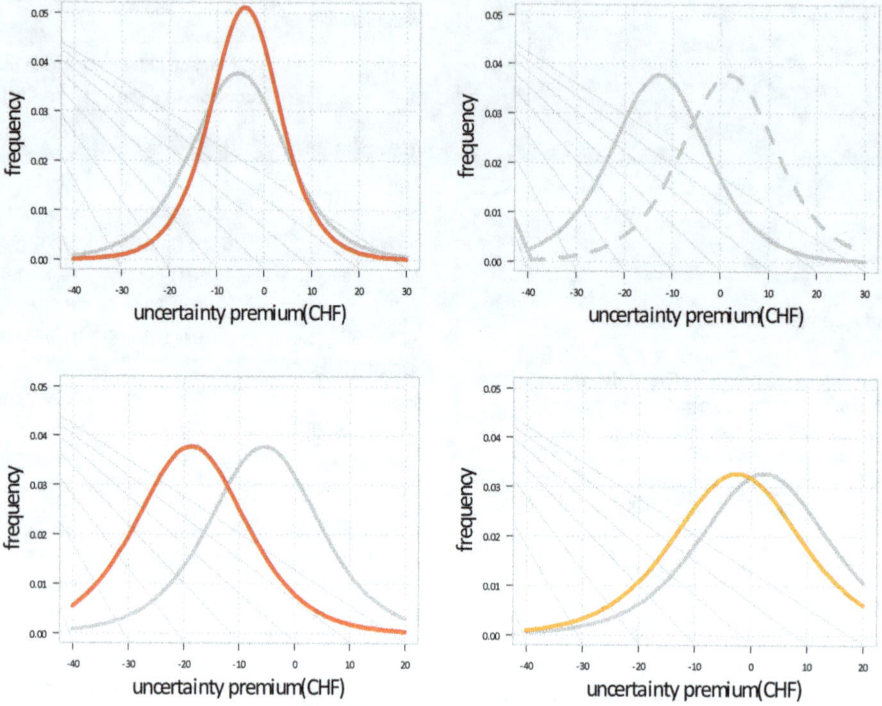

FIGURE 2 | Effect of sex, winning probability, increasing cocaine use, and cocaine in the hair on the participants' choice depicted by the distribution of the indifference points. Negative uncertainty premiums represent risk-prone behavior, while positive values indicate risk-averse behavior. [upper left] male (red) behavior shows smaller variability; [upper right] the change of the winning probability from 0.05 to 0.95 (pointed line) results in a shift toward risk-aversion; [lower left] increasing cocaine use (red) results in a shift toward risk-proneness; [lower right] high cocaine concentration in the hair (yellow) at the 95% quantile of all individuals results in a slight shift toward risk-proneness.

and the logarithm of average of coc_{tot} in the hair. Coc_{tot} was automatically selected because it showed a higher effect than cocaethylene and cumulative lifetime consumption of cocaine on risk taking. All the parameters were significant at $p < 0.001$ and the test for variance inflation resulted in values close to one, indicating no co-linearity.

Figure 2 (lower right) depicts the effect of cocaine concentrations in the hair on the probability distribution of the indifference point and indicates that high cocaine concentrations in the hair were associated with participants' negative *up*, indicating risk-prone behavior.

DISCUSSION

In this study, we report on differences in non-social decision-making without immediate feedback in cocaine users in comparison with a control group. Careful psychiatric diagnostic procedures ensured that cocaine users had few psychiatric co-morbidities and detailed toxicological hair analyses showed relatively sparse polysubstance use. Importantly, we used the GLM analysis approach as a technique to identify demographic, task-related, and cocaine-related variables with the highest explanatory power for risk-taking. Our study yielded the following major findings: (I) Cocaine users, as a group, are more prone to risky decisions in a lottery task in comparison to a matched control group without regular drug use. (II) Risky decisions are associated with male sex, self-reported increase in cocaine use, higher amounts of cocaine in the hair and younger age. More specifically, (III) *increasers* made significantly more risky decisions in the lotteries than the other groups as they chose less favorable options with a higher probability for losing in the lottery task, depicted by a negative indifference point. Moreover, (IV) higher concentrations of cocaine in the hair and cumulative lifetime consumption of cocaine across all user groups were associated with risky decisions, whereas potentially confounding factors like attention, working memory, long-term memory, symptoms of depression and ADHD had no significant effect. Taken together, our results indicate that cocaine users who increased their consumption in the last 12 months show deficits in the processing of risky information and exhibit increased risk-taking in comparison to the other groups of cocaine users and controls.

To our knowledge, the effect of cocaine use on *risky decisions without feedback* has not yet been investigated with an experimental economic analysis approach. One study examined *risky decisions with immediate feedback* in the game of dice task that presents choices between different lotteries with known expected utility. In congruence with our results, cocaine users made a significantly reduced number of safe bets although they only gambled with hypothetical monetary gains (Gorini et al., 2014).

TABLE 3 | Correlation-matrix with *r*-values for cardinal variables.

	C	*up*	*p*	coc_{lt}	coc_{eth}	coc_{tot}	Age	RVP	LNST	$RAVLT_{sum}$	$RAVLT_7$	SWM
C	1.00											
up (lot)	**0.46**	1.00										
p	−0.26	0.07	1.00									
coc_{lt}	0.01	0.04	−0.07	1.00								
coc_{eth}	−0.11	0.04	0.00	**0.40**	1.00							
coc_{tot}	−0.07	0.03	−0.02	**0.48**	**0.87**	1.00						
Age	−0.10	0.01	0.00	0.27	0.20	0.25	1.00					
RVP	0.06	−0.03	0.03	**−0.44**	**−0.40**	−0.32	−0.30	1.00				
LNST	0.02	0.04	0.04	**−0.33**	−0.21	−0.32	**−0.34**	0.33	1.00			
$RAVLT_{sum}$	0.07	0.00	0.01	**−0.42**	−0.23	−0.27	−0.18	**0.49**	**0.34**	1.00		
$RAVLT_7$	0.07	−0.01	0.03	**−0.43**	−0.24	−0.30	−0.15	**0.42**	0.31	**0.91**	1.00	
SWM	−0.02	−0.01	−0.04	0.24	0.26	0.32	0.10	**−0.43**	−0.36	−0.28	−0.18	1.00

BDI, Beck Depression Inventory; ADHD, attention-deficit hyperactivity disorder; C, choice behavior; Coctot, cocaine, benzoylecgonine, norcocaine in hair sample; Coceth, ethylcocaine in hair sample; CCQ, cocaine craving questionnaire; p, probability of the uncertain alternative, RVP A′, Rapid Visual Processing task A′; LNST, Letter Number Sequencing Task; RAVLT sum, Rey Auditory Verbal Learning Test (Σtrials 1-5); RAVLT7, Rey Auditory Verbal Learning Test (trial 7); SWM, Spatial Working Memory; up, uncertainty premium. Significant correlations ($p < 0.01$) are shown in bold.

TABLE 4 | Analysis of deviance table (type II analysis).

	LR Chi^2	*df*	*p*(>Chisq)
p	79.8	1	**0.01**
CCQ	0.02	1	0.89
BDI	1.22	1	0.26
ADHD	0.01	1	0.98
Age	5.46	1	**0.02**
coc_{eth}	44.33	1	**0.01**
coc_{lt}	1.70	1	0.19
coc_{tot}	14.04	1	**0.01**
INC	61.52	4	**0.01**
RVP A′	2.11	1	0.15
LNST	2.54	1	0.11
$RAVLT_{sum}$	2.85	1	0.09
RAVLT7	0.36	1	0.53
SWM	0.16	1	0.69
up^*SEX	364.31	2	**0.01**

Deviance measures the explanatory power of the model components. The interaction of SEX and risk premium had the biggest influence, followed by the probability of the lottery p, INC, coc_{eth}, and coc_{tot}. BDI, Beck Depression Inventory; ADHD, attention-deficit hyperactivity disorder; Coctot, cocaine, benzoylecgonine, norcocaine in hair sample; Coc_{eth}, ethylcocaine in hair sample; CCQ, cocaine craving questionnaire; INC, factor group, p, probability of the uncertain alternative, RVP A′, Rapid Visual Processing task A′; LNST, Letter Number Sequencing Task; RAVLT sum, Rey Auditory Verbal Learning Test (Σtrials 1–5); RAVLT7, Rey Auditory Verbal Learning Test (trial 7); SWM, Spatial Working Memory; up, uncertainty premium. Significant p-values are shown in bold.

TABLE 5 | Parameter estimation for a model based on cocaine use patterns.

	Estimate	SE	*z*-value	Significance
(Intercept)	2.51	0.36	6.87	***
p	−2.41	0.27	−8.75	***
Age	−0.05	0.01	−5.11	***
Group (increasers)	1.08	0.22	4.97	***
Group (decreasers)	−0.13	0.20	−0.65	
Group (steady use)	−0.15	0.23	−0.64	
Group (control)	−0.15	0.52	−0.29	
up^*SEXf	0.14	0.01	9.81	***
up^*SEXm	0.19	0.02	10.57	***

p, probability of the uncertain alternative; SEXf, female sex, SEXm, male sex; up, uncertainty premium. $^{***}p < 0.001$.

Moreover, several previous studies have shown that cocaine users exhibit disadvantageous decision-making in *ambiguous decisions with immediate feedback* that require adequate processing of reward and punishment contingencies as measured by the IGT (Bechara et al., 2002; Verdejo-Garcia et al., 2007; Vadhan et al., 2009; Kjome et al., 2010; Balconi et al., 2014) and by the Balloon Analogue Risk Task (Canavan et al., 2014): However, some studies also report no significant effect of cocaine use on performance in either the IGT (Bolla et al., 2003; Hulka et al., 2014) or the Balloon Analogue Risk Task (Gorini et al., 2014). The reasons for these inconsistent results remain unclear. It has been suggested that dependent cocaine users fail to incorporate ongoing feedback to guide future behaviors, make impulsive decisions that are based on immediate reward (Bechara et al., 2002) and fail to learn from repeated mistakes because of an insensitivity to future consequences (Bechara, 2001).

Our results indicate that risky decisions in cocaine users can also be observed without feedback, indicating an additional and more basic mechanism than the failure to learn from immediate mistakes. Zack and Poulos (2009) proposed that "...the placing of the bet, execution of the play, and anticipation of its outcome may induce a subjective state (suspense/thrill) quite apart from the outcome itself (win/lose). Thus, in gambling,

TABLE 6 | Parameter estimation for a model based on cocaine in the hair.

	Estimate	SE	z value	
(Intercept)	0.88	0.16	5.59	***
p	−2.36	0.27	−8.82	***
Log (coc_{tot}+1)	0.091	0.027	3.38	***
up*SEXf	0.13	0.014	9.32	***
up*SEXm	0.18	0.017	10.68	***

Coc_{tot}, cocaine, benzoylecgonine, norcocaine in hair sample; p, probability of the uncertain alternative; SEXf, female sex, SEXm, male sex; up, uncertainty premium. $^{***}p < 0.001$.

it is possible to subjectively *like* the state of *wanting.* This is not unique to gambling; it is seen in seduction or striptease, as well as in activities like hunting. In each case, the subject enjoys the state of pursuit *per se.* [...]. One likely subjective correlate of such pursuit is arousal." In the present study participants received no feedback on the outcome of their decisions, however, they gambled with real money as they were informed that they would receive a monetary gain at the end of the study. Our results indicate that even without the feedback of "you win!" or "you lose!" cocaine users and controls make significantly different risky decisions. Regarding possible basic mechanisms of this finding, neurophysiological studies in monkeys reveal that dopamine neurons show phasic activations related predominantly, but not exclusively, to feedback (reward and punishment), but also without feedback to risk, expectancy of reward, and the salience of the stimulus: the activations increase with reward value, probability and their multiplied product, expected value (Schultz, 2010). Dopamine has been widely implicated in reinforcement, reward, and pleasure (Schultz, 2015). In addition, Panksepp (1998) characterized dopamine as the "seeking-system" and similarly Berridge (2007) have argued that dopamine is more strongly involved in the "wanting"—i.e., the moment before and without the feedback—than in the "liking" of a result. Dopamine therefore drives the ability to recognize a stimulus as a signal for future reward and to elicit approach behavior even without direct reward. Here, we focused on this "wanting" aspect of gambling behavior in cocaine users. Interestingly, dopamine plays a similar role in pathological gambling to its role in psychostimulant addiction: chronic exposure to both gambling and psychostimulants is believed to induce profound and long lasting changes in brain function, where sensitization of dopamine pathways are considered to play a critical underlying role in the pathological effect (Robinson and Berridge, 2001). Importantly, Zack and Poulos (2009) highlighted that the signals for uncertain reward in gambling lead to dynamic changes in dopamine release, much like that induced by psychostimulant drugs. They hypothesize that these changes in dopamine release may reinforce gambling behavior regardless of its outcome. Our results may be in accordance with this hypothesis. Following this line of thought, reward-predicting stimuli may induce a pseudo-cocaine-state of "wanting" in cocaine users leading to risk-prone behavior and the ignorance of the long-term negative consequences, due to sensitization of dopamine pathways.

It has been suggested that hypothetical monetary gains might not always offer enough incentive for gambling behavior in cocaine users, therefore—in contrast to most previous studies (Bechara and Damasio, 2002; Kjome et al., 2010; Balconi et al., 2014; Canavan et al., 2014; Gorini et al., 2014)—our participants gambled with real money. However, rewards have been shown to lose some of their value when they are delayed, even though their objective reward value is the same (Ainslie, 1975). This effect might be increased in cocaine users, since they display a highly stable preference for smaller, immediate rewards compared to larger but delayed rewards (Hulka et al., 2014, 2015). However, our results indicate that the expected reward of a monetary payment at the end of the study was large enough to motivate "wanting"—behavior in cocaine users.

There are some limitations inherent to the present study. Firstly, it is impossible to substantiate whether the differences in risky decisions in cocaine users are due to a predisposition, to cocaine-induced neuroplasticity, or to an interaction of both, given that we assessed risk-taking behavior only cross-sectionally and only at the follow-up of the $ZuCo^2St$. Secondly, our results indicate that an increase in substance use is associated with a high level of risk-taking. Importantly, these results have no prognostic value so far as risk-taking was measured only at the follow-up study. Thus, it is possible that risk-taking did increase in line with cocaine use and therefore might not be valid as a prognostic marker for the development of addiction. However, this finding is interesting for future research in the context of the question of why some users get addicted while others don't, but it remains to be shown whether risk-taking could be a predictor for the development of an addiction. Thirdly, the group size was relatively modest, mainly due to our strict inclusion criteria. However, we have measured relatively pure cocaine users with very little psychiatric and no medical comorbidities, which is also an advantage. Finally, stepwise regression procedures of the kind we employed have been criticized (Henderson and Denison, 1989; Sribney, 2011). Sribney (2011) gave a helpful overview on the problems of stepwise regression analyses—e.g., in the presence of collinearity or outliers. Importantly, a GLM analysis is only a model for reality and will never depict cause/effect relationships, only possible (statistically significant) associations.

In conclusion, our results indicate that even in risky decisions without direct feedback cocaine users differ in their behavior, exhibiting risk-proneness. Interestingly, users who have increased their consumption over a period of 1 year show deficits in the processing of risky information. Considering that real world financial risks do often come with an expected value and delayed feedback this evidence strengthens the point that cocaine use could add to mismanagement and should be avoided by decision makers. Importantly, Bechara (2005) has proposed that drug users with impaired decision-making might be more vulnerable to embarking on a downward-spiraling path, because poor decision-making leads to addiction. Following this argument, future prospective studies should analyse whether neurocognitive development depicted by risky decisions could serve as a marker for addictive disorders and success of treatment.

AUTHOR CONTRIBUTIONS

AW wrote the first draft of the manuscript and contributed to the cooperation and design of the study. The risk task was designed by HH and AW. LH and MV obtained the data. The data were analyzed by HRH as well as AW and LH. AW, LH, MV, and HH were involved in the revision of the manuscript. BQ designed the study, interpreted the results, wrote and revised the manuscript, and bears responsibility for data acquisition and analyses.

ACKNOWLEDGMENTS

The study was supported by grants from the Swiss National Science Foundation (SNSF; grant No. PP00P1-123516/1 and PP00P1-146326/1) and the Olga Mayenfisch Foundation. We are grateful to Daniela Jenni, Kathrin Küpeli, Franziska Minder, and Katrin H. Preller for excellent support of recruitment and assessment of the participants.

REFERENCES

Ainslie, G. (1975). Specious reward: a behavioral theory of impulsiveness and impulse control. *Psychol. Bull.* 82, 463–496. doi: 10.1037/h0076860

Anderson, G. (2013). *Did Cocaine Use by Bankers Cause the Global Financial Crisis? The Guardian [Online].* Available online at: http://www.theguardian.com/business/shortcuts/2013/apr/15/cocaine-bankers-global-financial-crisis

Anderson, S., Harrison, G. W., Lau, M. I., and Rutstrom, E. E. (2007). Valuation using multiple price list formats. *Appl. Econ.* 39, 675–682. doi: 10.1080/00036840500462046

APA (1994). *American Psychological Association. Diagnostic and Statistical Manual of Mental Disorders: DSM-IV.* Washington, DC: American Psychiatric Association (APA).

Balconi, M., Finocchiaro, R., and Campanella, S. (2014). Reward sensitivity, decisional bias, and metacognitive deficits in cocaine drug addiction. *J. Addict. Med.* 8, 399–406. doi: 10.1097/ADM.0000000000000065

Bechara, A. (2001). Neurobiology of decision-making: risk and reward. *Semin. Clin. Neuropsychiatry* 6, 205–216. doi: 10.1053/scnp.2001.22927

Bechara, A. (2005). Decision making, impulse control and loss of willpower to resist drugs: a neurocognitive perspective. *Nat. Neurosci.* 8, 1458–1463. doi: 10.1038/nn1584

Bechara, A., and Damasio, H. (2002). Decision-making and addiction (part I): impaired activation of somatic states in substance dependent individuals when pondering decisions with negative future consequences. *Neuropsychologia* 40, 1675–1689. doi: 10.1016/S0028-3932(02)00015-5

Bechara, A., Dolan, S., and Hindes, A. (2002). Decision-making and addiction (part II): myopia for the future or hypersensitivity to reward? *Neuropsychologia* 40, 1690–1705. doi: 10.1016/S0028-3932(02)00016-7

Beck, A. T., Ward, C. H., Mendelson, M., Mock, J., and Erbaugh, J. (1961). An inventory for measuring depression. *Arch. Gen. Psychiatry* 4, 561–571. doi: 10.1001/archpsyc.1961.01710120031004

Berridge, K. C. (2007). The debate over dopamine's role in reward: the case for incentive salience. *Psychopharmacology (Berl).* 191, 391–431. doi: 10.1007/s00213-006-0578-x

Bolla, K. I., Cadet, J. L., and London, E. D. (1998). The neuropsychiatry of chronic cocaine abuse. *J. Neuropsychiatry Clin. Neurosci.* 10, 280–289. doi: 10.1176/jnp.10.3.280

Bolla, K. I., Eldreth, D. A., London, E. D., Kiehl, K. A., Mouratidis, M., Contoreggi, C., et al. (2003). Orbitofrontal cortex dysfunction in abstinent cocaine abusers performing a decision-making task. *Neuroimage* 19, 1085–1094. doi: 10.1016/S1053-8119(03)00113-7

Bolla, K. I., Funderburk, F. R., and Cadet, J. L. (2000). Differential effects of cocaine and cocaine plus alcohol on neurocognitive performance. *Neurology* 54, 2285–2292. doi: 10.1212/WNL.54.12.2285

Bush, D. M. (2008). The U.S. Mandatory guidelines for federal workplace drug testing programs: current status and future considerations. *Forensic Sci. Int.* 174, 111–119. doi: 10.1016/j.forsciint.2007.03.008

Canavan, S. V., Forselius, E. L., Bessette, A. J., and Morgan, P. T. (2014). Preliminary evidence for normalization of risk taking by modafinil in chronic cocaine users. *Addict. Behav.* 39, 1057–1061. doi: 10.1016/j.addbeh.2014.02.015

Charness, G., Uri, G., and Alex, I. (2013). Experimental methods: eliciting risk preferences. *J. Econ. Behav. Organ.* 87, 43–51. doi: 10.1016/j.jebo.2012.12.023

Cooper, G. A., Kronstrand, R., Kintz, P., and Society of Hair, T. (2012). Society of Hair Testing guidelines for drug testing in hair. *Forensic Sci. Int.* 218, 20–24. doi: 10.1016/j.forsciint.2011.10.024

EMCDDA (2014). *European Monitoring Centre for Drugs and Drug Addiction. European Drug Report 2014. Trends and developments.* Luxembourg: Publications Office of the European Union.

Fehr-Duda, H. (2006). Gender, financial risks, and probability weights. *Theory Decis.* 60, 283–313. doi: 10.1007/s11238-005-4590-0

Fox, E., Sudderth, E. B., Jordan, M. I., and Willsky, A. S. (2011). Bayesian nonparametric inference of switching dynamic linear models. *IEEE Trans. Signal Process.* 59, 1569–1585. doi: 10.1109/TSP.2010.2102756

Gorini, A., Lucchiari, C., Russell-Edu, W., and Pravettoni, G. (2014). Modulation of risky choices in recently abstinent dependent cocaine users: a transcranial direct-current stimulation study. *Front. Hum. Neurosci.* 8:661. doi: 10.3389/fnhum.2014.00661

Helmstaedter, C., Lendt, M., and Lux, S. (2001). *Verbaler Lern- und Merkfähigkeitstest.* Göttingen: Beltz.

Henderson, D., and Denison, D. R. (1989). Stepwise regression in social and psychological research. *Psychol. Rep.* 64, 251–257. doi: 10.2466/pr0.1989.64.1.251

Hoelzle, C., Scheutler, F., Uhl, M., Sachs, H., and Thieme, D. (2008). Application of discriminant analysis to differentiate between incorporation of cocaine and its congeners into hair and contamination. *Forensic Sci. Int.* 176, 13–18. doi: 10.1016/j.forsciint.2007.07.020

Hulka, L. M., Eisenegger, C., Preller, K. H., Vonmoos, M., Jenni, D., Bendrick, K., et al. (2014). Altered social and non-social decision-making in recreational and dependent cocaine users. *Psychol. Med.* 44, 1015–1028. doi: 10.1017/S0033291713001839

Hulka, L. M., Vonmoos, M., Preller, K. H., Baumgartner, M. R., Seifritz, E., Gamma, A., et al. (2015). Changes in cocaine consumption are associated with fluctuations in self-reported impulsivity and gambling decision-making. *Psychol. Med.* 45, 3097–3110. doi: 10.1017/S0033291715001063

Iversen, L., Gibbons, S., Treble, R., Setola, V., Huang, X. P., and Roth, B. L. (2013). Neurochemical profiles of some novel psychoactive substances. *Eur. J. Pharmacol.* 700, 147–151. doi: 10.1016/j.ejphar.2012.12.006

Jovanovski, D., Erb, S., and Zakzanis, K. K. (2005). Neurocognitive deficits in cocaine users: a quantitative review of the evidence. *J. Clin. Exp. Neuropsychol.* 27, 189–204. doi: 10.1080/13803390490515694

Kjome, K. L., Lane, S. D., Schmitz, J. M., Green, C., Ma, L., Prasla, I., et al. (2010). Relationship between impulsivity and decision making in cocaine dependence. *Psychiatry Res.* 178, 299–304. doi: 10.1016/j.psychres.2009.11.024

Koob, G. F., and Volkow, N. D. (2010). Neurocircuitry of addiction. *Neuropsychopharmacology* 35, 217–238. doi: 10.1038/npp.2009.110

Langsrud, Y. (2003). ANOVA for unbalanced data: use Type II instead of Type III sums of squares. *Stat. Comput.* 13, 163–167. doi: 10.1023/A:1023260610025

McCullagh, P., and Nelder, J. A. (1989). *Generalized Linear Models,* 2nd Edn. London: Chapman & Hall.

Montgomery, D. C. (1999). Experimental design for product and process design and development. *J. R. Stat. Soc. Series D* 48, 159–177. doi: 10.1111/1467-9884.00179

Nnadi, C. U., Mimiko, O. A., Mccurtis, H. L., and Cadet, L. (2005). Neuropsychiatric effects of cocaine use disorders. *J. Natl. Med. Assoc.* 97, 1504–1515.

Nutt, D., King, L. A., Saulsbury, W., and Blakemore, C. (2007). Development of a rational scale to assess the harm of drugs of potential misuse. *Lancet* 369, 1047–1053. doi: 10.1016/S0140-6736(07)60464-4

Olesen, J., Gustavsson, A., Svensson, M., Wittchen, H. U., and Jonsson, B. (2012). The economic cost of brain disorders in Europe. *Eur. J. Neurol.* 19, 155–162. doi: 10.1111/j.1468-1331.2011.03590.x

Panksepp, J. (1998). *Affective Neuroscience: The Foundations of Human and Animal Emotions*. Oxford: Oxford University Press.

Pennings, E. J. M., Leccese, A. P., and De Wolff, F. A. (2002). Effects of concurrent use of alcohol and cocaine. *Addiction* 97, 773–783. doi: 10.1046/j.1360-0443.2002.00158.x

Platt, M. L., and Huettel, S. A. (2008). Risky business: the neuroeconomics of decision making under uncertainty. *Nat. Neurosci.* 11, 398–403. doi: 10.1038/nn2062

Preller, K. H., Hulka, L. M., Vonmoos, M., Jenni, D., Baumgartner, M. R., Seifritz, E., et al. (2014). Impaired emotional empathy and related social network deficits in cocaine users. *Addict. Biol.* 19, 452–466. doi: 10.1111/adb.12070

Preller, K. H., Ingold, N., Hulka, L. M., Vonmoos, M., Jenni, D., Baumgartner, M. R., et al. (2013). Increased sensorimotor gating in recreational and dependent cocaine users is modulated by craving and attention-deficit/hyperactivity disorder symptoms. *Biol. Psychiatry* 73, 225–234. doi: 10.1016/j.biopsych.2012.08.003

Quednow, B. B., and Herdener, M. (2016). Human pharmacology for addiction medicine: from evidence to clinical recommendations. *Prog. Brain Res.* 224, 227–250. doi: 10.1016/bs.pbr.2015.07.017

Quednow, B. B., Kuhn, K. U., Hoenig, K., Maier, W., and Wagner, M. (2004). Prepulse inhibition and habituation of acoustic startle response in male MDMA ('ecstasy') users, cannabis users, and healthy controls. *Neuropsychopharmacology* 29, 982–990. doi: 10.1038/sj.npp.1300396

Ritz, M. C., Lamb, R. J., Goldberg, S. R., and Kuhar, M. J. (1987). Cocaine receptors on dopamine transporters are related to self-administration of cocaine. *Science* 237, 1219–1223. doi: 10.1126/science.2820058

Robinson, T. E., and Berridge, K. C. (2001). Incentive-sensitization and addiction. *Addiction* 96, 103–114. doi: 10.1046/j.1360-0443.2001.9611038.x

Robinson, T. E., and Kolb, B. (2004). Structural plasticity associated with exposure to drugs of abuse. *Neuropharmacology* 47(Suppl. 1), 33–46. doi: 10.1016/j.neuropharm.2004.06.025

Roesler, M., Retz, W., Retz-Junginger, P., Thome, J., Supprian, T., Nissen, T., et al. (2004). Instrumente zur diagnostik der Aufmerksamkeitsdefizit-/Hyperaktivitätsstörung (ADHS) im Erwachsenenalter. *Nervenarzt* 75, 888–895. doi: 10.1007/s00115-003-1622-2

Schubert, R., and Brown, M. (1999). Financial decision-making: are women really more risk-averse? *Am. Econ. Rev.* 89, 386–391.

Schultz, W. (2010). Dopamine signals for reward value and risk: basic and recent data. *Behav. Brain Funct.* 6:24. doi: 10.1186/1744-9081-6-24

Schultz, W. (2015). Neuronal reward and decision signals: from theories to data. *Physiol. Rev.* 95, 853–951. doi: 10.1152/physrev.00023.2014

Searle, S. R. (1987). *Linear Models for Unbalanced Data*. New York, NY: John Wiley & Sons.

Shafir, E. (2008). "Desicion making," in *MIT Encyclopedia of the Cognitive Sciences*, eds R. A. Wilson and F. C. Keil (Cambridge, MA: MIT Press), 220–223.

Soar, K., Mason, C., Potton, A., and Dawkins, L. (2012). Neuropsychological effects associated with recreational cocaine use. *Psychopharmacology (Berl).* 222, 633–643. doi: 10.1007/s00213-012-2666-4

Sribney, B. (2011). *What are Some of the Problems with Stepwise Regression [Online]. StataCorp*. Available online at: http://www.stata.com/support/faqs/statistics/stepwise-regression-problems/ (Accessed March 13, 2016).

Strauss, E., Sherman, E. M. S., and Spreen, O. A. (2006). *Compendium of Neuropsychological Tests: Administration, Norms, and Commentary*. Oxford, UK: Oxford University Press.

Sussner, B. D., Smelson, D. A., Rodrigues, S., Kline, A., Losonczy, M., and Ziedonis, D. (2006). The validity and reliability of a brief measure of cocaine craving. *Drug Alcohol Depend.* 83, 233–237. doi: 10.1016/j.drugalcdep.2005.11.022

Tversky, K. (1992). Advances in prospect theory: cumulative representation of uncertainty. *J. Risk Uncertain.* 5, 297–323. doi: 10.1007/BF00122574

Vadhan, N. P., Hart, C. L., Haney, M., Van Gorp, W. G., and Foltin, R. W. (2009). Decision-making in long-term cocaine users: effects of a cash monetary contingency on Gambling task performance. *Drug Alcohol Depend.* 102, 95–101. doi: 10.1016/j.drugalcdep.2009.02.003

Verdejo-Garcia, A., Benbrookb, A., Funderburkc, F., Davidb, P., Cadetd, J. L., and Bolla, K. (2007). The differential relationship between cocaine use and marijuana use on decision-making performance over repeat testing with the Iowa Gambling Task. *Drug Alcohol Depend.* 90, 2–11. doi: 10.1016/j.drugalcdep.2007.02.004

Vonmoos, M., Hulka, L. M., Preller, K. H., Jenni, D., Baumgartner, M. R., Stohler, R., et al. (2013a). Cognitive dysfunctions in recreational and dependent cocaine users: role of attention-deficit hyperactivity disorder, craving and early age at onset. *Br. J. Psychiatry* 203, 35–43. doi: 10.1192/bjp.bp.112.118091

Vonmoos, M., Hulka, L. M., Preller, K. H., Jenni, D., Schulz, C., Baumgartner, M. R., et al. (2013b). Differences in self-reported and behavioral measures of impulsivity in recreational and dependent cocaine users. *Drug Alcohol Depend.* 133, 61–70. doi: 10.1016/j.drugalcdep.2013.05.032

Vonmoos, M., Hulka, L. M., Preller, K. H., Minder, F., Baumgartner, M. R., and Quednow, B. B. (2014). Cognitive impairment in cocaine users is drug-induced but partially reversible: evidence from a longitudinal study. *Neuropsychopharmacology* 39, 2200–2210. doi: 10.1038/npp.2014.71

Wagner, F. A., and Anthony, J. C. (2002). From first drug use to drug dependence; developmental periods of risk for dependence upon marijuana, cocaine, and alcohol. *Neuropsychopharmacology* 26, 479–488. doi: 10.1016/S0893-133X(01)00367-0

Wechsler, D. A. (1997). *Wechsler Memory Scale, 3rd Edn. Manual.* San Antonio, TX: Psychological Corporation.

Zack, M., and Poulos, C. X. (2009). Parallel roles for dopamine in pathological gambling and psychostimulant addiction. *Curr. Drug Abuse Rev.* 2, 11–25. doi: 10.2174/1874473710902010011

13

Psychological Disorders and Ecological Factors Affect the Development of Executive Functions

Rafika Zebdi[1], Louise Goyet[2], Charlotte Pinabiaux[3] and Bahia Guellaï[4]**

[1] Laboratoire EvaCliPsy (EA CLIPSYD 4430), Université Paris Ouest Nanterre La Défense, Nanterre, France, [2] Laboratoire Paragraphe (EA 349), Université Paris 8 Vincennes-Saint-Denis, Saint-Denis, France, [3] Laboratoire CHArt (EA 4004), Université Paris Ouest Nanterre La Défense, Nanterre, France, [4] Laboratoire Ethologie, Cognition, Développement, Université Paris Ouest Nanterre La Défense, Nanterre, France

Edited by:
Rodrigo Grassi-Oliveira,
Pontifícia Universidade Católica do Rio Grande do Sul, Brazil

Reviewed by:
Breno Satler Diniz,
Universidade Federal de Minas Gerais, Brazil
Maicon Rodrigues Albuquerque,
Universidade Federal de Minas Gerais, Brazil
Bruno Kluwe Schiavon,
University of Zürich, Brazil

***Correspondence:**
Rafika Zebdi
zebdi.r@gmail.com;
Bahia Guellaï
bahia.guellai@gmail.com

The links between deficits in executive functions (EFs) (e.g., mental flexibility, inhibition capacities, etc.) and some psychological disorders (e.g., anxiety and depressive disorders) have been investigated in the past decades or so. Observations evidenced that some deficits in working memory, planning, and mental flexibility were highly correlated with anxiety and depressive disorders. The majority of studies focused on adults' population, whereas it seems important to adopt a developmental perspective to fully understand the dynamic relation of these EF/psychological disorders. We suggest to focus on the following two axes in future research: (i) relations between EF and anxiety traits through development and (ii) the possible role of external factors such as parent–child relationships on the development of EF.

Keywords: psychological disorders, development, parenting, executive functions, children

INTRODUCTION

One possible short definition of executive functions (EFs) is that they are adaptive, goal-directed behaviors that enable individuals to override more automatic responses (1, 2). EFs reflect a cognitive function that incorporates a set of abilities, which aims to coordinate and control processes such as planning skills. From a developmental perspective, EFs play an important role in the development of learning and in socio-cognitive abilities (3, 4). Although the study of EF in adulthood has long been a field of active research, little is known about early EF development. One of the reasons for this gap is the lack of age-appropriate EF tasks. Nonetheless, some studies evidenced that the first 5 years of life play a critical role in the development of EF (5, 6). Early work on infants and primates suggests that the prefrontal cortex (PFC) is operative since birth in humans and in other species (7–11). In fact, children are born with the potential to develop these skills. Despite growing interest in the development of EF, it is not clear whether this development is associated with psychological factors and/or external ones. Indeed, some clinical studies evidenced that EF deficits can be impaired by specific psychological factors such as anxiety depression and stress in adults (12, 13), whereas other studies evidenced that ecological factors such as socioeconomic status (SES) could impact EF.

In the present paper, we propose to explore the possible links between the development of EF, psychological disorders, and ecological factors based on the following two axes: (i) the links between EF and psychological factors such as anxiety disorders and (ii) the possible role of ecological factors such as macro- and micro-environmental characteristics on the development of EF.

RELATIONS BETWEEN EXECUTIVE FUNCTIONS AND ANXIETY DISORDERS

In this section, we present how psychological disorders such as anxiety can affect the development of EF in adults and adolescents. The links between EF and anxiety are more and more explored since the last decades or so (14–17). Nonetheless, the relations between EF and anxiety from a developmental perspective are far from being established and clear. Still, we do not know much about the developmental trajectory of this link and the factors that could play a role.

Deficits in some aspects of EF such as attention and memory are frequently reported in studies on anxiety disorders in adults. The main anxiety disorders explored in these studies are obsessive–compulsive disorder (OCD), posttraumatic stress disorder (PTSD), social anxiety disorder (SAD), generalized anxiety disorder (GAD), and panic disorder at a given age (children, teenagers, or adults).

Goussé et al. (18) found that adults with OCD symptoms have specific deficits in spatial working memory and planning. Memory, attention, and processing speed are also impaired in these adult populations (19). The dysfunction of EF, attention, verbal, and visual memory has been reported as being associated with PTSD in adults (20). Olff et al. (21) also indicate that PTSD patients have poorer flexibility and set shifting, planning, and working memory than trauma-exposed controls. Other studies have also shown deficits in EF in patients with SAD, such as poorer cognitive flexibility (22, 23). There are also links between panic disorders and deficits in EF in adults (24).

These relations between anxiety disorders and deficits in EF in adults can be in part explained by external factors. Indeed, stressful life events can cause temporary changes in PFC functioning, which negatively affects EF and results in impaired ability for cognitive inhibition (25).

Interestingly, the relations between anxiety disorders and EF impairment are present earlier than adulthood, but results are mixed. For example, teenagers (i.e., a non-clinical population), who present anxiety symptoms such as GAD, have been reported with deficits in EF in some studies (26). A study by Yang et al. (27) showed that children and adolescents with PTSD related to a natural disaster have deficits only in the emotional control domain compared with controls exposed to the same disaster. Other studies evidenced no links between GAD and EF in clinical adults' samples (14, 28). How can we explain those mixed results? One way would be to take a developmental perspective. For example, children with OCD symptoms showed deficits in mental set shifting supporting the frontal–striatal dysfunction hypothesis of OCD diagnosis in children as well as in adults (29). Van den Heuvel et al.'s (30) study supports the hypothesis that decreased dorsal prefrontal–striatal responsiveness is associated with impaired planning capacity in OCD patients. Because the described frontal–striatal dysfunction in OCD is independent of state anxiety and disease symptom severity, they concluded that executive impairment is a core feature in OCD.

Other studies exist but they considered a broader range of disorders called "internalizing problems" that encompass anxiety disorders and depression. Riggs et al. (31) conducted a prospective study with 6- to 9-year-old children in regular classrooms over a period of 2 years. They found that proficient inhibitory control and sequencing ability were predictive of reduction of internalizing problems. Besides, some studies with children and adolescents with internalizing disorders have evidenced impaired performance on several aspects of the EF especially linked to anxiety profiles (29, 32, 33). For example, children with OCD have impaired perceptual organization ability under time pressure compared to a control population.

Longitudinal studies are needed to explore the developmental aspect of EF, but their existence is very sparse so far. Indeed, such studies demand a very large data collection with large samples and a lot of time for delayed results. Besides, in this particular area, the lack of developmental studies may be also explained by two factors: (1) late interest in studying the link between EF and psychological disorders through development trajectories (4) and (2) differences of conceptual models of anxiety disorders that are not easily understandable from a neuropsychological perspective (17). Until now the psychological models of anxiety have only been less integrated to neuroscience research (17, 34–36). Theoretical progress is necessary to fill the gap between neurobiological data, self-assessment, and clinical data. Sharp et al. (17) suggested the creation of transdiagnostics anxiety constructs that are particularly useful to connect the psychophysiological data and the psychological models of anxiety. More precisely, some studies evidenced both heightened right-lateralized activity and left-lateralized activity across a wide range of DSM anxiety disorders such as GAD, panic disorder, SAD, and OCD (37, 38). It is an important point as authors (17) suggest to disentangle between the anxious apprehension and the anxious arousal during the examination of anxiety with regard to other constructs such as EF to avoid confusion (39).

THE POSSIBLE ROLE OF ECOLOGICAL FACTORS ON THE DEVELOPMENT OF EF

Based on Bronfenbrenner's ecological systems theory (40), it might be hypothesized that some external factors could play a role in the development of EF. This hypothesis identifies some environmental factors with which an individual interacts, such as the macrosystem that refers to the cultural contexts, or SES in which individuals live, and the microsystem that describes the groups that directly influence the child's development (e.g., family members and language). Thus, in this section, we review possible links between the development of EF and some macro- and micro-environmental factors. Given its physiological characteristics such as longer maturation, the PFC is especially sensitive to ecological factors (41, 42). Therefore, EFs are thought to develop as a result of a dynamic interaction between the child's PFC and the external environment (43, 44). The link between characteristics of the child's environment, as well as the quality of parent–child relationships, and child's cognitive development has received growing interest in the past decades or so (45).

Ecological influences may be conceptualized at different levels including the macro-environments (i.e., cultural context, for example, SES), and the micro-environments (i.e., the family setting and parent–child relationships) (46, 47). Thus, microenvironmental factors such as parents "scaffolding" (48) means that a child reach higher levels of comprehension and skill acquisition, thanks to adults' support. At the beginning, they are dependent on adult support, and then they become more independent of the way they acquire new knowledge. Thus, this support could help children to improve their executive function skills (learning to coordinate and control processes) before they must perform by their own. It is important for children to develop these skills through social relations. Indeed, social partners will teach them to cope with stress, to face issues, and to provide opportunities for directing their own actions (decision making) without any adult's control. It was shown that adverse environments resulting from neglect, abuse, violence, stress, and SES of the family may expose children to toxic stress, which disrupts brain architecture and impairs and seriously delays the development of EF (49, 50). Also, stress, lack of sleep, loneliness, or lack of exercise each could impair EF (51).

Macro-Environmental Factors and the Development of EF

An important macro-environmental factor that seems to play a role on the development of EF is the characteristics of the family setting such as SES. Some studies demonstrated that family SES is associated with children's working memory and cognitive control (52–55). More recently, Sarsour et al. (56) studied the independent and interactive associations between family SES and single parenthood to predict child EF. Single parent and family SES were associated with children' inhibitory control and cognitive flexibility such that children from low SES families who were living with one parent performed less well on EF tests than children from similarly low SES who were living with two parents. Interestingly, this study demonstrates interactions between different external factors and children EF. Moreover, mediation models help us to better understand the interaction between macro-environmental and the development of EF: the links between SES and EF are at least partially explained by associated variations in parenting behaviors (57). Besides, the level of stress, associated with a negative affectivity, has also been pointed out for its mediation role between macro-environmental factors and the development of EF (58).

Micro-Environmental Factors and the Development of EF

The Case of Bilingualism

An important aspect in the child's micro-environment is the language used at home and more specifically the fact that children may grow up in a mono- or bi-lingual environment. Some studies evidenced enhanced abilities of bilingual children to coordinate the executive control components required in performing complex tasks (59, 60). This link appears to be present early in the development as an advantage for bilingual 7- to 12-month-old infants on inhibitory control and attention over monolingual infants of the same age has been evidenced (61, 62). Therefore, it seems that executive control develops earlier in bilingual children than in comparable monolinguals (63, 64). This advantage continues to be present later in the development as bilingual adults still outperform monolinguals on EF tasks (65–67). Therefore, the mastery of two languages provides bilingual speakers cognitive benefits over monolinguals, particularly on cognitive flexibility and selective attention. To the best of our knowledge, only one study explored the effect of the bilingualism factor on EF longitudinally showing a task-specific advantage in inhibitory control in bilingual toddlers (68). Another micro-environmental factor that influences the development of EF is the role of parenting.

The Role of Parenting

Vygotsky (69) accounted that the interaction with a more competent social partner, such as the parent, fosters children's higher order cognitive functions. From this socio-constructivist point of view, the development of EF can be considered as a transfer from inter- to intra-personal regulation. The link between quality of parent–infant interactions and subsequent child's EF has been explored only recently.

Three dimensions of parenting have been associated with the development of EF (70): scaffolding, sensitivity, and mind-mindedness. Most of the studies have focused on scaffolding. This large concept refers to how parental guidance enables children to achieve level of problem solving, which they could not have reached on their own. Hughes and Ensor (71) showed that maternal scaffolding was more predictable of the development of EF at 2–4 years than imitation model or than more global positive or negative models. In another study, Bernier et al. (72) explored the relationship between scaffolding (measured as autonomy support), sensitivity, and mind-mindedness on the one hand and conflict EF[1] and impulse control on the other hand. Parenting habits were observed during free play and problem solving sessions at 12, 18, and 23 months and were correlated with several measures of EF at 18 and 26 months in 80 mother–child dyads. Independent of maternal education and general cognitive ability, they found that (1) sensitivity at 12 months was predictive of the development of conflict EF at 26 months; (2) mind-mindedness at 12 months was predictive of working memory at 18 months and of increase in EF skills between 18 and 23 months; and (3) scaffolding at 12 months was predictive of working memory and categorization at 18 months and conflict EF at 26 months. In another study, Bernier et al. (73) investigated the link between maternal interactive behavior, paternal interactive behavior, and child attachment security between 1 and 2 years of age, and child EF at 2 and 3 years. The results suggest that parental behavior and child attachment are related to child performance on EF tasks especially on cognitive flexibility components. These findings suggest that parent–child relationships may play an important

[1] Factors including measures of working memory, set shifting, and inhibition control.

role in children's developing self-regulatory capacities. More recently, Bernier et al. (74) confirmed this predictive role of attachment security at 2 years on the development of EF at 5–6 years.

The following two explanations can be made: (1) parenting provides the child with the social context in which to practice emerging regulatory skills and (2) parenting may affect brain structures involved in EF, especially the response to stress system, as it has been demonstrated in studies with animals (75). Indeed, Wagner et al. (76) evidenced that children with poorer EF had higher levels of salivary cortisol (i.e., related to stress level), and their parents reported higher parenting stress. Hence it seems that parenting and other psychological factors such as stress are important to understand the development of EF.

CONCLUSION

The idea of the present review was to explore the relations between EF and factors such as anxiety disorders and parenting through development. Much of the early influences on later EF dysfunctions appear to be transmitted through the quality of parent–child interaction during early childhood (57) and may also depend on the development of frontal brain areas and the stress response system. Interestingly, the studies reporting relationships between parenting practice and the development of EF have pointed out impacts only on some specific aspects of EF, namely, working memory and cognitive flexibility (71–73, 77). Possible hypothesis can be proposed to explain the link between EF, anxiety, and some ecological factors: (1) parenting is the main factor that impact EF development; (2) SES and bilingual environments are two important side factors playing a role in the development of EF as they are related to parental practices; and (3) poorer parenting behaviors together with a poor environment could impact EF development and predict anxiety symptoms. Interestingly, these possible scenarios are linked together. Future studies should explore the neural and social mechanisms underlying the links between parent–child relationships and the development of EF. Here, we also highlight the links between some anxiety disorders and deficits in EF. Future clinical research should take into account the transdiagnosic anxiety construct (17). It is possible that different levels of anxiety apprehension and anxiety arousal could explain results observed in previous research on the link between anxiety and EF. If these two dimensions are taken into account in a transdiagnosis construct, we could precise which dimension is associated with which aspect of EF independent of the DSM diagnosis. Investigating this axis of research would also help clarifying the pathogenesis of diverse forms of anxiety and the potential deficits in EF through development. In that sense, it would be interesting to explore the multifactorial dimensions (i.e., internal and external factors: anxiety and parent–child relationships) on the development of EF. Innovative tools, providing the support for children to develop these EF skills at home, in early care units, and in education programs, will offer new perspectives to explore the influence of children environment, parenting behavior, and clinical profiles on early development of EF. Furthermore, if we have to take into account the developmental timetable, ecological and external factors, and the variability of the clinical symptomatology, new studies should investigate the development of EF from a longitudinal perspective with infants' population and the impact of this factors on EF (cognitive) development. These new directions of research could also help to promote clinical and neuropsychological tests and to set up remediation tools for very young children.

AUTHOR CONTRIBUTIONS

All the authors participated to writing of the paper. RZ and BG contributed equally to the writing.

REFERENCES

1. Lezak MD. *Neuropsychological Assessment*. 3rd ed. New York: Oxford University Press (1995).
2. Mesulam MM. The human frontal lobes: transcending the default mode through contingent encoding. In: Stuss DT, Knight RT, editors. *Principles of Frontal Lobe Function*. Oxford: Oxford University Press (2002). p. 8–30.
3. Lyon GR, Krasnegor NG, McMenamin S. Attention, memory, and executive function. *J Dev Behav Pediatr* (1996) 17(4):278. doi:10.1097/00004703-199608000-00014
4. Roy A, Le Gall D, Roulin JL, Fournet N. Les fonctions exécutives chez l'enfant: approche épistémologique et sémiologie clinique. *Rev Neuropsychol* (2013) 4(4):287–97. doi:10.3917/rne.044.0287
5. Welsh MC, Pennington BF. Assessing frontal lobe functioning in children: views from developmental psychology. *Dev Neuropsychol* (1988) 4:199–230. doi:10.1080/87565648809540405
6. Welsh MC, Pennington BF, Groisser DB. A normative-developmental study of executive function. *Dev Neuropsychol* (1991) 7:131–49. doi:10.1080/87565649109540483
7. Diamond A. Development of the ability to use recall to guide action, as indicated by infants' performance on AB. *Child Dev* (1985) 56:868–83. doi:10.2307/1130099
8. Diamond A. Developmental time course in human infants and infant monkeys, and the neural bases of inhibitory control in reaching. *Ann N Y Acad Sci* (1990) 608:637–76. doi:10.1111/j.1749-6632.1990.tb48913.x
9. Diamond A. The development and neural bases of memory functions as indexed by the AB and delayed response tasks in human infants and infant monkeys. *Ann N Y Acad Sci* (1990) 608:267–317. doi:10.1111/j.1749-6632.1990.tb48900.x
10. Diamond A, Goldman-Rakic PS. Evidence for involvement of prefrontal cortex in cognitive changes during the first year of life: comparison of performance of human infant and rhesus monkeys on a detour task with transparent barrier. *Neuroscience* (1985) 11:832.
11. Diamond A, Goldman-Rakic PS. Comparison of human infants and rhesus monkeys on Piaget's AB task: evidence for dependence on dorsolateral prefrontal cortex. *Exp Brain Res* (1989) 74:24–40. doi:10.1007/BF00248277
12. Moritz S, Birkner C, Kloss M, Jahn H, Hand I, Haasen C, et al. Executive functioning in obsessive-compulsive disorder, unipolar depression, and schizophrenia. *Arch Clin Neuropsychol* (2002) 17:477–83. doi:10.1093/arclin/17.5.477
13. Han G, Helm J, Lucha C, Zahn-Waxler C, Hastings PD, Klimes-Dougan B. Are executive functioning deficits concurrently and predictively associated with depressive and anxiety symptoms in adolescents? *J Clin Child Adolesc Psychol* (2016) 45(1):44–58. doi:10.1080/15374416.2015.1041592
14. Airaksinen E, Larsson M, Forsell Y. Neuropsychological functions in anxiety disorders in population-based samples: evidence of episodic memory dysfunction. *J Psychiatr Res* (2005) 39:207–14. doi:10.1016/j.jpsychires.2004.06.001
15. Barrett LF. The conceptual act theory: a précis. *Emot Rev* (2014) 6(4):292–7. doi:10.1177/1754073914534479

16. Eysenck MW, Derakshan N, Santos R, Calvo MG. Anxiety and cognitive performance: attentional control theory. *Emotion* (2007) 7:336–53. doi:10.1037/1528-3542.7.2.336
17. Sharp PB, Miller GA, Heller W. Transdiagnostic dimensions of anxiety: neural mechanisms, executive functions, and new directions. *Int J Psychophysiol* (2015) 98(2):365–77. doi:10.1016/j.ijpsycho.2015.07.001
18. Goussé V, Delorme R, Chabane N, Perez-Diaz F, Flavie M, Mouren-Siméoni MC, et al. Fonctions exécutives dans le trouble obsessionnel compulsif: effet de l'âge de début des troubles. *Lencéphale* (2005) 31(6):666–71. doi:10.1016/S0013-7006(05)82424-8
19. Castaneda AE, Tuulio-Henriksson A, Marttunen M, Suvisaari J, Lönnqvist J. A review on cognitive impairments in depressive and anxiety disorders with a focus on young adults. *J Affect Disord* (2008) 106(1):1–27. doi:10.1016/j.jad.2007.06.006
20. Ferreri F, Lapp LK, Peretti CS. Current research on cognitive aspects of anxiety disorders. *Curr Opin Psychiatry* (2011) 24(1):49–54. doi:10.1097/YCO.0b013e32833f5585
21. Olff M, Polak AR, Witteveen AB, Denys D. Executive function in posttraumatic stress disorder (PTSD) and the influence of comorbid depression. *Neurobiol Learn Mem* (2014) 112:114–21. doi:10.1016/j.nlm.2014.01.003
22. Fujii Y, Kitagawa N, Shimizu Y, Mitsui N, Toyomaki A, Hashimoto N, et al. Severity of generalized social anxiety disorder correlates with low executive functioning. *Neurosci Lett* (2013) 543:42–6. doi:10.1016/j.neulet.2013.02.059
23. Frick A, Howner K, Fischer H, Eskildsen SF, Kristiansson M, Furmark T. Cortical thickness alterations in social anxiety disorder. *Neurosci Lett* (2013) 536:52–5. doi:10.1016/j.neulet.2012.12.060
24. Hovland A, Pallesen S, Hammar Å, Hansen AL, Thayer JF, Tarvainen MP, et al. The relationships among heart rate variability, executive functions, and clinical variables in patients with panic disorder. *Int J Psychophysiol* (2012) 86(3):269–75. doi:10.1016/j.ijpsycho.2012.10.004
25. Thayer JF, Hansen AL, Saus-Rose E, Johnsen BH. Heart rate variability, prefrontal neural function, and cognitive performance: the neurovisceral integration perspective on self-regulation, adaptation, and health. *Ann Behav Med* (2009) 37(2):141–53. doi:10.1007/s12160-009-9101-z
26. Tempesta D, Mazza M, Serroni N, Moschetta FS, Di Giannantonio M, Ferrara M, et al. Neuropsychological functioning in young subjects with generalized anxiety disorder with and without pharmacotherapy. *Prog Neuro-psychopharmacol Biol Psychiatry* (2013) 45:236–41. doi:10.1016/j.pnpbp.2013.06.006
27. Yang R, Xiang YT, Shuai L, Qian Y, Lai KY, Ungvari GS, et al. Executive function in children and adolescents with posttraumatic stress disorder 4 and 12 months after the Sichuan earthquake in China. *J Child Psychol Psychiatry* (2014) 55(1):31–8. doi:10.1111/jcpp.12089
28. Smitherman TA, Huerkamp JK, Miller BI, Houle TT, O'Jile JR. The relation of depression and anxiety to measures of executive functioning in a mixed psychiatric sample. *Arch Clin Neuropsychol* (2007) 22:647–54. doi:10.1016/j.acn.2007.04.007
29. Shin MS, Choi H, Kim H, Hwang JW, Kim BN, Cho SC. A study of neuropsychological deficit in children with obsessive-compulsive disorder. *Eur Psychiatry* (2008) 23(7):512–20. doi:10.1016/j.eurpsy.2008.03.010
30. Van den Heuvel OA, Veltman DJ, Groenewegen HJ, Witter MP, Merkelbach J, Cath DC, et al. Disorder-specific neuroanatomical correlates of attentional bias in obsessive-compulsive disorder, panic disorder, and hypochondriasis. *Arch Gen Psychiatry* (2005) 62(8):922–33. doi:10.1001/archpsyc.62.8.922
31. Riggs NR, Blair CB, Greenberg MT. Concurrent and 2-year longitudinal relations between executive function and the behavior of 1st and 2nd grade children. *Child Neuropsychol* (2004) 9(4):267–76. doi:10.1076/chin.9.4.267.23513
32. Beers SR, De Bellis MD. Neuropsychological function in children with maltreatment-related posttraumatic stress disorder. *Am J Psychiatry* (2002) 159(3):483–6. doi:10.1176/appi.ajp.159.3.483
33. Toren P, Sadeh M, Wolmer L, Eldar S, Koren S, Weizman R, et al. Neurocognitive correlates of anxiety disorders in children: a preliminary report. *J Anxiety Disord* (2000) 14(3):239–47. doi:10.1016/S0887-6185(99)00036-5
34. Lang PJ. Fear reduction and fear behavior: problems in treating a construct. In: Schlien J, editor. *Research in Psychotherapy III*. Washington, DC: APA (1968). p. 90–103.
35. Lang PJ. Anxiety: toward a psychophysiological definition. In: Akiskal HS, Webb WL, editors. *Psychiatric Diagnosis: Exploration of Biological Predictors*. New York: Spectrum (1978). p. 365–89.
36. Kozak MJ, Miller GA. Hypothetical constructs versus intervening variables: a reappraisal of the three-systems model of anxiety assessment. *Behav Assess* (1982) 14:347–58.
37. Heller W, Nitschke JB. The puzzle of regional brain activity in depression and anxiety: the importance of subtypes and comorbidity. *Cogn Emot* (1998) 12:421–47. doi:10.1080/026999398379664
38. Nitschke JB, Heller W, Miller GA. Anxiety, stress, and cortical brain function. In: Borod JC, editor. *The Neuropsychology of Emotion*. New York, NY: Oxford University Press (2000). p. 298–319.
39. Moser JS, Moran TP, Schroder HS, Donnellan MB, Yeung N. On the relationship between anxiety and error monitoring: a meta-analysis and conceptual framework. *Front Hum Neurosci* (2013) 7:466. doi:10.3389/fnhum.2013.00466
40. Bronfenbrenner U. Ecological systems theory. In: Vasta R, editor. *Annals of Child Development. Six Theories of Child Development: Revised Formulations and Current Issues*. London: Jessica Kingsley Publishers (1992). p. 187–249.
41. Diamond A. Normal development of prefrontal cortex from birth to young adulthood: cognitive functions, anatomy, and biochemistry. In: Stuss DT, Knight RT, editors. *Principles of Frontal Lobe Function*. London: Oxford University Press (2002). p. 466–503.
42. Diamond A. The early development of executive functions. In: Bialystock E, Craik FIM, editors. *Lifespan Cognition: Mechanisms of Change*. Oxford, England: Oxford University Press (2006). p. 70–95.
43. Calkins SD, Fox NA. Self-regulatory processes in early personality development: a multilevel approach to the study of childhood social withdrawal and aggression. *Dev Psychopathol* (2002) 14:477–98. doi:10.1017/S095457940200305X
44. Diamond A. All or none hypothesis: a global-default mode that characterizes the brain and mind. *Dev Psychol* (2009) 45:130–8. doi:10.1037/a0014025
45. Garon N, Bryson SE, Smith IM. Executive function in preschoolers: a review using an integrative framework. *Psychol Bull* (2008) 134:31–60. doi:10.1037/0033-2909.134.1.31
46. Baumeister RF, Vohs KD. Sexual economics: sex as female resource for social exchange in heterosexual interactions. *Pers Soc Psychol Rev* (2004) 8:339–63. doi:10.1207/s15327957pspr0804_2
47. Hertzman C, Boyce T. How experience gets under the skin to create gradients in developmental health. *Annu Rev Public Health* (2010) 31:329–47. doi:10.1146/annurev.publhealth.012809.103538
48. Vygotski LS. *Myslenie i rec'. French translation: Pensée et langage*. In: Sève F, editor. Paris: Messidor/Éditions Sociales (1934).
49. McClelland MM, Tominey SL. The development of self-regulation and executive function in young children. *Zero to Three J* (2014) 35:2–8.
50. Starcke K, Wiesen C, Trotzke P, Brand M. Effects of acute laboratory stress on executive functions. *Front Psychol* (2016) 7:461. doi:10.3389/fpsyg.2016.00461
51. Diamond A. Executive functions. *Annu Rev Psychol* (2013) 64:135–68. doi:10.1146/annurev-psych-113011-143750
52. Farah MJ, Shera DM, Savage JH, Betancourt L, Giannetta JM, Brodsky NL, et al. Childhood poverty: specific associations with neurocognitive development. *Brain Res* (2006) 1110:166–74. doi:10.1016/j.brainres.2006.06.072
53. Noble KG, Farah MJ, McCandliss BM. Socio-economic background modulates cognition-achievement relationships in reading. *Cogn Dev* (2006) 21(3):349–68. doi:10.1016/j.cogdev.2006.01.007
54. Noble KG, McCandliss BD, Farah MJ. Socioeconomic gradients predict individual differences in neurocognitive abilities. *Dev Sci* (2007) 10:464–80. doi:10.1111/j.1467-7687.2007.00600.x
55. Noble KG, Norman MF, Farah MJ. Neurocognitive correlates of socioeconomic status in kindergarten children. *Dev Sci* (2005) 8:74–87. doi:10.1111/j.1467-7687.2005.00394.x
56. Sarsour K, Sheridan M, Jutte D, Nuru-Jeter A, Hinshaw S, Boyce WT. Family socioeconomic status and child executive functions: the roles of language, home environment, and single parenthood. *J Int Neuropsychol Soc* (2011) 17:120–32. doi:10.1017/S1355617710001335
57. Rhoades BL, Greenberg MT, Lanza ST, Blair C. Demographic and familial predictors of early executive function development: contribution of a person-centered perspective. *J Exp Child Psychol* (2011) 108(3):638–62. doi:10.1016/j.jecp.2010.08.004

58. He Z-H, Yin W-G. Family environments and children's executive function: the mediating role of children's affective state and stress. *J Genet Psychol* (2016) 177(5):143–55. doi:10.1080/00221325.2016.1218322
59. Bialystok E. Coordination of executive functions in monolingual and bilingual children. *J Exp Child Psychol* (2011) 110:461–8. doi:10.1016/j.jecp.2011.05.005
60. Morales J, Yudes C, Gómez-Ariza CJ, Bajo MT. Bilingualism modulates dual mechanisms of cognitive control: evidence from ERPs. *Neuropsychologia* (2015) 66:157–69. doi:10.1016/j.neuropsychologia.2014.11.014
61. Kovács AM, Mehler J. Cognitive gains in 7-month-old bilingual infants. *Proc Natl Acad Sci U S A* (2009) 106:6556–60.
62. Kovács ÁM, Mehler J. Flexible learning of multiple speech structures in bilingual infants. *Science* (2009) 5940:611–2. doi:10.1126/science.1173947
63. Adi-Japha E, Berberich-Artzi J, Libnawi A. Cognitive flexibility in drawings of bilingual children. *Child Dev* (2010) 81(5):1356–66. doi:10.1111/j.1467-8624.2010.01477.x
64. Bialystok E. Global-local and trail-making tasks by monolingual and bilingual children: beyond inhibition. *Dev Psychol* (2010) 46:93–105. doi:10.1037/a0015466
65. Bialystok E, Craik FI, Klein R, Viswanathan M. Bilingualism, aging, and cognitive control: evidence from the Simon task. *Psychol Aging* (2004) 19(2):290. doi:10.1037/0882-7974.19.2.290
66. Costa A, Hernández M, Sebastián-Gallés N. Bilingualism aids conflict resolution: evidence from the ANT task. *Cognition* (2008) 106:59–86. doi:10.1016/j.cognition.2006.12.013
67. Prior A, MacWhinney B. A bilingual advantage in task switching. *Biling Lang Cognit* (2010) 13:253–62. doi:10.1017/S1366728909990526
68. Cristina Crivello C, Kuzyk O, Rodrigues M, Friend M, Zesiger P, Poulin-Dubois D. The effects of bilingual growth on toddlers' executive function. *J Exp Child Psychol* (2016) 141:121–32. doi:10.1016/j.jecp.2015.08.004
69. Vygotsky L. Interaction between learning and development. In: Gauvain M, Cole M, editors. *Readings on the Development of Children.* New York: Scientific (1978). p. 34–41.
70. Carlson SM. Executive function in context: development, measurement, theory, and experience. *Monogr Soc Res Child Dev* (2003) 68(3):138–51. doi:10.1111/j.1540-5834.2003.06803012.x
71. Hughes CH, Ensor RA. How do families help or hinder the emergence of early executive function? *New Dir Child Adolesc Dev* (2009) 123:35–50. doi:10.1002/cd.234
72. Bernier A, Carlson SM, Whipple N. From external regulation to self-regulation: early parenting precursors of young children's executive functioning. *Child Dev* (2010) 81(1):326–39. doi:10.1111/j.1467-8624.2009.01397.x
73. Bernier A, Carlson SM, Deschênes M, Matte-Gagné C. Social factors in the development of early executive functioning: a closer look at the caregiving environment. *Dev Sci* (2012) 15(1):12–24. doi:10.1111/j.1467-7687.2011.01093
74. Bernier A, Beauchamp MH, Carlson SM, Lalonde G. A secure base from which to regulate: attachment security in toddlerhood as a predictor of executive functioning at school entry. *Dev Psychol* (2015) 51(9):1177–89. doi:10.1037/dev0000032
75. Gunnar MR, Fisher PA. The early experience, stress, and prevention network. Bringing basic research on early experience and stress neurobiology to bear on preventative interventions for neglected and maltreated children. *Dev Psychopathol* (2006) 18:651–77. doi:10.1017/S0954579406060330
76. Wagner S, Müller C, Helmreich I, Huss M, Tadić A. A meta-analysis of cognitive functions in children and adolescents with major depressive disorder. *Eur Child Adolesc Psychiatry* (2015) 24:5–19. doi:10.1007/s00787-014-0559-2
77. Bibok MB, Carpendale JIM, Müller U. Parental scaffolding and the development of executive function. *New Dir Child Adolesc Dev* (2009) 123:17–34. doi:10.1002/cd.233

14

Brain Oscillatory Correlates of Altered Executive Functioning in Positive and Negative Symptomatic Schizophrenia Patients and Healthy Controls

Barbara Berger[1†], Tamas Minarik[1†], Birgit Griesmayr[2], Renate Stelzig-Schoeler[3], Wolfgang Aichhorn[3] and Paul Sauseng[1]*

[1] Department of Psychology, Biological Psychology, Ludwig-Maximilians University, Munich, Germany, [2] Department of Psychology, University of Salzburg, Salzburg, Austria, [3] University Clinic for Psychiatry and Psychotherapy, Christian-Doppler-Clinic, Paracelsus-Medical Private University, Salzburg, Austria

Edited by:
Leandro Fernandes Malloy-Diniz, Universidade Federal de Minas Gerais, Brazil

Reviewed by:
Evangelia G. Chrysikou, University of Kansas, USA
Dawei Li, Duke University, USA

***Correspondence:**
Paul Sauseng
paul.sauseng@lmu.de

† These authors have contributed equally to this work.

Working Memory and executive functioning deficits are core characteristics of patients suffering from schizophrenia. Electrophysiological research indicates that altered patterns of neural oscillatory mechanisms underpinning executive functioning are associated with the psychiatric disorder. Such brain oscillatory changes have been found in local amplitude differences at gamma and theta frequencies in task-specific cortical areas. Moreover, interregional interactions are also disrupted as signified by decreased phase coherence of fronto-posterior theta activity in schizophrenia patients. However, schizophrenia is not a one-dimensional psychiatric disorder but has various forms and expressions. A common distinction is between positive and negative symptomatology but most patients have both negative and positive symptoms to some extent. Here, we examined three groups—healthy controls, predominantly negative, and predominantly positive symptomatic schizophrenia patients—when performing a working memory task with increasing cognitive demand and increasing need for executive control. We analyzed brain oscillatory activity in the three groups separately and investigated how predominant symptomatology might explain differences in brain oscillatory patterns. Our results indicate that differences in task specific fronto-posterior network activity (i.e., executive control network) expressed by interregional phase synchronization are able to account for working memory dysfunctions between groups. Local changes in the theta and gamma frequency range also show differences between patients and healthy controls, and more importantly, between the two patient groups. We conclude that differences in oscillatory brain activation patterns related to executive processing can be an indicator for positive and negative symptomatology in schizophrenia. Furthermore, changes in cognitive and especially executive functioning in patients are expressed by alterations in a task-specific fronto-posterior connectivity even in the absence of behavioral impairment.

Keywords: positive and negative symptomatic schizophrenia, brain oscillations, executive functions, working memory, fronto-parietal network, theta, gamma

INTRODUCTION

Schizophrenia is a complex disorder comprised of widespread affective, cognitive, and behavioral disturbances and disruptions. The most widely used sub-classification of schizophrenia is the division into positive (hallucinations and delusions or confused thoughts and speech) and negative (anhedonia and withdrawal) symptomatology. Further core characteristics of the disorder are cognitive deficits such as disrupted memory processes, executive functioning, and attention. Such cognitive disturbances are usually equally present in patients showing predominantly negative or positive symptoms.

At the cortical level, patients suffering from schizophrenia (SZ) show large scale structural changes and alterations in the functional architecture of the brain. The condition is associated with significant gray and white matter volume losses (Kiriakopoulos et al., 2008; Huhlshoff Pol et al., 2002; Roalf et al., 2015; van Erp et al., 2015). Furthermore, fMRI studies indicate altered hemodynamic responses in distributed brain regions among SZ patients from sensory areas (Haenschel et al., 2009) to regions associated with higher-cognitive functioning (for a review see Ettinger et al., 2015). Electrophysiological studies also revealed dysfunctional electrophysiological activity in various parts of the cortex (Haenschel and Linden, 2011; Uhlhaas and Singer, 2015). The widespread structural and haemodynamic changes are a hallmark of schizophrenia. Yet the PFC seems to be disproportionately affected regarding structural but also functional changes (Wen et al., 2011; Zhou et al., 2015), and appears to contribute to patients' cognitive impairment (WM loss, attention deficit, impaired executive functioning, etc.).

Indeed several studies confirmed that dysactivation in the PFC is correlated with WM and executive functioning deficits (see Teffer and Semendeferi, 2012 for reviews; Etkin et al., 2013). In patients suffering from schizophrenia hypofrontality is most often reported where SZ patients display a pronounced decrease in prefrontal activation compared to healthy control participants while performance is usually but not necessarily affected (e.g., Carter et al., 1997; Callicott et al., 2003). Furthermore, Kerns et al. (2005) show that patients display reduced activity in the anterior cingulate cortex (ACC) during cognitive tasks, and that this reduction is associated with impaired conflict monitoring. In a meta-analysis by Glahn et al. (2005) clear support for hypofrontality in patients as compared to healthy controls was found. But the opposite seems to hold true in many cases; where patients consistently show increased activation (hyperfrontality) in prefrontal regions during working memory operations. Such hyperfrontality is normally interpreted as a compensatory mechanism (Callicott et al., 2003; Manoach, 2003). For example, Karlsgodt et al. (2007) found a strong positive association between the amount of prefrontal activation and performance. Manoach et al. (2000), on the other hand, report an increased prefrontal activation in SZ patients while performance was significantly impaired as compared to healthy controls. Taken together these studies indicate a less than uniform picture about frontal activation in patients with SZ during working memory task performance. What becomes clear, however, is that aberrant frontal activation during cognitive task performance and executive control is prominent in patients and might reflect general dysfunctions due to the disorder as well as mechanisms to compensate for those.

Thus, investigating WM, attention, executive control, and altered activity in the PFC seem to be a key factor for understanding the cognitive deficits associated with SZ. However, the above mentioned studies do not tell the entire story. Converging evidence suggests not only overall activation/deactivation as measured with brain imaging techniques but also transient and sustained EEG oscillatory mechanisms are crucial for understanding brain functioning in healthy as well as patient populations (Voytek and Knight, 2015). The exact timing of neuronal activity is important for information processing (e.g., O'Keefe and Recce, 1993; Singer and Gray, 1995) and rhythmic activity ranging from below 1 Hz to well above 100 Hz provide a time frame for neuronal synchrony (e.g., Buzsaki and Wang, 2012). Slow oscillations (e.g., theta 4–7 Hz) are associated with co-ordinating processes that span larger networks sometimes distributed across several cortical areas. Frontal theta oscillations—consistently found to originate in the ACC (e.g., Tsujimoto et al., 2006) are sensitive to task difficulty and prominent during maintenance and manipulation of information, during sustained attention and during unspecific processes of cognitive resource allocation (e.g., Gevins et al., 1997; Sauseng et al., 2007, 2010; Mitchell et al., 2008; Berger et al., 2014; Cavanagh and Frank, 2014). By contrast, gamma oscillations are mainly reported in connection to local information processing and co-ordination of activity in rather small networks. Gamma frequency oscillations are positively correlated with the BOLD signal and the firing of local neuronal assemblies (e.g., Roux and Uhlhaas, 2014).

A series of studies emphasizes that WM and attention deficits in patients with schizophrenia are accompanied by alterations in brain oscillatory activity. Gamma band-specific changes in the PFC are some of the most often reported oscillatory correlates of SZ, usually exhibiting lowered resting-state and task specific gamma activity (e.g., Cho et al., 2006; Basar-Eroglu et al., 2007; Gandal et al., 2012; Senkowski and Gallinat, 2015). However, contradicting findings also exist where SZ patients displayed stronger PFC gamma activity both during resting and cognitive operations in comparison to healthy control subjects (see e.g., Moran and Hong, 2011 or Senkowski and Gallinat, 2015 for a review). The dysregulation of GABAergic inhibitory neurotransmission—and hence imbalance between inhibition and excitation—is thought to underlie prefrontal gamma band changes. It might be one potential key mechanism responsible for many of the cognitive deficits in schizophrenia (Dasklakis et al., 2007; Uhlhaas and Singer, 2010; Lisman, 2012).

Another brain oscillatory pattern commonly found in SZ is increased low frequency brain activity in particular at theta, but also at delta frequencies (see Lisman, 2012 for a review). However, findings are also reported in the opposite direction where patients suffering from SZ display significantly less theta power than healthy control subjects (e.g., Koychev et al., 2012). This frontal—and especially medial frontal—slow frequency aberration in patients with SZ is well in line with their experienced deficits in WM and attention processes and might either portray the impairment itself or alternatively, a compensatory mechanism to employ prefrontal resources to counter the deficit in cognitive processing. The controversial results regarding theta increase or decrease, however, are somewhat difficult to explain as the neurobiological mechanisms behind low frequency changes in SZ are less well identified than the ones behind fast frequencies. Furthermore, it is unclear whether low and high frequency changes are related or whether they are manifestations of two entirely separate neurobiological mechanisms (Uhlhaas and Singer, 2014).

Recent research identified local oscillatory and interregional coupling mechanisms driving allocation of attention and WM operations (Sauseng et al., 2005, 2010; Mizuhara and Yamagutchi, 2007; Wang et al., 2009; Ishii et al., 2014). Thereby, fronto-parietal neural synchronization seems to play a major role for executive functions. Given that executive control and WM operations are described as deficient in patients with SZ, it would make sense if the underlying neural correlates were affected by the disorder as well. And indeed, as Griesmayr et al. (2014) could show theta coherence between frontal and posterior cortical brain areas seems to be strongly decreased during a WM task in SZ patients as compared to healthy controls. In line with this, in a PET study, Meyer-Lindenberg et al. (2001) found aberrant fronto-posterior connectivity patterns as well as hypofrontality located in the ACC during a WM task in patients suffering from schizophrenia as compared to control subjects. Additionally, Popov et al. (2015) found decreased fronto-parietal connectivity (indexed by ACC theta phase to inferior parietal gamma amplitude coupling) in patients during increased demand for executive control. These findings are well in line with work demonstrating a general dysconnectivity in schizophrenia (see Uhlhaas and Singer, 2010; Schmitt et al., 2011). Rogasch et al. (2014), for instance, present evidence for dysconnectivity between task-dependently interacting cortical and subcortical areas in SZ as compared to healthy controls. Furthermore, they conclude that the inability to generate gamma oscillations in the PFC seems to be linked to higher positive symptomatology and cognitive impairment.

Findings highlighting specific symptoms being differentially linked to altered functional brain activity indicate that patients suffering from predominantly positive or predominantly negative symptoms might have differentially affected electrophysiological correlates of cognitive and especially executive functioning. This might also explain some of the above discussed controversial fMRI/EEG results. Lisman and Buzsaki (2008) for example argue that dysregulations of theta and gamma oscillations could result in very different symptoms; the former is responsible for confusion in the order of thoughts or percepts while the latter for memory deficits. Herrmann and Demiralp (2005) found that negative symptoms correlate with a decrease in gamma activity, whereas increased gamma activity was linked to positive symptoms such as hallucinations. Despite their high value for understanding the disorder itself, it might be a critical issue that most of the electrophysiological studies differentiating between positive and negative symptomatology look at the resting state activity in patients and healthy controls only. Importantly, however, in order to link findings regarding neural correlates of executive control and working memory deficits in SZ patients with their dysfunctional neuronal processes, it is vital to investigate patients during the execution of such a task. More specifically, we wanted to investigate and compare patients with predominantly positive and predominantly negative symptomatology regarding central executive difficulties in working memory. Additionally, the aim of this study was to investigate potential brain oscillatory signatures of central executive dysfunctioning at fast as well as slow EEG frequencies.

For this purpose we examined the difference between patients with predominantly negative symptoms, patients with predominantly positive symptoms and healthy control subjects that were tightly matched in gender, age and highest level of education during executing a visuo-spatial delayed-match-to-sample working memory task with high executive function demand while EEG was recorded. We investigated whether the two patient groups and healthy controls display differences in neuronal processing in the theta and gamma frequency bands in the ACC as well as the posterior parietal cortex (right and left BA40). As outlined above these frequency bands seem to be critically involved in complex working memory operations and the specified regions of interest are crucial for fronto-parietal executive control processes. Finally, we wanted to know whether patients and control subjects differ in terms of fronto-parietal communication during a working memory task with high central executive load. Our study aims at understanding alterations of working memory related brain oscillatory activity in patients suffering from schizophrenia predominated by different symptomatologies (negative and positive). Thereby we are trying to fill a gap in the understanding of this complex disorder as, to our knowledge, there is no research that has investigated these schizophrenia sub-populations in such a manner.

MATERIALS AND METHODS

The here reported data are a reanalysis of part of the data previously published by Griesmayr et al. (2014). In comparison to this earlier publication, however, the analyzed sample was divided according to symptomatology; i.e., patients suffering from predominantly positive symptomatic and predominantly negative symptomatic schizophrenia. Moreover, in the current paper data were analyzed in EEG source space in order to identify the effects in specific regions crucially implicated in the fronto-parietal control network.

Participants

Twenty-seven patients meeting ICD 10- criteria for schizophrenia participated in the study. Patients were recruited from the in- and outpatient facilities of the "Christian-Doppler Klinik Salzburg." They had normal or corrected to normal vision and intact color vision. None of the patients showed a history of neurological illness or had alcohol or substance abuse within the last month prior to study participation. Further criteria for participation were that pharmacological treatment was stable and that they did not have acute florid symptomatology. Seven participants had to be excluded from data analysis because they could not finish the task ($n = 3$), the EEG was too heavily contaminated with artifacts ($n = 4$). Severity of clinical symptomatology was assessed with the PANSS (Positive and Negative Syndrome Scale; Kay et al., 1987) by trained psychiatrists. The obtained scores were used to classify patients either as "predominantly negative symptomatic" or "predominantly positive symptomatic" (later referred to as NEG and POS, respectively) which resulted in the two patient sub-groups (NEG and POS) with 10 patients each (see **Table 1** for details and statistical comparisons). The two patient groups were matched according to age, gender, and highest education level. The diagnostic subgroups of the NEG and POS groups were paranoid schizophrenia (NEG: $n = 7$; POS: $n = 9$), undifferentiated schizophrenia (NEG: $n = 1$) and schizoaffective disorder (NEG: $n = 1$; POS: $n = 2$). Patients received treatment with atypical (NEG: $n = 9$; POS: $n = 5$), typical (POS: $n = 2$), and combined atypical and typical (NEG: $n = 1$; POS: $n = 3$) antipsychotics. Additionally, some participants received low doses of benzodiazepines (POS: $n = 3$) and/or antidepressants (NEG: $n = 5$; POS: $n = 3$). The mean chlorpromazine equivalent for NEG was 321.67 mg/day (SD = 257.92) and for POS 806.68 mg/day (SD = 326.87) (see Möller et al., 2000; Woods, 2003; see **Table 1** for statistical comparisons).

The 10 healthy control participants (later referred to as CON group) are a sub-set of the 21 healthy controls used by Griesmayr et al. (2014). They were matched to the two patient groups according to age, gender and level of highest education. Prior to testing they completed the Brief Symptom Inventory (Franke, 2000) which screens for clinically relevant psychological stress symptoms and the Structured Clinical Interview (SCI-I) to check for any mental disorders. Moreover, participants were excluded if they had any neurological diseases or first-degree relatives with a psychiatric disorder as well as when they reported alcohol or substance abuse within the last month prior to study participation.

All participants gave a written informed consent and were monetarily reimbursed for participation. The study was approved by the ethics committee of the Federal State of Salzburg and conducted in agreement with the Declaration of Helsinki.

Experimental Procedure

Participants performed a visuo-spatial delayed-match-to-sample working memory task in a dimly lit room. The stimuli were presented centrally on a computer screen with Presentation® 0.71. The memory set was presented at the beginning of each trial for 700 ms as a 6 × 6 matrix (visual angle of 9.2° × 9.2°) in which either one (load 1) or three (load 3) colored squares were presented. Additionally, if the squares were green, participants simply needed to retain their position for a delay period of 2000 ms (retention task); while if the squares were red they needed to mentally rotate their positions around a vertical line in the middle of the matrix (manipulation task) during the delay interval. During the 2000 ms delay period a mask was presented to prevent afterimages. Thereafter, a probe matrix was presented in which one or three (depending on load) gray squares were presented for a further 2000 ms. Participants then needed to indicate by mouse button press whether the square locations in the probe matrix matched the memory set or not (or the mentally rotated version thereof, depending on task). For non-match trials one of the squares in the probe matrix was shifted for one location. Between trials participants saw a fixation cross (duration jittered between 2100 and 2500 ms; see **Figure 1** for depiction of trial structure and stimulus example). Participants were instructed to answer as correctly as possible.

In total 224 trials were presented which resulted in 56 trials per condition—retention load 1 (RETL1), retention load 3 (RETL3), manipulation load 1 (MANL1), and manipulation load 3 (MANL3)—of which half were match and half were non-match. Trials were presented in randomized order and a practice block was carried out before the start of the actual experiment.

EEG Recording

Data were recorded from 28 Ag-AgCl ring electrodes (Easycap®) mounted according to the international 10–20 system: Fp1, Fp2, F7, F3, Fz, F4, F8, FC3, FCz, FC4, T3, C3, Cz, C4, T4, CP5, CPz, CP6, T5, P3, Pz, P4, T6, PO3, PO4, O1, Oz, O2; against two reference electrodes placed on the earlobes. The ground electrode was placed on the forehead and eye movements were recorded with an electrode each above and next to the right eye. The EEG signal was registered between 0.016 and 80 Hz with a sampling rate of 1000 Hz and a notch-filter set at 50 Hz using a BrainAmp MR+ amplifier (Brain Products®). Impedances were kept below 15 kΩ.

Data Analysis

Behavioral Data Analysis

For behavioral data analysis IBM SPSS Statistics 22 was used. The accuracy (percentage of correctly performed trials) was analyzed using Wilcoxon Signed Rank test to examine the difference in performance comparing low-load and high-load conditions, as well as, the retention and the manipulation task, irrespective of the group of participants. The impact of the participants' group on the accuracy was further tested with a series of Kruskal-Wallis tests.

EEG Data Analysis Pre-processing

For EEG data analysis Brain Vision Analyzer 2.0 (Brain Products®) and in-house Matlab R2014b scripts (Math Works®) were used and statistical analyses were performed with IBM SPSS Statistics 22 and Matlab. Data were first offline re-referenced to digitally linked earlobes and high-pass filtered with a low cut-off at 1 Hz (48 db/Oct Butterworth Zero Phase IIR Filter as implemented in BrainVision Analyzer 2.0). In order to remove horizontal and vertical eye movements and blinks, independent component analysis (ICA) ocular correction was applied to the filtered raw EEG data. Remaining artifacts were removed by visual inspection. Then data were segmented (from 1000 ms pre-stimulus onset to 3000 after stimulus onset, in respect to the memory set) for every condition separately as the focus of the analysis was on the delay interval; i.e., when participant retained the location of the square(s) or mentally rotated them. On average this resulted in 45.97 (SD = 4.82) artifact free trials for RETL1, 46.7 (SD = 5.02) for RETL3, 44.4 (SD = 4.77) for

TABLE 1 | Demographic and clinical characteristics (*p*-values represent the significance of the performed Kruskal–Wallis tests between groups, except gender, and education, which were tested with chi-square tests).

	Controls	Negative symptomatic sub-group	Positive symptomatic sub-group	*p*-values
N	10	10	10	
Age	33.50 ± 2.87	31.60 ± 2.59	32.80 ± 2.43	$p = 0.925$
Gender (male/female)	6/10	7/10	8/10	$p = 0.621$
PANSS overall	–	78.66 ± 23.91	77.11 ± 20.91	$p = 0.880$
PANSS neg.sympt.	–	24.67 ± 3.03	14.56 ± 1.51	$p = 0.015$
PANSS pos.sympt.	–	16.67 ± 2.12	21.67 ± 2.78	$p = 0.138$
Education				$p = 0.312$
Higher degree	3	3	0	
A-levels	5	4	3	
Apprenticeship/professional school	1	1	3	
Elementary school	1	2	4	
Colrpromazine (mg/day)	–	321.67 ± 257.92	806.68 ± 326.87	$p = 0.002$

MANL1 and 47.57 (SD = 4.13) for MANL3. An estimation of the electrophysiological activity at source space was then calculated using the LORETA algorithm implemented in Brain Vision Analyzer 2.0 (see Pascual-Marqui et al., 1994). The algorithm transforms the scalp-level EEG data into a time series of current source density in pre-defined regions of interest (ROIs) in 3D-source space for each single trial. The ROIs were specified in line with the fronto-parietal network hypothesis outlined in the introduction; this resulted in one ROI in the bilateral ACC and one in the right BA40 (posterior parietal cortex bordering the IPS) and one in the left BA40.

Instantaneous Amplitude

To obtain the instantaneous amplitude of theta and gamma frequencies in these regions, two individual continuous complex Morlet wavelet transformations were calculated for slow and fast frequencies, respectively. For slow frequencies a 5-cycle Morlet wavelet was used to analyse the frequency range from 3 to 15 Hz in 13 frequency steps. For fast frequencies a 10-cycle Morlet wavelet transform was calculated from 30 to 80 Hz in 6 frequency steps. Any further analysis was done using in-house Matlab R2014b scripts (Math Works®). In order to account for outliers we used a conventional cut-off of ±3.29 standard deviations for every subject and every data point across trials. Values that exceeded this individual cut-off were set to the value representing ±3.29 times the standard deviation. This was done to attenuate the impact of extreme values without having to remove the whole trial. For the calculation of changes in the instantaneous amplitude of theta and gamma oscillations during the 2000 ms retention/manipulation interval the instantaneous amplitude values were first averaged across trials. The power values of both, theta and gamma frequencies were decibel transformed (see (Cohen and Ridderinkhof, 2013) for more details) according to a baseline period from 500 to 200 ms prior to stimulus onset. Decibel conversion was used in order to ensure comparability between all frequencies, conditions, groups or subjects and time points as it brings all data to the same scale. Frequency bins between 4 and 8 Hz were averaged to obtain a theta band, and frequency bins between 30 and 50 Hz and between 50 and 80 Hz were averaged into a slow and a fast gamma band, respectively. Finally, the decibel transformed amplitude values for the three frequency bands were averaged into four time windows of 500 ms each between stimulus-offset and probe-onset. For statistical comparisons the average decibel transformed amplitude values for each time window were exported for each condition (RETL1, RETL3, MANL1, and MANL3) and each individual subject and analyzed in IBM SPSS Statistics 22 with a mixed-model ANOVA with the three within-subject factors: task (RET, MAN), load (L1, L3), and time window (1–4; Time); and the between-subject factor: group (NEG, POS, CON). This statistical procedure was repeated for each frequency band and each ROI separately. *Post-hoc* tests were Bonferroni corrected and when assumption of sphericity was not met data were Huynh-Feldt corrected.

Phase Synchronization

In order to obtain theta phase values for calculations of the phase locking value (PLV) the phase of theta (center frequency of 6; 5 cycles complex continuous Morlet wavelet) was estimated between −pi and +pi in Brain Vision Analyzer 2.0 and then exported into Matlab to be further analyzed using in-house scripts. To assess whether theta phase estimated from the ACC is locked to the theta phases as obtained from the right and left BA40 the PLV was calculated according to Lachaux et al. (1999). The PLV is a measure of interregional phase synchronization by assessing the inter-trial variability of phase differences between signals from two distinct sources at any given time point. The PLV can range from zero to one, where a value of 1 indicates perfect stability of phase differences between the two signals across trials, and a value of 0 indicates completely random distribution of phase differences. First, the theta phase differences were calculated between two ROIs (frontal and right or left parietal) for every time point in every trial (2000 ms of delay period) for every condition and every participant separately. Then the values across trials were averaged and finally the data within the 2000 ms delay period were again averaged into four time windows of 500 ms each (see instantaneous amplitude). For

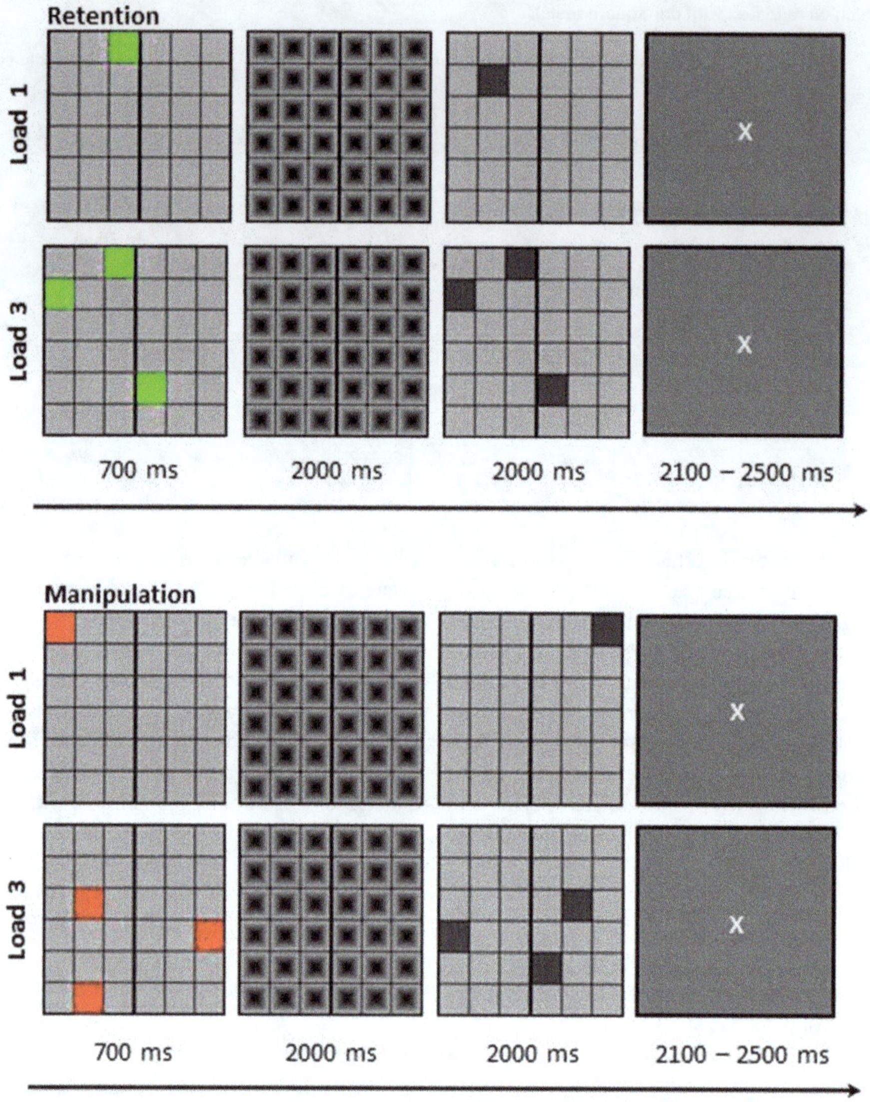

FIGURE 1 | Schematic depiction of the visuo-spatial delayed match to sample working memory task. Participants had to either retain the positions of the colored squares (Retention) or mirror their positions around the vertical line (Manipulation). The load was either one item (L1) or three items (L3). Figure taken with permission from Griesmayr et al. (2014).

statistical analysis the PLV values were analyzed in IBM SPSS Statistics 22 with a mixed-model ANOVA with the three within-subject factors: condition (RET, MAN), load (L1, L3), and time window (1–4); and the between-subject factor: group (NEG, POS, CON) for the right and the left BA40 separately.

RESULTS

Behavioral Results

The analysis of the behavioral data showed that the accuracy was significantly lower in the high-load (L3) than in the low-load (L1) condition in the retention task ($Mdn_{L1} = 98.21$, $Mdn_{L3} = 97.32$), $Z = -2.38$, $p = 0.017$, and in the manipulation task ($Mdn_{L1} = 96.43$, $Mdn_{L3} = 83.04$), $Z = -4.79$, $p < 0.001$. Further analysis showed that the accuracy was affected not only by the load, but also by the task. That is the accuracy was significantly lower in the manipulation task at low-load, $Z = -2.71$, $p = 0.007$ and at high load $Z = -4.79$, $p < 0.001$ in comparison to the retention task.

Importantly, the performed analysis on the accuracy between the three groups (negative symptomatic, positive symptomatic patients, and healthy controls) revealed no significant effect in either of the tasks at neither load. More specifically, the accuracy of the NEG, POS, and CON groups showed no significant difference in the retention task at low-load (L1), $H_{(2)} = 3.28$, $p = 0.19$, and at high-load (L3), $H_{(2)} = 3.28$, $p = 0.19$, or in the manipulation task at low-load (L1), $H_{(2)} = 0.34$, $p = 0.846$, and at high-load, $H_{(2)} = 1.02$, $p = 0.602$.

In sum the behavioral result suggest that accuracy was influenced by load and also by task. Participants performed better in the low-load conditions and in the retention task. Importantly, the three groups showed similar behavior performance, i.e., the control group performed no better than the patient groups (see **Table 2** for accuracy values).

Instantaneous Amplitude

ACC Theta

Analysis of the task-specific instantaneous theta amplitude values in the ACC revealed a main effect of Task, $F_{(1, 27)} = 10.85$, $p = 0.003$, indicating that the manipulation task was associated with higher theta amplitude in the ACC than the retention task. Furthermore, the main effect of Load was also significant, $F_{(1, 27)} = 9.59$, $p = 0.005$, because of the higher theta amplitude in the high-load (L3) condition. In addition, the also significant main effect of Time (1–4), $F_{(1.88, 50.7)} = 10.94$, $p < 0.001$, was the result of the attenuation of the theta amplitude increase (as to baseline) over the course of the delay period.

In addition, interaction effects [Load × Time, $F_{(2.6, 70.18)} = 10.69$, $p < 0.001$; Task × Time interaction, $F_{(2.57, 68.74)} = 8.2$, $p < 0.001$] indicate that theta stays higher over the course of the whole delay period for the more difficult conditions (i.e., higher load and manipulation task). Finally, a Task × Load × Time × Group four-way interaction effect also reached significance, $F_{(5.95, 80.31)} = 2.55$, $p = 0.026$. Further testing showed that in the control group the theta power increase (as to baseline) showed consistent attenuation over the course of the delay period for the retention task in general and for the low-load condition of the manipulation task [main effect of Time $F_{RetL1(3, 27)} = 8.87$, $p < 0.001$; $F_{RetL3(3, 27)} = 17.94$, $p < 0.001$; $F_{ManL1(3, 27)} = 13.41$, $p < 0.001$]; whereas it did not drop over time in the high-load manipulation condition [Time $F_{ManL3(3, 27)} = 0.9$; $p = 0.455$]. The negative symptomatic group showed a pattern similar to the controls in the low-load retention condition [Time $F_{RetL1(1.3, 11.8)} = 5.84$, $p = 0.026$] but with a less pronounced attenuation of theta power. However, theta power was sustained not only in the manipulation high-load but also in the low-load and retention high-load condition [Time $F_{RetL3(1.8, 16.3)} = 0.31$, $p = 0.715$; $F_{ManL3(1.4, 12.9)} = 0.1$, $p = 0.845$; $F_{ManL1(3, 27)} = 2.48$, $p = 0.083$]. The positive symptomatic group displayed rather sustained theta power over the course of the delay period in all conditions except low-load retention condition [Time $F_{RetL1(3, 27)} = 8.62$, $p < 0.001$; $F_{RetL3(3, 27)} = 2.22$, $p = 0.109$; $F_{ManL1(3, 27)} = 2.99$, $p = 0.052$; $F_{ManL3(1.8, 16.6)} = 1.29$, $p = 0.300$]; with the high-load manipulation condition showing even a slight steady increase over the delay period (see **Figure 2**).

Overall, these results suggest that ACC theta amplitude was increased in the high-load condition and in the manipulation task and that theta amplitude was particularly pronounced during the early time windows of the delay period. Furthermore, the decrease over the course of the delay period was smaller in the high-load condition and in the manipulation task.

ACC Gamma

The only effect that was significant in the analysis of the low-gamma band, was a main effect of Time, $F_{(2.56, 66.47)} = 5.79$,

TABLE 2 | Mean accuracy with standard error across groups, conditions, and load.

	Retention		Manipulation	
	Load 1	*Load 3*	*Load 1*	*Load 3*
CON	95.18 ± 3.25	93.04 ± 3.41	93.57 ± 2.58	81.79 ± 3.73
NEG	98.39 ± 0.62	97.50 ± 1.07	96.07 ± 0.95	83.22 ± 1.49
POS	97.14 ± 0.48	93.22 ± 2.01	94.64 ± 1.38	79.82 ± 2.61
Total	96.90 ± 1.10	94.58 ± 1.37	94.76 ± 1.01	81.61 ± 1.56

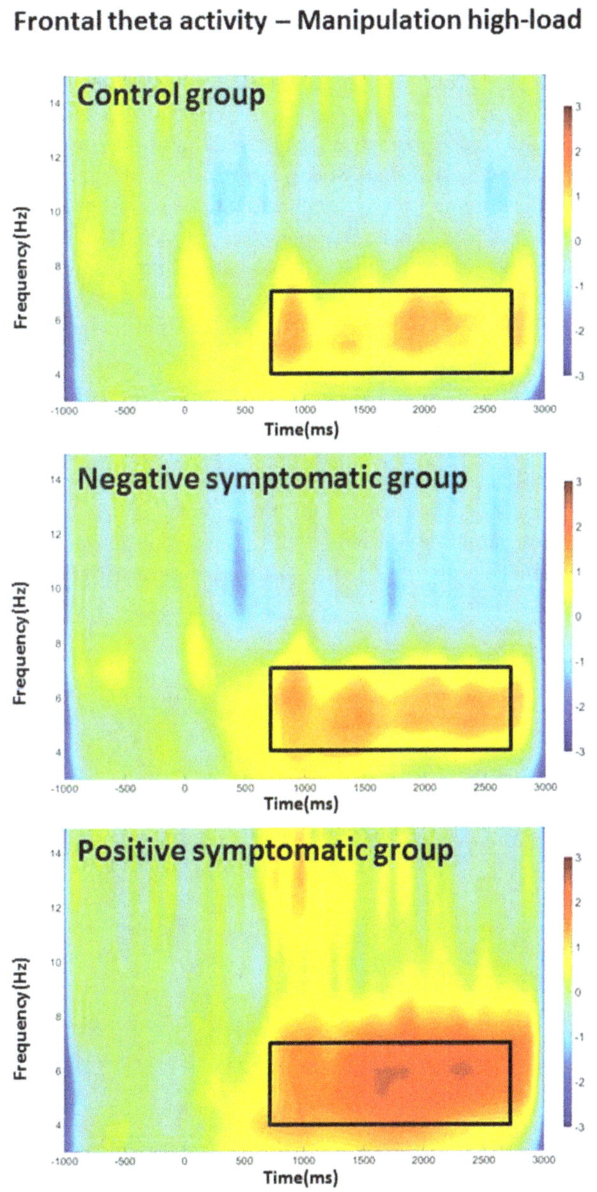

FIGURE 2 | Frontal theta band activity for the high-load manipulation condition for all three groups. The frequency of interest (4–7 Hz) and time period of interest (delay period) are indicated with a frame.

$p = 0.002$, indicating higher gamma power during the second part of the delay period, irrespective of task, load and group.

The analysis in the high gamma range revealed a main effect of Time, $F_{(1.92,\ 51.85)} = 5.82$, $p = 0.006$, which was driven by the increase of gamma power over the course of the delay period. Furthermore, central to our hypothesis, a marginally significant Load × Group interaction effect was found, $F_{(2,\ 27)} = 3.1$, $p = 0.061$ (see **Figure 3**). *Post-hoc* ANOVAs performed separately on low-load and high-load trials showed that whilst in the low-load condition, no significant main effect or interaction involving Group emerged, in the high-load condition a main effect of Group reached significance, $F_{(1,\ 27)} = 3.48$, $p = 0.045$. Importantly, the Bonferroni corrected ($p_{crit} < 0.017$) pairwise comparisons showed a significant difference only between positive and negative symptomatic groups, $t_{(18)} = 2.65$, $p = 0.016$, indicating higher gamma power in the negative symptomatic group than in the positive symptomatic group at high-load. In fact, further *post-hoc* repeated-measures ANOVA carried out on the positive and negative symptomatic group data separately suggested that, whereas in the negative symptomatic group the gamma power significantly increased from low-load to high-load conditions, $F_{(1,\ 9)} = 6.29$, $p = 0.034$, there was no difference in the positive symptomatic group gamma power across the same conditions (see **Figure 3**).

To summarize the above results, in the lower gamma frequency range the only significant finding suggested amplitude increase over the delay period. Similarly, high gamma amplitude also increased over the delay period; but importantly, amplitude was differentially affected by the factor group in the high- and low-load conditions. Whereas, in the low-load condition there was no difference among the groups, in the high-load condition gamma power was significantly higher in the negative symptomatic group than in the positive symptomatic group.

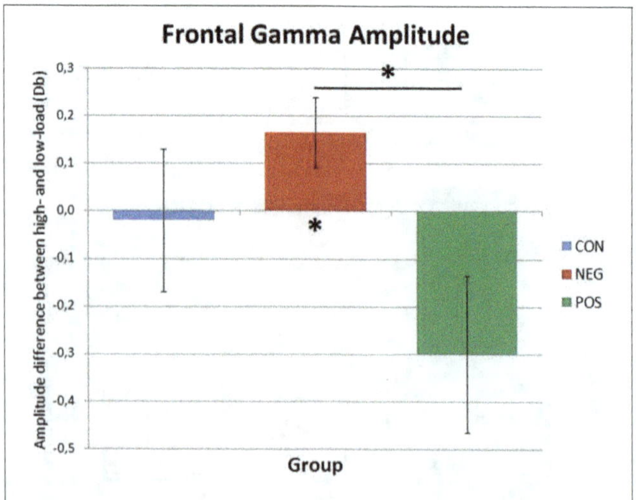

FIGURE 3 | Frontal gamma amplitude differences between high-load and low-load conditions for the three groups. While the positive symptomatic group shows decreased gamma power in the ACC in the high-load condition, the negative symptomatic group displays a marked increase. The healthy control subjects do not differ from either patient group. Significant differences are indicated by asterisks ($p < 0.05$).

BA40 Theta

Theta power in the right parietal ROI was modulated by several factors as a series of main and interaction effects showed. The strongly significant main effect of Time, $F_{(2.39,\ 64.62)} = 11.57$, $p < 0.001$, reflected the fact that theta amplitude was higher in the earlier time windows and showed a decrease over the course of the delay period.

Importantly, the results also indicated significant Time × Group, $F_{(4.79,\ 64.62)} = 2.60$, $p = 0.035$, and Task × Group interaction effects, $F_{(2,\ 27)} = 3.55$, $p = 0.043$. The former suggests that the decrease of theta power over the delay period was further modulated by the Group factor. Additional separate ANOVAs for each group individually revealed that there is no significant effect of Time in the healthy controls and the positive symptomatic group but a strongly significant main effect of Time in the negative symptomatic group $F_{(3,\ 9)} = 13.73$, $p < 0.001$; showing a decrease of theta power over the course of the delay period in the right BA40.

Furthermore, the above-mentioned significant Task × Group interaction effect was primarily driven by the fact that while the control group had increased theta power in the manipulation task compared to the retention task (irrespective of load), $F_{(1,\ 9)} = 7.21$, $p = 0.025$, the positive symptomatic group displayed a marginally significant decrease in the manipulation as compared to the retention task $F_{(1,\ 9)} = 3.88$, $p = 0.08$, and the negative symptomatic group displayed no significant difference.

Finally, the analysis of the left parietal ROI also showed a significant main effect of Time, $F_{(2.22,\ 59.87)} = 31.65$, $p < 0.001$ and a marginally significant main effect of Load, $F_{(1,\ 27)} = 4.16$, $p = 0.051$. The main effect of time indicated that over the course of the delay period theta power decreased.

To sum up, theta power in the right parietal ROI decreased over the delay period. This decrease was only significant in the negative symptomatic group but not in the other two groups. In addition, theta power was higher in the manipulation task compared to the retention task in the control group but not different between the two tasks in the patient groups.

BA40 Gamma

No significant effects were found in the lower gamma band in the right BA40 and in the lower and high gamma band in the left BA40.

In the high gamma band the interaction effect Task × Load × Time was marginally significant $F_{(2.99,\ 80.76)} = 2.7$, $p = 0.052$ and the four-way interaction Task × Load × Time × Group reached a significant level $F_{(5.98,\ 80.76)} = 3.99$, $p = 0.002$ in the right BA40. Further investigation of the Task × Load × Time effect showed that while there was no task-dependent difference in right BA40 gamma power in the retention task (low- and high-load) and the high-load condition of the manipulation task; there was a marginally significant increase in the low-load condition of the manipulation task $F_{(2.2,\ 63.7)} = 2.94$, $p = 0.055$.

In order to explain the four-way interaction separate ANOVAs for the four conditions (RETL1, RETL3, MANL1, and MANL3) were run. No significant effects were found for the low-load and high-load retention and low-load manipulation conditions. In the high-load manipulation condition the controls displayed an increase in gamma amplitude over time, while the negative symptomatic group showed a decrease. The positive symptomatic group showed a pattern where there is a decrease in the early delay period and then an increase in the later time windows.

Phase Synchronization

The PLV of the theta frequency band between the ACC and right BA40 showed a highly significant Group effect, $F_{(1, 27)} = 14.85$, $p < 0.001$. Further *post-hoc* tests revealed that the control group had significantly higher PLV than the negative ($p = 0.001$), and also the positive symptomatic groups ($p < 0.001$), whereas the PLV did not differ significantly between the two patient groups ($p = 0.654$).

In addition to this main effect, a significant Load × Time × Group, $F_{(6, 81)} = 2.28$, $p = 0.044$ three-way interaction effect was found (see **Figure 4**). Investigation of this three-way interaction indicated that the controls and positive symptomatic group displayed the same amount of theta phase synchronization over time for the low-load and high-load conditions while the negative symptomatic group showed a significant Load × Time interaction $F_{(3, 27)} = 5.88$, $p = 0.003$ indicating that there is a rather transient increase in phase synchronization in the low-load condition in the first half of the delay period. The high-load condition, on the other hand, shows a more sustained increase of phase synchronization over the course of the delay period.

Overall, these results indicate significantly stronger fronto-posterior theta phase synchronization in the healthy controls as compared to the patient groups.

DISCUSSION

Executive functions have previously been shown to employ a network of cortical structures spanning prefrontal areas, in particular the ACC, and right posterior parietal regions. This network is strongly involved in working memory and operations requiring cognitive control. Both, executive functions as well as the underlying neuronal network have been found to be compromised in schizophrenia. However, little is known about what it is exactly that underlies those dysfunctions. Furthermore, even less is known about the brain oscillatory correlates of the complex and highly diverse symptomatology of schizophrenia (i.e., negative and positive symptomatology) and its relation to executive functioning.

In this article we examined schizophrenia patients with predominantly negative symptomatology, with predominantly positive symptomatology and healthy control subjects. We recorded EEG while they performed a visuo-spatial delayed match to sample working memory task with varying load and varying need to employ executive functions. We investigated the delay period of the WM task and compared the three groups in respect to performance and brain oscillatory activity. We investigated areas of the fronto-parietal executive control network (ACC and right BA40 as well as left BA40) by looking at local amplitude changes of theta and gamma oscillations; two frequencies repeatedly found to be strongly implicated in visual working memory operations in these areas. Moreover, we investigated communication within this network by analysing phase synchrony in the theta frequency between the frontal and the parietal regions of interest. We hypothesized that patients would show a different pattern of functional cortical activation as compared to healthy controls. Furthermore, we expected the two patient groups to display differences in brain oscillatory correlates of executive functioning, given that their different symptomatologies greatly differ in their behavioral expression.

A very robust finding in this study is that sustained phase synchronization in the theta frequency between the ACC and the right (but not the left) BA40 was significantly disrupted in the patient groups as compared to controls (see **Figure 4**). Similar results were also obtained on scalp level by Griesmayr et al. (2014) where the 21 patients—as one sample—were compared with 21 matched healthy control subjects. Moreover, these findings are very well in line with the dysconnectivity theory of schizophrenia (e.g., Uhlhaas and Singer, 2010; Rogasch et al., 2014) stating that global cortical communication is disrupted in patients suffering from SZ. During working memory operations that require executive functions it is repeatedly found that theta oscillations in prefrontal areas are synchronized with theta oscillations in posterior parietal regions. This long-range communication is said to underlie (top–down) executive control from frontal areas interacting with local posterior information processing (e.g., Sauseng et al., 2005; Wu et al., 2007; Sauseng et al., 2008). Given that executive functions are often impaired in SZ, it stands to reason that such long-range theta coherence should also be disrupted. In our case, however, this pattern of dysconnectivity in SZ patients was not related to impaired task execution, i.e., patients did do just as well as the healthy control subjects.

In addition to theta long-range synchronization, the patients were also distinguishable from the healthy control subjects by the amount of local theta power difference between the retention and the manipulation tasks in the right BA40. While the healthy controls showed a markedly higher theta activity in the right posterior ROI in the manipulation task as compared to the retention task, the patient groups displayed no such load-dependent increase during the delay period. Posterior theta activity has been found to increase during working memory operations (e.g., Osipova et al., 2006; see Roux and Uhlhaas, 2014 for a review) and increasing load and has been linked to determining WM capacity (e.g., Moran et al., 2010). Hence, an increase in posterior theta activity from the retention to the manipulation task is not surprising. Such a task/load-dependent increase was also found in the ACC for all three groups; where theta power was significantly higher for the high-load and manipulation task as compared to low-load and retention task. What is curious, however, is that while patients displayed such task-dependent increase in theta power in the ACC, they did not show this pattern of increasing theta power in the BA40. Moreover, the positive symptomatic group was distinct from the healthy controls and the negative symptomatic group by the pattern of ACC theta activity mainly in the manipulation high-load condition (see **Figure 2**). The positive symptomatic patient group seemed to employ generally more sustained frontal theta activity in all conditions over time and even displayed an increase over the course of the delay period in the most difficult (high-load manipulation) condition. Given that frontal theta increase is

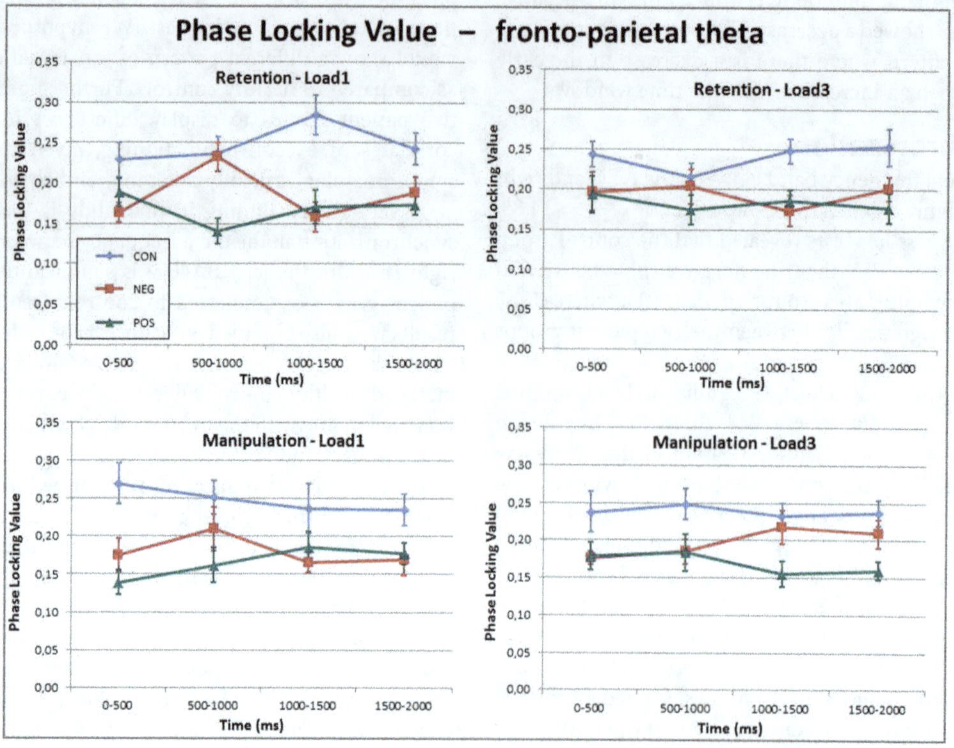

FIGURE 4 | Theta phase synchronization between the ACC and the BA40 indexed by phase locking values (PLVs) for all three groups in the four conditions over the delay period. While the phase synchronization is fairly constant over time and between conditions, the healthy control subjects display a generally higher phase synchronization than the two patient groups.

a strong indicator for executive control (e.g., Gevins et al., 1997) this might hint at the employment of some sort of compensatory mechanism which recruits more executive processing power to successfully complete the task at hand.

Interestingly, we also found an effect in the high gamma frequency range in the ACC differentiating the two patient groups (see **Figure 3**). While gamma power did not differ between the three groups in the low-load conditions, the negative symptomatic patient group displayed significantly stronger gamma power than the positive symptomatic group in the high-load conditions. In fact, while local gamma power in the ACC increased from the low- to the high-load condition in the negative symptomatic group, the positive symptomatic group showed no difference between the two conditions. This finding suggests that local frontal information processing represented by gamma oscillatory activity seems to be aberrant in SZ and might be a key factor in differentiating the neural underpinnings of the different symptomatologies of the disorder. It is a finding well in line with the suggestion by Rogasch et al. (2014) that decreased prefrontal gamma activity is strongly linked to positive symptomatology. Furthermore, such differences between the patient groups might play a major role in explaining contradictory findings in literature where some authors find decreased frontal gamma in SZ while others find the opposite pattern (see Senkowski and Gallinat, 2015 for a review).

Another, although less robust effect indicated that theta power was attenuated over the time course of the delay period in the right parietal area in the negative symptomatic group whereas it stayed constant in the positive symptomatic group and in healthy control participants indicating consistent engagement with the to-be-retained information. As the area is thought to be strongly involved in visuospatial processing (Moscovitch et al., 1995) and there is evidence suggesting that the theta frequency band is particularly relevant in such processing (Romei et al., 2011), the disproportionate reduction of theta power could have a negative impact on visuospatial working memory. However, this different pattern in the negative symptomatic group does not necessarily reflect impairment: Firstly, their behavioral performance was not impaired as compared to the other two groups; and secondly, they seem to show a generally slightly different oscillatory pattern in this task than controls and positive symptomatic patients. This might partly reflect parallel mechanisms to compensate for the comprised parietal theta activity (see for instance the ACC gamma activity differences between negative symptomatic and the other two groups). To draw any clear conclusions further studies would be needed to investigate the exact nature and relevance of this effect more in depth.

In the current study we only found local and fronto-parietal coupling results in the right but not the left parietal ROI. This might be because of the material type (i.e., strictly spatial information processing) or the required attention network.

The right parietal region is strongly linked to visuospatial processing and moreover to sustained attention to spatial locations (e.g., Smith et al., 1996; Malhotra et al., 2009; Jackson et al., 2011). A right hemispheric dominance for visuospatial processing, representation and working memory has been shown in both, primates and humans with neuropsychological and neuroimaging techniques as well as in neurostimulation studies (e.g., Pisella et al., 2011; for reviews see Oleksiak et al., 2011; Pisella, 2016). However, we want to point out that the role of the right parietal cortex in visuospatial cognition is not yet fully understood and that visual working memory processing and attention is not exclusively right lateralised (e.g., Cowan et al., 2011 for color processing; Majerus et al., 2010 for faces; Popov et al., 2015 for executive functioning).

Generally, our results suggest that patients suffering from schizophrenia display altered oscillatory patterns during executive processes indicated by disrupted fronto-parietal theta synchronization in the executive network and local right parietal theta activity, indicating differential local neural processes. Importantly, local ACC gamma and to a lesser extent right parietal and ACC theta also have differential patterns between positive and negative symptomatic SZ patients, but long-range fronto-parietal coupling did not distinguish the two patient groups but only patients and healthy controls. It is important to point out that our data mainly identified neuronal processes inherent to patients suffering from predominantly negative symptomatology which was the group the most distinguishable from both, the healthy controls and the positive symptomatic group in local neuronal processing (see group effects in ACC gamma and right BA40 theta). That this group stands out is not surprising given that the two patient groups only differ significantly in the negative symptoms (see **Table 1**) while their positive symptomatology scores are not significantly different. The fact that the performance between groups was not different points toward the aberrant neuronal processing displayed by the negative symptomatic group really being partly of a compensatory nature; however, from our data we cannot make any definite conclusions about the meaning of different oscillatory patterns or suggestions regarding causality. Given that aberrant gamma oscillations are linked to a dysregulation of GABAergic inhibitory neurotransmission, the differential findings in the gamma frequency band between the two patient groups might have potential implications for medication treatment of the SZ subgroups in the future.

We argue that the set of results might have very distinct origins and functions. The pattern of dysconnectivity in SZ which we also found in this study might be explained by general white matter loss in patients (e.g., Roalf et al., 2015), irrespective of symptomatology. However, diffusion tensor imaging studies would be needed to confirm such a claim. With regards to the local effects we found in right parietal and ACC theta power and frontal gamma power, this might reflect either on local disruptions (in the case of parietal theta activity) or alternatively, compensatory mechanisms in order to counter processing deficits. The increased frontal gamma and theta activity in the negative symptomatic group and positive symptomatic group, respectively, fits nicely with findings suggesting an increase in frontal activity as compensatory mechanism (i.e., hyperfrontality) as gamma activity has been found to reflect local neuronal spiking and frontal theta activity is strongly linked to executive functions.

It is important to emphasize that the above findings are unlikely to represent only dysfunctional neural processes. Disruption of a neural network may also trigger compensatory mechanisms. Thus, in particular the here described local differences between SZ patients and healthy controls, as well as, between the negative and positive symptomatic patient groups can represent local disruption or local compensation mechanisms. Considering that the negative and positive patient groups' behavioral performance was at the level of the healthy controls, the presence of such compensatory mechanisms is more than likely. However, it is also important to note that in the present study the healthy control sample was a tight match to the patient sample. While most studies comparing SZ patients and healthy controls report that patients perform markedly worse than healthy controls, the non-existent group difference in our study might indicate that no other factors (e.g., general cognitive abilities) contributed to the differences in brain oscillatory activity we found.

Furthermore, it is relevant to point out that the negative and positive patient groups received various psychopharmacological medications, which could potentially influence oscillatory processes; especially as there was a significant difference between the two patient groups. Hence it cannot be excluded that our results may be affected by these medications. However, the impact of medications on oscillatory processes is most likely generic and not task-specific. The presented results were specific to executive functions in a working memory task and do not reflect on generally altered oscillatory patterns as investigated in studies looking at resting EEG activity. It might also be worth mentioning that during the baseline period in our task there was no significant difference in either frequency band between groups. Moreover, it was found that prefrontal theta and gamma changes are not associated with psychopharmacological treatment in first-episode SZ patients (e.g., Minzenberg et al., 2010) and that deficits are not just due to lack of concentration, distracting positive symptoms or medication effects (e.g., Kraguljac et al., 2013).

Finally, we want to highlight that our analysis was strictly hypothesis driven. That is we did only analyse regions and frequency bands that are strongly implicated in fronto-parietal executive functions and visual working memory operations that are easily accessible with EEG source localization; i.e., the ACC and BA40. We cannot exclude, however, that other regions might play an important role and show distinct patterns in patients and controls, and more to the point, between the two patient groups. This would need to be further investigated with a more exploratory approach and potentially wider range of cognitive tasks and neuroimaging methods. In addition, in order to be able to make definite claims our results would need to be investigated further with a much larger sample of patients and healthy controls.

CONCLUSION

In conclusion, our results indicate that indeed, the fronto-parietal executive functions network as indexed by theta phase synchronization is comprised in SZ. Moreover, local frontal and right parietal activity in the theta and gamma frequency ranges can distinguish between patients with predominantly negative and predominantly positive symptomatology; and are especially able to differentiate patients with negative symptomatology from patients with positive symptoms and healthy controls. Finally, task-related theta and gamma oscillations can be highly beneficial for understanding the multifaceted nature of SZ and how its various cognitive dysfunctions and symptoms emerge—even in the absence of behavioral impairment—and so in furthering its treatment.

AUTHOR CONTRIBUTIONS

BB and TM share the first authorship for this paper and contributed equally. BB, data collection, data analysis, writing manuscript; TM, data analysis, writing manuscript; BG, implementation of experiment, data collection, writing manuscript; RS, WA, implementation of experiment, writing manuscript; PS, implementation of experiment, data analysis, writing manuscript.

REFERENCES

Basar-Eroglu, C., Brand, A., Hildebrandt, H., Kedzior, K. K., Mathes, B., and Schmiedt, C. (2007). Working memory related gamma oscillations in schizophrenia patients. *Int. J. Psychophysiol.* 64, 39–45. doi: 10.1016/j.ijpsycho.2006.07.007

Berger, B., Omer, S., Minarik, T., Sterr, A., and Sauseng, P. (2014). Interacting memory systems - does EEG alpha activity respond to semantic long-term memory access in a working memory task? *Biology* 4, 1–16. doi: 10.3390/biology4010001

Buzsaki, G., and Wang, X.-J. (2012). Mechanisms of gamma oscillations. *Annu. Rev. Neurosci.* 35, 203–225. doi: 10.1146/annurev-neuro-062111-150444

Callicott, J. H., Mattay, V. S., Verchinski, B. A., Marenco, S., Egan, M. F., and Weinberger, D. R. (2003). Complexity of prefrontal cortical dysfunction in schizophrenia: More than up or down. *Am. J. Psychiatry* 160, 2209–2215. doi: 10.1176/appi.ajp.160.12.2209

Carter, C. S., Mintun, M., Nichols, T., and Cohen, J. D. (1997). Anterior cingulate gyrus dysfunction and selectrive attentino deficit in schizophrenia: [15 O]H2O PET study during single-trial stroop task performance. *Am. J. Psychiatry* 154, 1670–1675. doi: 10.1176/ajp.154.12.1670

Cavanagh, J. G., and Frank, M. J. (2014). Frontal theta as a mechanism for cognitive control. *Trends Cogn. Sci.* 18, 414–421. doi: 10.1016/j.tics.2014.04.012

Cho, R. Y., Konecky, R. O., and Carter, C. S. (2006). Impairments in frontal cortical γ synchrony and cognitive control in schizophrenia. *Proc. Natl. Acad. Sci. U.S.A.* 103, 19878–19883. doi: 10.1073/pnas.0609440103

Cohen, M. X., and Ridderinkhof, K. R. (2013). EEG source reconstruction reveals frontal-parietal dynamics of spatial conflict processing. *PLoS ONE* 8:e57293. doi: 10.1371/journal.pone.0057293

Cowan, N., Li, D., Moffitt, A., Becker, T. M., Martin, E. A., Saults, J. S., et al. (2011). A neural region of abstract working memory. *J. Cogn. Neurosci.* 23, 2852–2863. doi: 10.1162/jocn.2011.21625

Dasklakis, Z. J., Fitzgerald, P. B., and Christensen, B. K. (2007). The role of cortical inhibition in the pathophysiology and treatment of schizophrenia. *Brain Res. Rev.* 56, 427–442. doi: 10.1016/j.brainresrev.2007.09.006

Etkin, A., Gyurak, A., and O'Hara, R. (2013). A neurobiological approach to the cognitive deficits of psychiatric disorders. *Dialogues Clin. Neurosci.* 15, 419–429.

Ettinger, U., Mohr, C., Gooding, D. C., Cohen, A. S., Rapp, A., Haenschel, C., et al. (2015). Cognition and brain function in schizotypy: a selective review. *Schizophr. Bull.* 41, 417–426. doi: 10.1093/schbul/sbu190

Franke, G. H. (2000). *BSI. Brief Symptom Inventory von L. R. Derogatis Deutsche Version*. Göttingen: Beltz.

Gandal, M. J., Edgar, J. C., Klook, K., and Siegel, S. J. (2012). Gamma synchrony: towards a translational biomarker for the treatment resistant symptoms of schizophrenia. *Neuropharmacology* 62, 1504–1518. doi: 10.1016/j.neuropharm.2011.02.007

Gevins, A., Smith, M. E., McEvoy, L., and Yu, D. (1997). High-resolution EEG mapping of cortical activation related to working memory: effects of task difficulty, type of processing, and practice. *Cereb. Cortex* 7, 374–385. doi: 10.1093/cercor/7.4.374

Glahn, D. D., Ragland, J. D., Abramoff, A., Barrett, J., Laird, A. R., Bearden, C. E., et al. (2005). Beyond hypofrontality: a quantitative meta-analysis of functional neuroimaging studies of working memory in schizophrenia. *Hum. Brain Mapp.* 25, 60–69. doi: 10.1002/hbm.20138

Griesmayr, B., Berger, B., Stelzig-Schoeler, R., Aichhorn, W., Bergmann, J., and Sauseng, P. (2014). EEG theta phase coupling during executive control of visual working memory investigated in individuals with schizophrenia and in healthy controls. *Cogn. Affect. Behav. Neurosci.* 14, 1340–1355. doi: 10.3758/s13415-014-0272-0

Haenschel, C., Bittner, R. A., Waltz, J., Haertling, F., Wibral, M., Singer, W., et al. (2009). Cortical oscillatory activity is critical for working memory as revealed by deficits in early-onset schizophrenia. *J. Neurosci.* 29, 9481–9489. doi: 10.1523/JNEUROSCI.1428-09.2009

Haenschel, C., and Linden, D. (2011). Exploring intermediate phenotypes with EEG: working memory dysfunction in schizophrenia. *Behav. Brain Res.* 216, 481–495. doi: 10.1016/j.bbr.2010.08.045

Herrmann, C. S., and Demiralp, T. (2005). Human EEG gamma oscillations in neuropsychiatric disorders. *Clin. Neurophysiol.* 116, 2719–2733. doi: 10.1016/j.clinph.2005.07.007

Huhlshoff Pol, H. E., Schnack, H. G., Bertens, M. G., van Haren, N. E., van der Tweel, I., Staal, W. G. et al. (2002). Volume changes in gray matter in patients with schizophrenia. *Am. J. Psychiatry* 159, 244–250. doi: 10.1176/appi.ajp.159.2.244

Ishii, R., Canuet, L., Ishihara, T., Aoki, Y., Ikeda, S., Hata, M., et al. (2014). Frontal midline theta rhythm and gamma power changes during focused attention on mental calculation: an MEG beamformer analysis. *Front. Hum. Neurosci.* 8:406. doi: 10.3389/fnhum.2014.00406

Jackson, M. C., Morgan, H. M., Shapiro, K. L., Mohr, H., and Linden, D. E. J. (2011). Strategic resource allocation in the human brain supports cognitive coordination of object and spatial working memory. *Hum. Brain Mapp.* 32, 1330–1348. doi: 10.1002/hbm.21112

Karlsgodt, K. H., Glahn, D. C., van Erp, T. G. M., Therman, S., Huttunen, M., Manninen, M., et al. (2007). The relationship between performance and fMRI signal during working memory in patients with schizophrenia, unaffected co-twins, and control subjects. *Schizophr. Res.* 89, 191–197. doi: 10.1016/j.schres.2006.08.016

Kay, S. R., Fiszbein, A., and Opler, L. A. (1987). The positive and negative syndrome scale (PANSS) for schizophrenia. *Schizophr. Bull.* 13, 261–276. doi: 10.1093/schbul/13.2.261

Kerns, J. G., Cohen, J. D., MacDonald, A. W. III, Johnson, M. K., Stenger, V. A., Aizenstein, H., et al. (2005). Decreased conflict- and error-related activity in the anterior cingulate cortex in subjects with schizophrenia. *Am. J. Psychiatry* 162, 1833–1839. doi: 10.1176/appi.ajp.162.10.1833

Kiriakopoulos, M., Bargiotas, T., Barker, G. J., and Frangou, S. (2008). Diffusion tensor imaging in schizophrenia. *Eur. Psychiatry* 23, 255–273. doi: 10.1016/j.eurpsy.2007.12.004

Koychev, I., El-Deredy, W., Mukherjee, T., Haenschel, C., and Deakin, J. F. W. (2012). Core dysfunction in schizophrenia: electrophysiology trait biomarkers. *Acta Psychiatr. Scand.* 126, 59–71. doi: 10.1111/j.1600-0447.2012.01849.x

Kraguljac, N. V., Srivastava, A., and Lahti, A. C. (2013). Memory deficits in schizophrenia: a selective review of functional magnetic resonance imaging (FMRI) studies. *Behav. Sci. (Basel)* 3, 330–347. doi: 10.3390/bs3030330

Lachaux, J.-P., Rodriguez, E., Martinerie, J., and Varela, F. J. (1999). Measuring phase synchrony in brain signals. *Hum. Brain Mapp.* 8, 194–208.

Lisman, J. (2012). Excitation, inhibition, local oscillations, or large-scale loops: what causes the symptoms of schizophrenia? *Curr. Opin. Neurobiol.* 22, 537–544. doi: 10.1016/j.conb.2011.10.018

Lisman, J., and Buzsaki, G. (2008). A neural coding scheme formed by the combined function of gamma and theta oscillations. *Schizophr. Bull.* 34, 974–980. doi: 10.1093/schbul/sbn060

Majerus, S., D'Argembeau, A., Perez, T. M., Belayachi, S., van der Linden, M., Collette, F., et al. (2010). The commonality of neural networks of verbal and visual short-term memory. *J. Cogn. Neurosci.* 22, 2570–2593. doi: 10.1162/jocn.2009.21378

Malhotra, P., Coulthard, E. J., and Husain, M. (2009). Role of right posterior parietal cortex in maintaining attention to spatial locations over time. *Brain* 132, 645–660. doi: 10.1093/brain/awn350

Manoach, D. S. (2003). Prefrontal cortex dysfunction during working memory performance in schizophrenia: reconciling discrepant findings. *Schizophr. Res.* 60, 285–298. doi: 10.1016/S0920-9964(02)00294-3

Manoach, D. S., Gollub, R. L., Benson, E. S., Searl, M. M., Goff, D. C., Halpern, E., et al. (2000). Schizophrenic subjects show aberrant fMRI activation of dorsolateral prefrontal cortex and basal ganglia during working memory performance. *Biol. Psychiatry* 48, 99–109. doi: 10.1016/S0006-3223(00)00227-4

Meyer-Lindenberg, A., Poline, J. B., Kohn, P. D., Holt, J. L., Egan, M. F., Weinberger, D. R., et al. (2001). Evidence for abnormal cortical functional connectivity during working memory in schizophrenia. *Am. J. Psychiatry* 158, 1809–1817. doi: 10.1176/appi.ajp.158.11.1809

Minzenberg, M. J., Firl, A. J., Yoon, J. H., Gomes, G. C., Reinking, C., and Carter, C. S. (2010). Gamma oscillatory power is impaired during cognitive control independent of medication status in first-episode schizophrenia. *Neuropsychopharmacology* 35, 2590–2599. doi: 10.1038/npp.2010.150

Mitchell, D. J., McNaughton, N., Flanagan, D., and Kirk, I. J. (2008). Frontal-midline theta from the perspective of hippocampal "theta". *Prog. Neurobiol.* 86, 156–185. doi: 10.1016/j.pneurobio.2008.09.005

Mizuhara, H., and Yamagutchi, Y. (2007). Human cortical circuits for central executive function emerge by theta phase synchronization. *Neuroimage* 36, 232–244. doi: 10.1016/j.neuroimage.2007.02.026

Möller, H.-J., Müller, W. E., and Volz, H.-P. (2000). *Psychopharmakotherapie. Ein Leitfaden für Klinik und Praxis.* Stuttgart: Kohlhammer.

Moran, L. V., and Hong, L. E. (2011). High vs low frequency neural oscillations in schizophrenia. *Schizophr. Bull.* 37, 659–663. doi: 10.1093/schbul/sbr056

Moran, R. J., Campo, P., Maestu, F., Reilly, R. B., Dolan, R. J., and Strange, B. A. (2010). Peak frequency in the theta and alpha bands correlates with human working memory capacity. *Front. Hum. Neurosci.* 4:200. doi: 10.3389/fnhum.2010.00200

Moscovitch, M., Kapur, S., Köhler, S., and Houle, S. (1995). Distinct neural correlates of visual long-term memory for spatial location and object identity: a positron emission tomography study in humans. *Proc. Natl. Acad. Sci. U.S.A.* 92, 3721–3725. doi: 10.1073/pnas.92.9.3721

O'Keefe, J., and Recce, M. L. (1993). Phase relationship between hippocampal place units and the EEG theta rhythm. *Hippocampus* 3, 317–330. doi: 10.1002/hipo.450030307

Oleksiak, A., Postma, A., van der Ham, I. J., Klink, P. C., and van Wezel, R. J. (2011). A review of lateralization of spatial functioning in nonhuman primates. *Brain Res. Rev.* 67, 56–72. doi: 10.1016/j.brainresrev.2010.11.002

Osipova, D., Takashima, A., Oostenveld, R., Fernández, G., Maris, E., and Jensen, O. (2006). Theta and gamma oscillations predict encoding and retrieval of declarative memory. *J. Neurosci.* 26, 7523–7531. doi: 10.1523/JNEUROSCI.1948-06.2006

Pascual-Marqui, R. D., Michel, C. M., and Lehmann, D. (1994). Low resolution electromagnetic tomography: a new method for localizing electrical activity in the brain. *Int. J. Psychophysiol.* 18, 49–65. doi: 10.1016/0167-8760(84)90014-X

Pisella, L. (2016). Visual perception is dependent on visuospatial working memory and thus on the posterior parietal cortex. *Ann. Phys. Rehabil. Med.* doi: 10.1016/j.rehab.2016.01.002. [Epub ahead of print].

Pisella, L., Alahyane, N., Blangero, A., Thery, F., Blanc, S., and Pelisson, D. (2011). Right-hemispheric dominance for visual remapping in humans. *Philos. Trans. R. Soc. Lond. B. Biol. Sci.* 366, 572–585. doi: 10.1098/rstb.2010.0258

Popov, T., Wienbruch, C., Meissner, S., Miller, G. A., and Rockstroh, B. (2015). A mechanism of deficient interregional neural communication in schizophrenia. *Psychophysiology* 52, 648–656. doi: 10.1111/psyp.12393

Roalf, D. R., Gur, R. E., Verma, R., Parker, W. W., Quarmley, M., Ruparel, K., et al. (2015). White matter microstructure in schizophrenia: Associations to neurocognitive and clinical symptomatology. *Schizophr. Res.* 161, 42–49. doi: 10.1016/j.schres.2014.09.026

Rogasch, N. C., Daskalakis, Z. J., and Fitzgerald, P. B. (2014). Cortical inhibition, excitation, and connectivity in schizophrenia: a review of insights from transcranial magnetic stimulation. *Schizophr. Bull.* 40, 685–696. doi: 10.1093/schbul/sbt078

Romei, V., Driver, J., Schyns, P. G., and Thut, G. (2011). Rhythmic TMS over right parietal cortex causally links distinct brain frequencies to global visual processing. *Curr. Biol.* 21, 334–337. doi: 10.1016/j.cub.2011.01.035

Roux, F., and Uhlhaas, P. J. (2014). Working memory and neural oscillations: alpha-gamma versus theta-gamma codes for distinct WM information? *Trends Cogn. Sci.* 18, 16–25. doi: 10.1016/j.tics.2013.10.010

Sauseng, P., Griesmayr, B., Freunberrger, R., and Klimesch, W. (2010). Control mechansims in working memory: A possible function of EEG theta oscillations. *Neurosci. Biobehav. Rev.* 34, 1015–1022. doi: 10.1016/j.neubiorev.2009.12.006

Sauseng, P., Hoppe, J., Klimesch, W., Gerloff, C., and Hummel, F. C. (2007). Dissociation of sustained attention from central executive functions: local activity and interregional connectivity in the theta range. *Eur. J. Neurosci.* 25, 587–593. doi: 10.1111/j.1460-9568.2006.05286.x

Sauseng, P., Klimesch, W., Gruber, W., and Birbaumer, N. (2008). Cross-frequency phase synchronization: a brain mechanism of memory matching and attention. *Neuroimage* 40, 308–317. doi: 10.1016/j.neuroimage.2007.11.032

Sauseng, P., Klimesch, W., Schabus, M., and Doppelmayr, M. (2005). Fronto-parietal EEG coherence in theta and upper alpha reflect central executive functions of working memory. *Int. J. Psychophysiol.* 57, 97–703. doi: 10.1016/j.ijpsycho.2005.03.018

Schmitt, A., Hasan, A., Gruber, O., and Falkai, P. (2011). Schizophrenia is a disorder or disconnectivity. *Eur. Arch. Psychiatry* 261, s150–s154. doi: 10.1007/s00406-011-0242-2

Senkowski, D., and Gallinat, J. (2015). Dysfunctional prefrontal gamma-band oscillations reflect working memory and other cognitive deficits in schizophrenia. *Biol. Psychiatry* 77, 1010–1019. doi: 10.1016/j.biopsych.2015.02.034

Singer, W., and Gray, C. M. (1995). Visual feature integration and the temporal correlation hypothesis. *Annu. Rev. Neurosci.* 18, 555–586. doi: 10.1146/annurev.ne.18.030195.003011

Smith, E. E., Jonides, J., and Koeppe, R. A. (1996). Dissociating verbal and spatial working memory using PET. *Cereb. Cortex* 6, 11–20. doi: 10.1093/cercor/6.1.11

Teffer, K., and Semendeferi, K. (2012). Human prefrontal cortex: evolution, development, and pathology. *Prog. Brain Res.* 195, 191–218. doi: 10.1016/B978-0-444-53860-4.00009-X

Tsujimoto, T., Shimazu, H., and Isomura, Y. (2006). Direct recording of theta oscillations in primate prefrontal and anterior cingulate cortices. *J. Neurophysiol.* 95, 2987–3000. doi: 10.1152/jn.00730.2005

Uhlhaas, P. J., and Singer, W. (2010). Abnormal neural oscillations and synchrony in schizophrenia. *Nat. Rev. Neurosci.* 11, 100–113. doi: 10.1038/nrn2774

Uhlhaas, P. J., and Singer, W. (2014). Oscillations and neuronal dynamics in schizophrenia: the search for basic symptoms and translational opportunities. *Biol. Psychiatry* 77, 1001–1009. doi: 10.1016/j.biopsych.2014.11.019

Uhlhaas, P. J., and Singer, W. (2015). Oscillations and neuronal dynamics in schizophrenia: the search for basic symptoms and translational opportunities. *Biol. Psychiatry* 77, 1001–1009. doi: 10.1016/j.biopsych.2014.11.019

van Erp, T. G. M., Hibar, D. P., Rasmussen, J. M., Glahn, D. C., Pearlson, D., Andreassen, O. A., et al. (2015). Subcortical brain volume abnormalities in 2028 individuals with schizophrenia and 2540 healthy controls via the ENIGMA consortium. *Mol. Psychiatry* 2015, 1–7. doi: 10.1038/mp.2015.63

Voytek, B., and Knight, R. T. (2015). Dynamic network communication as a unifying neural basis for cognition, development, aging, and disease. *Biol. Psychiatry* 77, 1089–1097. doi: 10.1016/j.biopsych,.2015.04.016

Wang, L., Liu, X., Guise, K. G., Knight, R., Ghajar, J., and Fan, J. (2009). Effective connectivity of the fronto-parietal network during attention control. *J. Cogn. Neurosci.* 22, 543–553. doi: 10.1162/jocn.2009.21210

Wen, W., Yong, H., and Sachdev, P. (2011). Structural brain networks and neuropsychiatric disorders. *Curr. Opin. Psychiatry* 24, 219–225. doi: 10.1097/YCO.0b013e32834591f8

Woods, S. W. (2003). Chlorpromazine equivalent doses for the newer atypical antipsychotics. *J. Clin. Psychiatry* 64, 663–667. doi: 10.4088/JCP.v64n0607

Wu, X., Chen, X., Li, Z., Han, S., and Zhang, D. (2007). Binding of verbal and spatial information in human working memory involves large-scale neural synchronization at theta frequency. *Neuroimage* 35, 1654–1662. doi: 10.1016/j.neuroimage.2007.02.011

Zhou, Y., Fan, L., Qiu, C., and Jiang, T. (2015). Prefrontal cortex and the dysconnectivity hypothesis of schizophrenia. *Neurosci. Bull.* 31, 207–219. doi: 10.1007/s12264-014-1502-8

15

Against Explanatory Minimalism in Psychiatry

*Tim Thornton**

College of Health and Wellbeing, University of Central Lancashire, Preston, UK

Edited by:
Derek Strijbos,
Radboud University, Netherlands

Reviewed by:
Daniel Douglas Hutto,
University of Wollongong, Australia
Dawa Ometto,
Utrecht University, Netherlands

***Correspondence:**
Tim Thornton
tthornton1@uclan.ac.uk

The idea that psychiatry contains, in principle, a series of levels of explanation has been criticized not only as empirically false but also, by Campbell, as unintelligible because it presupposes a discredited pre-Humean view of causation. Campbell's criticism is based on an interventionist-inspired denial that mechanisms and rational connections underpin physical and mental causation, respectively, and hence underpin levels of explanation. These claims echo some superficially similar remarks in Wittgenstein's *Zettel*. But attention to the context of Wittgenstein's remarks suggests a reason to reject explanatory minimalism in psychiatry and reinstate a Wittgensteinian notion of levels of explanation. Only in a context broader than the one provided by interventionism is that the ascription of propositional attitudes, even in the puzzling case of delusions, justified. Such a view, informed by Wittgenstein, can reconcile the idea that the ascription mental phenomena presupposes a particular level of explanation with the rejection of an *a priori* claim about its connection to a neurological level of explanation.

Keywords: Campbell, levels of explanation, intentionality, mechanism, rationality, Wittgenstein

INTRODUCTION

Psychiatry deals with phenomena that range between large-scale higher order social phenomena (e.g., poverty, cultural norms), person level phenomena (e.g., trauma, symptoms such as delusions and syndromes such as depression), and the sub-personal level phenomena (e.g., genes, neurones). It advances explanations that invoke a variety of factors across the scale and both proximal and distal. It is tempting to think that this apparent heterogeneity could be simplified, in principle at least, by fitting it into a picture of different levels of explanation – whether ontological or epistemological – which relate together in some general ways.

The actual applicability of this picture to present psychiatry has been contested (1). Typically, psychiatry trades across levels. This paper, however, describes a principled attack on the very idea of levels of explanation in favor of a form of explanatory minimalism. Put roughly, causal explanation can trade across putative levels because causation is brute and answers to no *a priori* conditions of intelligibility. That being so, the very idea of a "level of explanation" – which depends on such *a priori* assumptions about intelligibility – is undermined. Or so John Campbell argues in a number of papers (2–4).

Having set out Campbell's argument for explanatory minimalism for psychiatry, I compare it to some similar sounding remarks from Wittgenstein's collection *Zettel* (5). Like Campbell, Wittgenstein denies the necessity for mechanisms to mediate (apparently) causal connections and also denies the assumption that rational connections between mental phenomena need be mediated by underlying neurological mechanisms. But Wittgenstein's remarks are aimed at undermining mechanistic accounts of the intentional directedness of mental states, not at denying that there is a characteristic level of explanation for mental phenomena. The problem lies not with the idea of levels of explanation but with an unwarranted metaphysical assumption about how they relate.

The final section builds on Wittgenstein's account of the normative connections between mental phenomena and argues that Campbell's explanatory minimalism is insufficient for psychiatry because it provides no account of what constitutes states as mental states, which plays an important role in psychiatric explanation.

BACKGROUND: LEVELS OF EXPLANATION

There are two dominant approaches to the idea of levels of explanation: ontological and epistemological. Both attempt to shed light on the idea of levels of explanation by characterizing the differences between the levels and also the constraining relations between them.

The ontological view is part of a traditional reductionist picture of the world. On this picture, sciences of the mind, such as psychiatry and psychology, can in principle be reduced to biology (which might be construed as physiology or evolutionary biology), biology to chemistry, and chemistry to physics. Oppenheim and Putnam expressed this view in their classic 1958 paper "Unity of science as working hypothesis."

> It is not absurd to suppose that psychological laws may eventually be explained in terms of the behaviour of individual neurons in the brain; that the behaviour of individual cells – including neurons – may eventually be explained in terms of their biochemical constitution; and that the behaviour of molecules – including the macromolecules that make up living cells – may eventually be explained in terms of atomic physics. If this is achieved, then psychological laws will have, *in principle*, been reduced to laws of atomic physics... [Ref. (6): p. 407]

Oppenheim and Putnam go on to argue that the unity of science is served by "microreductions." These are reductions in which:

> The objects in the universe of discourse of [the reduced science or theory] are wholes which possess a decomposition into proper parts all of which belong to the universe of discourse of [the reducing science or theory] [ibid: 407].

In fact, they argue more strongly that microreduction is the *only* method seriously available for the unity of science [ibid: 408]. They then go on to explore the consequences of this view by examining the preconditions for successfully attaining unity via microreduction. Since microreduction is construed as the only serious possibility for the unity of science, and since its success rests on a number of other things being the case, the goal of unification has a number of presuppositions:

> 1. There must be several levels.
> 2. The number of levels must be finite.
> 3. There must be a unique lowest level ...
> 4. Anything of any level except the lowest must possess a decomposition into things belonging to the next lowest level ... [ibid: 409].

This list suggests the following view of nature and the constraining relations between levels of explanation. The world is made up of basic building blocks or atoms, which display regularities that can be described in the law statements of the most basic science. The basic atoms also combine to form larger structures that display characteristic regularities of their own. These can in turn be codified in the law statements of higher level sciences. But the higher level regularities do not emerge out of nothing. They can be explained as the consequences of the more basic patterns of behavior of atoms. So, the structure of the world and the structure of science can be seen as two isomorphic hierarchies of levels.

The picture suggests three interrelated mutually reinforcing views of the levels of explanation. First, they correspond to different disciplines within science. Second, higher levels contain objects that are constituted from lower level objects. Third, higher level objects are larger than lower level objects. These views fit together on the assumptions that different sciences study objects at different scales and that objects only interact with other objects at the same level. However, these assumptions have been criticized (7).

There is, however, another and quite different approach to levels of explanation, which has been influential. It is based not on the size and composition but rather degree of abstraction to higher order causal processes. This is Marr's threefold epistemological distinction between:

> *Computational theory*: What is the goal of the computation, why is it appropriate, and what is the logic of the strategy by which it can be carried out?
> *Representation and algorithm*: How can this computational theory be implemented? In particular, what is the representation for the input and output, and what is the algorithm for the transformation?
> *Hardware Implementation*: How can the representation and algorithm be realized physically? [Ref. (8): p. 25]

This hierarchy does not concern different ontological levels but rather different ways of understanding the same ontology. The highest, most abstract level concerns the function of a system. It might be carried out by a variety of different algorithms at the middle level. Finally, the same algorithm might be realized in different physical ways at the lowest level. Thus, the higher levels are multiply realizable by lower levels. Determining the computational level is a matter of determining the goals of a system independently of its physical or neurological properties.

Although Marr's epistemic approach seems appropriate for its original application to vision, where the goals of the system can be theorized about independent of algorithm and physiological realization, it is less clear that it applies to psychiatry. As Dominic Murphy argues, actual practice in psychiatry is to determine the functions of systems in part with a view of what the lower level physiology could sustain. "[O]ur understanding of realisation feeds back into and constrains our understanding of the abstract demands of cognition" [Ref. (1): p. 105].

Neither, however, does the ontological view of levels of explanation fit psychiatry because "causes described in genetic vocabulary will be related to effects described in terms of behavioural tests, for example, and generalisations will cross levels" [ibid: 108]. Thus, according to Murphy, there are different systems operating at different levels, unlike the epistemic view, but the different levels interact, unlike the ontological view.

Murphy's argument starts from a relaxed approach to the nature of levels – "I have little to say about what levels of explanation actually are" [ibid: 103] – and then argues that they do not apply to psychiatry. Whatever they are, psychiatric explanation typically crosses them. Such an argument, however, leaves open the response that it merely reflects the current imperfect state of psychiatry. It is tempting to think that Oppenheim and Putnam's picture reflects how reality must be structured even if, for contingent reasons, causal generalizations can link different levels. Equally, the fact that knowledge of physical realization informs more abstract theories of function need not conflict with the idea that there are, in principle, different levels of abstraction applicable to a completed psychiatry. These possibilities remain because Murphy's arguments do not, explicitly at least, undermine the intelligibility of the concept of levels of explanation. By contrast, according to John Campbell, the very idea of a level of explanation is a reflection of a mistaken pre-Humean view of causation. There is less to explanation than the requirement to fit a specific level would require.

CAMPBELL'S CRITICISM OF LEVELS OF EXPLANATION IN PSYCHIATRY

To characterize his target, Campbell gives the example of a discussion of thought insertion by Christopher Frith (9). Frith claims that whether or not inappropriate firings of dopamine neurons are found in subjects who experience thought insertion, this fact could not be used to explain their experiences. It would shed no light on why that kind of symptom, rather than another, was produced by inappropriate firings of dopamine neurons. To shed light, Frith assumes that we need an account pitched at a particular level: in Frith's case that of a sub-personal but still cognitive model of mechanisms supposedly responsible for thought insertion.

Campbell suggests that the assumption that there is a right level of explanation that clarifies things in the way Frith desires is the result of a pre-Humean view of causal explanation. Although often forgotten, Hume successfully argued that there need be no intelligible connection between cause and effect. That is implicit in his rejection of any logical connection to analyze the apparently necessitating relation between cause and effect. Causal connections are merely brute facts to be discovered by experience.

Resisting the idea that the right kind of cause and effect have to be intelligibly, rather than merely brutely related also undercuts the motivation for the levels of explanation picture on both approaches: ontological and epistemic.

> We naturally seek a certain kind of intelligibility in nature; we naturally try to find explanations that will show the world to conform to reason, to behave as it ought. Hume's point is that there are no such intelligible connections to be found. This point has generally been accepted by philosophers thinking about causation. Hume's comments nonetheless do leave us in an uncomfortable position, because we do tend to look for explanations that make the phenomena intelligible to reason. We are prone to relapse, to think that after all we must be able to find intelligibility in the world. This tendency survives, I suspect, in the idea of 'levels of explanation'. The idea is that within certain levels of explanation, we will find a particular kind of intelligibility. [T]he lesson from Hume is that there is no more to causation than arbitrary connections between independent variables of cause and effect. We have to resist the demand for intelligibility [Ref. (2): p. 201].

This is not just a restatement of Murphy's claim that, in psychiatry, explanations may cross levels. Rather, the very idea of levels of explanation, understood as causation operating under some constraint of intelligibility, is itself undercut. This applies to both ontological and epistemic versions as both assume that causation is governed by *a priori* constraints, whether degree of abstraction or composition.

This leaves, however, the issue of shedding some light on the nature of causal connections (if not *a priori* light on particular causal connections). In (non-mental) cases of causation, the notion of *mechanism* plays a central role in empirical research. Searching out the way in which causal influence is transmitted has been an important part of scientific practice. "It would seem a kind of madness if someone were to acknowledge that there is a causal link, but propose that there may be no mechanism linking the two" [Ref. (3): p. 138]. But if science has usefully explored the mechanisms that mediate causal influence, there must be some paradigmatic mechanisms that stand in need of no further explanation and the transmission of motion by impulse, in Hume's billiard ball example, is one such prototype.

Nevertheless, the idea that there *must* be such a mechanism is a kind of synthetic *a priori* claim which, Campbell suggests, should be rejected in line with Hume's argument. He adopts the interventionist model defended most extensively by James Woodward in *Making Things Happen* according to which for X to be a cause of Y is for intervening on X to be away of intervening on Y (10). The rejection of the necessity of a mechanism and the adoption of an interventionist approach opens up the possibility of a causal connection – in accord with interventionism – where there is no mechanism. In the case of psychiatry, however, the key issue is causation in the absence of a *mental* mechanism, whatever that is taken to be.

Just as we find it natural to expect there to be a mechanism underpinning material causal connections – even if this assumption lacks any genuine *a priori* justification – so Campbell also suggests that in the case of mental causation we expect there to be a rational connection between propositional attitudes. The rational link between two propositional attitudes is our paradigm of a mental causal mechanism. So, if one hears someone explain that they believe that Tranmere Rovers won their most recent football match because they heard it on the BBC, which they take to be trustworthy, no further inquiry is needed as to why the beliefs about what they hear and trust cause the belief about the result. Again, however, while the idea that mental causation is underpinned by rational connections is natural and compelling, it lacks *a priori* justification.

> [T]here is an analogy between:
> 1 the idea that propositional attitude ascriptions depend on the ascription of rationality to the subject, and
> 2 the idea that all causal interactions between pieces of matter must be comprehensible in mechanistic terms.
>
> Both ideas express an insight – that we find it extremely puzzling when we encounter causal relations among propositional attitudes that are not broadly rational, just as we find it extremely puzzling when we encounter causal interactions between physical objects that are not mechanistic, and that involve spooky 'action-at-a-distance'. Both ideas express a natural impulse of philosophers – to elevate this kind of point into a kind of synthetic *a priori* demand that reason makes on the world. This impulse has to be resisted [Ref. (3): p. 142].

In both cases, there is a genuine insight. As a matter of custom and habit, we find an absence of material mechanisms and an absence of rational connections between mental states puzzling. But in both cases, it is a characteristic philosophical error to promote this natural expectation into a justified *a priori* claim that the world must respect. Mere custom and habit cannot rationally sustain any such demand on how the world must be.

The rejection of the necessity for rational connections between causally related mental states looks to ease a central problem for the philosophy of psychiatry: explaining delusions. There need be nothing genuinely mysterious about a causal connection, which lacks a rational connection (the expected mental mechanism).

> Suppose you believe:
> 1 that this man is stroking his chin, and
> 2 that this man believes you need to shave.
>
> What is it for the first belief to be a cause of the second? On the interventionist analysis, it is for the intervention on the first belief to be a way of changing whether you have the second belief. So if some external force changed your belief that this man is stroking his chin, you would no longer believe that he believes you need to shave. There is no appeal to rationality here, no appeals to mechanism [Ref. (3): p. 143].

The causal connection between one state and another is underpinned in interventionist terms based on the idea that if intervening on the first belief is a stable way of bringing about a change in the second then this is sufficient for there to be a causal connection between them.

Spelling this idea out involves a little more complexity, however. Given a scanner capable of yielding a complete microphysical description of the human body and a longitudinal study of schizophrenia in a population, Campbell suggests that it might be possible to form a disjunctive characterization of the set of microphysical states that are nomically sufficient for schizophrenia. But that function from physical states to illness would lack any concise expression and would not be couched in terms of variables, which could be affected by local intervention. This point reflects the pragmatic aspect to interventionism: not every nomically sufficient state counts as a cause.

For propositional attitudes to count as causes of delusions, Campbell suggests two conditions have to be met. There should be "systematic relations between cause variables and the subsequent delusion" and there should be a correlation between a change of the cause and a change of the effect [Ref. (3): p. 146]. More generally for the causal explanation of mental states, the causal variables, which he calls "control variables," should have large, specific, and systematic correlations with their effects akin to the way the controls of a car systematically control its behavior. These conditions do not require a rational connection, however. To repeat Campbell's phrase, there need be "no appeal to rationality here."

> The classical philosophical approach has been to regard propositional attitudes as part of a 'conceptual scheme' that we bring to bear in describing the ordinary world. This conceptual scheme is taken to have strong *a priori* constraints on its applicability. In particular, as we have seen, rationality is taken to be a norm with which the scheme has to comply. The appeal I have just been making to the notion of a control variable is intended to replace this invocation of rationality. [I]t is the fact that we have control variables, not the fact that we have rationality, which means that we are 'at the right level' to talk of beliefs and desires [Ref. (3): p. 147].

The phrase "at the right level" occurs in inverted commas to flag the fact that the notion of the right explanatory level has been undercut. Without a pre-Humean insistence on the intelligibility of causal relations, there is no more to the notion of being at the right level than that there is a causal relation tracked through the idea of control variables.

With the idea of control variables replacing an *a priori* requirement for rationality in mental causation, psychiatric explanation of delusions is in principle in the same predicament as the explanation of any other belief. Causal explanation has been achieved once one has an understanding of the variables necessary for changing the delusional belief entertained. The apparently principled problem of attempting to fit primary delusions into some sort of rational framework is replaced by a practical problem of charting the variables that affect them. But is that minimal approach enough for psychiatric explanation?

WITTGENSTEIN ON CAUSATION AND MECHANISM

Campbell suggests a mutually supportive analogy between the denial that mental causation requires rational mediation and that physical causation requires a mechanism. The latter denial echoes some remarks by Wittgenstein in *Zettel*. In this section, I will outline the context of Wittgenstein's discussion, outline a key disanalogy and hence begin to suggest a reason to reject explanatory minimalism in psychiatry.

The later Wittgenstein makes a number of comments both explicitly and implicitly on the connection between mind and body. Throughout his various discussions of propositional attitudes, he denies the possibility of an explanation of meaning or forming an intentional mental state via an appeal to brain states. This accords with his criticisms of causal and dispositional explanations of rule following in the *Philosophical Investigations* (11). As the discussions of both real and ideal machines imply, the attempt to explain rules by appeal to mechanisms is either question begging or fails to sustain their normativity [ibid §§193–4]. Thus, no account could be given in which thought processes might be read off from brain processes.

Such considerations might be thought to motivate the following claim in *Zettel*:

> No supposition seems to me more natural than that there is no process in the brain correlated with associating or with thinking; so that it would be impossible to read off thought-processes from brain-processes. I mean this: if I talk or write there is, I assume, a system of impulses going out from my brain and correlated with my spoken or written thoughts. But why should the *system* continue further in the direction of the centre? Why should this order not proceed, so to speak, out of chaos? [Ref. (5): §608]
> It is thus perfectly possible that certain psychological phenomena *cannot* be investigated physiologically, because physiologically nothing corresponds to them [ibid: §609].

These passages could be interpreted as merely denying that the systematicity of thought can be explained as resulting from an underlying systematicity in the brain. In other words, they could be interpreted as a denial of reductionist explanations of meaning and mental content.

This interpretation would also be consistent with another passage:

> Imagine the following phenomenon. If I want someone to take note of a text that I recite to him, so that he can repeat it to me later, I have to give him paper and pencil; while I am speaking he makes lines, marks, on the paper; if he has to reproduce the text later he follows those marks with his eyes and recites the text. But I assume that what he has jotted down is not *writing*, it is not connected by rules with the words of the text; yet without those jottings he is unable to reproduce the text; and if anything in it is altered, if part of it is destroyed, he sticks in his 'reading' or recites the text uncertainly or carelessly, or cannot find the words at all. – This *can* be imagined! – What I called jottings would not be a *rendering* of the text, not so to speak a translation with another symbolism. The text would not be *stored up* in the jottings. And why should it be stored up in our nervous system? [ibid: §612]

This passage does not say that the marks on paper do not form a system. It is just that they do not form a system of the same sort as writing. That is why they are not a *rendering* of the text. They are not connected by *rules* to words. But in that case, what is their connection to the text supposed to be? Given that this is supposed to be an analogy for the connection between the nervous system and our linguistic abilities, one suggestion is that the marks are connected to written or spoken words *causally* rather than via shared meaning. If this were the case, while the internal system could not be used to *reduce* mental content, it could still play a necessary causal role.

But in fact, Wittgenstein goes further than this. He suggests that there need be *no* cause of a memory in the nervous system. Nothing need be stored "up there" in any form. There need be no physiological regularity or order causing psychological order. Mental order could proceed out of chaos:

> The case would be like the following – certain kinds of plants multiply by seed, so that a seed always produces a plant of the same kind as that from which it was produced – but *nothing* in the seed corresponds to the plant which comes from it; so that it is impossible to infer the properties or structure of the plant from those of the seed that it comes out of – this can only be done from the *history* of the seed. So an organism might come into being even out of something quite amorphous, as it were causelessly; and there is no reason why this should not really hold for our thoughts, and hence for our talking and writing [ibid: §608].
> I saw this man years ago: now I have seen him again, I recognise him, I remember his name. And why does there have to be a cause of this remembering in my nervous system? Why must something or other, whatever it may be, be stored up there *in any form*? Why *must* a trace have been left behind? Why should there not be a psychological regularity to which *no* physiological regularity corresponds? If this upsets our concepts of causality then it is high time they were upset [ibid: §610].

These two passages are pitched against a model of levels of explanation in which a psychological regularity corresponds to a regularity at a lower level. That is, they run counter to the assumption in both Putnam and Oppenheim's ontological, but also Marr's epistemological, accounts of the constraints operating between levels of explanation. By contrast with Campbell, Wittgenstein does not reject the idea that there is a characteristic level of explanation for mental happenings.

Using terminology not in widespread use when Wittgenstein wrote these remarks, they amount to the claim that plants' development do not supervene on their seeds' microstructure. Given contemporary understanding of RNA, this might seem a bizarre possibility. But the denial is of a *modal* claim: that the plant *must* be determined by something in the seed's structure. Wittgenstein denies this assumption, natural though it currently seems.

Like Campbell, Wittgenstein denies that the psychological regularity has to be mediated by one at the neurological or physical level. Furthermore, like Campbell, he suggests an analogical denial. What we might have taken to be a causal physical connection – in the seed and tree example – also need not be mediated by any mechanism. (The analogy is with psychological regularity depending on the physical level.) There is a difference between Wittgenstein and Campbell, however, in that Wittgenstein here assumes the very connection between causation and mechanism that Campbell denies in favor of interventionism. Wittgenstein asks:

> Why should there not be a natural law connecting a starting and a finishing state of a system, but not covering the intermediary state? (Only one must not think of *causal efficacy*.) [ibid: §613]

This passage assumes that the denial of an intervening mechanism implies a denial of causal efficacy. Given that the natural law would sustain the kind of intervention conditionals, then a particular kind of seed producing a particular kind of plant would count as a causal connection according to Campbell. But this looks merely like a difference of terminology. Both Campbell and Wittgenstein can grant a law-like connection. Campbell's account suggests it should count as "causal" while Wittgenstein denies it "causal efficacy." Both deny that there need be an intermediate mechanism. But aside from its causal status, the metaphysical facts are agreed.

Despite that, however, there is a fundamental difference. Wittgenstein's remarks are aimed at removing the tension of reconciling a connection made at the mental level in mental and, according to him, non-causal terms with assumptions about underlying causal mechanisms at a physiological level. Campbell's, by contrast, suggest that transitions at the mental level can, when explanatory, be causal. I will now explore the significance of this difference.

THE ROLE OF AN APPEAL TO RATIONALITY IN WITTGENSTEIN'S DISCUSSION OF INTENTIONALITY

In order to see the difference between Campbell and Wittgenstein, it will be helpful to start with what they share. There are two particularly clear examples in the *Philosophical Investigations* where Wittgenstein, like Campbell, rejects an appeal to underlying mechanisms to explain a connection at the mental level. But, by contrast with Campbell, he goes on to suggest a different account of the mental connection. It is this that suggests Wittgenstein's commitment to a characteristically mental level of explanation.

One example concerns the ability to read out loud, of what reading comprises. He considers the temptation to identify the ability with a mechanism through the example of a comparison between an expert reader and a beginner who can only read words by laboriously spelling them out.

> Now we would, of course, like to say: What goes on in the practised reader and in the beginner when they utter the word *can't* be the same. And if there is no difference in what they are currently conscious of, there must be one in the unconscious workings of their minds, or, again, in the brain. – So we'd like to say: There are, at any rate, two different mechanisms here! And what goes on in them must distinguish reading from not reading. – But these mechanisms are only hypotheses, models to explain, to sum up, what you observe [Ref. (11): p. §156].

Rejecting the hypothetical mechanism – whether an unconscious mental mechanism or physiological one – as well as conscious experiences of being guided or feelings of familiarity, he stresses instead the relation between the text and spoken words, however, mediated. Whatever mediating processes there may be are not what is meant by "reading."

A second example concerns the intentional directedness of having someone in mind.

> "I am thinking of N." "I am speaking of N."
> How do I speak *of* him? I say, for instance, "I must go and see N. today" – But surely that is not enough! After all, when I say "N.", I might mean various people of this name. – "Then there must surely be a further link between my words and N., for otherwise I would *still* not have meant him." Certainly such a link exists. Only not as you imagine it: namely, by means of a mental *mechanism* [ibid: §689].

In the surrounding discussion, various putative explanatory connections are considered and rejected including the idea that no such connection exists, that it is created in being verbally avowed (and that both are true!), and that it is connected to what would, counter-factually, have been reported. Wittgenstein's discussion fits a meta-philosophical injunction: "The point is not to explain a language-game by means of our experiences, but to take account of a language-game" [ibid: §655]. But it also accords with a brief assertion in the middle of an earlier discussion of the intentional directedness of propositional attitudes: "It is in language that an expectation and its fulfilment make contact" [ibid: §445].

This terse comment picks up the idea that avowals and descriptions of expectations and other propositional attitudes reuse the same fragments of language as descriptions of the events that would satisfy them (12). To be able to form such a propositional attitude requires the contingent ability to fit one's avowals and actions into the rational pattern articulated in language. The criticism of underlying mechanisms is made against the background account that psychological order has a rational linguistically mediated structure.

This suggests a fundamental contrast with Campbell's view. Although both Campbell and Wittgenstein reject mechanisms, Wittgenstein's rejection goes hand in hand with a normative and rationalistic view at the mental level which Campbell, at least in the series of papers so far discussed, downplays. In the final section, I will outline the consequences of this disagreement for causal explanation in psychiatry. But first I will briefly summarize how Wittgenstein's views of meaning and mental content suggest a picture of levels of explanation.

A WITTGENSTEINIAN VIEW OF LEVELS OF EXPLANATION

I began by outlining the two dominant approaches to thinking about levels of explanation, both ontological and epistemic. Both approaches not only suggest ways of distinguishing levels but both also suggest constraining relations of either composition, in the ontological case, or realization, in the epistemological approach. Wittgenstein's discussion of mental phenomena in, especially, his *Philosophical Investigations* sets out some of the key differences between normative meaning-related or intentional connections and causal connections. But his remarks in *Zettel* run counter to the assumptions, particularly in Putnam and Oppenheim, of the constraining relations between the psychological and the neurological.

In other words, Wittgenstein's remarks suggest a middle ground between Campbell, on the one hand, and Putnam and Oppenheim, on the other hand. Thinking that there are distinct forms of intelligibility need not imply an *a priori* view of a constraining relation between them. Putnam and Oppenheim assume a series of levels of explanation but then impose a reductionist view of their relations. Campbell rejects the intelligibility of levels of explanation in the first place. Wittgenstein, however, suggests that grasping events or states as mental phenomena presupposes fitting them into a normative and rational linguistic structure but denies that this necessitates connections to a non-normative pattern of causal relations. This suggests that to understand a state to be a state of expectation, for example, involves relating it in a characteristic way to events that would satisfy or fulfill it and hence to presuppose a particular *a priori* pattern of intelligibility. But Wittgenstein denies the need, *a priori* at least, to connect this to any underlying pattern of neurological cause and effect.

The denial of an *a priori* connection to underlying neurology is not the same as denying an *a posteriori* connection. The remarks in *Zettel* do not contradict the possibility of neurological and psychiatric research establishing local connections between medical interventions and psychological effects. Instead, they caution merely against assuming that a pattern at one level must be relatable to a pattern at a lower level.

INFLATING EXPLANATORY MINIMALISM IN PSYCHIATRY

Earlier I reported Campbell's claim that:

> [I]t is the fact that we have control variables, not the fact that we have rationality, which means that we are 'at the right level' to talk of beliefs and desires [Ref. (3): p. 147].

I asked whether the resulting picture of explanatory minimalism was sufficient for psychiatric explanation. It is not sufficient because it provides no account of what constitutes a state as a belief, or a desire or even a delusion. In the absence of that, however, psychiatric explanation would miss a key feature of the phenomena it aims to illuminate.

In an earlier paper, Campbell himself endorses the role of rationality as a presupposition for holding propositional attitudes. He suggests two general reasons for this. The less important one is as follows.

> One simple reason for thinking that rationality is critical here is that unless you assume the other person is rational, it does not seem possible to say what the significance is of ascribing any particular propositional state to the subject. If you tell me that someone rational thinks that it is raining, then given that the person is rational and does not want to get wet, I know what kinds of behavior to expect. If, however, the person is not at all rational, then saying they have the belief has no implications at all for how they will behave [Ref. (13): p. 89].

Campbell's focus is on the *ascription* of propositional attitudes to others. The imputation of rationality goes hand-in-hand with an ascription of propositional attitudes. The argument in the passage seems to concern what follows from the ascription. Without the assumption that the subject is also rational, it is not clear what can be inferred from the ascription of particular mental states to them. But this argument surely broadens. Without a rational pattern, the very idea that the subject has some determinate mental state is undermined (14–16).

There is a second connection, however, which Campbell thinks is the more important. It concerns the connection between rationality, belief, and meaning. Understanding others' utterances and hence ascribing beliefs to them is only possible against a background assumption of rationality. There is a balance between possible irrationality and the ascription of meaning.

> The finding of irrationality can always be traded for a finding of mistranslation. And we should always translate so as to find the subject rational in the use of a term by the lights of the subject's own understanding of the term [ibid: 90].

This sketch of the connection between interpretation and the ascription of belief echoes Wittgenstein's suggestion of a linguistic mediation of mental states and their intentional objects. The very idea of having propositional attitudes presupposes a harmony between the meaning of utterances, the mental states held, and the pattern of actions they rationalize.

Thus, the claim that control variables, rather than rationality, constitutes the "right level" to talk of beliefs and desires fails to address a prior constitutive question. What is it about some particular causes and effects, described using the interventionist model of causation, which constitutes them as intentional mental states in the first place? Given its broad application to causation in the non-mental as well as mental world, talk of control variables alone is insufficient to address this question. But introducing issues of language, interpretation, and rationality suggests that there is a particular level of explanation which is of central importance to psychiatry when it addresses the meaning and content of psychological phenomena.

In the example described above, Campbell argues that for the belief that this man is stroking his chin to cause the belief that this man believes you need to shave all that is needed is a suitable interventionist counterfactual relation rather than an appeal to rationality. But without some further background conditions, of which rationality is one plausible candidate, the ascription of determinate mental states is illicit.

It may seem, however, that defending the role of a rational connection between utterance, mental state, and behavior is particularly difficult in the case of psychiatric explanation. After all, psychiatry investigates phenomena that appear to resist rational understanding. While this is true and puzzling, however, it does not threaten the connection itself.

Consider Campbell's discussion of Capgras in the earlier paper (13). He uses the link between meaning and rationality to suggest a problem with the interpretation of characteristic expressions of the delusion. The characteristic type of utterance associated with the delusion is: "That woman is not my wife!." But that sentence might be used to make a number of different claims. It might, for example, be used to flag the discovery of illegality in a past wedding ceremony. The most plausible interpretation in the context of the expression of the Capgras delusion is something like: This [demonstrated] woman is not that [remembered] woman. But such an interpretation is put under strain because, typically, the subject of the delusion does not attempt to carry out any of the paradigmatic or canonical forms of checking appropriate for such a claim: for example, discussing past events and checking memories. They do not do what they ought to do to check such a thought. Given the link between meaning, mental content, and rationality, this apparent failure of rationality undermines such an interpretation.

Campbell himself goes on to try a partial accommodation of the delusion within rational space by suggesting it might be a deviant hinge or framework proposition since, if it were, it would be rational not to subject it to testing. It is unclear whether this approach can work as it is unclear what understanding there can be of a framework proposition which is not shared (17). But the difficulties Campbell highlights seem genuine. Does a subject who makes a paradigmatic Capgras utterance but does nothing else different really believe that their partner is an imposter? Likewise, does the Cotard utterance "I am dead" really express the impossible belief that the subject is dead? The difficulty seems fundamental to such cases.

In a more recent paper, Campbell seems more pessimistic about fitting delusions into any sort of rational pattern. He considers a delusion in which the subject thinks that her mother's thoughts were inserted into her mind via raindrops and the air conditioner. He points out that the structure of this delusion could not be used to teach what is meant by "rationality." But further:

> The trouble is not even that the patient is not rational. We have no idea what a rational way of going on would be, once one has accepted that thoughts are being inserted into one's mind. How must the world be, for that to happen? Would it make sense to argue with this patient that, by her own lights, it is not the raindrops in the air conditioning that should be blamed, but rather the electrical sockets all around? We have departed so far from the ordinary world that we have no idea what stands fast and what has to go [Ref. (3): p. 141].

Again, these seem to be genuine and substantial difficulties in working out what the subject actually thinks. But Campbell offers a particular interpretation of the difficulty. He says:

> We should not appeal to the idea that there are *a priori* constraints on causal relations among propositional attitudes. We have to accept that the propositional attitudes are one thing and the causal relations among them are another. If propositional attitudes do not conform to rationality, that is puzzling. But we cannot legislate in advance that this cannot happen [ibid: 140].

This seems an unjustified response, however. The problem is not merely that there are contingent breakdowns in the expected rational connections between identifiable propositional attitudes. Rather, in the case of delusion, the nature of the supposed propositional attitudes themselves is, and continues to be, puzzling. Hence, for example, attempts to suggest that the delusion may be a propositional attitude of imagination rather than belief [e.g., Ref. (18)]. It is not that the bizarre quality of delusions threatens the general connection between meaning, mental state, and rationality but instead that the general connection helps to illuminate what is so puzzling about delusion. The connection to rationality is not arbitrary: it helps justify the claim that a state is a mental state or that an utterance expresses a particular propositional attitude.

CONCLUSION

Given the heterogeneity of the factors that feature in explanations in psychiatry, it is tempting to assume that, in principle, they can be related within an ordered hierarchy of levels of explanation. There is reason, however, to doubt that this picture fits contemporary psychiatry. But that leaves open the response that that is a reflection merely on the current state of psychiatric research and that a completed psychiatry would form an ordered hierarchy.

More radically, John Campbell has argued in recent papers that the very idea of levels of explanation presupposes a discredited pre-Humean view of causation. He claims that although the assumption that physical causation is mediated by mechanisms and that psychological causation is mediated by rational relations have both been fruitful neither need to be true. With their rejection as synthetic *a priori* claims about the world, the idea of levels of explanation also falls away to leave an explanatory minimalism.

Comparing Campbell's remarks with some superficially similar remarks in Wittgenstein's *Zettel* suggests an objection to explanatory minimalism. The very idea of a state being a mental state presupposes broader connections. Rationality is one such candidate. If so, explanation in psychiatry inflates from Campbell's minimalism and introduces an appropriate level of explanation at which mentality comes into view. But it is possible to hold on to the necessity of such general levels of explanation while rejecting *a priori* claims about how different levels of explanation must relate to each other.

REFERENCES

1. Murphy D. Levels of explanation in psychiatry. In: Kendler KS, Parnas J, editors. *Philosophical Issues in Psychiatry*. Baltimore, MD: Johns Hopkins University Press (2008). p. 102–25.
2. Campbell J. Causation in psychiatry. In: Kendler KS, Parnas J, editors. *Philosophical Issues in Psychiatry*. Baltimore, MD: Johns Hopkins University Press (2008). p. 199–216.
3. Campbell J. What does rationality have to do with psychological causation? Propositional attitudes as mechanisms and as control variables. In: Bortolotti L, Broome M, editors. *Psychiatry as Cognitive Neuroscience*. Oxford: Oxford University Press (2009). p. 137–50.
4. Campbell J. Causation and mechanisms in psychiatry. In: Fulford KWM, Davies M, Gipps R, Graham G, Sadler J, Stanghellini G, et al., editors. *Oxford Handbook of Philosophy and Psychiatry*. Oxford: Oxford University Press (2013). p. 935–49.
5. Wittgenstein L. *Zettel*. Oxford: Blackwell (1981).
6. Oppenheim P, Putnam H. Unity of science as a working hypothesis. In: Boyd R, Gasper P, Trout JD, editors. *Philosophy of Science*. London: MIT Press (1991). p. 405–27.
7. Craver C. *Explaining the Brain*. Oxford: Oxford University Press (2007).
8. Marr D. *Vision*. San Francisco, CA: W.H.Freeman (1982).
9. Frith C. *The Cognitive Neuropsychology of Schizophrenia*. Hove: Lawrence Erlbaum (1992).
10. Woodward. *Making Things Happen*. Oxford: Oxford University Press (2003).
11. Wittgenstein L. *Philosophical Investigations*. Oxford: Blackwell (1953).
12. Arrington RL. Making contact in language: the harmony between thought and reality. In: Arrington RL, Glock H-J, editors. *Wittgenstein's Philosophical Investigations*. London: Routledge (1991). p. 175–202.
13. Campbell J. Rationality, meaning, and the analysis of delusion. *Philos Psychiatr Psychol* (2001) **8**:89–100. doi:10.1353/ppp.2001.0004
14. Davidson D. *Inquiries into Truth and Interpretation*. Oxford: Oxford University Press (1984).
15. Dennett D. *The Intentional Stance*. Cambridge, MA: MIT Press (1987).
16. Hopkins J. Wittgenstein, Davidson, and radical interpretation. In: Hahn F, editor. *The Library of Living Philosophers: Donald Davidson*. Chicago: Open Court Hopkins (1999). p. 255–85.
17. Thornton T. Why the idea of framework propositions cannot contribute to an understanding of delusion. *Phenomenol Cogn Sci* (2008) **7**:159–75. doi:10.1007/s11097-007-9079-6
18. Currie G. Imagination, delusion and hallucinations. *Mind Lang* (2000) **15**:168–83. doi:10.1111/1468-0017.00128

16

Executive Function is Selectively Impaired in Old Age Bipolar Depression

Leonardo Caixeta[1,2], Vânia L. D. Soares[2], Renata T. Vieira[2], Cândida D. Soares[2], Victor Caixeta[1], Sandra B. Ferreira[2] and Tales A. Aversi-Ferreira[3,4]*

[1] Bipolar Disorder Unit, Hospital das Clínicas, School of Medicine, Federal University of Goiás, Goiania, Brazil, [2] Unit of Neuropsychiatry, Neuropsychology and Behavior Neurology (UNCO), Federal University of Goiás, Goiania, Brazil, [3] Federal University of Alfenas, Alfenas, Brazil, [4] System Emotional Science, School of Medicine and Pharmaceutical Sciences, University of Toyama, Toyama, Japan

Edited by:
Debora Marques Miranda, Universidade Federal de Minas Gerais, Brazil

Reviewed by:
Timo Partonen, National Institute for Health and Welfare, Finland
Maria Aparecida Bicalho, Universidade Federal de Minas Gerais, Brazil

***Correspondence:**
Leonardo Caixeta
leonardocaixeta1@gmail.com

Background: Little is known about the cognitive signature of bipolar disorder (BD) in elderly brains. The neuropsychological features of depressive elderly with early-onset BD are largely unknown. This issue is relevant because cognitive impairment can produce an additional impact on the already compromised functionality of elderly with BD. The aim of this study is to assess executive functions (EFs) in the depressive phase of elderly outpatients with early-onset BD.

Methods: Forty-nine elderly outpatients with early-onset BD were assessed with several neuropsychological tests for EF in the depressive phase of the disorder.

Results: Executive dysfunction is very common in old age bipolar depression. Thirteen patients (26.5%) had a pseudodementia presentation. The worst performances were observed in the following tests: Trail Making B, Stroop Test 3, Backward Digit Span and Wisconsin Card Sorting Test.

Conclusion: Executive dysfunction profile in elderly BD is complex and heterogeneous, but most cases display difficulties in working memory, inhibitory control, mental flexibility, and information processing speed. The performance of elderly with bipolar depression in executive assessment can be divided into two main categories: (1) Single EF domain impairment; and (2) Multiple EF domain impairment with or without a pseudodementia syndrome. Executive dysfunction in old age bipolar depression may be explained by lack of sufficient mental energy to run those cognitive processes that require larger amounts of effort to be performed.

Keywords: aging, bipolar disorder, elderly patients, executive dysfunctions, neuropsychology

INTRODUCTION

Bipolar disorder (BD) in the elderly is a growing public health concern and a major cause of disability (Sajatovic et al., 2015). Despite considerable knowledge accumulated in recent decades points to the presence of cognitive impairment in BD (Tsitsipa and Fountoulakis, 2015), few consistent data exist on the neuropsychology of old age patients with BD. Studies with very selective samples and multiple age groups suggest that higher age in BD is associated with greater neurocognitive deficits (Kessler et al., 2013). Some authors state that elderly patients with BD have significant cognitive disabilities and that BD with late onset is associated with more severe cognitive impairment than early-onset BD (Schouws et al., 2007, 2009), but all these studies were done in euthymic BD. There is a lack of knowledge especially in relation to the neuropsychology of bipolar depression in late life (Rise et al., 2016).

Little is known about the cognitive signature of BD in elderly brains. This issue is relevant because cognitive impairment can produce an additional impact on the already compromised functionality of elderly with BD (Rise et al., 2016). Besides that, the identification of specific cognitive profiles in BD can perhaps help differentiate subgroups and pave the way to the identification of possible endophenotypes (Volkert et al., 2016). Finally, a comprehensive mapping of cognitive domains impaired in BD can add some insights into the physiopathology of the disorder and the many mechanisms by which cognitive symptoms may relate to behavior alterations. For instance, in the young adult it is known that cognitive deficits in BD are directly related to the daily losses presented by these patients in social adaptation or even in suicide behavior (Malloy-Diniz et al., 2009).

Among the most disputed issues in contemporary cognitive neuropsychiatry is the deterioration of executive functions (EF) and the neurocircuitry disruption that support these disabilities. EFs impact affective-emotional, motivational, and social skills. Executive dysfunction may represent an important contributor to the cognitive, functional and social impairments usually observed in adults (Tsitsipa and Fountoulakis, 2015) and elderly (Schouws et al., 2009) with BD.

The aim of this study is to assess EFs in the depressive phase of elderly outpatients with early-onset BD.

MATERIALS AND METHODS

Participants

We have selected 49 consecutive elderly outpatients diagnosed by the same senior psychiatrist (LC) as a BD according to DSM-5 criteria, from the BD program in a university hospital (Hospital das Clínicas at the Federal University of Goiás) in Central Brazil, from August 2013 to 2015. All subjects provided written informed consent, as required by the ethical committee of Federal University of Goiás. The hospital's catchment area involves a population of approximately 1500 elderly. We calculated a sample size of 50.33 patients with a sampling error of approximately 2.13% at a 95% confidence level. Originally, 157 elderly bipolar patients were enrolled in the service. Of these, 91 were eliminated by the exclusion criteria (44 patients with late-onset BD – type VI; 42 with dementia; 3 alcoholics; and 2 with psychostimulant use). Thus, 66 patients were eligible for the study, but 17 refused or could not undergo neuropsychological evaluation, leaving, therefore, 49 patients to compose the definitive sample.

Inclusion criteria were: age 60–90 years old; the onset of BD prior to the age of 40 years (definition of 'early-onset' BD [Schouws et al., 2009]); any ethnicity; portuguese speaking Brazilian outpatients; followed at least during 1 year in our service with serial (monthly) psychiatric assessment in order to rule out primary dementia cases. We have included any degree of cognitive and functional impairment. We have excluded from our search elderly bipolar patients who began their disease late in life (BD type VI), since this subtype has a strong association with neurological disease and structural damage to the brain (Ng et al., 2008), what could interfere in the neuropsychological performance. The same senior psychiatrist (LC) made the diagnosis of BD and assessed the diagnosis for the depressive phase of BD.

According to international recommendations (Burdick et al., 2015), it was excluded subjects taking high-dose anticholinergics, topiramate, clozapine, tricyclics, benzodiazepines, psycho-stimulants, and those who had electroconvulsivetherapy within past 6 months. Medication titration could not be done in the week of neuropsychological assessment. Patients with general clinical conditions which could impact cognitive performance were also not included in our sample: delirium, untreated hypothyroidism, severe anemia, AIDS, any kind of encephalopathy.

Laboratory Testing and Neuroimaging

All patients were submitted to laboratory screening and neuroimaging exams according international recommendations (Knopman et al., 2001) in order to rule out systemic or neurological causes of cognitive impairment and primary dementias with structural brain damage.

Neuropsychological Assessment

Neuropsychological assessment of the patients was carried out by three senior clinical neuropsychologists (VLDS, CDS, SBF).

Patients were evaluated during the depressive phase. Total assessment was divided into three sessions of 30 min each within a period of 3 days in order to prevent mental fatigue. All patients were submitted to the most frequently used tests for assessing EFs in aging (Faria et al., 2015), consisting of subtests from standard test batteries validated for Portuguese use in Brazilian patients: (1) Trail Making Test Form A (TMT-A): attention, information processing speed; (2) Trail Making Test Form B (TMT-B): mental flexibility, information processing speed; (3) Stroop Test: inhibitory control; (4) Digits Forward and Backward subtests (WAIS-R): working memory; (5) Wisconsin Card Sorting Test (WCST): mental flexibility; (6) Verbal Fluency Test (Animals category): verbal fluency and information processing speed; (7) Verbal Fluency or Letter Fluency Test – FAS: verbal fluency, information processing speed and active search for specific information in memory.

Statistical Analysis

Clinical data were statistically analyzed using conventional descriptive methods. Quantitative variables were described as means and standard deviations, while categorical variables were described using frequency and percentages.

When describing neuropsychological performance in depressive bipolar elderly, we transformed raw scores for all individual neuropsychological tests (except WCST) into Z-scores using the distribution of the older adult controls' database (i.e., controls' performance on any test has mean of 0 and SD of 1). For WCST was used T-score; scores were considered abnormal based on Brazilian norms and validation of these instruments in Brazilian population (Zimmermann et al., 2015).

RESULTS

The mean age of BD patients was 69.1 years (60–88, ±7.0). Most patients were female ($n = 31$; 62.2%). The mean schooling was 10.8 years (±4.2).

Table 1 shows the descriptive analysis (mean, standard deviation) of the neuropsychological assessment.

Of patients, 28 (57.1%) scored −2SDs (moderate impairment) on at least one EF test measure, and 49 (100%) scored lowest than −1SD on at least one EF test measure or, in other words, none of the patients had a normal performance in all EF tests.

Forty patients (81.6% of total sample) presented a more extensive and severe dysexecutive profile, involving many EFs. From these, thirteen patients (26.5%) had a pseudodementia presentation.

Nine patients (18.3%) had a mild executive dysfunction (affecting, for example, only one executive domain, such as working memory or mental flexibility).

The mean of WCST (24.4) according *T*-score is in the diagnostic category of "moderately-to-severely impaired range" (Heaton et al., 1993). No patient was able to complete all categories of WCST perfectly.

Twenty-three patients (46.9%) had scores lowest than −1SD on VFT-animals and 22 (44.8%) on FAS. On average, patients had difficulty in verbal fluency tasks as indicated by negative *Z*-scores, but the mean does not exceed the adopted *Z*-score cutoff. On average, performance on VFT (Animals category) was worse than FAS (−0.86 versus −0.69, respectively).

DISCUSSION

Our data support the notion that executive dysfunction is very common in elderly with BD, since all the sample had performance below average in at least one EF test. Moreover, we report new data concerning executive dysfunction in BD elderly outpatients in the depressive phase, since studies are focused on euthymic or manic elderly (Young et al., 2006; Schouws et al., 2007, 2009; Samamé et al., 2013). It is not clear whether bipolar and unipolar old age depression have similar or different cognitive profiles, but our data, when compared to the cognitive profile described in the literature for unipolar depression in the elderly (Dybedal et al., 2013; Pantzar et al., 2014), show similarity in executive dysfunction between both forms of depression. Xu et al. (2012) studying adults state that bipolar and unipolar patients have a similar pattern of cognitive impairment during the state of acute depressive episode.

It is remarkably difficult to make definite statements about the neuropsychology of BD, since it depends on the BD type, age considered, medications in use, and mood state at the time of neuropsychological assessment (Tsitsipa and Fountoulakis, 2015). Even in a relatively homogeneous sample as ours, in which we have specifically arranged elderly, BD patients, in the depressive phase, the cognitive profile is not uniform. Notwithstanding all the sample presented with some degree of executive dysfunction, it was found a large span of executive performance among subjects, as indicated by the high variability between minimum and maximum scores, and varying from mild executive dysfunction (affecting, for example, only one executive domain, such as selective attention or working memory), until a more extensive and severe dysexecutive profile (involving many EFs, such as mental flexibility, mental engagement, self-control, self-monitoring, many attention domains and working memory). Therefore, BD elderly patients can indeed reach a level of cognitive dysfunction in their depressive phase compatible with a dementia syndrome (depressive pseudodementia). Based on our data, we can divide patients' performance in neuropsychological assessment into two main categories: (1) Single EF domain impairment; and (2) Multiple EF domain impairment. The

TABLE 1 | Statistical description of executive function tests in elderly with bipolar depression ($n = 49$).

Tests	Minimum	Maximum	Mean	Standard deviation
Stroop Test 1	−6.05	6.24	1.17	2.30
Stroop Test 2	−0.02	7.52	2.02	2.01
Stroop Test 3	−5.19	1.55	−1.05	1.42
Errors Stroop 1	0	1.00	0.04	0.20
Errors Stroop 2	0	6.00	0.23	0.98
Errors Stroop 3	0	15.00	1.79	3.17
TMT-A	−8.08	8.05	1.30	3.38
TMT-A errors	0	4.00	0.19	0.77
TMT-B	−10.44	1.06	−2.02	2.40
TMT-B errors	0	26.00	8.84	8.44
VF Digit Span	−1.85	1.34	−0.55	0.48
VB Digit Span	−2.54	0.10	−1.17	0.55
VFT – Animals category	−2.39	1.66	−0.86	0.81
VFT – FAS	−2.31	1.89	−0.69	1.00
WCST	15	49.00	24.42	9.27

TMT, Trail Making Test; VF Digit Span, Visual Forward Digit Span; VB Digit Span, Visual Backward Digit Span; VFT, Verbal Fluency Test; WCST, Wisconsin Card Sorting Test. For all tests (except WCST) was used Z-score. For WCST was used T-score.

second one can present with or without a pseudodementia syndrome.

One of the most impaired functions in the elderly with BD in our sample was mental flexibility, assessed by TMT-B and WCST. These two tests also recruit working memory, selective attention, mental engagement and are sensitive to impulsive behavior (Faria et al., 2015). As these functions are related to the dorsolateral prefrontal areas in the brain, we can assume that in depressive phase of BD elderly the neural circuits involving this topography are somewhat affected. In fact, some authors (Brooks et al., 2010) have found dorsolateral prefrontal hypometabolism using positron emission tomography associated with impaired performance on executive tasks among older adults with BD.

Inhibitory control is a core member of the EFs and generally refers to the capacity to actively inhibit or delay a dominant response to achieve a goal. Inhibitory control is impaired in BD elderly as showed by poor performance in Stroop Test 3 seen in our sample. The ability to inhibit an automatic behavior and perform a controlled behavior is associated to ventral-fronto-striatal circuitry (Durston et al., 2002), therefore we can suggest that this network is somewhat impaired in the depressive phase of BD. Penfold et al. (2015) also found inferior prefrontal hypoactivation (using MRI) in medication-free adults with bipolar depression during response inhibition test. The weakening of inhibitory control can contribute to some aspects of social and functional impairment seen in BD, and can explain in part how depressive BD meet the day-to-day demands of conflict, delay, and compliance challenges.

Information processing speed is impaired in our sample of old age bipolar depression as suggested by TMT-B poor performances. Processing speed was also one of the most impaired cognitive functions in many studies dealing with BD in adults (Xu et al., 2012; Kessler et al., 2013). In fact, some authors (Volkert et al., 2016) suggest that reduced psychomotor speed could serve as a potential endophenotype for BD.

Working memory was also importantly impaired in our sample, as demonstrated by Digits Backward subtest of WAIS-R. Information storage by verbal working memory (measured in Digits Forward) and verbal content processing in working memory (measured in Digits Backward) are EFs highly sensitive to depressive mood states.

Verbal fluency was not importantly impaired in most cases of our sample, suggesting that the neural circuits involved in this cognitive function generally are not impacted by depressive state in bipolar elderly. In adults this finding might be different, since some authors have found important deficits in verbal fluency among depressive bipolar patients (Xu et al., 2012).

Executive dysfunction in elderly in the depressive phase of BD may be associated with lack of sufficient mental energy to run those cognitive processes that require larger amounts of effort to be performed. For instance, patients in our sample had more difficult in TMT-B than TMT-A, and in Stroop Test 3 than the other phases, suggesting that, as cognitive demand increases, their cognitive reserve is overpowered and, as a consequence, they cannot keep up with the growing executive demands. According to this hypothesis, this cognitive impairment would be reversible, returning to normal cognitive functioning as soon as patients switch their depressive state into an euthymic (normal mood) phase. Follow-up studies are required to test if this executive dysfunction in BD elderly is really transitory and completely dependent upon the affective phase of BD. One study has addressed cognitive outcomes in longitudinal assessment of old age euthymic BD (type I and II) and concluded that they did not exhibit accelerated cognitive decline over 2 years (Gildengers et al., 2012). Another study performs a systematic review about the neurocognitive dysfunction in BD and concluded that cognitive dysfunction is an enduring component and represents a core primary characteristic of BD, rather than being secondary to the mood state or medication, but they add that this core deficit can be confounded (either increased or attenuated) by the disease phase, in other words, depression may produce a temporary increase in the total amount of cognitive deficits seen in BD, which is in accordance with our view (Tsitsipa and Fountoulakis, 2015).

As a methodological limitation of our study, despite having restricted our sample only to the depressive phase of BD, this mood state in itself is very heterogeneous, varying from mild to severe depression. Future studies must try to control this variable.

In summary, executive dysfunction was very common in BD elderly patients in our sample, notwithstanding it was not severe in most of the cases. BD seems to contribute with additional burden to the aging process in the brain. Trail Making B, Stroop Test 3, Backward Digit Span and WCST represent a useful selection of tests sensitive to the specific executive dysfunction presented in old age bipolar depression. These tests seem more suitable than global screening cognitive measures frequently used in samples of elderly patients with cognitive impairment (e.g., the Mini-Mental State Examination; MMSE), which are likely not applicable in BD context due to low sensitivity (Burdick et al., 2015). The general pattern of specific executive deficits presented by our sample may suggest anomalous prefrontal-subcortical activation in elderly with BD. These cognitive findings can help understand some social and functional impairments seen in this disorder and indicate therapeutic targets as well as insights into its neurophysiopathology.

AUTHOR CONTRIBUTIONS

LC conception or design of the work; data collection; data analysis and interpretation; drafting the article. VS data collection; data analysis and interpretation. CS data collection; data analysis and interpretation. RV data collection; data analysis and interpretation; drafting the article. SF data collection; data analysis and interpretation. VC data collection; data analysis and interpretation. TA-F data collection; data analysis and interpretation; drafting the article.

ACKNOWLEDGMENT

TA-F thanks to CNPq-Brazil for Scholarship in Productivity Research.

REFERENCES

Brooks, J. O. III, Bearden, C. E., Hoblyn, J. C., Woodard, S. A., and Ketter, T. A. (2010). Prefrontal and paralimbic metabolic dysregulation related to sustained attention in euthymic older adults with bipolar disorder. *Bipolar Disord.* 12, 866–874. doi: 10.1111/j.1399-5618.2010.00881.x

Burdick, K. E., Ketter, T. A., Goldberg, J. F., and Calabrese, J. R. (2015). Assessing cognitive function in bipolar disorder: challenges and recommendations for clinical trial design. *J. Clin. Psychiatry* 76, e342–e350. doi: 10.4088/JCP.14cs09399

Durston, S., Thomas, K. M., Yang, Y., Ulug, A. M., Zimmerman, R. D., and Casey, B. J. (2002). A neural basis for the development of inhibitory control. *Dev. Sci.* 5, F9–F16. doi: 10.1111/1467-7687.00235

Dybedal, G. S., Tanum, L., Sundet, K., Gaarden, T. L., and Bjølseth, T. M. (2013). Neuropsychological functioning in late-life depression. *Front. Psychol.* 4:381. doi: 10.3389/fpsyg.2013.00381

Faria, C. A., Alves, H. V. D., and Charchat-Fichman, H. (2015). The most frequently used tests for assessing executive functions in aging. *Dement. Neuropsychol.* 9, 149–155. doi: 10.1590/1980-57642015DN92000009

Gildengers, A. G., Chisholm, D., Butters, M. A., Anderson, S. J., Begley, A., Holm, M., et al. (2012). Two-year course of cognitive function and instrumental activities of daily living in older adults with bipolar disorder: evidence for neuroprogression? *Psychol. Med.* 43, 801–811. doi: 10.1017/S0033291712001614

Heaton, K. R., Chelune, G. J., Talley, J. L., Kay, G. G., and Curtiss, G. (1993). *Wisconsin Card Sorting Test Manual.* Odessa: Psychological Assessment Resources.

Kessler, U., Schoeyen, H. K., Andreassen, O. A., Eide, G. E., Hammar, Å., Malt, U. F., et al. (2013). Neurocognitive profiles in treatment-resistant bipolar I and bipolar II disorder depression. *BMC Psychiatry* 13:105. doi: 10.1186/1471-244X-13-105

Knopman, D. S., DeKosky, S. T., Cummings, J. L., Chui, H., Corey-Bloom, J., Relkin, N., et al. (2001). Practice parameter: diagnosis of dementia (an evidence-based review). Report of the Quality Standards Subcommittee of the American Academy of Neurology. *Neurology* 56, 1143–1153.

Malloy-Diniz, L. F., Neves, F. S., Abrantes, S. S., Fuentes, D., and Corrêa, H. (2009). Suicide behavior and neuropsychological assessment of type I bipolar patients. *J. Affect. Disord.* 112, 231–236. doi: 10.1016/j.jad.2008.03.019

Ng, B., Camacho, A., Lara, D. R., Brunstein, M. G., Pinto, O. C., and Akiskal, H. S. (2008). A case series on the hypothesized connection between dementia and bipolar spectrum disorders: bipolar type VI? *J. Affect. Disord.* 107, 307–315. doi: 10.1016/j.jad.2007.08.018

Pantzar, A., Laukka, E. J., Atti, A. R., Fastbom, J., Fratiglioni, L., and Bäckman, L. (2014). Cognitive deficits in unipolar old-age depression: a population-based study. *Psychol. Med.* 44, 937–947. doi: 10.1017/S0033291713001736

Penfold, C., Vizueta, N., Townsend, J. D., Bookheimer, S. Y., and Altshuler, L. L. (2015). Frontal lobe hypoactivation in medication-free adults with bipolar II depression during response inhibition. *Psychiatry Res.* 23, 202–209. doi: 10.1016/j.pscychresns.2014.11.005

Rise, I. V., Haro, J. M., and Gjervan, B. (2016). Clinical features, comorbidity, and cognitive impairment in elderly bipolar patients. *Neuropsychiatr. Dis Treat.* 17, 1203–1213. doi: 10.2147/NDT.S100843

Sajatovic, M., Strejilevich, S. A., Gildengers, A. G., Dols, A., Al Jurdi, R. K., Forester, B. P., et al. (2015). A report on older-age bipolar disorder from the International Society for Bipolar Disorders Task Force. *Bipolar Disord.* 17, 689–704. doi: 10.1111/bdi.12331

Samamé, C., Martino, D. J., and Strejilevich, S. A. (2013). A quantitative review of neurocognition in euthymic late-life bipolar disorder. *Bipolar Disord.* 15, 633–644. doi: 10.1111/bdi.12077

Schouws, S. N., Comijs, H. C., Stek, M. L., Dekker, J., Oostervink, F., Naarding, P., et al. (2009). Cognitive impairment in early and late bipolar disorder. *Am. J. Geriatr. Psychiatry* 17, 508–515. doi: 10.1097/JGP.0b013e31819e2d50

Schouws, S. N., Zoeteman, J. B., Comijs, H. C., Stek, M. L., and Beekman, A. T. (2007). Cognitive functioning in elderly patients with early-onset bipolar disorder. *Int. J. Geriatr. Psychiatry* 22, 856–861. doi: 10.1002/gps.1751

Tsitsipa, E., and Fountoulakis, K. N. (2015). The neurocognitive functioning in bipolar disorder: a systematic review of data. *Ann. Gen. Psychiatry* 14:42. doi: 10.1186/s12991-015-0081-z

Volkert, J., Haubner, J., Kazmaier, J., Glaser, F., Kopf, J., Kittel-Schneider, S., et al. (2016). Cognitive deficits in first-degree relatives of bipolar patients: the use of homogeneous subgroups in the search of cognitive endophenotypes. *J. Neural. Transm. (Vienna)* 123, 1001–1011. doi: 10.1007/s00702-016-1581-y

Xu, G., Lin, K., Rao, D., Dang, Y., Ouyang, H., Guo, Y., et al. (2012). Neuropsychological performance in bipolar I, bipolar II, and unipolar depression patients: a longitudinal, naturalistic study. *J. Affect. Disord.* 136, 328–339. doi: 10.1016/j.jad.2011.11.029

Young, R. C., Murphy, C. F., Heo, M., Schulberg, H. C., and Alexopoulos, G. S. (2006). Cognitive impairment in bipolar disorder in old age: literature review and findings in manic patients. *J. Affect. Disord.* 92, 125–131. doi: 10.1016/j.jad.2005.12.042

Zimmermann, N., Cardoso, C. O., Trentini, C. M., Grassi-Oliveira, R., and Fonseca, R. P. (2015). Brazilian preliminary norms and investigation of age and education effects on the Modified Wisconsin Card Sorting Test, Stroop Color and Word test and Digit Span test in adults. *Dement. Neuropsychol.* 9, 120–127. doi: 10.1590/1980-57642015DN92000006

17

Enhancing Executive Function and Neural Health in Bipolar Disorder through Reasoning Training

Erin E. Venza[1†], Sandra B. Chapman[1†], Sina Aslan[1,2], Jennifer E. Zientz[1], David L. Tyler[3] and Jeffrey S. Spence[1]*

[1] Center for BrainHealth, The University of Texas at Dallas, Dallas, TX, USA, [2] Advance MRI, LLC, Frisco, TX, USA, [3] Private Practice, Dallas, TX, USA

Edited by:
Leandro Fernandes Malloy-Diniz, Universidade Federal de Minas Gerais, Brazil

Reviewed by:
Mahesh Menon, University of British Columbia, Canada
Jonathan K. Wynn, University of California, Los Angeles, USA

***Correspondence:**
Sandra B. Chapman
schapman@utdallas.edu

† These authors have contributed equally to this work.

Cognitive deficits in executive function and memory among individuals with bipolar disorder (BD) are well-documented; however, only recently have efforts begun to address whether such cognitive deficits can be ameliorated through cognitive training. This pilot study examined the effects of a top–down, cognitive reasoning training program in adults with BD on both brain and cognitive measures. Twenty-seven participants (11 males, 16 females), aged 21–70 years old, completed the study. Participants completed neurocognitive testing and functional magnetic resonance imaging (fMRI) before and after training, consisting of 8 h (2 h/week) of training in small groups. The training delivered information processing strategies that were implemented and applicable to a variety of daily living contexts. Results indicated that participants showed significant gains in the primary outcome measure of complex abstraction, also referred to as gist reasoning, as well as in untrained domains of executive function and memory. We found a significant increase in resting cerebral blood flow (CBF) in left inferior frontal gyrus after cognitive training. We also found that resting CBF in the right frontal middle gyrus correlated positively with performance on the measure of complex abstraction. This feasibility study provides promising evidence that short-term reasoning training can enhance cognitive performance and brain health in adults with BD. These data motivate further efforts to explore adjuvant therapeutics to improve cognitive performance and underlying brain systems in bipolar, as well as other psychiatric disorders. Clinicaltrials.gov Identifier: NCT02843282, http://www.clinicaltrials.gov/ct2/show/NCT02843282

Keywords: bipolar disorder, cerebral blood flow, cognition, cognitive training, executive function, frontal networks, memory

INTRODUCTION

Bipolar disorder (BD), a mental illness with recurring episodes of mania and depression, can have far-reaching detrimental effects on the everyday function and living of those with the diagnosis. In addition to causing distressing shifts in mood and energy level, we now know that patients with BD experience cognitive deficits, not only during mood episodes but also in remission (van Gorp et al., 1998; Quraishi and Frangou, 2002; Martinez-Aran et al., 2004). A meta-analysis of cognitive deficits in adult euthymic patients with BD (i.e., neither depressed nor manic) consistently found deficits in executive function and verbal learning, with variance in deficits across other areas of cognition, such as memory, abstraction, set-shifting, sustained attention, and inhibition (Robinson and Ferrier, 2006). Robinson's study also suggested such cognitive deficits in euthymic individuals with BD are consistent across cultures (Robinson and Ferrier, 2006).

Imaging studies also reveal underlying neural abnormalities, including changes in brain blood flow and activation. For instance, O'Connell et al. (1995) examined cerebral blood flow (CBF) in BD and identified decreased CBF in prefrontal cortex during unipolar and bipolar depression, with schizophrenic and manic bipolar individuals exhibiting even greater hypofrontality. Benabarre et al. (2005) further supported this finding of hypofrontality by correlating poorer performance in executive function and memory with low perfusion in the frontal region. Resting state functional imaging studies of individuals with BD demonstrate abnormal activation in the prefrontal and cingulate cortices (Blumberg et al., 2003; Phillips et al., 2003, 2008; Kronhaus et al., 2006; Green et al., 2007). Other studies, including a quantitative meta-analysis review of functional magnetic resonance imaging studies in BD, extend previous evidence of attenuated activation of the left inferior frontal gurus (IFG) across emotional and cognitive tasks (Phillips et al., 2008; Chen et al., 2011). Whereas cognitive and brain abnormalities in both symptomatic and asymptomatic individuals with BD are well-documented, available clinical interventions continue to be limited to pharmacological and/or psychological counseling regimens to manage symptoms. These approaches will continue to be a vital aspect of BD treatment; however, additive benefits may be derived from protocols that directly address the common cognitive sequelae.

Emerging research has examined whether individuals with BD benefit from non-pharmacological approaches to improve the cognitive symptom complex of BD, such as cognitive training, with promising results suggesting an array of potential gains in performance (Deckersbach et al., 2010; Preiss et al., 2013; Torrent et al., 2013). Previously reported studies have implemented cognitive training alone or in conjunction with other symptom management and therapeutic interventions (e.g., mood management and psychoeducation) (Deckersbach et al., 2010; Preiss et al., 2013; Torrent et al., 2013; Demant et al., 2015). The cognitive training portion of these studies targeted specific processing deficits in BD, such as memory, executive function, and attention. Studies by Deckersbach et al. (2010) and Preiss et al. (2013) resulted in significant cognitive and mood improvement after training, specifically with gains on measures of executive function and reductions in reported depressive symptoms. On the other hand, similarly well-constructed studies to address cognitive and psychosocial deficits in BD failed to find significant improvement in cognitive function (Torrent et al., 2013; Demant et al., 2015). While cognitive gains were not reported, the Torrent et al. (2013) participants did exhibit significantly improved scores on a functional outcome measure. These studies, while varied in results, support the rationale for investigating component-specific cognitive training with individuals with BD.

Based on this foundation of evidence that targeting specific cognitive processes may benefit individuals with BD, we were interested in testing whether a top–down strategy-based cognitive training of integrative processes could reap brain and cognitive gains as has been uncovered in other populations (Gamino et al., 2010; Vas et al., 2011, 2016a; Mudar et al., 2013; Cook et al., 2014; Chapman et al., 2015). We were particularly interested in measuring the benefits of gist-reasoning training, which we will refer to as 'reasoning training,' in this population since prior work has shown reasoning training to generalize to other cognitive domains more than targeting specific processes, albeit in different populations (Gamino et al., 2010; Vas et al., 2011, 2016a; Mudar et al., 2013; Cook et al., 2014; Chapman et al., 2015). Evidence from a series of studies from our lab has found that strategy-based reasoning training (described below) improved cognitive functions in both primary and secondary measures across several different populations including individuals with mild cognitive impairment (MCI), traumatic brain injury (TBI), as well as healthy adults and teenagers (Gamino et al., 2010; Anand et al., 2011; Vas et al., 2011, 2016a; Chapman and Mudar, 2014; Chapman et al., 2015, 2016; Mudar et al., 2016). Randomized trials comparing reasoning training to a new learning intervention in adults with TBI in chronic stages post-injury showed significant gains in abstraction, memory, executive functions of working memory and switching, non-verbal reasoning, and daily function (Vas et al., 2011). A larger randomized trial in adults with TBI found similar improvements in measures of executive function, memory and daily function (Vas et al., 2015). In this latter study, the reasoning training was shown to significantly improve psychological health with reduced depression and stress-related symptoms. A comparison of reasoning training versus a new learning intervention in adults with MCI also resulted in significant improvements in executive function and memory measures in the reasoning group (Mudar et al., 2016). A more recent study with healthy adults examined both cognitive and neural changes after reasoning training and found significant improvements in a number of frontally mediated executive functions (Chapman et al., 2015). More notably, this integrative cognitive training induced a number of brain changes at rest, including increased global and regional CBF in the default mode network and central executive network, greater connectivity in these same regions, and increased white matter integrity in the left uncinate (Chapman et al., 2015).

Previous cognitive training approaches with BD have focused largely on targeting specific cognitive processes and measuring improvement through cognitive batteries alone. Additionally, previous training protocols (e.g., cognitive remediation) have tended to require a lengthy time commitment, sometimes up to 24 weeks. In contrast, strategy-based, integrative processes can be trained over a relatively short time-span with training in ways to incorporate strategies into daily life routines. Based on principles of experience-driven plasticity, the likelihood of increased usage throughout daily life may increase chances of achieving spill-over affects into other cognitive domains, maximizing treatment efforts. For instance, in the aforementioned studies which trained reasoning, participants showed improvements in the primary outcome measure, as well as generalized cognitive benefits in other secondary outcome measures of memory and executive functioning skills (Vas et al., 2011, 2015; Chapman et al., 2015).

To date, no known study has investigated the effectiveness of a reasoning training program in individuals with BD. Additionally, of the cognitive trainings completed within the BD population, none have coupled neurocognitive and imaging measures. Therefore, the current phase I pilot trial fills a void by providing preliminary evidence of cognitive and neural benefits from a cognitive training program in individuals with BD. The current study had three major objectives. First, we proposed that a reasoning program, Strategic Memory Advanced Reasoning Training (SMART), would not only improve performance on the primary domain of complex abstraction, but would also show transfer effects to untrained domains of executive function and memory. Our second major goal was to determine whether training induced neuroplasticity changes as measured by resting CBF using pseudo-continuous arterial spin labeling (pCASL) magnetic resonance imaging (MRI). Recent studies demonstrate that CBF is reflective of neuronal health (Chen et al., 2013). Lastly, we were interested in whether the cognitive gains would be linked to specific brain blood flow changes to elucidate possible mechanisms of improvement.

MATERIALS AND METHODS

Participants

A total of 27 adults with a diagnosis of BD I or II between the ages of 21 and 70 (see **Table 1**) participated in this study. Participants were recruited at the University of Texas Southwestern Medical Center, through psychiatrist referral, flyers and website advertising. All participants were native English speakers, had a minimum of high school education, and provided written consent in accordance with the Institutional Review Board (IRB) of our academic institutions: The University of Texas at Dallas and The University of Texas Southwestern Medical Center. Participants underwent a telephone screen with a research clinician, including a brief medical questionnaire covering their history, current medications and any pre-existing conditions. After the participant met the requirements covered by the phone screen, they were asked to complete a neurocognitive testing battery, including the Mini Mental State Exam (MMSE). The inclusion of partially (in addition to fully) remitted individuals served to confirm sufficient sample size and was based on evidence suggesting that residual affective symptoms have no major effects on objective cognitive function (Burdick et al., 2012). If subjects scored $\geq$26 on the MMSE and $\leq$17 on the Hamilton Depression Rating Scale (HAM-D), they were invited to continue with the intervention portion of the study. In addition, participants were administered a standard MRI prescreening form to assess the presence of contraindications for MRI compatibility (e.g., non-removable metal within/on the body, claustrophobia, pregnancy, non-correctable vision problems, head trauma, and CNS disease). Diagnosis of BD and euthymic state was confirmed with collaborating psychiatrist. When the participant was not a patient of the collaborating psychiatrist, written approval was obtained from the treating psychiatrist confirming the following: participant was between ages 21 and 70; participant had a diagnosis of BDI or BDII; participant was in a euthymic, rather than manic or depressive, state; participant had been stable on medications for at least 3 months; and participant was believed to be appropriate for the study. All patients were taking mood stabilizing medications and reported remaining on a consistent dose of medications throughout the study (see **Table 1**).

Procedure

This was a phase I, non-randomized, pilot intervention study examining the neurocognitive and brain changes from a reasoning training program, SMART, in euthymic individuals with BD. Outcome measures were administered at baseline (pre-training, T1) and within 2 weeks after completing the training sessions (post-training, T2). All 27 participants received SMART in small groups of 5–7 people. Groups were led by the same licensed speech-language pathologist. Groups met for 2 h once a week for 4 weeks (total training of 8 h). Groups were formed in order of enrollment and schedule alignment.

Reasoning Training

Strategic Memory Advanced Reasoning Training equips participants with meta-cognitive strategies of Strategic Attention, Integrative Reasoning, and Innovation as a guide for engaging in deeper-level innovative thinking across real-life activities (Chapman and Kirkland, 2014). Strategic Attention targets the ability to filter irrelevant information in order to focus on the important information. Integrative Reasoning targets the ability to abstract meanings from specific key details (be it from a book, medical or legal advice, a movie, conversation, meeting, or other daily interaction), and to interpret within a broader context of world knowledge to create global themes and take away messages that remain relevant to the information or task at hand. Innovation targets perspective-taking, fluency, and novel idea generation in topics or areas of life that have become stagnant.

At the end of each session, participants were given homework assignments that required use of the strategies.

TABLE 1 | Subject characteristics.

Participant demographic	(Mean ± SD)
Total participants (*n*)	**27**
Age at study entry (years)	45.8 ± 12.9
Gender (M/F)	11/16
Education (years)	16.0 ± 1.8
Age of onset (years)	34.0 ± 12.3
Duration of illness (years)	11.8 ± 9.7
Mini Mental State Examination (MMSE)	27.7 ± 1.2
Hamilton Depression Rating Scale (HAMD)	5.9 ± 3.6
Medications (*n*)	**27**
Lithium	8
Anticonvulsant	13
Antipsychotic	17
Antianxiety	4
Antidepressant	7
Benzodiazepines	4

Homework was discussed in the initial portion of the following session, and each participant reported completing the assignments. Exercises utilized a variety of materials, varying in complexity (e.g., articles, artwork, podcasts, current events, TED Talks, etc.) in multiple modalities. Emphasis was put on application of strategies to other contexts (e.g., personal relationships, work environment, and daily responsibilities). The three strategies were presented in sessions one and two, leaving sessions three and four for (1) participant demonstration of how they were incorporating the strategies in their daily lives, (2) participant-generated exercises that required implementation of the strategies (exhibiting further understanding of material), and (3) feedback, questions, and broader conversations focusing on how to practically and independently implement the strategies in daily life, as this was the final goal.

Outcome Measures

Neurocognitive Measures

A battery of neurocognitive measures was administered on a non-training day at two time periods, i.e., baseline/pre-training (T1) and within 2 weeks after training (T2). Cognitive assessment measures were completed in individual, face-to-face testing sessions. All test batteries were pencil and paper measures administered by a trained research clinician (see **Table 2**).

The primary outcome measure of complex abstraction was evaluated using the Test of Strategic Learning (TOSL) (Chapman et al., 2002). Complex abstraction is also referred to as gist reasoning. The TOSL is an assessment that has been previously utilized as a criterion-referenced measure of ability to abstract meaning from complex information in typically developing youth (Chapman et al., 2012; Motes et al., 2014), healthy adults (Anand et al., 2011; Vas et al., 2016a), adults with MCI (Mudar et al., 2016), and adults and youth with TBI (Vas et al., 2011, 2015, 2016a; Cook et al., 2014). Recent evidence supports TOSL as both a sensitive and specific metric of complex abstraction ability (Vas et al., 2016b). Participants read a complex text (approximately 600 words). To evaluate complex abstraction, participants are then instructed to generate a high-level summary of the text. Another subtest of TOSL assesses the ability to recall key facts from the text. The TOSL complex abstraction measure has a manualized objective scoring system where each abstracted idea in the summary receives one point and verbatim or paraphrased ideas do not receive any points, the final score then reflects the total

TABLE 2 | Brief description of outcome variables (scaled scores used if not otherwise specified below).

Variable	Measure	Description
Primary outcome measure		
Complex abstraction	Test of Strategic Learning (TOSL) (Chapman et al., 2002)	Participant synthesizes information into overview. Score: number of abstracted ideas
Secondary outcome measures		
Concept formation	Similarities (Wechsler, 1997a)	Participant explains what pairs of words have in common
Problem solving	D-KEFS Card Sorting Task (Delis et al., 2001)	Participant sorts six cards into two groups of three based on eight different sorting rules
Verbal fluency	Controlled Oral Word Association (COWA) (Benton et al., 1994; Spreen and Strauss, 1998)	Participant says as many words/minute as they can that begin with the given letter
Memory	Logical memory (Wechsler, 1997b)	Participant orally recalls (immediate and delayed) details of a short story read aloud
	Memory for key facts/details (TOSL) (Chapman et al., 2002)	Participant recalls (after probe) specific important facts/details from the text. Score: 0–24
	Rey Auditory Verbal Learning Test (RAVLT) (Rey, 1964; Schmidt, 1996; Spreen and Strauss, 1998)	Participants are given a list of 15 unrelated words repeated over five different trials and are asked to recall. After an interference list is given, the client must again recall the original list of 15 words and then again after 30 min. Score: 0–15 per trial
Working memory	Digits backward (Wechsler, 1997b)	Participant orally recalls number strings in backward order
Inhibition	D-KEFS Color-Word Task, Condition 3 (Delis et al., 2001)	Participant names the color of the ink a work is printed in versus reading the word (color word different than color ink)
Switching	Trails B	Participant alternately connects a set of numbers and letters in ascending alphabetical order
	D-KEFS Color-Word Task, Condition 4 (Delis et al., 2001)	Participant alternates from reading color of printed word and stating ink color of printed word. Score: total time to complete
Daily function	Quality of life in bipolar disorder (Michalak and Murray, 2010)	A 56-item self-report questionnaire on 12 domains of quality of life: Physical, Sleep, Mood, Cognition, Leisure, Social, Spirituality, Finances, Household, Self-esteem, Independence and Identity and two optional domains (Work and Education). Score: 56–280, higher score is associated with higher quality of life

number of accurately abstracted ideas from the text. Different versions of the TOSL were administered at pre- and post-testing.

Secondary outcome measures included tests of executive function (verbal reasoning, problem solving, switching, verbal fluency), memory (including recall for details from TOSL text), complex attention, and quality of life (see **Table 2**). Recall for details from TOSL text yields a maximum possible score of 24. The Quality of Life in Bipolar Disorder (QoL.BD) was created by the Collaborative Research Team to study psychosocial issues in BD (Michalak and Murray, 2010). The QoL.BD scale is the only quality of life questionnaire specifically designed for individuals with BD. The full version has 56 questions within 10 basic domains: physical, sleep, mood, cognition, leisure, social, spirituality, finances, household, self-esteem, and two optional domains (work and education).

MRI Experiment

Magnetic resonance imaging investigations were performed on 12 participants (six males/six females), as the rest of the participants exhibited contraindications for MRI compatibility (non-removable metal within/on the body and claustrophobia). Imaging was performed on a 3 Tesla MR system (Philips Medical System, Best, The Netherlands). A body coil was used for radiofrequency (RF) transmission and an 8-channel head coil with parallel imaging capability was used for signal reception. The MRI scans of participants were performed at rest with their eyes open and on a non-training day. We used a pCASL sequence to measure CBF at rest (Aslan et al., 2010) as well as a high resolution T1 weighted image as an anatomical reference. The details of imaging parameters and their processing techniques are provided below.

Imaging parameters for pCASL experiments were: single-shot gradient-echo EPI, field-of-view (FOV) = 240 × 240, matrix = 80 × 80, voxel size = 3 mm × 3 mm, 27 slices acquired in ascending order, slice thickness = 5 mm, no gap between slices, labeling duration = 1650 ms, time interval between consecutive slice acquisitions = 35.5 ms, TR/TE = 4020/14 ms, SENSE factor 2.5, number of controls/labels = 30 pairs, RF duration = 0.5 ms, pause between RF pulses = 0.5 ms, labeling pulse flip angle = 18°, bandwidth = 2.7 kHz, echo train length = 35, and scan duration 4.5 min. The hypercapnia BOLD imaging parameters were: single shot gradient echo EPI sequence, TR/TE/flip = 2000 ms/25 ms/80°, 43 axial slices, slice thickness = 3.5 mm, FOV = 220 mm × 220 mm, matrix size = 64 × 64 and scan duration = 7 min. The high resolution T1 weighted image parameters were: Magnetization Prepared Rapid Acquisition of Gradient Echo (MPRAGE) sequence, TR/TE = 8.3/3.8 ms, shot interval = 2100 ms, inversion time = 1100 ms, flip angle = 12°, 160 sagittal slices, voxel size = 1 mm × 1 mm × 1 mm, FOV = 256 mm × 256 mm × 160 mm, and duration 4 min.

MRI Analysis

The pCASL MRI data underwent routine processing (Aslan et al., 2010). PCASL image series were realigned to the first volume for motion correction (SPM5's realign function, University College London, UK). All datasets were within the applied motion threshold of 3 mm translation and 3° rotation. An in-house MATLAB (MathWorks, Natick, MA, USA) program was used to calculate the difference between averaged control and label images. The difference image was then corrected for imaging slice delay time to yield CBF-weight image, which was normalized to the brain template from Montreal Neurological Institute (MNI). Lastly, the absolute CBF was estimated in the units of mL blood/min/100 g of brain tissue (Aslan et al., 2010). The absolute whole brain blood flow values were calculated by averaging all the voxels in the absolute CBF (aCBF) map. In voxel based analyses (VBA), the individual aCBF maps were spatially smoothed [with full-width half-maximum (FWHM) of 4 mm] to account for small differences in sulci/gyri location across subjects.

Statistical Analyses

Each neurocognitive measure was considered a dependent variable in a standard linear model. We did not omit subjects whose baseline measures were not paired with their respective post-training measures from lack of follow-up. Thus, the intent-to-treat analyses necessitated the use of a mixed model with time as a within-subject fixed factor and subjects themselves as a random factor. Temporal contrasts, which estimated mean change across the two measurement times, were of primary interest; and all hypotheses were one-sided. That is, we expected only improvements post-training. Given the inclusion of partially (in addition to fully) remitted individuals with BD, we included, in another set of models, the depression measure HAM-D as a covariate with possible interactions temporally. In these models temporal contrasts were conditional on the mean HAM-D estimate across subjects. In addition, we included age as a covariate as well as indicators for the presence or absence of concurrent antipsychotic and anticonvulsive medications to assess any potential effects on the neurocognitive measures. Finally, we applied the Benjamini-Hochberg method to control the false discovery rate (FDR) due to the large number of statistical tests on the neurocognitive battery.

For the voxel-based imaging analyses, each subject had paired measurements pre- and post-training. Thus, voxel level analyses were paired t-tests. Statistical inference, however, was at the cluster level using AFNI's *3dclustsim* bootstrap method conditional on a cluster-defining threshold ($p = 0.05$) applied to all voxel-level statistics. At this threshold, contiguous clusters of voxels exceeding 1,449 (11,592 mm^3) in number (volume) were significant at a 0.05 level, corrected for multiple clusters. We also implemented a VBA with age adjusted TOSL scores as a covariate to find potential brain regions where changes in CBF are associated with changes in complex abstraction as measured by TOSL. In this case cluster-level inference proceeded as just described, except that the cluster-defining threshold was $p = 0.005$ and the cluster size threshold for a corrected inference level of 0.01 was 263 voxels (2,104 mm^3).

RESULTS

Neurocognitive Measures

All 27 participants completed 8 h of training. **Table 3** summarizes results for primary and secondary outcomes. Most significant changes include measures of executive function and memory. Executive function measures WAIS Similarities (concept formation) ($p = 0.004$) and DKEFS Card Sorting (problem solving) ($p = 0.001$) improved significantly from pre- to post-training. Immediate memory recall improved on TOSL memory for details ($p = 0.002$). RAVLT scores improved across trials ($p = 0.008$), at a short delay ($p < 0.001$), and at long delay ($p = 0.020$). Our primary measure of complex abstraction did show improvement from pre- to post-training, although not based on the FDR criterion. This is similarly true for Trails B, Digits Backward, and Color-Word (inhibition). When HAM-D was included as a covariate, results were consistent.

MRI Experiment

CBF was measured by pCASL MRI in BD participants' pre- and post-cognitive training. The global CBF did not change significantly from T1 to T2; 51.2 ± 9.8 mL/100 g/min and 52.3 ± 7.8 mL/100 g/min, respectively ($p = 0.40$). The VBA was conducted on relative CBF maps, which included dividing the aCBF maps by the whole brain aCBF. In a prior investigation, we had shown that such technique improves sensitivity of regional differences by reducing physiological variations (Aslan et al., 2010). **Figure 1** shows the VBA results between T1 and T2. The BD group showed a significant increase in blood flow in left IFG after cognitive training (T1 < T2). However, no change was detected in the reverse contrast (T1 > T2). **Table 4** summarizes these findings.

TABLE 3 | Summary of results for each cognitive domain (mean, standard error).

	Pre-training	Post-training	*p*-value
Primary outcome measure			
Complex abstraction			
TOSL	2.35 (0.32)	3.04 (0.32)	0.040
Secondary outcome measures			
Executive function			
WAIS, similarities	12.63 (0.40)	13.61 (0.41)	0.004**
DKEFS card sorting: correct sorts	11.70 (0.42)	13.56 (0.42)	<0.001**
DKEFS card sorting: description	11.74 (0.43)	12.96 (0.43)	0.001**
DKEFS card sorting: recognition	11.56 (0.47)	12.89 (0.47)	0.007**
Trails B	73.44 (5.43)	66.86 (5.48)	0.052
Verbal fluency	11.30 (0.61)	11.82 (0.61)	0.121
Memory			
Logical memory, immediate	13.85 (0.59)	13.30 (0.59)	0.812
Logical memory, delay	11.89 (0.72)	12.26 (0.72)	0.278
TOSL – memory for details	13.26 (1.00)	16.37 (0.98)	0.002**
RAVLT, trial 5	11.96 (0.48)	12.74 (0.48)	0.008**
RAVLT, short delay	9.74 (0.65)	11.44 (0.65)	<0.001**
RAVLT, long delay	9.70 (0.68)	10.93 (0.68)	0.019*
Complex attention			
Digits backward	6.78 (0.36)	7.30 (0.36)	0.039
D-KEFS color-word, condition #3	10.12 (0.54)	11.04 (0.54)	0.023
D-KEFS, color-word, condition #4	11.04 (0.37)	11.46 (0.37)	0.092
Everyday function questionnaires			
Quality of life in bipolar disorder	176.93 (6.90)	183.93 (7.00)	0.095

**FDR = 0.10; **FDR = 0.05.*

Neural Correlates of Brain and Cognition

Whole brain voxel-wise correlation analysis between complex abstraction (i.e., TOSL Complex abstraction score and CBF maps, T2–T1) showed significant correlation to right middle frontal CBF; MNI coordinates: [+42 +30 +22], *t*-score of 7.6 and cluster size = 263 voxels (2,104 mm^3, FWE cluster-level $p < 0.01$), shown in **Figure 2**.

DISCUSSION

This feasibility study is the first known attempt to investigate both cognitive (i.e., executive function, memory, complex attention) and brain (i.e., CBF) changes in response to a top–down, strategy-based cognitive training protocol in BD. The novel aspects of this pilot trial are testing a cognitive training protocol (SMART) and brain measurement (CBF) that have previously shown promise in studies focused on harnessing cognitive and neural plasticity. As stated above, SMART teaches top–down, metacognitive strategies that can be utilized in everyday life and its efficacy is supported by prior evidence of improved executive function and frontoparietal networks in other clinical and healthy populations (Chapman et al., 2015, 2016; Vas et al., 2015; Mudar et al., 2016). Previous neurobehavioral interventions in BD have focused largely on improving the psychological health with only more recent focus on targeting the cognitive deficits that have now been well-documented (Deckersbach et al., 2010; Preiss et al., 2013; Torrent et al., 2013; Demant et al., 2015). Additionally, recent technological advancements in resting state MRI allow measurement of neuroplasticity changes with CBF, which is beginning to show promise as one potential objective neural marker of enhanced brain health. This potential measurement of neuroplasticity change is derived from a well-accepted coupling between healthy neural activity and cerebrovascular flow (Raichle and Gusnard, 2002; Chapman et al., 2016), as well as accumulating evidence that different forms of interventions show increased CBF with concomitant improvement in cognitive functions (Takeuchi et al., 2013; Chapman and Mudar, 2014; Chapman et al., 2015, 2016; Vas et al., 2016a).

Three major findings emerged from this pilot study. First, we found that a strategy-based reasoning training, delivered over 4 weeks with 2 h each week for a total of 8 h, improved complex abstraction abilities in adults with BD. Moreover, the training showed generalized benefits to other cognitive domains that were not specifically trained, including specific executive functions (i.e., concept abstraction and problem solving) and memory

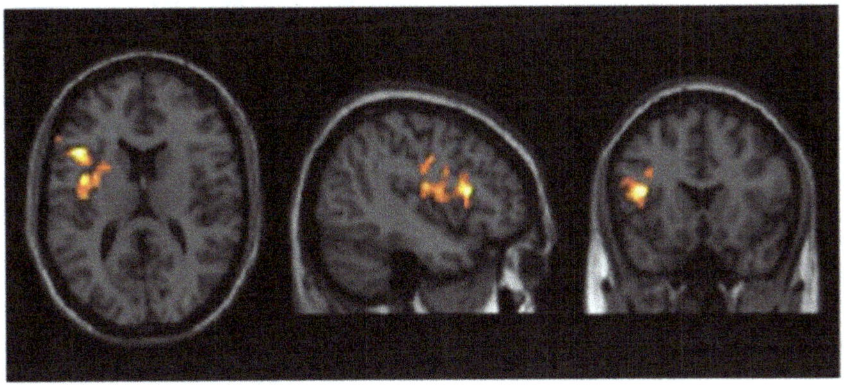

FIGURE 1 | Results of cerebral blood flow (CBF) voxel based comparison superimposed on T1 image. Bipolar disorder (BD) participants showed a CBF increase in left inferior frontal gyrus from T1 to T2 after cognitive training, $p < 0.05$ (FWE cluster corrected) and $k \geq 11{,}592$ mm^3.

TABLE 4 | Cerebral blood flow (CBF) regions that showed significant blood flow change at rest in bipolar disorder (BD) group from T1 to T2.

			MNI			
Brain regions	**BA**	**Cluster size (mm^3)**	***X***	***Y***	***Z***	***T*-value**
Pre-Training < Post-Training						
Left Inferior Oper. Frontal G	13/45/6/44	11,752	−42	18	14	6.79
Pre-Training > Post-Training						
None						

FWE cluster level, corrected p < 0.05, voxel threshold at p = 0.05 and K = 11,592 mm^3.

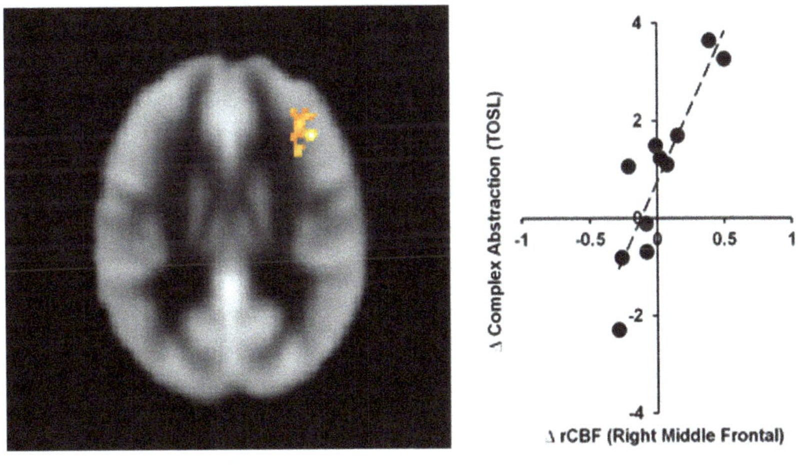

FIGURE 2 | Bipolar disorder group showed significant association between gains in regional CBF and behavioral measures. The BD group's TOSL complex abstraction score difference showed significant association to right middle frontal CBF increase at T2, cluster-level $p < 0.01$ (FWE corrected).

(word lists at immediate and delayed periods and details from complex information). Secondly, we found significant pre to post increases in CBF in the left prefrontal cortex, namely in the left inferior frontal gyrus (LIFG), a region of the brain associated with semantic and cognitive control processes (Poldrack et al., 1999; Gold et al., 2006; Badre and Wagner, 2007; Danker et al., 2008; Race et al., 2009). Third, we found a positive correlation between enhanced cognition (complex abstraction) and increased resting CBF in the right prefrontal cortex, supporting the potential for the training to positively impact both brain and cognition; in other words, enhance brain health.

Our findings of improved executive functions in BD with SMART concur with recent evidence from other trainings that impairments in executive function in BD can be mitigated with cognitive training (Deckersbach et al., 2010; Preiss et al., 2013). The trainings in these two prior studies trained a broad-base of specific processes whereas our training taught strategies to deal with complex information and contexts encountered in everyday life. Additionally, we found significant improvement on memory measures, a cognitive domain which has not previously shown to be enhanced in other cognitive training studies with BD. These findings support SMART training as an integrative, top–down process that promotes not only synthesizing and abstraction of information, but can also potentially promote deeper encoding and recall of information. Current results add to prior evidence that cognitive training of higher-order integrative functions, which equip individuals with strategies to employ throughout their daily routine after training has ended, could be a beneficial intervention, when used to complement standard of care therapeutic approaches in BD.

Since both our training and the Preiss et al. (2013) study took only 8 h of training, we propose that short-term cognitive interventions may be worth the cost in terms of time and money since they appear to provide benefits in mitigating cognitive deficits in BD. Moreover, the present results add to the emerging evidence that neurotherapeutic management and overall life functionality in BD may be improved when the cognitive deficits are addressed along with the psychiatric symptoms of depression (Deckersbach et al., 2010). The current results suggest the degree of depressive symptoms was not a contributing factor that impacted response to cognitive training, a promising finding which suggests these psychiatric problems are not necessarily a limiting factor to treatment benefit. Treatment of psychiatric disorders, e.g., BD, and other brain disorders has far too long been siloed with sole focus on only one domain of brain health rather than taking into account other aspects of brain health, both cognitive and psychological health. For example, the psychiatric symptoms in BD tend to be the sole focus of management without addressing the co-occurring cognitive deficits. In a contrasting focus, in acquired brain injury the key focus has been on remediating executive functions without concern for the co-morbid psychiatric problems, such as depression and anxiety which are being identified (Didehbani et al., 2013; Max et al., 2015). The potential for cognitive training to show spillover effects to improving psychological health benefits is intriguing. In a previous study, we found that SMART training in adults with TBI showed not only cognitive gains but also psychological benefits that were manifested by a significant reduction of depressive and stress-related symptoms that continued to improve 3 months after the training ceased (Vas et al., 2016a). Unfortunately, we failed to measure post-treatment psychological health in BD in the present study. Nonetheless, Deckersbach et al. (2010) showed that cognitive training was associated with a decrease in residual depressive symptoms as well-increased occupational and overall psychosocial functioning immediately and at 3 month follow up.

In addition to improvement on neurocognitive measures, imaging results showed increased regional brain blood flow in the left prefrontal cortex. There is considerable controversy as to whether increased CBF is associated with improved brain function (Sojkova et al., 2008) or compensatory reaction. Much of the controversy arises in activation studies, but less so in resting state CBF studies. For example, activation studies have measured both increases and decreases in BOLD signal during mental activation tasks. What is important to note, however, is that this change is a transient effect and is typically restored to baseline level when the brain returns to resting state (Raichle and Gusnard, 2002). Therefore, as a tightly regulated system, resting CBF is remarkably consistent and an important biomarker (Raichle and Gusnard, 2002). Additionally, results from a growing number of studies reveal that resting state CBF may represent a promising neural marker of brain response to distinct interventions across clinical populations (Mozolic et al., 2010; Vas et al., 2015). These studies identify a correlation between increased CBF and improved cognitive function with healthy agers and those with brain injury (Takeuchi et al., 2013; Chapman et al., 2015, 2016; Vas et al., 2015). We propose that the increased resting CBF in the present study of individuals with BD reflects a similar improvement. Specifically within the frontal lobe, we found a significant increase in resting CBF in the LIFG (which showed a significant gain from pre- to post-training). Other researchers have supported the pivotal role of the LIFG as being associated with cognitive control processes, such as executive function (Poldrack et al., 1999; Gold et al., 2006; Badre and Wagner, 2007; Danker et al., 2008; Race et al., 2009). What is intriguing and perhaps strengthens the present results, is that we also previously reported increased resting CBF in the LIFG at post SMART training in other populations (Chapman et al., 2015; Vas et al., 2015).

Thirdly, we found a significant association between increased CBF in the right middle frontal gyrus (MFG) and improved complex abstraction. We speculate that the reasoning training engaged cognitive control to facilitate processing of complex information that also involved fine-tuning of attentional systems to inhibit less important information with concomitant improvement in prefrontal cortex (Chapman et al., 2016). Supporting this plausible explanation, Corbetta et al. (2008) have shown the right MFG to be a potential modulator between attention networks. Additionally, the right frontal cortex has previously been associated with increased CBF being linked to higher complex abstraction performance (Chiu Wong et al., 2006).

Whereas the current results require further examination in larger clinical trials, the capacity to induce increased resting CBF in the prefrontal cortex of individuals with BD as a result of integrative cognitive training could have beneficial clinical implications. This is the first known study to investigate brain changes in response to cognitive training in BD with findings suggesting improvement to brain areas that might be compromised by the disease, such as the prefrontal cortex (Blumberg et al., 2003; Phillips et al., 2003, 2008; Kronhaus et al., 2006; Green et al., 2007). In sum, we propose that the increased health of the frontal regions, as manifested by elevated CBF, could be a result of experience-driven neural plasticity where the concerted cognitive effort recruited and improved the health of this neural system.

Limitations and Future Directions

This study has a number of strengths, which include utilization of brain and neurocognitive outcome measures, as well as implementation of a novel cognitive training intervention for individuals with BD. We also note a number of limitations which make us interpret our findings cautiously. The major limitations include the lack of either a waitlist or active control group and the fact that the same clinician trained and tested participants. With regard to the first limitation of no control group, we cannot rule out the possibility of practice effects; however, we do not feel that practice effects account for the gains across measures, especially given the convergence of gains in cognition and increased CBF. Additionally, in prior studies testing efficacy of SMART, which included active control or wait-list control groups, we found similar executive function and neural benefits from the reasoning training as compared to the control groups. Specifically, studies with traumatic brain injury populations demonstrated similar gains in areas of complex abstraction, executive function, and memory after training; whereas the control group exhibited no significant gains in any cognitive domains (Vas et al., 2011; Cook et al., 2014). Studies examining SMART training with healthy individuals, both adolescent and adult, resulted in significantly improved ability in measures of executive function including complex abstraction and memory, while the control group showed no significant gains in any cognitive domains (Gamino et al., 2010; Chapman et al., 2015). Similarly, in a population at-risk for Alzheimer's, Mudar et al. (2013) found significant improvements following the SMART protocol on measures of abstraction, executive function, and memory relative to the active control group, which showed no such significant gains except for the D-KEFS sorting test. Regarding the second potential limitation of clinician bias, two clinicians, who were unaware of time of testing (i.e., pre or post) scored the key measures independently to minimize experimenter bias. Moreover, participants' pre- to post-responses were not paired for scoring so that no comparison between pre and post response could bias change scores. We failed to find significant differences between scores of the two raters. Alternate versions of primary and secondary measures were used, when available, at pre- and post-testing to also help reduce practice effect. We recognize that future studies should include a control group as well as blind the examiners to group membership. Nonetheless, we do not feel that these two factors fully explain the current findings and believe the current results offer a promising pattern of findings that motivate a more in-depth trial.

Another potential weakness, but also strength, is the limited range of depressive symptoms. As our participants had relatively low depression scores, it would be interesting to consider whether patients with greater levels of depressive symptoms would show different degrees of benefit, perhaps more or perhaps less. The fact that the degree of affective symptoms did not affect results leaves the question open as to whether those with more serious levels of symptomatology might still benefit. A recent review concluded that cognitive effects of lithium, anticonvulsants, and antipsychotics on cognition in BD are still unknown, primarily due to flawed research methodology, small sample sizes, and inconsistent findings (Vreeker et al., 2015). In this current study, however, we did assess the potential effects of anticonvulsants and antipsychotics. Neither medication type nor its interaction with time were significantly different for any behavioral measure. With a larger sample size, we could also more clearly examine effects of medications, such as anti-psychotics and mood stabilizers, as well as dosage effects. We find the strength of the current results encouraging for conducting a larger trial to confirm these findings and consider other questions such as treatment earlier in the disease course, perhaps after the first episode of depression. Additional weaknesses are the relatively small sample size, a lack of post-testing in psychological health, testing at extended periods post-treatment to evaluate whether the gains persisted and the failure to consider occupational functionality.

The cognitive gains from the current study replicate previous findings of training-specific gains, as well as generalized improvement in cognitive skills in various clinical populations that underwent reasoning training (Anand et al., 2011; Vas et al., 2011, 2015; Mudar et al., 2016). We propose that these preliminary data motivate a larger, randomized study. A larger sample size would also allow better assessment as to what, if any, distinct effect depressive symptoms had regarding training benefits. Future investigations should also include indicators of level of engagement and long-term follow-up assessments (e.g., 6 and 12 months post) to evaluate maintenance of gains, as well as earlier in the disease course.

CONCLUSION

The impact of cognitive training protocols is a particularly important line of research in BD. The potential to strengthen mental capabilities, and executive functions, in particular, may be a tangible path to motivate a productive life style course in populations with psychiatric disorders where the cognitive sequela has been relatively unexplored. Strengthening neural circuits through cognitive training in individuals with psychiatric disease may provide one promising adjuvant to the pharma-interventions to supplement individuals' capacity with psychiatric disease to achieve higher levels of success in personal and occupational goals, as has been suggested by Fisher et al. (2009).

AUTHOR CONTRIBUTION

All authors listed, have made substantial, direct and intellectual contribution to the work, and approved it for publication.

ACKNOWLEDGMENTS

The authors acknowledge the generous support of the Dunlap family, which made this study possible. We also thank William

L. Thorton at The University of Texas Southwestern for his collaboration, as well as Audette Rackley, Molly Keebler, Jillian Hill, Nellie Caulkins, Alison Perez, and the rest of the cognitive training team at The Center for BrainHealth for their support and contribution to this study. Finally, we whole-heartedly thank the participants of this study.

REFERENCES

Anand, R., Chapman, S. B., Rackley, A., Keebler, M., Zientz, J., and Hart, J. (2011). Gist reasoning training in cognitively normal seniors. *Int. J. Geriatr. Psychiatry* 26, 961–968. doi: 10.1002/gps.2633

Aslan, S., Xu, F., Wang, P. L., Uh, J., Yezhuvath, U. S., van Osch, M., et al. (2010). Estimation of labeling efficiency in pseudocontinuous arterial spin labeling. *Magn. Reson. Med.* 63, 765–771. doi: 10.1002/mrm.22245

Badre, D., and Wagner, A. D. (2007). Left ventrolateral prefrontal cortex and the cognitive control of memory. *Neuropsychologia* 45, 2883–2901. doi: 10.1016/j.neuropsychologia.2007.06.015

Benabarre, A., Vieta, E., Martínez-Arán, A., Garcia-Garcia, M., Martín, F., Lomeña, F., et al. (2005). Neuropsychological disturbances and cerebral blood flow in bipolar disorder. *Aust. N. Z. J. Psychiatry* 39, 227–234. doi: 10.1080/j.1440-1614.2004.01558.x

Benton, A. L., Hamsher, K. D., and Sivan, A. B. (1994). *Multilingual Aphasia Examination: Manual of Instructions*. Iowa City, IA: AJA Associates Inc.

Blumberg, H. P., Leung, H.-C., Skudlarski, P., Lacadie, C. M., Fredericks, C. A., Harris, B. C., et al. (2003). A functional magnetic resonance imaging study of bipolar disorder: state-and trait-related dysfunction in ventral prefrontal cortices. *Arch. Gen. Psychiatry* 60, 601–609. doi: 10.1001/archpsyc.60.6.601

Burdick, K. E., Braga, R. J., Nnadi, C. U., Shaya, Y., Stearns, W. H., and Malhotra, A. K. (2012). Placebo-controlled adjunctive trial of pramipexole in patients with bipolar disorder: targeting cognitive dysfunction. *J. Clin. Psychiatry* 73, 103–112. doi: 10.4088/JCP.11m07299

Chapman, S. B., Aslan, S., Spence, J., Keebler, M. W., DeFina, L. F., Didehbani, N., et al. (2016). Distinct brain and behavioral benefits from cognitive versus physical training: a randomized trial in aging adults. *Front. Hum. Neurosci.* 10:338. doi: 10.3389/fnhum.2016.00338

Chapman, S. B., Aslan, S., Spence, J. S., Hart, J. J. Jr, Bartz, E. K., Didehbani, N., et al. (2015). Neural mechanisms of brain plasticity with complex cognitive training in healthy seniors. *Cereb. Cortex* 25, 396–405. doi: 10.1093/cercor/bht234

Chapman, S. B., Gamino, J. F., and Mudar, R. A. (2012). "Higher-order strategic gist reasoning in adolescence," in *The Adolescent Brain: Learning, Reasoning, and Decison Making*, eds V. Reyna, S. B. Chapman, M. R. Dougherty, and J. Confrey (Washington, DC: American Psychological Association), 123–151.

Chapman, S. B., and Kirkland, S. (2014). *Make Your Brain Smarter: Increase Your Brain's Creativity, Energy, and Focus*. New York City, NY: Simon and Schuster.

Chapman, S. B., and Mudar, R. A. (2014). Enhancement of cognitive and neural functions through complex reasoning training: evidence from normal and clinical populations. *Front. Syst. Neurosci.* 8:69. doi: 10.3389/fnsys.2014.00069

Chapman, S. B., Zientz, J., Weiner, M., Rosenberg, R., Frawley, W., and Burns, M. H. (2002). Discourse changes in early Alzheimer disease, mild cognitive impairment, and normal aging. *Alzheimer Dis. Assoc. Disord.* 16, 177–186. doi: 10.1097/00002093-200207000-00008

Chen, C. H., Suckling, J., Lennox, B. R., Ooi, C., and Bullmore, E. T. (2011). A quantitative meta-analysis of fMRI studies in bipolar disorder. *Bipolar Disord.* 13, 1–15. doi: 10.1111/j.1399-5618.2011.00893.x

Chen, J. J., Rosas, H. D., and Salat, D. H. (2013). The relationship between cortical blood flow and sub-cortical white-matter health across the adult age span. *PLoS ONE* 8:e56733. doi: 10.1371/journal.pone.0056733

Chiu Wong, S. B., Chapman, S. B., Cook, L. G., Anand, R., Gamino, J. F., and Devous, M. D. Sr. (2006). A SPECT study of language and brain reorganization three years after pediatric brain injury. *Prog. Brain Res.* 157, 173–394. doi: 10.1016/S0079-6123(06)57011-6

Cook, L. G., Chapman, S. B., Elliott, A. C., Evenson, N. N., and Vinton, K. (2014). Cognitive gains from gist reasoning training in adolescents with chronic-stage traumatic brain injury. *Front. Neurol.* 5:87. doi: 10.3389/fneur.2014.00087

Corbetta, M., Patel, G., and Shulman, L. (2008). The reorienting system of the human brain: from environment to theory of mind. *Neuron* 58, 306–324. doi: 10.1016/j.neuron.2008.04.017

Danker, J. F., Gunn, P., and Anderson, J. R. (2008). A rational account of memory predicts left prefrontal activation during controlled retrieval. *Cereb. Cortex* 18, 2674–2685. doi: 10.1093/cercor/bhn027

Deckersbach, T., Nierenberg, A. A., Kessler, R., Lund, H. G., Ametrano, R. M., Sachs, G., et al. (2010). RESEARCH: cognitive rehabilitation for bipolar disorder: an open trial for employed patients with residual depressive symptoms. *CNS Neurosci. Ther.* 16, 298–307. doi: 10.1111/j.1755-5949.2009.00110.x

Delis, D. C., Kaplan, E., and Kramer, J. H. (2001). *Delis-Kaplan Executive Function System (D-KEFS)*. San Antonio, TX: Psychological Corporation.

Demant, K. M., Vinberg, M., Kessing, L. V., and Miskowiak, K. W. (2015). Effects of short-term cognitive remediation on cognitive dysfunction in partially or fully remitted individuals with bipolar disorder: results of a randomised controlled trial. *PLoS ONE* 10:e0127955. doi: 10.1371/journal.pone.0127955

Didehbani, N., Cullum, C. M., Mansinghani, S., Conover, H., and Hart, J. (2013). Depressive symptoms and concussions in aging retired NFL players. *Arch. Clin. Neuropsychol.* 28, 418–424. doi: 10.1093/arclin/act028

Fisher, M., Holland, C., Merzenich, M. M., and Vinogradov, S. (2009). Using neuroplasticity-based auditory training to improve verbal memory in schizophrenia. *Am. J. Psychiatry* 166, 805–811. doi: 10.1176/appi.ajp.2009.08050757

Gamino, J. F., Chapman, S. B., Hull, E. L., and Lyon, G. R. (2010). Effects of higher-order cognitive strategy training on gist-reasoning and fact-learning in adolescents. *Front. Psychol.* 1:188. doi: 10.3389/fpsyg.2010.00188

Gold, B. T., Balota, D. A., Jones, S. J., Powell, D. K., Smith, C. D., and Andersen, A. H. (2006). Dissociation of automatic and strategic lexical-semantics: functional magnetic resonance imaging evidence for differing roles of multiple frontotemporal regions. *J. Neurosci.* 26, 6523–6532. doi: 10.1523/jneurosci.0808-06.2006

Green, M. J., Cahill, C. M., and Malhi, G. S. (2007). The cognitive and neurophysiological basis of emotion dysregulation in bipolar disorder. *J. Affect. Disord.* 103, 29–42. doi: 10.1016/j.jad.2007.01.024

Kronhaus, D. M., Lawrence, N. S., Williams, A. M., Frangou, S., Brammer, M. J., Williams, S. C. R., et al. (2006). Stroop performance in bipolar disorder: further evidence for abnormalities in the ventral prefrontal cortex. *Bipolar Disord.* 8, 28–39. doi: 10.1111/j.1399-5618.2006.00282.x

Martinez-Aran, A., Vieta, E., Colom, F., Torrent, C., Sanchez-Moreno, J., Reinares, M., et al. (2004). Cognitive impairment in euthymic bipolar patients: implications for clinical and functional outcome. *Bipolar Disord.* 6, 224–232. doi: 10.1111/j.1399-5618.2004.00111.x

Max, J. E., Lopez, A., Wilde, E. A., Bigler, E. D., Schachar, R. J., Saunders, A., et al. (2015). Anxiety disorders in children and adolescents in the second six months after traumatic brain injury. *J. Pediatr. Rehabil. Med.* 8, 345–355. doi: 10.3233/PRM-150352

Michalak, E. E., and Murray, G. (2010). Development of the QoL. BD: a disorder-specific scale to assess quality of life in bipolar disorder. *Bipolar Disord.* 12, 727–740. doi: 10.1111/j.1399-5618.2010.00865.x

Motes, M. A., Gamino, J. F., Chapman, S. B., Rao, N. K., Maguire, M. J., Brier, M. R., et al. (2014). Inhibitory control gains from higher-order cognitive strategy training. *Brain Cogn.* 84, 44–62. doi: 10.1016/j.bandc.2013.10.007

Mozolic, J. L., Hayaska, S., and Laurienti, P. J. (2010). A cognitive training intervention increases resting cerebral blood flow in healthy older adults. *Front. Hum. Neurosci.* 4:16. doi: 10.3389/neuro.09.016.2010

Mudar, R., Chiang, H.-S., Eroh, J., Rackley, A., Venza, E., Martin-Cook, K., et al. (2013). "Benefits of cognitive training in individuals with mild cognitive impairment," in *Poster Presentation - Cognitive Neuroscience Society Annual Meeting*, San Francisco, CA.

Mudar, R. A., Chapman, S. B., Rackley, A., Eroh, J., Chiang, H. S., Perez, A., et al. (2016). Enhancing latent cognitive capacity in mild cognitive impairment with gist reasoning training: a pilot study. *Int. J. Geriatr. Psychiatry* doi: 10.1002/gps.4492 [Epub ahead of print].

O'Connell, R. A., Van Heertum, R. L., Luck, D., Yudd, A. P., Cueva, J. E., Billick, S. B., et al. (1995). Single-photon emission computed tomography of the brain in acute mania and schizophrenia. *J. Neuroimag.* 5, 101–104. doi: 10.1111/jon199552101

Phillips, M. L., Drevets, W. C., Rauch, S. L., and Lane, R. (2003). Neurobiology of emotion perception I: the neural basis of normal emotion perception. *Biol. Psychiatry* 54, 504–514. doi: 10.1016/S0006-3223(03)00168-9

Phillips, M. L., Ladouceur, C. D., and Drevets, W. C. (2008). A neural model of voluntary and automatic emotion regulation: implications for understanding the pathophysiology and neurodevelopment of bipolar disorder. *Mol. Psychiatry* 13, 833–857. doi: 10.1038/mp.2008.65

Poldrack, R. A., Wagner, A. D., Prull, M. W., Desmond, J. E., Glover, G. H., and Gabrieli, J. D. E. (1999). Functional specialization for semantic and phonological processing in the left inferior prefrontal cortex. *Neuroimage* 10, 15–35. doi: 10.1006/nimg.1999.0441

Preiss, M., Shatil, E., Cermakova, R., Cimermanova, D., and Ram, I. (2013). Personalized cognitive training in unipolar and bipolar disorder: a study of cognitive functioning. *Front. Hum. Neurosci.* 7:108. doi: 10.3389/fnhum.2013.00108

Quraishi, S., and Frangou, S. (2002). Neuropsychology of bipolar disorder: a review. *J. Affect. Disord.* 72, 209–226. doi: 10.1016/S0165-0327(02)00091-5

Race, E. A., Shanker, S., and Wagner, A. D. (2009). Neural priming in human frontal cortex: multiple forms of learning reduce demands on the prefrontal executive system. *J. Cogn. Neurosci.* 21, 1766–1781. doi: 10.1162/jocn.2009.21132

Raichle, M. E., and Gusnard, D. A. (2002). Appraising the brain's energy budget. *Proc. Natl. Acad. Sci. U.S.A.* 99, 10237–10239. doi: 10.1073/pnas.172399499

Rey, A. (1964). *L'examen Clinique en Psychologie [The clinical psychological examination]*. Paris: Presses Universitaires de France.

Robinson, L. J., and Ferrier, I. N. (2006). Evolution of cognitive impairment in bipolar disorder: a systematic review of cross-sectional evidence. *Bipolar Disord.* 8, 103–116. doi: 10.1111/j.1399-5618.2006.00277.x

Schmidt, M. (1996). *Rey Auditory Verbal Learning Test: A Handbook*. Los Angeles, CA: Western Psychological Services.

Sojkova, J., Beason-Held, L., Zhou, Y., An, Y., Kraut, M. A., Ye, W., et al. (2008). Longitudinal cerebral blood flow and amyloid deposition: an emerging pattern? *J. Nucl. Med.* 49, 1465–1471. doi: 10.2967/jnumed.108.051946

Spreen, O., and Strauss, E. (1998). *A Compendium of Neuropsychological Tests: Administration, Norms, and Commentary*. New York, NY: Oxford University Press.

Takeuchi, H., Taki, Y., Nouchi, R., Hashizume, H., Sekiguchi, A., Kotozaki, Y., et al. (2013). Effects of working memory training on functional connectivity and cerebral blood flow during rest. *Cortex* 49, 2106–2125. doi: 10.1016/j.cortex.2012.09.007

Torrent, C., del Mar Bonnin, C., Martínez-Arán, A., Valle, J., Amann, B. L., González-Pinto, A., et al. (2013). Efficacy of functional remediation in bipolar disorder: a multicenter randomized controlled study. *Am. J. Psychiatry* 170, 852–859. doi: 10.1176/appi.ajp.2012.12070971

van Gorp, W. G., Altshuler, L., Theberge, D. C., Wilkins, J., and Dixon, W. (1998). Cognitive impairment in euthymic bipolar patients with and without prior alcohol dependence. *A preliminary study. Arch. Gen. Psychiatry* 55, 41–46. doi: 10.1001/archpsyc.55.1.41

Vas, A., Chapman, S., Aslan, S., Spence, J., Keebler, M., Rodriguez-Larrain, G., et al. (2016a). Reasoning training in veteran and civilian traumatic brain injury with persistent mild impairment. *Neuropsychol. Rehabil.* 26, 502–531. doi: 10.1080/09602011.2015.1044013

Vas, A., Spence, J., Eschler, B., and Chapman, S. (2016b). Sensitivity and specificity of abstraction using gist reasoning measure in adults with traumatic brain injury. *J. Appl. Biobehav. Res.*

Vas, A. K., Chapman, S. B., and Cook, L. G. (2015). Language impairments in traumatic brain injury: a window into complex cognitive performance. *Handb. Clin. Neurol.* 128, 497–510. doi: 10.1016/b978-0-444-63521-1.00031-5

Vas, A. K., Chapman, S. B., Cook, L. G., Elliott, A. C., and Keebler, M. (2011). Higher-order reasoning training years after traumatic brain injury in adults. *J. Head Trauma Rehabil.* 26, 224–239. doi: 10.1097/HTR.0b013e31821 8dd3d

Vreeker, A., van Bergen, A. H., and Kahn, R. S. (2015). Cognitive enhancing agents in schizophrenia, and bipolar disorder. *Eur. Neuropsychopharmacol.* 25, 969–1002. doi: 10.1016/j.euroneuro.2015.04.014

Wechsler, D. (1997a). *Manual for the Wechsler Adult Intelligence Scale-III*. San Antonio, TX: Psychological Corporation.

Wechsler, D. (1997b). *Wechsler Memory Scale (WMS-III)*. San Antonio, TX: Psychological Corporation.

18

Balancing Automatic-Controlled Behaviors and Emotional-Salience States: A Dynamic Executive Functioning Hypothesis

Bruno Kluwe-Schiavon[1,2], Thiago W. Viola[3], Breno Sanvicente-Vieira[2], Leandro F. Malloy-Diniz[4,5] and Rodrigo Grassi-Oliveira[2,3]**

[1] Experimentelle und Klinische Pharmakopsychologie, Psychiatrische Universitätsklinik Zürich, Zürich, Switzerland, [2] Developmental Cognitive Neuroscience Lab, Graduate Program in Psychology, Pontifical Catholic University of Rio Grande do Sul (PUCRS), Porto Alegre, Brazil, [3] Developmental Cognitive Neuroscience Lab, Graduate Program in Pediatrics and Child Health, Pontifical Catholic University of Rio Grande do Sul (PUCRS), Porto Alegre, Brazil, [4] Department of Mental Health, School of Medicine, Federal University of Minas Gerais, Belo Horizonte, Brazil, [5] LUMINA Neurosciences and Mental Health Institute, Belo Horizonte, Brazil

Edited by:
Alexandre Heeren,
Harvard University, USA

Reviewed by:
Caroline Gurvich,
Monash University, Australia
Chrissie Ferreira De Carvalho,
Federal University of Bahia (UFBA),
Brazil

***Correspondence:**
Bruno Kluwe-Schiavon
brunokluwe@gmail.com
Rodrigo Grassi-Oliveira
rodrigo.grassi@pucrs.br

Recently, there has been growing interest in understanding how executive functions are conceptualized in psychopathology. Since several models have been proposed, the major issue lies within the definition of executive functioning itself. Theoretical discussions have emerged, narrowing the boundaries between "hot" and "cold" executive functions or between self-regulation and cognitive control. Nevertheless, the definition of executive functions is far from a consensual proposition and it has been suggested that these models might be outdated. Current efforts indicate that human behavior and cognition are by-products of many brain systems operating and interacting at different levels, and therefore, it is very simplistic to assume a dualistic perspective of information processing. Based upon an adaptive perspective, we discuss how executive functions could emerge from the ability to solve immediate problems and to generalize successful strategies, as well as from the ability to synthesize and to classify environmental information in order to predict context and future. We present an executive functioning perspective that emerges from the dynamic balance between automatic-controlled behaviors and an emotional-salience state. According to our perspective, the adaptive role of executive functioning is to automatize efficient solutions simultaneously with cognitive demand, enabling individuals to engage such processes with increasingly complex problems. Understanding executive functioning as a mediator of stress and cognitive engagement not only fosters discussions concerning individual differences, but also offers an important paradigm to understand executive functioning as a continuum process rather than a categorical and multicomponent structure.

Keywords: executive functions, cognitive control, self-regulation, neuropsychology, automatic process, reasoning, stress, psychological

INTRODUCTION

The conceptualizations of executive functions have emerged from the observation of patients who had suffered frontal lobe lesions and became unable to manipulate, integrate, and respond to internal and external stimulus in the same way they used to do (Jurado and Rosselli, 2007; Goldstein et al., 2014). Throughout the last few decades, a range of models have emerged and executive functions has become a multifaceted mental concept that includes more than 30 different components (Barkley, 2001, 2012). Although these components were assumed to be interrelated, their exact relationship has not been clearly elucidated. After more than 40 years of studies, there is no consensus regarding the definition of executive functions. The concept previously included a variety of behaviors that were broadly accepted as "high-order cognitive processes," such as inhibitory control, attention shifting, working memory, goal-directed behavior, and strategic planning [for an extended review of definitions please see (Goldstein et al., 2014)].

Based upon recent neuroscientific findings and theories of cognitive sciences, this article questions this hierarchical characteristic, as well as the multicomponent categorical approaches, commonly attributed to executive functions, by presenting a novel and testable dynamic executive functioning hypothesis. Consequently, different from the majority of reviews on this topic (Miyake et al., 2000; Collette et al., 2005; Jurado and Rosselli, 2007; Tirapu-Ustarroz et al., 2008a,b; Kluwe-Schiavon et al., 2012; Goldstein et al., 2014), it is not the aim of this article to perform an updated overview concerning the theoretical models of executive functions, nor discuss current evidences for the reliability of unitary or multiple components models, and we do not aim to describe the subcomponents that were mostly accepted as "executive".

In order to accomplish our goal, the article is organized into three sections. In the first section, we briefly discuss the hierarchical and categorical framework that supports the majority of the models of executive functions, especially dual-processing models. In the second section, we highlight a selection of neuroscientific evidences to discuss stress as a core factor behind executive functioning phylogeny, particularly, that stress should be included in executive functioning models as a continuous variable leading to different levels of homeostasis disturbance and, as a consequence, cognitive engagement. The third section introduces the executive functioning hypothesis, elucidating similarities and differences between this perspective and some of the current theoretical models in the field. In this section, we also discuss that the so-called "executive" behaviors (e.g., set-shifting, cognitive flexibility, inhibition, and updating) that could be comprehended as consequences of a permanent adaptive switching between reflexive, conditioned, and goal-oriented behaviors, instead of core individual, but interrelated, cognitive components. Finally, the fourth section of the article discusses subsequent testing of our executive functioning hypothesis and future perspectives.

THE HIERARCHICAL FRAMEWORK OF EXECUTIVE FUNCTIONS

In an extensive review regarding executive functions, Goldstein et al. (2014) clarified that the first hypotheses concerning the role of prefrontal cortex (PFC) in human cognition were based upon the theoretical backgrounds of selective attention and multi-store memory models. These models suggested different linear schemas, such as the Bottleneck theory of attention from Donald Broadbent or the three component model from Richard Atkinson and Richard Shiffrin, in order to explain how environmental information are perceived, buffered, and retrieved for conscious awareness (Atkinson and Shiffrin, 1971; Goldstein et al., 2014). Although these models were able to distinguish automatic and controlled cognitive processes, they did not completely explain how information could be deliberatively selected or inhibited during demanding attentional tasks. To fill this gap, the term "cognitive control" was introduced in Posner and Snyder (1975) to describe the capacity to manage thoughts and emotions, allowing people to adapt behaviors across situations according their goals (Goldstein et al., 2014).

Together with previous studies from Alexander Luria, these dual-processing models - and subsequent models, such as the Supervisory Attentional System (SAS) from Norman and Shallice (1983) - were crucial to including the PFC as the main brain structure involved in cognitive control, which was capable of managing and regulating automatic behaviors (Luria, 1970; Norman and Shallice, 1983).

The differences between automatic and controlled processes driven by the cognitive revolution in psychology [for a review, please see (Miller, 2003)] favored a hierarchical and categorical approach, in which cognitive processes were organized as independent, but inter-related components according to their main functions, and aimed to decode the information processing pathway between a stimulus and behavioral response. The multicomponent working memory model proposed by Alan Baddeley and Graham Hitch (Baddeley, 2012) could be viewed as an example of this hierarchical and categorical reasoning, in which three distinct slave systems are coordinated by a central executive. However, according to Baddeley (2012), even though the central executive is the most complex component of working memory, it could be seen as a homunculus that represents a marker of issues requiring explanation. Although Baddeley (2012) suggested that in due course the homunculus might be pensioned off, several models remain convinced that the PFC is the "final frontier of neuropsychology" at the "center of human nature" (Stuss, 2011), and that executive functions "are at the heart of all socially useful, personally, enhancing, constructive, and creative activities" (Lezak, 1982). In other words, hierarchical and categorical approaches have often referred to executive functions as a homunculus that inhibits our instincts and guides our rational behavior.

This categorical approach can be widely observed in the executive functions multicomponent models. Examples include the four-component model hypothesized by (Lezak, 1995), as well as the three core functions summarized by Diamond (2013). The four-component model suggests that executive functions consist of those capacities that enable a person to engage successfully in independent, purposive, and self-serving behavior (Lezak et al., 2012), such as volition, planning, purposeful action, and effective performance (Goldstein et al., 2014). Similarly, Diamond (2013) suggested that executive functions can be described as a family of top down mental processes recruited when automatic, instinct or intuition would be insufficient to cope with an ongoing demand. Diamond relies upon the assumption that there is a general agreement regarding three core executive functions: behavioral/cognitive inhibition (including selective attention), working memory, and cognitive flexibility (Diamond, 2013). These functions encourage individuals to not act impulsively, hold information to solve problems, and apply different approaches to a problem when facing new rules or priorities (Diamond, 2013).

In general, both models were based upon clinical experience and observation and they became expressive frameworks in the neuropsychological field. According to our perspective, the three main contributions of these models are: (i) hierarchical and multicomponent approaches make it easier to define some behaviors that seem to represent cognitive processes that could not be classified as general automatic responses caused by a stimulus (e.g., planning and cognitive flexibility); (ii) the possibility to develop specific tasks to assess each component independently (even theoretically considering that they are interrelated), which fits with one of the main aims of neuropsychology as a clinical field, to assess and treat patients with brain injury or disease; and (iii) the possibility to provide an explanation as to how executive dysfunction affects all aspects of behavior differently from specific cognitive deficits (Lezak et al., 2012). However, multicomponent models of executive functions are still based upon the traditional framework of "cognitive control" proposed by Posner and Snyder (2004), in which the PFC plays an "executive" role over goal-oriented behaviors (Pribram, 1973) and emotional self-regulation (for a review on this topic please see (Peterson and Welsh, 2014). To explain such control medical imaging technologies, developmental research, experimental psychology, and neurosciences have rescued dual-processes theories to describe the so-called "cold" and "hot" cognitive information processing systems (Sahlin et al., 2010; Zelazo and Carlson, 2012).

Once more, many dualistic models have been proposed to characterize these systems for an extensive review see (Evans, 2008). Usually, System 1 (or Type 1) demands stronger activation of subcortical structures and could be defined as unconscious, rapid, automatic, and allowed parallel information processing; while System 2 (or Type 2) demands stronger activation of cortical structures and could be defined as conscious, slow, deliberative, and mostly responsible for serial information processing (Kahneman, 2011; Noël et al., 2013). The idea of an "emotional versus rational" thinking or neural system has found support in several studies and has been extensively used to describe cognitive changes associated with psychiatric disorders and/or neurodevelopment. Some inhibition dysfunction theories of addiction, for example, suggest that chronic drug use reduces self-control, which is needed to inhibit the hedonic impulse to take the rewarding drug again [for a review about models of addiction please see (Emcdda, 2014)]. According to the dual-processing framework of addiction, the neuroplasticity induced by addictive drugs triggered by epigenetic mechanisms impacts proteins in an intracellular level, modifying neurotransmitter signaling in various neuronal circuits leading to an imbalance between those areas that are associated with emotions and reward (e.g., orbitofrontal cortex, ventral striatum, and the limbic system) – usually recruited during situations with stronger affective salience (e.g., facing conditioned drug cues or stress) – and those areas that are associated with more purely cognitive processing and the activation of the dorsolateral parts of the PFC (Volkow and Baler, 2014). Moreover, the imbalance between "hot" and "cold" brain systems has also been used to describe and explain risk-taking behaviors during adolescence, such as unprotected sex, criminal behavior, drug use and abuse, and accidents (Gladwin et al., 2011). Beyond social and environmental factors, neurodevelopmental researchers emphasized that the relatively early maturation of the "hot" affective-motivational bottom-up system and the more slowly developing "cold" top-down control system could explain impulsive behaviors due to the difficulty in delaying gratification (Benningfield et al., 2014), weighing of risks and benefits of a set of actions (Pripfl et al., 2013), and use of ongoing outcomes of these actions to monitor their own performance (Kluwe-Schiavon et al., 2016).

Although dual-process models have explained important issues, especially regarding decision-making, there are studies suggesting that these models might be outdated (Reyna and Brainerd, 2011; Gladwin and Figner, 2014). First, some authors argue that dual-processing models cannot supply and predict mechanisms for developmental reversals in cognition during development, such as increased reasoning biases from childhood to adulthood (Kahneman and Tversky, 2000; Reyna and Brainerd, 2011). Second, the boundaries between "hot" and "cold" executive functions are not clear and, considering previous theories regarding cognitive automaticity, it is not even clear if there are such boundaries (Bargh, 1992; Moors and De Houwer, 2006). Consequently, it became hard to investigate how individual factors (e.g., personality traits or mood), developmental factors (e.g., age and life experiences) and/or contextual factors (e.g., healthy or financial decisions and social interactions) – could influence the "warmth" of a task (Peterson and Welsh, 2014), thus requiring research to use decompositional approaches (Moors and De Houwer, 2006). In fact, it is true that earlier dual-processing models argued that a process is neither fully controlled nor automatic (Bargh, 1992). Despite many studies have discussed that "hot" and "cold" executive functions are supported by an integrated neural network, and, therefore, might be all interrelated (Zimmerman et al., 2016), in practice current studies still assume significantly different concepts. Finally, the third point is that dualistic conceptions (as well as the central executive homunculus of Baddeley) were thought to be didactically used to describe and explain complex behaviors. However, the exception has become the rule and these dualistic conceptions are replicated and measured as two independent categories instead of two poles of the same gradient. In other words, it is acceptable that "cold" executive functions are measured with tasks that demand planning, working memory, and concept formation, while "hot" executive functions are measured with tasks that demand social cognition, empathy, and emotion regulation (Zimmerman et al., 2016). In the next section we briefly highlight a selection of studies that support the idea that an executive functioning model should be thought of as a frontal-subcortical circuit, in which emotions (here stress) directly modulate the cognitive processes and vice-versa.

NEUROSCIENTIFIC FINDINGS TOWARD EXECUTIVE FUNCTIONING

The idea that executive functions are not exclusive related to frontal-cortical areas, but would involve frontal–subcortical neuronal circuits is not new (Leh et al., 2010). Based upon an evolutionary perspective, Ardila (2008) emphasized that executive functions are mediated by dynamic and flexible neuronal networks, questioning the central role of PFC in the executive functions and, afterward, discussing how the executive functions may have evolved in our species. Nonetheless, questioning the central role of PFC in relation to executive functions goes beyond suggesting that executive functions involve subcortical networks, but in fact this also allow us to question the hierarchical perspective in which PFC exerts control over impulses and should be taken as the center of rationality. Note that we do not intend to argue here that the PFC does not exert a key role in cognitive and response inhibition, but that there are enough evidences suggesting that the relationship between cognition and emotion could be more complex than the old-fashioned reasoning that the first (e.g., central executive, superego, or PFC) should control the second (e.g., impulses, id, or limbic system). In this sense, here we focus on those studies which suggested that some level of stress is necessary to motivate the organism to act and allocate cognitive resources to controlled processes, such as problem solving, monitoring, and updating. After a certain level of stress, the cognitive resources are reallocated in favor of more automatic processes, decreasing working memory span and, in the last instance, increasing response inhibition and unconditioned behaviors, such as fight or flight responses. Additionally, we mainly focus upon acute stress research since in the biological and psychological fields the term has been commonly used to describe external events capable of disrupting organism stability or homeostasis.

The executive functioning hypothesis is supported by studies that suggest that the PFC, especially medial areas, coordinates the brain circuits that mediate emotional responses (Hermans et al., 2014; McKlveen et al., 2015). This idea was deeply investigated under the somatic marker hypothesis, which demonstrated that the ventromedial PFC and its projections to the orbitofrontal cortex are involved in both emotional response and cognition (Bar-On et al., 2003; Li et al., 2010). The somatic marker hypothesis suggested that body signals (somatic markers) are represented and regulated in the ventromedial PFC, since these somatic markers were not found in people with lesions in this area, which are also correlated with poorer performance on decision-making tasks (Dunn et al., 2006). Additionally, the orbitofrontal cortex is known to show an increased activity in response to stress and it also is implicated in many cognitive functions, such as working memory. In this sense, pre-clinical research has hypothesized that acute stress can enhance working memory performance by selectively increasing glutamatergic signaling in PFC pyramidal neurons (Yuen et al., 2009). However, the extent to which stress can have a positive or negative effect on specific cognitive functions remains unclear. Barsegyan et al. (2010), for example, demonstrated that acute stress triggers working memory impairment and concurrent enhancement of memory consolidation. Interesting, the authors emphasized the interaction of glucocorticoid receptors and catecholaminergic activity, suggesting that working memory impairment and enhancement of memory consolidation shared a common neural influence within the medial PFC via a common activation of the noradrenergic signaling pathway (Barsegyan et al., 2010).

These data reinforce the idea that the medial PFC is an important integrator of the neuroendocrine and autonomic systems, acting as a coordinator of stress responses. In addition, these data also indicate that stress can be considered as a stimulus that allocates energetic systems to respond to an ongoing or anticipated challenge. McKlveen et al. (2015) discussed that this allocation of energetic systems may occur mostly via hypothalamic-pituitary-adrenal axis (HPA-axis) activation that culminate in the release of glucocorticoids and catecholamines, which in turn leads to several alterations in different brain systems in order to promote adaptive behaviors. As an example of allocation of energy systems, Hermans et al. (2014) have shown that acute stress shifts the phasic activation of locus coeruleus toward a tonic mode of activity, guiding attentional resources for potentially salient information. This allocation of energy resources could explain different behavior patterns observed during stress.

In this regard, two meta-analyses were performed to investigate the effects of psychosocial stress on executive functions (Shields et al., 2016) and the effects of stress on decisions made under uncertainty (Starcke and Brand, 2016). In the first, the authors found that acute stress impaired working memory and cognitive flexibility in humans. Furthermore, Shields et al. (2016) suggested that within inhibition, stress impaired cognitive inhibition (selectively attending to or ignoring information) but enhanced response inhibition. Concerning decision-making, Starcke and Brand (2016) found that stress had significant effects only in those situations in which increased reward seeking and risk taking is disadvantageous and discussed that this finding could be explained by two mechanisms: the first suggests that acute stress should increase the reliance on immediate and high rewards via alterations in dopamine release at the cost of considering potential losses; while the second mechanism suggests that stress may lead to unsystematic decisions without considering all of the options and may generally impair executive control via reductions of prefrontal functioning (Shields et al., 2016). Taken together, their findings are in agreement with the current perspective that stress reallocates limited executive resources in adaptive ways to facilitates adaptive decisions, although the authors highlight that it is not clear what executive function receives these reallocated resources and why (Shields et al., 2016).

It is also hypothesized that stress-induced shifts in cognitive functions occur because two different large-scale neuronal networks (salience network and executive control network) may compete for limited resources, and as proposed by Hermans et al. (2014), regulate externally directed attention. This model goes further than the majority of "hot" and "cold" dualistic perspectives because it introduces a dynamic interaction between the delay between stressor onset and task performance, and also because it considers the prefrontal areas as the key structures supporting this "competition." In a second meta-analysis, Shields et al. (2015) investigated the effects of acute cortisol administration on executive functions, focusing upon working memory inhibition and set-shifting shifting. After separating the genomic effects of cortisol (slow-acting effects caused by the modulation of gene expression) from its non-genomic effects (rapid-acting effects without the modulation of gene expression) by controlling for the delay between cortisol administration and cognitive testing, the authors found interesting and divergent effects of the hormone in cognition according to different time-windows post-administration. The authors suggested that the non-genomic effects of cortisol significantly impair working memory between 15 and 73 min post-administration, but begins to improve working memory after this period. However, the same effects of cortisol improve inhibition from 15 to 135 min post-administration, but begins to impair inhibition after this period, and no effects where found related to set-shifting (Shields et al., 2015). This data is in accordance with the idea that stress levels modulate the allocation of cognitive resources in a dynamic perspective, increasing inhibitory control and decreasing working memory capacity, which we hypothesized could facilitate the organism to engage in a logic deliberative reasoning to solve the problem. Nevertheless, if this strategy was not sufficient to solve the problem, individuals might use the working memory as an automatic adaptive cognitive mechanism to guide behavior, demanding less logic deliberative reasoning. Moreover, this meta-analysis emphasized that the time course difference between salience network and executive control network to reach the peak and then return to the baseline could also be an important feature to comprehend different effects of stress in the executive functions. In the acute phase, neural resources are allocated toward the salience network and the executive control network is actively suppressed, while in the recovery phase, this effect is reversed.

Here we argue that, at a primary level, a minimum amount of stress is required in order to motivate the organism to act and cognitively engage in problem solving by decreasing working memory capacity. Unfortunately, there are few studies directly investigating these effects and the majority of evidences in this direction are based upon clinical studies suggesting that stress could decrease the threshold to act. For example, some authors suggest that schizophrenia is primarily a frontostriatal disorder (Liu et al., 2011), in which executive functions deficits and deterioration are a central aspect of the disease [for a review see (Kluwe-Schiavon et al., 2013)]. In this sense, recent findings in schizophrenia have reconceptualised context processing as a function of proactive and reactive cognitive control (Aron, 2011). Proactive control can be comprehended as a form of default mode activated by goal-relevant information before the occurrence of cognitively demanding events, to optimally bias attention, perception, and action systems in a goal-driven manner; while reactive control is recruited only after the detection of a high-interference event, favoring attentional control and response inhibition (Anticevic et al., 2013). The proactive control depends upon the updating and maintenance of contextual information, which in turn, are associated with Gamma-aminobutyric Acid (GABA) and glutamate neurotransmitter mechanisms and *N*-methyl-D-aspartate (NMDA) receptor functioning. There are evidences suggesting that in schizophrenia, the connectivity between dorsolateral PFC and other cognitive control related brain regions are associated with dopamine and GABAergic signaling impairments, which support the information representation in dorsolateral PFC (Barch and Ceaser, 2012). Thus, such dysfunction in dopamine and GABAergic signaling may explain, in part, some of the behavior difficulties observed in schizophrenia related to proactive control, such as engaging in a conversation or planning. The notion of proactive control fits an executive functioning perspective because when facing a minimum level of stress, patients diagnosed with schizophrenia may have difficulties in allocating executive functioning resources necessary to properly engage in adaptive behavior.

Therefore, it seems unlikely that a "hot" vs. "cold" dichotomy will remain as a source of hypotheses for research in cognitive and experimental neuroscience. Although these dual-processes models have contributed to the understanding of information processing and brain disorders (Volkow and Baler, 2014), research questions centerd upon a categorical epistemological base seem to defy recent findings in the field (Morris and Cuthbert, 2012). Current interdisciplinary efforts to integrate "hot" and "cold" processes is timely and important since psychological scientists have previously assumed that adaptive behavior in real-world contexts involves continuous interactions between emotional and cognitive processes (Peterson and Welsh, 2014).

Taken together, our main goal here is to highlight that although the literature converges toward a dynamic role of PFC as a coordinator of stress adaptation, executive functions literature appears to be mostly focused upon hierarchical and categorical approaches. More than inter-related components that exert control over emotional salience, we propose that executive functioning should be comprehended as the main processes behind the allocation of cognitive resources in the face of a challenge. In this sense, instead of looking for energization, one can investigate the amount of stress that is needed to motivate the organism to act; instead of looking for problem solving or inhibitory control, one can investigate how long the organism can keep the executive control network engaged without shifting energy resources for working memory and salience network during a mild, moderate, or severe stress challenge. Instead of looking for cognitive flexibility, one can investigate how fast the organism can retrieve and adapt conditioned behavior schemas to cope with a new scenario. This dynamic perspective considers executive functioning as continuum process that could be used to identify how adaptable the organism is to an unpredictable environment.

A DYNAMIC EXECUTIVE FUNCTIONING HYPOTHESIS

Our dynamic executive functioning hypothesis emerged from a fundamental question raised by Barkley (2001), "Why did humans develop executive functions?" Taking an evolutionary perspective, we argue that executive functioning emerged from: (a) the ability to solve immediate problems and generalize successful strategies; and (b) the ability to synthesize and organize environmental information in view of identifying uniformities that allow predictions about nature and future. From our perspective, these abilities are intrinsically related with two fundamental assumptions that are omitted by the majority of executive functions models. The first is a motivational feature that refers to the necessity of an existent problem to be solved, in other words, a motivational variable that might stress the organism and instigate the goal-oriented behavior. The second refers to the optimization of future solutions based upon previous experience, which is an ontogenetic assumption based upon the combination of the ability to generalize successful strategies along development and the ability to predict problems. The first assumption instigates the necessity to include a motivational variable derived from an internal or external stressful event capable of disturbing the organism homeostasis. Thus, this motivational aspect should be comprehended as a continuum that represents levels of homeostasis disturbance. The second assumption suggests that executive functions could be considered a "cyclical" process (that is why we refer to it as executive "functioning"), in which the main goal is to automatize efficient solutions that were cognitively demanding in the past, enabling individuals to allocate cognitive resources to the executive control network to solve new complex problems.

Here we proposed a schematic model to illustrate that the executive functioning could be comprehended as a balance between the salient network and the executive control network (**Figure 1A**). Differently from the majority of dual-processing models in which the strongest activation of salient network necessarily culminates in the weakness of cognitive executive control network, our theoretical hypothesis suggests that the strength and the direction of the relationship between these two networks would be indicative of optimal or impaired executive functioning. In optimal executive functioning, the organism

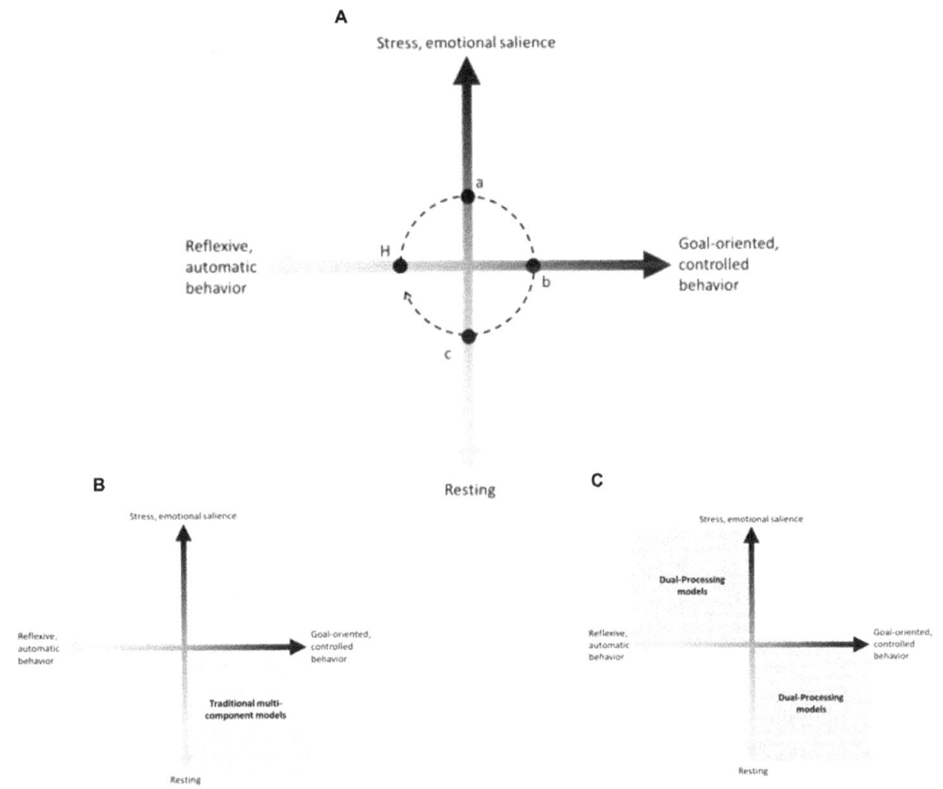

FIGURE 1 | Dynamic executive functioning hypothesis. (A) Dynamic executive functioning hypothesis: our theoretical hypothesis suggests that organisms tend to maintain a homeostatic state (H). Stress occurs, when any environmental demand gradually triggers goal-oriented behaviors, firstly using habitual responses and adapting it to adjust to the new demand. In an optimal executive functioning, when the ongoing behavior is insufficient to respond to environmental demands the emotional salience network reaches a peak (a), the organism would be able to inhibit disruptive automatic behaviors such as fight or flight responses and to use the available information (emotional salience and previous behaviors) to successfully respond to the environmental demand, decreasing the emotional salience and decoding the new contingencies (b). Once the new contingencies are decoded, the organism would repeatedly use the successful behavior (c) to completely solve the environmental demand and, then, returning to the homeostatic state (H). **(B)** Traditional multicomponent models. **(C)** Dual-processing models.

should be able to quickly adjust the ongoing behavior when faced with a stressful event. To do so, the organism should retrieve previous successful strategies and should be flexible enough to adapt these strategies if necessary. The executive functioning lies in the amount of stress necessary to motivate problem solving and the amount of cognitive effort demanded to solve the problem. If the organism is not sufficiently sensitive to identify potentially stressful events and to initiate an adaptive response in time, this would suggest a failure in updating environmental information. If the problem-solving demands a greater amount of cognitive effort that does not correspond to the difficulty level of the task, this results in a failure in monitoring the ongoing behavior or in a lack of cognitive flexibility. If the organism is not able to maintain the ongoing goal-oriented behavior with a certain level of stress, or if the organism shifts to habitual (or reflexive) responses, even with a minor increase of the stress levels, this would suggest a failure in inhibitory control.

In this perspective, traditional executive components (i.e., updating, monitoring, problem solving, cognitive flexibility, and control inhibition) could not be accessed without taking into account their role in the entire adaptive process and the optimization of cognitive effort due to a perceived stress. In this sense, different from the majority of traditional multi-component models of executive functions that emphasized high-order quality of the cognitive processes, or the majority of dual-processing models that expanded the traditional models investigating the "mirrored" features (**Figures 1B,C**), the dynamic executive functioning hypothesis – based upon the salience and executive control neuronal networks proposed by Hermans et al. (2014) – intended to set aside these conceptual categorical borders commonly used to define executive behaviors, suggesting that an optimal adaptive process would consider the constant interaction between an emotional salience axis and executive controlled axis.

As shown in **Figure 1**, executive functioning would: (1) constantly monitor the environment, adjusting the ongoing behavior as soon as new demands are identified; and (2) promote the automation of successful behavioral strategies. The first point is in accordance with the first assumption presented in the beginning of this section. Considering that executive functioning is an adaptive process, it means that without any environmental demand the organism remain in a homeostatic state, for example the so-called Default Mode Network that usually is found when neuroimaging studies investigate participants at rest (Damoiseaux et al., 2006). However, even without a demand capable of triggering goal-oriented behaviors, people still need to monitor and perceive environmental changes, which is likely supported by the synchronicity found between the brain salience network and default mode network at rest, whose disruption falls over dysfunctional thinking (Orliac et al., 2013). The second point means that as soon as a new goal-oriented behavior achieves success in responding to environmental demand, it should be added to the repertoire of successful behavioral strategies of the organisms. This point refers directly to the second assumption also presented in the beginning of this section, which claims that executive functioning should be comprehended as a continuous adaptive process that enables the organism to save cognitive resources when faced with the same environmental demand. This aspect has a key evolutionary purpose since the organism would be able to retrieve previous information to solve similar environmental demands without allocating additional efforts to learn completely new strategies. Even though automaticity has been largely discussed and still lacks consensus, most views of automaticity share the assumption that training and repetition may lead to changes in effort and cognitive demands (Moors and De Houwer, 2006).

Furthermore, executive functioning could be exemplified in daily life situations, particularly, since when we face a new environmental demand (an important appointment or any unpredictable event) cognitive resources should be allocated to cope with that event. Indeed, even relatively low-level cognitive processes can be regulated through environmental stimulus, such as priming. Some authors have suggested that selective attention could be comprehended as a strategic self-regulatory process, since it allows that individuals focus their attention on the goal-relevant information (Fitzsimons and Bargh, 2004). Thus, it seems to be counterintuitive to think that an individual can be emotionally engaged with a certain task while no cognitive resources are allocated to cope with it, at least, on some basic attentional level.

To give another example of our executive functioning hypothesis, we propose a re-interpretation of the most popular example of prefrontal lobe lesion and executive dysfunction, Phineas Gage. The case was first published by Harlow (1868) and since then has inspired the executive functions research and modern hypotheses, such as the somatic marker (Damasio, 1995). Not surprisingly, great attention is given to the fact that the reliable and hardworking foreman miraculously survived after a serious accident in which a tamping iron went through his frontal lobe. Even more surprisingly is that approximately 3 months after the accident, Gage was recovered enough to travel and meet his family. However, in a later report, Harlow (1868) described that previous to his injury Gage "was looked upon by those who knew him as a shrewd, smart business man, very energetic and persistent in executing all his plans of operation," but afterward he was "no longer Gage." Although many executive functions models have focused on this point, to illustrate our hypothesis we briefly highlight a peculiar moment that may have happened few minutes before the accident.

According to some reports, Gage's task consisted of adding blasting powder and a fuse in a hole drilled into the rock, then using the tamping iron to pack sand into the hole above the powder. After "the powder and fuse had been adjusted in the hole, and he was in the act of 'tamping it in,' his attention was attracted by his men in the pit behind him" (...) "at the same instant dropping the iron upon the charge, it struck fire upon the rock, and the explosion followed" (Harlow, 1868). Within our perspective, the failure in maintaining the primary attentional focus on the task could also be described as an executive functioning failure. After a couple of months of performing the same tasks and procedures, it is possible that the individual became used to it, automating some behaviors. In the meantime, the emotional salience associated with the dangerousness of the task also decreased and the likelihood to commit a mistake gradually increased. In other words, it is possible that Gage was working in an automatic-resting state and was not able to update the new environmental demand in time. The same would have occurred with any individual working on an assembly line, or any other activity that requires repeating a series of procedures during a certain period.

On the contrary, during a lecture, teachers should be cognitively engaged to maintain the attentional focus on the topic, while delivering an informative but attractive speech. Their work require highly specialized knowledge and abilities; integrating a series of cognitive processes, such as perception, attention, memory, theory of mind, etc. The teachers in this example would be able to easily maintain low levels of stress and we could argue that they behave in a resting-control state, which is enough to keep them alert but not hypervigilant. The resting-control state is responsible for the majority of goal-oriented behaviors, and it is commonly described as the high-order cognitive abilities associated with traditional multi-component models of executive functions. Continuing with this example, after a 3-h lecture some arrogant students become bored, making noise and telling jokes. The teacher easily becomes stressed, but he/she maintains the same level of his/her lecture, while thinking about the available options to solve this annoyance. The teacher behaves in an "emotional salient-control" state, in which maintaining the executive functioning is extensively exhausting. After asking for respect and silence more than once, a laugh is heard and the teacher immediately yells at students to leave the class. The executive functioning was not enough to inhibit the response and for that reason it could illustrate an "emotional salient-automatic" behavior that solved the problem, but makes the teacher embarrassed. Without the arrogant and noisy students, the teacher relaxes and the lecture continues, now in a resting-automatic state. Although **Figure 1** suggests an adaptive process in which the organism goes through the same states, but in a specific direction (i.e., H, a, b, c), this example also shows that the executive functioning is constantly regulating the allocation of cognitive resources and emotional salience. The next time that the teacher faces a similar situation, he/she could utilize gist representations of the previous event, taking effective split-second decisions without reaching the peak of stress.

The theoretical hypothesis of executive functioning is not intended to go against any specific model or theory, but compile some important features already observed and deeply discussed by other models. Therefore, our goal is to integrate these features to suggest a more comprehensive executive functioning hypothesis, focusing on a continuous adaptive process. The similarities between different models of executive functions are evident when considering the key issues that these models seek to explain: How automatic responses are suppressed in favor of controlled responses? Are controlled responses effortful? If yes, in which way? How working memory capacity influences the suppression of automatic responses and the variability of controlled responses? What are the roles of executive functions in emotional, behavioral, and cognitive self-regulation? Considering these, some comparisons with previous models and theories could help to elucidate some features of our executive functioning perspective.

In this sense, Teuber (1972) was one of the first researchers to synthesize and discuss evidences that the PFC could anticipate consequences based upon sensory systems information, elucidating that emotional responses could be necessary to adequate cognitive functioning in some circumstances. His studies proposed an executive functions framework with a twofold gradient, including a vertical up–down gradient (related to emotional reactivity) and a horizontal back-to-front gradient (related to delay-response task) that modulates sensory systems in anticipation of future changes (Teuber, 1972). The two-fold gradient model from Teuber greatly influenced many future works, as well as the present hypothesis, because it emphasized that a certain level of emotional responses should be important to goal-oriented behaviors. Further studies from Fuster (2006), Stuss and Levine (2002), and Zelazo and Carlson (2012), for example, investigated the energizing effect of emotions in cognition and the self-regulatory aspects of executive functions.

Another important issue of our executive functioning hypothesis refers to the adaptive capacity of the organism to retrieve previous successful strategies. This idea was mostly based upon the model from Norman and Shallice (1983), which postulated that automatic responses should be suppressed in favor of more assertive ones. Initially, the idea of an automatic-controlled axis corroborates with the notion of an attentional control – described by Norman and Shallice (1983) as SAS – that emerged when routine schemas become unable to deal with non-routine circumstances. The major contribution of SAS to our perspective is based upon the idea that our attention could operate in different well-defined levels. Moreover, in accordance with the authors, the SAS indicates that individuals applied previously learned strategies to novel problems, highlighting that an executive functioning may be critical for adaptive behavior and the improvement of cognitive schemes for problem resolutions, as we discussed. By this token, it also has similarities with the theoretical and conceptual analysis of automaticity proposed by Moors and De Houwer (2006) by assuming that practice can lead to less effort in processing – something that some call automaticity – and that cognitive functioning works in a gradual manner. However, this model assumes that this dynamic process works through different features involved in automatic and controlled processes separately, and that the combination of some of these features that may influence types of behaviors/processes that we often call automatic, should in fact be considered an umbrella term for a range of features.

Interestingly, the capacity to improve previous cognitive schemes may be related to the capacity of self-monitoring and behavior inhibition since individuals might be able to anticipate future outcomes according with their own behavior (Barkley, 2001). Barkley (2001) also suggests that an executive functions model may take into account an evolutionary principle of gradualism. Therefore, executive functions may be understood as a continuum form of mental capacity that might be observed in other species, in which human beings show the higher capacity of mental representation concerning future perspectives and the ability to inhibit undesirable behaviors (Barkley, 2001). In this sense, the capacity to constantly update environmental contingencies and inhibit behaviors also seems to be a central aspect in our perspective since it allows the individual to transit by all behavioral states (**Figure 1**), predicting hypothetical futures based upon previous experiences and them inhibiting an automatic response in favor of a controlled one (SAS influence).

More recently, Asp et al. (2013) defined this monitoring/updating characteristic of inhibitory control as the False Tag Theory (FTT), suggesting that affective processes signalize inappropriate responses ("false tags"). In order to include affective processing, the authors also suggest that the capacity to "false tag" inappropriate responses has a limited resource, which can be taxed during periods of high cognitive work (Asp et al., 2013). In this sense, the FTT extended the Somatic Marker Theory (SMT) proposed by Damasio (1996), which elucidated that decision-making is an emotion-dependent process that is wrought through the repetition of experiences. However, FTT proposes how affective signaling could operate with cognitive processes, showing that if there is a concurrent requirement of both "false tagging" to perceptual and cognitive representations, there can be competition for the "false tagging" resource and the efficacy of each process may be decreased (Asp et al., 2013). For our perspective, it corroborates with the idea that cognitive processes are influenced by emotional salience, facilitating or biasing cognitive processes.

Finally, our executive functioning hypothesis is in accordance with the Hot-Cold Decision Triangle (Yang et al., 2012) and the Tri-dimensional Processing model (Varga and Hamburger, 2014). First, both models emerged as a criticism of standard dual-processing models, each one focusing on different arguments. Yang et al. (2012) discuss that effortlessly and effortful cognitive engagement are mediated by an emotional processing, the model suggests that optimal and healthier decisions are influenced by the extent to which System 1 overlaps System 2. Our perspective of executive functioning is different from the Hot-Cold Decision Triangle because their model assumes a prescriptive framework in which optimal decisions are made with less emotional engagement. Moreover, the Tri-dimensional Processing model also added an important issue concerning the continuous dimensions of information processing. However, the authors did not suggest it as an executive functioning outcome, derived from the interaction between automatic-controlled behaviors and emotional salience. This interaction was deeply discussed by Ernst (2014), who suggested that the efficient adaptive behavior would result from the balance between appetitive (striatum-dependent) and avoidant (amygdala-dependent) processes. In his model, PFC works as a "conductor" and regulates approach-avoidant behaviors according to environmental demands (Ernst, 2014).

FUTURE PERSPECTIVES

Instead of presenting a new model, the executive functioning hypothesis presented here should question the current hierarchical and categorical framework and be interpreted as an alternative perspective for future studies. An executive functioning perspective may favor novel discussions about which individual factors can mediate the balance between emotional salience and automatic-controlled behaviors. For example, the threshold of the amount of stress that someone could tolerate to maintain goal-oriented behaviors (emotional salient-controlled state) and not act impulsively (emotional salient-automatic state), may be influenced by personality traits and early experiences, as well as developmental stages and genetic background. Specifically, positive and negative urgency are individual characteristics that are marked by the ineffective control of decisions under extreme emotional states, and particularly, people react differently under different emotional states (Cyders and Smith, 2008). There are some individuals who react rashly to emotional states with positive valences (which means they present positive urgency), and there are people who can react rashly only under negative emotional states (which means they present negative urgency). It has been documented that a combination of personality factors contributes to positive and negative urgency (Gay et al., 2008). With regards to genetic factors, there are evidences suggesting that polymorphisms in the dopamine receptors and serotonin transporters genes are related to positive and negative urgency related to decision-making [for a review about positive and negative urgency and those consequences for behavior, see (Billieux et al., 2010).

Moreover, as reviewed by Peterson and Welsh (2014), an additional feature that should be clearly elucidated concerns the emotional-salience axis. Although dual-processing models theoretically assume that "cold" and "hot" are not independent features of executive functions, in practice the "thermal gradient" between them is still poorly understood. Future researches in experimental psychological should manipulate the "temperature" of a single task (Peterson and Welsh, 2014). Using an interesting approach combining behavioral economic and computational modeling, Summerfield et al. (2011) investigated the allocation of higher-order cognitive strategies by manipulating the volatility of the environment (i.e., the level of uncertainty when environment can change rapidly and without warning). On the other hand, a computational working memory model seems to fit the individual's behavior better during high-volatile (i.e., uncertainty) scenarios. Interesting, the authors suggested that the optimal (Bayesian) decision model predicted-related activity in more posterior regions of the medial PFC while anterior regions of the medial PFC actively respond when decisions are based on motivational information (Summerfield et al., 2011). Likewise, our recent work suggested that during scenarios in which participants have no knowledge about their own performance and lower emotional arousal responses (for more details see Huang et al., 2013), their behavior is mostly modulated by the use of the available information in the decision scenario. Conversely, if some feedback is provided, participants tend to use less or even no available information about the environmental risks (Kluwe-Schiavon et al., 2016). These data are in line with the idea that contingency learning, habitual behavior, and goal-directed behavior could be studied as a continuum modulated by the uncertainty of the environment. Furthermore, manipulating these variables – environmental volatility or the presence of feedback – in experimental contexts might be an effective way to understand behavioral and neural mechanisms behind updating previously learned schemas. Bearing in mind that our model considers an executive functioning that updates itself continuously, integrating both external and internal homeostatic changes, stress paradigms, such as the Trier Social Stress Test (TSST), seem to be a promising option. In this sense, it should be noted that a recent study showed that stressful situations mimicked by the TSST, elicited a stronger activation of the PFC associated with a risky decision-making process (Gathmann et al., 2014).

Additionally, one could question how our executive functioning hypothesis would account for dissociation between different components of executive functions that can be observed in health and mental illness (e.g., how would this hypothesis account for impaired reasoning and problem solving but intact working memory, or impaired working memory but intact inhibitory control). As supported by Summerfield et al. (2011), a dimensional perspective of executive functioning would be able to identify the amount of environmental volatility that someone may confront until goal-oriented responses shift to habitual responses. In this sense, it is still possible that someone could have an intact working memory and impaired problem solving, especially because according to our hypothesis, good performance in working memory could favor the individual to respond to the environmental demand based upon ongoing feedback, without necessarily allocating excessive cognitive resources to planning and problem solving. The same could occur with someone who has an impaired working memory but intact inhibitory control. In this case, someone that presents a decrease in working memory capacity (meaning that less information is retained in his/her memory span) could also present high behavioral variability, which is different from impulsivity or impairments in inhibitory control. It is possible that the same person would not have problems in inhibiting an automatic response when a high emotional-salient stimulus is shown. However, it is true that according to our hypothesis, it would be harder to explain someone who has an impaired working memory but has no difficulties in successfully planning goal-oriented behaviors. This point is important, once more, to illustrate that the current categorical multi-component view of executive functions is still focused on classifying which behaviors should represent cognitive flexibility or inhibitory control (Diamond, 2013), instead of understanding each behavior as a reflex of an adaptive process.

Finally, when we propose different axis we are not assuming consistently that there is a marked frontier between each axis, but we perform an estimation that is relative for understanding proposes. This criteria is similar to that suggested by Moors and De Houwer (2006) when they flagged one limitation of theories that use gradual models. In this sense, further studies could be done to clearly define emotional-salience states and automatic-controlled responses in order to measure it accurately. Based upon a behavioral perspective, it is possible to infer that automatic responses could be defined as those reflexive or conditioned responses. We hypothesized that automatic responses are more likely to occur in an environment with a very high or very low emotional-salience. Moors and De Houwer (2006) discussed that we can identify automaticity by viewing components/features that probably play a more significant role in less controlled processes (e.g., unconscious, unintentionally, or autonomous processing). This view indicated the need to use decompositional methods to investigate automaticity and highlighted that some combinations of different features can give us insight into the dynamics of cognitive control (Moors and De Houwer, 2006). On the other side of the automatic-controlled axis, controlled responses could be defined as those goal-oriented, non-conditioned responses that according to our hypothesis, are more likely to occur with middle-level emotional-salience. However, a clear definition of emotional-salience state is needed. For example, as discussed by Shields et al. (2016) and extensively described by McEwen et al. (2015), the effects of stress on executive functions goes beyond cortisol alone and the HPA-axis, since circulating proinflammatory cytokines can also have an impact on working memory (Marsland et al., 2006) and cognitive flexibility (Levandowski et al., 2016). Further studies should investigate multiple hormones and immune system processes in order to deeply understand the biological mechanisms behind the effects of stress on executive functions (Shields et al., 2016).

AUTHOR CONTRIBUTIONS

BK-S substantially contributed to the conception of the model and design of the work; AND, drafting the work and revising it critically for important intellectual content; AND final approval of the version to be published; AND agreement to be accountable for all aspects of the work in ensuring that questions related to the accuracy or integrity of any part of the work are appropriately discussed and resolved. TWV contributed to drafting the work and revising it critically for important intellectual content; AND final approval of the version to be published. BS-V substantially contributed to the conception of the model and design of the work; AND drafting the work. LM-D final approval of the version to be published; AND agreement to be accountable for all aspects of the work in ensuring that questions related to the accuracy or integrity of any part of the work are appropriately discussed and resolved. RG-O substantially contributed to the conception of the model and design of the work, AND final approval of the version to be published; AND agreement to be accountable for all aspects of the work in ensuring that questions related to the accuracy or integrity of any part of the work are appropriately discussed and resolved.

ACKNOWLEDGMENT

Coordenação de Aperfeiçoamento de Pessoal de Nível Superior (CAPES).

REFERENCES

Anticevic, A., Dowd, E. C., and Barch, D. M. (2013). "Cognitive and motivational neuroscience of psychotic disorders," in *Neurobiology of Mental Illness*, 4 Edn, eds D. S. Charney, J. D. Buxbaum, P. Sklar, and E. J. Nestler (New York, NY: Oxford University Press), 269–286.

Ardila, A. (2008). On the evolutionary origins of executive functions. *Brain Cogn.* 68, 92–99. doi: 10.1016/j.bandc.2008.03.003

Aron, A. R. (2011). From reactive to proactive and selective control: developing a richer model for stopping inappropriate responses. *Biol. Psychiatry* 69, e55–e68. doi: 10.1016/j.biopsych.2010.07.024

Asp, E., Manzel, K., Koestner, B., Denburg, N., and Tranel, D. (2013). Benefit of the doubt: a new view of the role of the prefrontal cortex in executive functioning and decision making. *Front. Neurosci.* 7:86. doi: 10.3389/fnins.2013.00086

Atkinson, R. C., and Shiffrin, R. M. (1971). The control of short-term memory. *Sci. Am.* 225, 82–90. doi: 10.1038/scientificamerican0871-82

Baddeley, A. (2012). Working memory: theories, models, and controversies. *Annu. Rev. Psychol.* 63, 1–29. doi: 10.1146/annurev-psych-120710-100422

Barch, D. M., and Ceaser, A. (2012). Cognition in schizophrenia: core psychological and neural mechanisms. *Trends Cogn. Sci.* 16, 27–34. doi: 10.1016/j.tics.2011.11.015

Bargh, J. A. (1992). The ecology of automaticity: toward establishing the conditions needed to produce automatic processing effects. *Am. J. Psychol.* 105, 181–199. doi: 10.2307/1423027

Barkley, R. A. (2001). The executive functions and self-regulation: an evolutionary neuropsychological perspective. *Neuropsychol. Rev.* 11, 1–29. doi: 10.1023/A:1009085417776

Barkley, R. A. (2012). *Executive Functions: What They Are, How They Work, and why they Evolved*. London: The Guilford Press.

Bar-On, R., Tranel, D., Denburg, N. L., and Bechara, A. (2003). Exploring the neurological substrate of emotional and social intelligence. *Brain* 126, 1790–1800. doi: 10.1093/brain/awg177

Barsegyan, A., Mackenzie, S. M., Kurose, B. D., Mcgaugh, J. L., and Roozendaal, B. (2010). Glucocorticoids in the prefrontal cortex enhance memory consolidation and impair working memory by a common neural mechanism. *Proc. Natl. Acad. Sci. U.S.A.* 107, 16655–16660. doi: 10.1073/pnas.1011975107

Benningfield, M. M., Blackford, J. U., Ellsworth, M. E., Samanez-Larkin, G. R., Martin, P. R., Cowan, R. L., et al. (2014). Caudate responses to reward anticipation associated with delay discounting behavior in healthy youth. *Dev. Cogn. Neurosci.* 7, 43–52. doi: 10.1016/j.dcn.2013.10.009

Billieux, J., Gay, P., Rochat, L., and Van Der Linden, M. (2010). The role of urgency and its underlying psychological mechanisms in problematic behaviours. *Behav. Res. Ther.* 48, 1085–1096. doi: 10.1016/j.brat.2010.07.008

Collette, F., Van Der Linden, M., Laureys, S., Delfiore, G., Degueldre, C., Luxen, A., et al. (2005). Exploring the unity and diversity of the neural substrates of executive functioning. *Hum. Brain Mapp.* 25, 409–423. doi: 10.1002/hbm.20118

Cyders, M. A., and Smith, G. T. (2008). Emotion-based dispositions to rash action: positive and negative urgency. *Psychol. Bull.* 134, 807–828. doi: 10.1037/a0013341

Damasio, A. R. (1995). *Descarte's Error: Emotion, Reason and the Human Brain*. New York, NY: G.P. Putnam.

Damasio, A. R. (1996). The somatic marker hypothesis and the possible functions of the prefrontal cortex. *Philos. Trans. R. Soc. B Biol. Sci.* 351, 1413–1420. doi: 10.1098/rstb.1996.0125

Damoiseaux, J. S., Rombouts, S. A., Barkhof, F., Scheltens, P., Stam, C. J., Smith, S. M., et al. (2006). Consistent resting-state networks across healthy subjects. *Proc. Natl. Acad. Sci. U.S.A.* 103, 13848–13853. doi: 10.1073/pnas.0601417103

Diamond, A. (2013). Executive Functions. *Annu. Rev. Psychol.* 64, 135–168. doi: 10.1146/annurev-psych-113011-143750

Dunn, B. D., Dalgleish, T., and Lawrence, A. D. (2006). The somatic marker hypothesis: a critical evaluation. *Neurosci. Biobehav. Rev.* 30, 239–271. doi: 10.1016/j.neubiorev.2005.07.001

Emcdda. (2014). *European Monitoring Centre for Drugs and Drug Addiction: European Drug Report: Trends and Developments*. Luxemburgo: Publications Office of the European Union.

Ernst, M. (2014). The triadic model perspective for the study of adolescent motivated behavior. *Brain Cogn.* 89, 104–111. doi: 10.1016/j.bandc.2014.01.006

Evans, J. S. B. T. (2008). Dual-processing accounts of reasoning, judgment, and social cognition. *Annu. Rev. Psychol.* 59, 255–278. doi: 10.1146/annurev.psych.59.103006.093629

Fitzsimons, G. M., and Bargh, J. A. (2004). "Automatic self-regulation," in *Handbook of Self-Regulation: Research, Theory, and Applications*, eds R. F. Baumeister and K. D. Vohs (London: The Guilford Press).

Fuster, J. M. (2006). The cognit: a network model of cortical representation. *Int. J. Psychophysiol.* 60, 125–132. doi: 10.1016/j.ijpsycho.2005.12.015

Gathmann, B., Schulte, F. P., Maderwald, S., Pawlikowski, M., Starcke, K., Schäfer, L. C., et al. (2014). Stress and decision making: neural correlates of the interaction between stress, executive functions, and decision making under risk. *Exp. Brain Res.* 232, 957–973. doi: 10.1007/s00221-013-3808-6

Gay, P., Rochat, L., Billieux, J., D'acremont, M., and Van Der Linden, M. (2008). Heterogeneous inhibition processes involved in different facets of self-reported impulsivity: evidence from a community sample. *Acta Psychol.* 129, 332–339. doi: 10.1016/j.actpsy.2008.08.010

Gladwin, T. E., and Figner, B. (2014). ""Hot" cognition and dual systems: introduction, criticisms, and ways forward," in *Frontiers of Cognitive Psychology Series: Neuroeconomics, Judgment and Decision Making*, eds E. A. Wilhelms and V. F. Reyna (London: Psychology Press), 157–181.

Gladwin, T. E., Figner, B., Crone, E. A., and Wiers, R. W. (2011). Addiction, adolescence, and the integration of control and motivation. *Dev. Cogn. Neurosci.* 1, 364–376. doi: 10.1016/j.dcn.2011.06.008

Goldstein, S., Naglieri, J., Princiotta, D., and Otero, T. (2014). "Introduction: a history of executive functioning as a theoretical and clinical construct," in *Handbook of Executive Functioning*, eds S. Goldstein and J. Naglieri (New York, NY: Springer), 3–12.

Harlow, J. (1868). Recovery from the passage of an iron bar throught the head. *Publications Massachusetts Med. Soc.* 2, 327–347.

Hermans, E. J., Henckens, M. J., Joels, M., and Fernandez, G. (2014). Dynamic adaptation of large-scale brain networks in response to acute stressors. *Trends Neurosci.* 37, 304–314. doi: 10.1016/j.tins.2014.03.006

Huang, Y., Wood, S., Berger, D. E., and Hanoch, Y. (2013). Risky choice in younger versus older adults: affective context matters. *Judgm. Decis. Mak.* 8, 179–187.

Jurado, M. B., and Rosselli, M. (2007). The elusive nature of executive functions: a review of our current understanding. *Neuropsychol. Rev.* 17, 213–233. doi: 10.1007/s11065-007-9040-z

Kahneman, D. (2011). *Thinking, Fast and Slow*. New York, NY: Farrar, Straus and Giroux.

Kahneman, D., and Tversky, A. (2000). *Choices, Values, and Frames*. Cambridge: Cambridge University Press.

Kluwe-Schiavon, B., Sanvicente-Vieira, B., Kristensen, C. H., and Grassi-Oliveira, R. (2013). Executive functions rehabilitation for schizophrenia: a critical systematic review. *J. Psychiatr. Res.* 47, 91–104. doi: 10.1016/j.jpsychires.2012.10.001

Kluwe-Schiavon, B., Viola, T. W., and Grassi-Oliveira, R. (2012). Modelos teóricos sobre construto único ou múltiplos processos das funções executivas. *Rev. Neuropsicol. Latinoamericana* 4, 29–34.

Kluwe-Schiavon, B., Viola, T. W., Sanvicente-Vieira, B., Pezzi, J. C., and Grassi-Oliveira, R. (2016). Similarities between adult female crack cocaine users and adolescents in risky decision-making scenarios. *J. Clin. Exp. Neuropsychol.* 38, 795–810. doi: 10.1080/13803395.2016.1167171

Leh, S. E., Petrides, M., and Strafella, A. P. (2010). The neural circuitry of executive functions in healthy subjects and Parkinson's disease. *Neuropsychopharmacology* 35, 70–85. doi: 10.1038/npp.2009.88

Levandowski, M. L., Hess, A. R., Grassi-Oliveira, R., and De Almeida, R. M. (2016). Plasma interleukin-6 and executive function in crack cocaine-dependent women. *Neurosci. Lett.* 628, 85–90. doi: 10.1016/j.neulet.2016.06.023

Lezak, M. D. (1982). The problem of assessing executive functions. *Int. J. Psychol.* 17, 281–297. doi: 10.1080/00207598208247445

Lezak, M. D. (1995). *Neurpsychological Assessment*. New York, NY: Oxford University Press.

Lezak, M. D., Howieson, D. B., Bigler, E. D., and Tranel, D. (2012). *Neuropsychological Assessment*. New York, NY: Oxford University Press.

Li, X., Lu, Z. L., D'argembeau, A., Ng, M., and Bechara, A. (2010). The iowa gambling task in fMRI images. *Hum. Brain Mapp.* 31, 410–423. doi: 10.1002/hbm.20875

Liu, K. C., Chan, R. C., Chan, K. K., Tang, J. Y., Chiu, C. P., Lam, M. M., et al. (2011). Executive function in first-episode schizophrenia: a three-year longitudinal study of an ecologically valid test. *Schizophr. Res.* 126, 87–92. doi: 10.1016/j.schres.2010.11.023

Luria, A. R. (1970). Functional organization of brain. *Sci. Am.* 222, 66–72. doi: 10.1038/scientificamerican0370-66

Marsland, A. L., Petersen, K. L., Sathanoori, R., Muldoon, M. F., Neumann, S. A., Ryan, C., et al. (2006). Interleukin-6 covaries inversely with cognitive performance among middle-aged community volunteers. *Psychosom. Med.* 68, 895–903. doi: 10.1097/01.psy.0000238451.22174.92

McEwen, B. S., Gray, J., and Nasca, C. (2015). Recognizing resilience: learning from the effects of stress on the brain. *Neurobiol. Stress* 1, 1–11. doi: 10.1016/j.ynstr.2014.09.001

McKlveen, J. M., Myers, B., and Herman, J. P. (2015). The medial prefrontal cortex: coordinator of autonomic, neuroendocrine and behavioural responses to stress. *J. Neuroendocrinol.* 27, 446–456. doi: 10.1111/jne.12272

Miller, G. A. (2003). The cognitive revolution: a historical perspective. *Trends Cogn. Sci.* 7, 141–144. doi: 10.1016/S1364-6613(03)00029-9

Miyake, A., Friedman, N. P., Emerson, M. J., Witzki, A. H., Howerter, A., and Wager, T. D. (2000). The unity and diversity of executive functions and their contributions to complex "frontal lobe" tasks: a latent variable analysis. *Cognit. Psychol.* 41, 49–100. doi: 10.1006/cogp.1999.0734

Moors, A., and De Houwer, J. (2006). Automaticity: a theoretical and conceptual analysis. *Psychol. Bull.* 132, 297–326. doi: 10.1037/0033-2909.132.2.297

Morris, S. E., and Cuthbert, B. N. (2012). Research domain criteria: cognitive systems, neural circuits, and dimensions of behavior. *Dialogues Clin. Neurosci.* 14, 29–37.

Noël, X., Brevers, D., and Bechara, A. (2013). A triadic neurocognitive approach to addiction for clinical interventions. *Front. Psychiatry* 4:179. doi: 10.3389/fpsyt.2013.00179

Norman, D. A., and Shallice, T. (1983). Attention to action - willed and automatic-control of behavior. *Bull. Psychon. Soc.* 21, 354–354.

Orliac, F., Naveau, M., Joliot, M., Delcroix, N., Razafimandimby, A., Brazo, P., et al. (2013). Links among resting-state default-mode network, salience network, and symptomatology in schizophrenia. *Schizophr. Res.* 148, 74–80. doi: 10.1016/j.schres.2013.05.007

Peterson, E., and Welsh, M. (2014). "The development of hot and cool executive functions: are we getting warmer?," in *Handbook of Executive Functions*, eds S. Goldstein and J. A. Naglieri (New York, NY: Springer).

Posner, M. I., and Snyder, C. R. (2004). Attention and Cognitive Control. *Cogn. Psychol.* 205–223.

Posner, M. I., and Snyder, C. R. R. (1975). "Attention and cognitive control," in *Information Processing and Cognition: The Loyola Symposium*, ed. R. L. Solso (Hillsdale, NJ: Lawrence Erlbaum Associates), 55–85.

Pribram, K. H. (1973). "The primate frontal cortex-executive of the brain," in *Psychophysiology of the Frontal Lobes*, eds K. H. Pribram and A. R. Luria (New York, NY: Academic Press), 293–314.

Pripfl, J., Neumann, R., Köhler, U., and Lamm, C. (2013). Effects of transcranial direct current stimulation on risky decision making are mediated by 'hot' and 'cold' decisions, personality, and hemisphere. *Eur. J. Neurosci.* 38, 3778–3785. doi: 10.1111/ejn.12375

Reyna, V. F., and Brainerd, C. J. (2011). Dual processes in decision making and developmental neuroscience: a fuzzy-trace model. *Dev. Rev.* 31, 180–206.

Sahlin, N.-E., Wallin, A., and Persson, J. (2010). Decision science: from Ramsey to dual process theories. *Synthese* 172, 129–143. doi: 10.1007/s11229-009-9472-5

Shields, G. S., Bonner, J. C., and Moons, W. G. (2015). Does cortisol influence core executive functions? A meta-analysis of acute cortisol administration effects on working memory, inhibition, and set-shifting. *Psychoneuroendocrinology* 58, 91–103. doi: 10.1016/j.psyneuen.2015.04.017

Shields, G. S., Sazma, M. A., and Yonelinas, A. P. (2016). The effects of acute stress on core executive functions: a meta-analysis and comparison with cortisol. *Neurosci. Biobehav. Rev.* 68, 651–668. doi: 10.1016/j.neubiorev.2016.06.038

Starcke, K., and Brand, M. (2016). Effects of stress on decisions under uncertainty: a meta-analysis. *Psychol. Bull.* 142, 909–933. doi: 10.1037/bul0000060

Stuss, D. T. (2011). Traumatic brain injury: relation to executive dysfunction and the frontal lobes. *Curr. Opin. Neurol.* 24, 584–589. doi: 10.1097/WCO.0b013e32834c7eb9

Stuss, D. T., and Levine, B. (2002). Adult clinical neuropsychology: lessons from studies of the frontal lobes. *Annu. Rev. Psychol.* 53, 401–433. doi: 10.1146/annurev.psych.53.100901.135220

Summerfield, C., Behrens, T. E., and Koechlin, E. (2011). Perceptual classification in a rapidly changing environment. *Neuron* 71, 725–736. doi: 10.1016/j.neuron.2011.06.022

Teuber, H. L. (1972). Unity and diversity of frontal lobe functions. *Acta Neurobiol. Exp.* 32, 615–65641.

Tirapu-Ustarroz, J., Garcia-Molina, A., Luna-Lario, P., Roig-Rovira, T., and Pelegrin-Valero, C. (2008a). Models of executive control and functions (I). *Rev. Neurol.* 46, 684–692.

Tirapu-Ustarroz, J., Garcia-Molina, A., Luna-Lario, P., Roig-Rovira, T., and Pelegrin-Valero, C. (2008b). Models of executive control and functions (II). *Rev. Neurol.* 46, 742–750.

Varga, A., and Hamburger, K. (2014). Beyond type 1 vs. type 2 processing: the tri-dimensional way. *Front. Psychol.* 5:993. doi: 10.3389/fpsyg.2014.00993

Volkow, N. D., and Baler, R. D. (2014). Addiction science: uncovering neurobiological complexity. *Neuropharmacology* 76(Pt B), 235–249. doi: 10.1016/j.neuropharm.2013.05.007

Yang, H., Carmon, Z., Kahn, B., Malani, A., Schwartz, J., Volpp, K., et al. (2012). The hot-cold decision triagle: a framework for healthier choices. *Mark. Lett.* 23, 457–472. doi: 10.1007/s11002-012-9179-0

Yuen, E. Y., Liu, W., Karatsoreos, I. N., Feng, J., Mcewen, B. S., and Yan, Z. (2009). Acute stress enhances glutamatergic transmission in prefrontal cortex and facilitates working memory. *Proc. Natl. Acad. Sci. U.S.A.* 106, 14075–14079. doi: 10.1073/pnas.0906791106

Zelazo, P. D., and Carlson, S. M. (2012). Hot and cool executive function in childhood and adolescence: development and plasticity. *Child Dev. Perspect.* 6, 354–360.

Zimmerman, D. L., Ownsworth, T., O'donovan, A., Roberts, J., and Gullo, M. J. (2016). Independence of hot and cold executive function deficits in high-functioning adults with autism spectrum disorder. *Front. Hum. Neurosci.* 10:24. doi: 10.3389/fnhum.2016.00024

19

Executive Dysfunctions: The Role in Attention Deficit Hyperactivity and Post-traumatic Stress Neuropsychiatric Disorders

*Lía Martínez[1], Edward Prada[1,2], Corina Satler[3], Maria C. H. Tavares[1] and Carlos Tomaz[1,4]**

[1] Laboratory of Neurosciences and Behavior, Department of Physiological Sciences, University of Brasilia, Brasilia, Brazil, [2] Faculty of Psychology, Social Sciences Department, Universidad Pontificia Bolivariana Seccional Bucaramanga, Bucaramanga, Colombia, [3] Faculty of Ceilandia, University of Brasilia, Brasilia, Brazil, [4] Neuroscience Research Program, University CEUMA, São Luis, Brazil

Edited by:
Leandro Fernandes Malloy-Diniz, Universidade Federal de Minas Gerais, Brazil

Reviewed by:
Mark Dust, Claremont Graduate University, USA
Giuliano Emerenciano Ginani, Uniamérica, Brazil

***Correspondence:**
Carlos Tomaz
ctomaz@unb.br
ctomaz@ceuma.br

Executive functions (EFs) is an umbrella term for various cognitive processes controlled by a complex neural activity, which allow the production of different types of behaviors seeking to achieve specific objectives, one of them being inhibitory control. There is a wide consensus that clinical and behavioral alterations associated with EF, such as inhibitory control, are present in various neuropsychiatric disorders. This paper reviews the research literature on the relationship between executive dysfunction, frontal-subcortical neural circuit changes, and the psychopathological processes associated with attention deficit hyperactivity disorder (ADHD) and post-traumatic stress disorder (PTSD). A revision on the role of frontal-subcortical neural circuits and their presumable abnormal functioning and the high frequency of neuropsychiatric symptoms could explain the difficulties with putting effector mechanisms into action, giving individuals the necessary tools to act efficiently in their environment. Although, neuronal substrate data about ADHD and PTSD has been reported in the literature, it is isolated. Therefore, this review highlights the overlapping of neural substrates in the symptomatology of ADHD and PTSD disorders concerning EFs, especially in the inhibitory component. Thus, the changes related to impaired EF that accompany disorders like ADHD and PTSD could be explained by disturbances that have a direct or indirect impact on the functioning of these loops. Initially, the theoretical model of EF according to current neuropsychology will be presented, focusing on the inhibitory component. In a second stage, this component will be analyzed for each of the disorders of interest, considering the clinical aspects, the etiology and the neurobiological basis. Additionally, commonalities between the two neuropsychiatric conditions will be taken into consideration from the perspectives of cognitive and emotional inhibition. Finally, the implications and future prospects for research and interventions in the area will be outlined, with the intention of contributing scientific reference information that encompasses the knowledge and understanding of executive dysfunction and its relationship with these treated disorders.

Keywords: ADHD, executive functions, inhibitory control, neuropsychiatric disorders, PTSD

INTRODUCTION

General Aspects of Executive Functions

Executive functions (EFs), also known as executive control or cognitive control, are a complex set of interrelated cognitive processes controlled by its top-down nature (Diamond, 2013) and mediated by dynamic behaviors in order to achieve goal-oriented behaviors that are essential for an individual to solve problems, resist interference, hold attention, learn, make decisions, plan, and regulate their behavior (including in new situations), among other skills necessary for everyday life (Diamond, 2013; Chung et al., 2014).

In the historical background, it has been found that although the term "EFs" was coined by Lezak, it was Luria - his direct predecessor - who first described it, even without mentioning it directly. He proposed a brain functioning model based on clinical findings, which consists of three functional units: (1) motivation arousal (reticular and limbic systems); (2) acquisition, processing, and storage of information (post-rolandic cortical areas); and (3) programming, monitoring, and verification of behavior [dependent on the activity of the prefrontal cortex (PFC); Ardila, 2008]. This complex brain system would be mediated by neuroanatomical and functional hierarchical regions, and would work together to regulate all behavior and mental processes (Jurado and Rosselli, 2007).

Regarding the classification of EFs, inhibition can be highlighted (inhibitory control, including self - behavioral inhibition - and control of interference, selective attention and cognitive inhibition), as well as working memory (WM), cognitive flexibility (also known as mental flexibility; Miyake et al., 2000), reasoning, problem solving, and planning (Collins and Koechlin, 2012; Lunt et al., 2012).

Fuster (2008) was one of the most recognized in the EFs study and was the one who proposed a general theory of the PFC and ideas about the importance of this area in the temporal structure of behavior. He suggested that EFs are cognitive skills that enable the organization of a sequence of actions in pursuit of a goal, and proposed the following cognitive skills as part of EFs: attention (alert, set, spatial attention, sustained attention, and control interference), memory, WM, planning, temporal integration, decision making, and inhibitory control.

Recently, there has been a consensus that three basic nuclei compose EFs: WM, cognitive flexibility, and inhibition of prepotent impulses (Hofmann et al., 2012; Diamond, 2013). WM refers to temporary maintenance and active control of information, avoiding distraction (Kane et al., 2001). For its part, cognitive flexibility is the ability to change and modify the course of thoughts or actions to multiple tasks that require it (Elliott, 2003), and inhibition is the ability to inhibit dominant or automatic responses when is necessary (Miyake et al., 2000). See **Figure 1**.

The focus of this study(revision) will be inhibitory control in EFs, describing and expanding its general characteristics, and the neuropsychiatric conditions of attention deficit hyperactivity disorder (ADHD) and post-traumatic stress disorder (PTSD), with special emphasis on cognitive and emotional perspectives. This paper reviews the research literature on the relationship between executive dysfunction, frontal-subcortical neural circuit changes, and psychopathological processes associated with ADHD and PTSD.

Neuroanatomy of Executive Functions

Executive Functions are closely linked to the activity of the frontal lobes, which establish a significant correlation on a clinical-anatomical level regarding clear evidence from case reports of patients with difficulties that arise after brain injuries to frontal areas, and which result in alterations called "executive dysfunction" or "frontal lobe dysfunction" (Elliott, 2003). But recently, with the advance of technology, various imaging methods [such as magnetic resonance imaging (MRI), functional magnetic resonance imaging (fMRI), and Positron emission tomography (PET)] there is evidence that executive functioning is associated with several distributed networks (Chung et al., 2014), which include not only the frontal regions of the cortex but the subcortical areas too (Collette et al., 2006; Bonelli and Cummings, 2007; Jurado and Rosselli, 2007; Marvel and Desmond, 2010).

The frontal lobe is anatomically shaped, in both human and non-human primates, by the dorsolateral PFC, the medial and cingulate PFC, and the orbital PFC (Fuster, 2002). These areas are involved in complex cognitive processes; the dorsolateral region in WM, the anterior and medial areas in desire and motivation, and the orbital region in inhibitory impulse control and interference (Fuster, 2002). See **Figure 2**.

Some authors have emphasized the "circuits," specifically the frontal-subcortical circuits, claiming that the dorsolateral prefrontal circuit is involved in the organization of information to facilitate a response; the anterior cingulate circuit is related to the conduct of motivation; and orbitofrontal circuit translates the limbic and emotional information into behavioral responses. For these authors, the deterioration of EFs resulting in apathy and impulsivity, for example, is a sign of dysfunction of the frontal-subcortical circuit (Bonelli and Cummings, 2007). Additionally, it is important to mention that the EFs, although closely linked with the PFC, do not rely only on this structure, but also on the intact functioning of the cortical-striatal dopaminergic system (Elliott, 2003). It is the neurobiological basis of EFs, occupying a favored place for "orchestrating all of these functions," as it has the ability to receive and send information to almost all sensory and motor brain systems (Arnsten and Li, 2005).

Bonelli and Cummings (2007) reported that neuropsychiatric expressions associated with neurodegenerative diseases are closely linked to impairments in neurocircuits generated from frontal connections with other brain areas, especially subcortical areas, since the effector mechanisms allowing the organism to act efficiently within its environment are disturbed. This supports the link that has been found between faiths and different psychopathological and behavioral disorders (Närhi et al., 2010; Biederman et al., 2011).

According to Jurado and Rosselli (2007) there are numerous neurodevelopmental and adult disorders for which alterations to the EFs have been identified, linked to the symptoms also

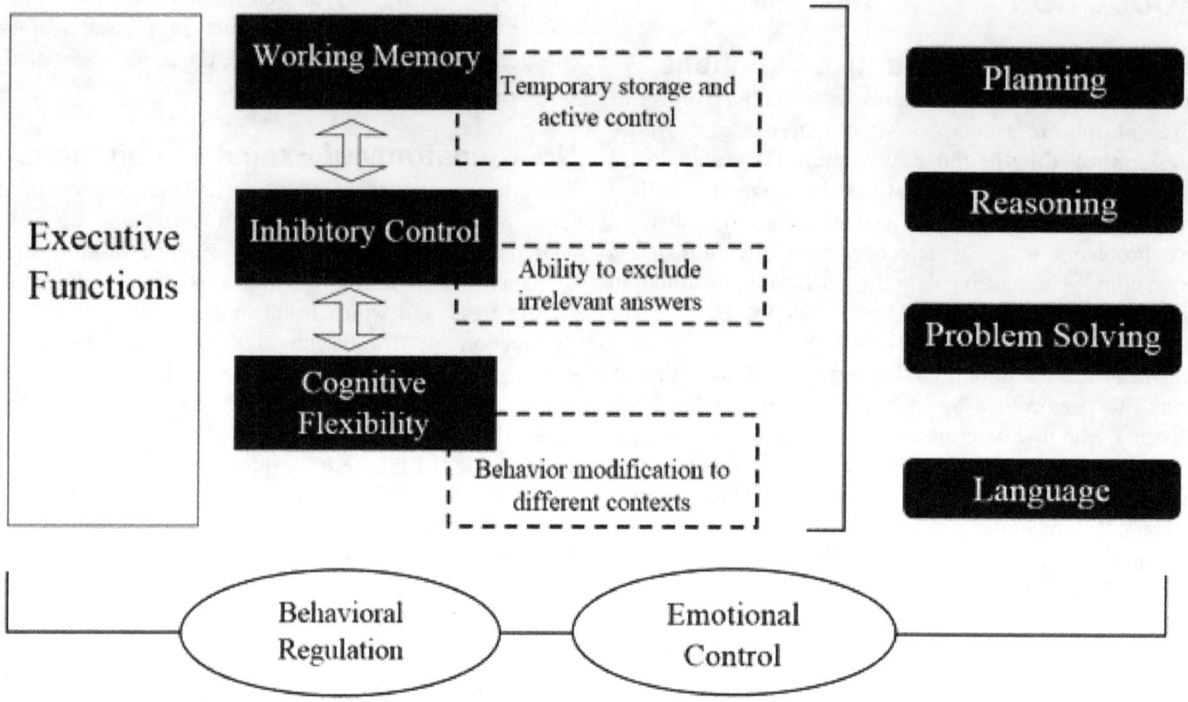

FIGURE 1 | Main components and characteristics of the EFs. Source: made by myself.

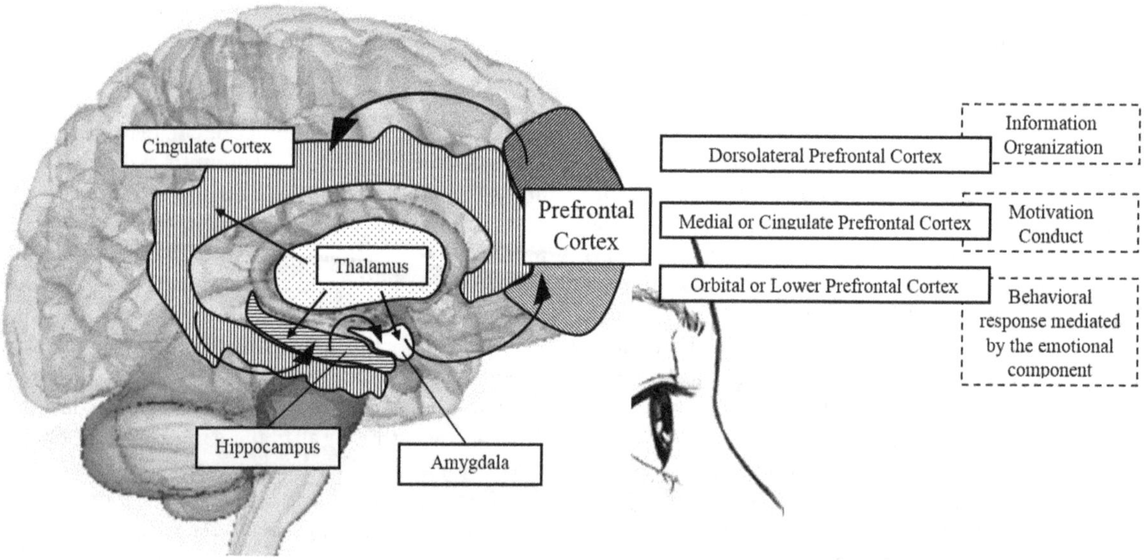

FIGURE 2 | Schematic representation of brain areas associated with the PFC and participation in shaping some components of EFs. Source: made by myself.

found in people with damaged frontal lobes, such as sustained and selective attention, impulsivity, hyperactivity, and deficits in warning systems, WM, the three mechanisms of inhibitory control (waiting, impulse, or interference control) and self-regulation of behavior, as well as perseveration, cognitive rigidity and planning difficulties, among others.

Inhibitory Control

Inhibitory control is considered an important EF due to its ability to control attention, behavior, thoughts and/or emotions, in order to override a strong internal or external predisposition to distraction, and to do so whenever appropriate or necessary according to the demands of the environment. The term "inhibition" refers to several different types of inhibition, such as response or motor inhibition, cognitive inhibition, interference control, motivational inhibition, and the automatic inhibition of attention (Diamond, 2013).

Inhibitory control refers to the mental processes responsible for intentional and voluntary control, involving the ability to resist interferences from irrelevant information and to erase previously relevant information that may create incentives in the short term, but that are not functional to solving a particular problem (Carlson and Wang, 2007). Motor inhibition is defined as the individual's ability to inhibit a behavioral response to a stimulus, i.e., the ability to inhibit a strong behavioral tendency (Diamond, 2006). On the other hand, cognitive inhibition refers to the suppression of irrelevant information in WM (Miyake et al., 2000). It has been found that failures in cognitive inhibition are associated with internalizing problems; on the contrary, the failures are related to behavioral inhibition outsourcing the problems and are based on the individual's ability to inhibit the behavioral response to a stimulus, specifically in tasks that require setting a plan and eliminating wrong answers (Diamond, 2013).

The existence of multiple inhibition types suggests the probability of an overlap between the different brain regions that underlie these inhibitory processes (Collette et al., 2001).

It is argued that the neural substrate of inhibitory control lies mainly in dorsolateral, orbitofrontal and ventromedial areas of the PFC (Fuster, 2002; Ditye et al., 2012), associated with the right prefrontal gyrus (Ditye et al., 2012). Thus, interactions between the right PFC, the basal ganglia, the primary motor regions and the medial temporal lobe are important for the expression of inhibitory control (Aron et al., 2004).

Neuroimaging studies that address inhibition processes have shown the involvement of several regions in the cingulate, prefrontal, parietal, and temporal areas (Collette et al., 2001). However, the exact role of the regions associated with inhibition processes is not completely defined, because the regions mentioned are quite heterogeneous (Collette et al., 2006). Some neuropsychiatric disorders are closely linked to defects in frontal-subcortical neurocircuits. These circuits participate in a variety of neuropsychiatric disorders such as Tourette's syndrome, Huntington's disease, obsessive-compulsive disorder, ADHD, schizophrenia and mood disorders, which occur as a result of changes in the orbitofrontal circuit and therefore in inhibitory control (Bonelli and Cummings, 2007).

ATTENTION DEFICIT DISORDER/HYPERACTIVITY

Characteristics, Prevalence, Diagnostic Criteria, and Comorbidity

Attention deficit hyperactivity disorder is one of the most common problems that develop during neurodevelopmental childhood, considered a disturbance and prevalent in approximately 5% of children and 2.5% of adults (American Psychiatric Association [APA], 2013).

According to several studies, it is estimated that up to 67% of these children will ontinue to exhibit symptoms in adulthood (Lundervold et al., 2011; Ranby et al., 2012). However, the prevalence data reported in the literature varies due to the range of diagnostic criteria and assessment methods used in the studies. With regard to symptoms, Sobanski et al. (2010) have postulated that hyperactivity behavior tends to decrease with age, while inattention increases.

Adolescents and adults with ADHD have a higher risk of failure in school, emotional problems, difficulties in social relationships and sometimes trouble with the law.

The American Psychiatric Association [APA] (2013) argues that many parents first observe excessive motor activity when the child is in early childhood, with symptoms that are difficult to distinguish from normal behavior, which can be variables before 4 years of age. Furthermore, ADHD is often identified at school when inattention becomes more pronounced and affects performance, stabilizing during early adolescence, but possibly worsening with the onset of antisocial behavior. Even so, for most individuals with ADHD the symptoms of motor hyperactivity become less noticeable during adolescence or adulthood, but difficulties associated with restlessness, inattention, planning and impulsivity may persist.

According to the American Psychiatric Association [APA] (2013) in its Diagnostic and Statistical Manual of Mental Disorders (DSM-5), ADHD is defined as a persistent pattern of behavior that manifests itself in various contexts (school/work, home, social, etc.) that interferes significantly with the development and functioning of the individual with the disorder. Thus, the APA states that the symptoms fall into two major predominant areas: inattention, and hyperactivity and impulsivity. Inattention manifests behaviorally with deviations at work, lack of persistence, difficulty maintaining attention, and disorganization, which are not due to a challenge or a lack of understanding; hyperactivity is reflected in excessive motor activity when it is not adequate; and impulsivity is evidenced by hasty actions that are taken without reflection, resulting from a desire for immediate reward or an inability to delay gratification. These characteristics are reflected in the established diagnostic criteria. See **Table 1**.

Regarding the diagnosis of ADHD, Arnett et al. (2013) believe that it must be mainly clinical, as there is no additional examination or neurobiological sign itself that is final; so it must be established based on clinical symptoms. Confirmation via questionnaires, neuropsychological tests and neuropsychological studies is needed for these patients, especially if they are validated by specific neuropsychological batteries that allow reassessments to control the patient's development regarding the indicated treatment.

It has been found that according to clinical research and the discussion in the DSM-5 (American Psychiatric Association [APA], 2013), comorbid disorders are common in individuals with ADHD. For example, oppositional defiant disorder coincides with ADHD in about half of children with combined prevalence and in about a quarter of predominantly inattentive children and adolescents; conduct disorder occurs in about a quarter of children and adolescents with combined

TABLE 1 | Summary of criteria and specific symptoms for the diagnosis of ADHD (American Psychiatric Association [APA], 2013).

Inattention	Hyperactivity/impulsivity
(1) Failure to pay attention to details or careless mistakes are made in schoolwork, work, or during other activities.	(1) Fidgets, claps hands or feet, or squirms in seat.
(2) Difficulty sustaining attention in tasks or recreational activities.	(2) Standing up in situations where they are expected to remain seated.
(3) Does not seem to listen when spoken to directly.	(3) Runs around or climbs in situations where it is not appropriate (may be limited to fidgeting in adolescents or adults).
(4) Does not follow instructions and fails to finish schoolwork, chores, or work duties.	(4) Is unable to play or engage in leisure activities quietly.
(5) Difficulty organizing tasks and activities	(5) Is "busy," acting as if impelled by a "motor."
(6) Avoids, dislikes, or lacks interest in starting tasks that require sustained mental effort.	(6) Talks excessively.
(7) Loses things necessary for tasks or activities.	(7) Responds unexpectedly or before a question has been concluded.
(8) Is easily distracted by external stimuli.	(8) Has difficulty taking turns.
(9) Forgets everyday activities.	(9) Disrupts or interferes with others (adolescents and adults may interfere or get ahead of what others are doing).
Combined	
Criteria for inattention (6+ symptoms) and hyperactivity-impulsivity (6+ symptoms) are met.	

The set of ADHD symptoms usually manifests before 12 years of age, presenting six or more of them (in older adolescents and adults aged 17 years of age, at least five symptoms are required) to diagnose any subtype of ADHD, maintained for a period exceeding 6 months, with an intensity that is incompatible with the level of development and has a direct negative impact on the social and academic/work activities of the individual.

presentation, depending on age and context; a lower percentage of children with ADHD have symptoms that meet criteria for disruptive mood dysregulation disorder; a specific learning disorder commonly occurs along with ADHD; anxiety disorders and major depressive disorders occur in a minority of individuals with ADHD, but more often than in the general population; intermittent explosive disorder occurs in a minority of adults with ADHD, but with levels above the general population; substance abuse disorders are present only in a minority of adults with ADHD, yet they are relatively more frequent among adults with ADHD than in the general population; and antisocial personality disorder and other personality disorders may be associated with ADHD in adults. Other disorders that may be comorbid with ADHD are obsessive-compulsive disorder, tic disorder and the autistic spectrum.

Cognitive Impairment in Attention Deficit Disorder/Hyperactivity

Attention deficit hyperactivity disorder has important cognitive consequences, especially in relation to EFs. Additionally, it is known that the disorder is not characterized by cognitive difficulties alone, but is also marked by an altered emotional level (recognition, regulation, and expression of emotions; Sobanski et al., 2010), a product of dysfunction in executive control processes; according to the DSM-5 (American Psychiatric Association [APA], 2013), this can generate a long-term impact on the operation and development of the individual.

The implications of ADHD, as well as being analyzed through measurements with neuropsychological and cognitive tests, is also studied using various neurological, neurophysiological and neuroimaging tests, with the electroencephalogram (EEG) having demonstrated its effectiveness. Recently, research related to the measurement of brain activity in individuals with ADHD showed a difference in activity patterns between children with and without ADHD, by evaluating electrophysiological variables such as reaction time (RT) in cognitive tasks (McLoughlin et al., 2014), in inhibitory control tasks (Bruckmann et al., 2012) and exposure to emotional stimuli (Singhal et al., 2012).

In general, the literature shows the existence of cognitive deficits in individuals with ADHD, such as deficits in attention, EFs, memory, and perception (Arnett et al., 2013). Thus, the deficit of individuals with ADHD, originated in dysfunction of the frontal lobes, specifically in the PFC, leading primarily to a delay or reduction of EFs, a basic prerequisite for the successful development of a variety of cognitive processes for achieving goals (Funahashi and Andreau, 2013).

A result of the alterations in the PFC, individuals with ADHD often have a syndrome associated with executive control disorders, mainly manifesting inhibitory difficulties in WM and planning (Willcutt et al., 2005), as well as productivity and creativity, and inability to abstract ideas and to anticipate the consequences of behavior, leading to increased impulsivity (Arnett et al., 2013); on the other hand, they also have significant difficulties modulating affective states and recognizing and understanding emotional information, which results in elevated levels of aggressiveness, irritability, or frustration (Martel and Nigg, 2006).

Neurobiology of Attention Deficit Disorder/Hyperactivity

Scientific studies demonstrate the involvement in ADHD of several neuroanatomical structures within the frontal cortex, especially the prefrontal area, the basal ganglia, and the posterior parietal cortex (Arnsten and Li, 2005).

Along with the PFC, the caudate nucleus and its associated circuitry play an important role in the pathogenesis of ADHD.

With MRI studies, structural abnormalities have been found in individuals with ADHD, related to reduced volumes of the left caudate nucleus and right anterior frontal cortex, indicating a reversal of the normal asymmetrical pattern. A bilateral reduction in the size of the putamen has also been found, as well as a reduction in the volume of the right globus pallidus (Cortese et al., 2012).

It is also known that through the use of neuroimaging techniques, structures such as the cerebellum show significantly lower measurements in children with ADHD (on average) throughout childhood and adolescence, compared with the same structures in children without the disorder; In addition, the right PFC is slightly larger in the general population, and its counterpart in the left hemisphere is more symmetrical in people with the disorder, affecting mental abilities such as inhibition of responses, planning behavior, selective focus and organization of information necessary for solving problems and using specific cognitive operations (memory, metacognition, learning, and reasoning; Doyle, 2006; Cortese et al., 2012). See **Figure 3**.

Studies using functional neuroimaging techniques with high spatial [single-photon emission computed tomography (SPECT), PET, and fMRI] temporal [event-related brain potentials (ERPs)] and spatiotemporal [magnetoencephalography (MEG)] resolutions show functional differences in the PFC and striatum in patients with ADHD compared to controls, indicating the existence of dysfunction in the frontostriatal network, which could explain the changes observed in processes such as response inhibition. Furthermore, they showed a decrease in gray matter in the frontal right turn and the rotation of the right posterior cingulate, and in the middle left white matter (Cortese et al., 2012).

Electroencephalogram studies show the existence of a relationship between clinical symptoms of ADHD and characteristics of brain activity, reporting the presence of increased theta activity in the EEG (Boutros et al., 2005).

Volkow et al. (2011) has also investigated the biochemical implications of ADHD, determining that the neurobiological basis of the disorder presents a dysfunction of dopaminergic, serotonergic and noradrenergic circuits, causing an alteration in some cognitive mechanisms. Castellanos (1997) proposed the unitary theory of dopamine transmission in ADHD, based on abnormalities in two dopaminergic regions: (a) hypoactivation cortical regions (anterior cingulate), which produces a cognitive deficit and (b) overactivity in subcortical regions (caudate nucleus), causing excessive motor levels.

Arnsten et al. (1996) suggested that there may be different abnormalities in two noradrenergic regions: an underactive cortical (dorsolateral prefrontal), which referred to primary care deficits (WM) and overactivity in the subcortical systems (locus coeruleus), resulting in over-alertness.

The genetic mechanisms of ADHD are polygenic and this study focused on those related to dopamine, a gene involved in ADHD that could be the D2 receptor gene located on chromosome 11 (11q22-23; Comings, 2001). Other associated genes include the transporter gene norepinephrine (NET1) and the dopamine receptor gene D1 (DRD1; Bobb et al., 2005).

In general, the various neurobiological implications of ADHD can explain and help to understand the effects that are mainly exhibited in cognitive processes, such as the EFs.

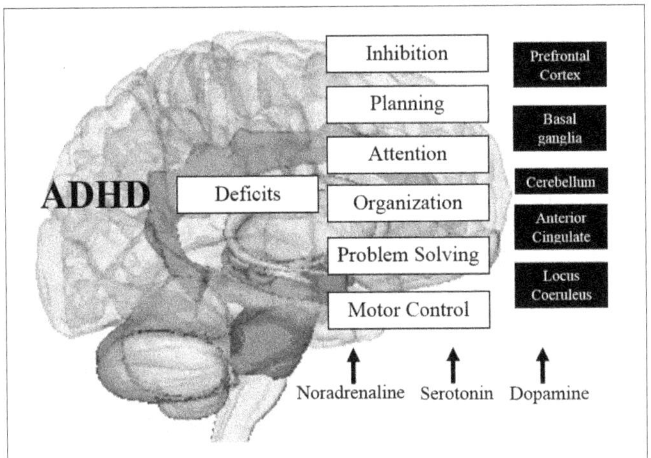

FIGURE 3 | Main altered brain structures in ADHD and their effects on cognitive components associated with EFs. Source: made by myself.

Inhibitory Control in Attention Deficit Disorder/Hyperactivity

One of the EFs most commonly affected in ADHD is inhibitory control (Doyle, 2006; Lange et al., 2010) and/or inability to inhibit responses associated with distracting stimuli (Arnsten and Li, 2005; Doyle, 2006).

Barkley (2006) argues that problems sustaining attention, such as ADHD, are the result of hypoactivity of the behavioral inhibition system, especially for poor interference control. He proposes a model (Barkley, 1997) in which he explains that the deficit in behavioral inhibition involves a delay or impairment in the development of four neuropsychological functions: the memory of non-verbal work, verbal WM, the self-regulation of emotion/motivation/activation, and reconstitution. The most important component of this model is the inhibition of behavior, which provides the basis for the neuropsychological skills mentioned; the other component of the model is the motor, which relates directly to the previous component and is mediated by the four EFs that control behavior.

Accordingly, Nigg (2001) shows clear evidence of the existence of a deficit in ADHD of different forms of executive inhibitory responses, but raises some doubts and questions about whether ADHD would be caused by a primary or secondary inhibitory disorder. To Nigg, although studies are consistent in the presence of an impulsive ADHD and disturbed behavior, the concept of inhibition should be refined, distinguishing between dependent inhibition of executive control and dependent inhibition of motivational Control; in turn, it suggests that the association between domains and deficits in ADHD is more related to inhibition on the strength of a major boost.

Attention deficit hyperactivity disorder is indeed associated with poor cognitive control, particularly inhibitory control (Willcutt et al., 2005; Chamberlain et al., 2011), this could explain why people with ADHD have slower RTs, suggesting the use of more time to inhibit prepotent responses in this population (Shen et al., 2011).

The inhibitory deficit in ADHD is associated with both structural and functional abnormalities in the frontostriatal and frontoparietal circuits, often revealing hypoactivation in prefrontal type tasks for go/no go, compared to the typical population (De La Fuente et al., 2013; Hart et al., 2013). Hervey et al. (2006) and Tamm et al. (2012) suggest that ADHD symptoms include poor performance on neuropsychological measures of inhibition, as well as associated measures (lack of foresight, lack of insight, difficulty delaying gratification, poor organization, poor sense of time, excessive responses).

Various studies of children with ADHD have identified alterations in sustained attention and inhibitory control, which leads to poor self-regulation and behavioral difficulties (Puentes-Rozo et al., 2008). These findings support the theory of the involvement of multioperational location systems in ADHD, including prefrontal and posterior cortical, reticular thalamic, striatal, limbic and mediated connections by specific neurotransmitter systems (Barkley, 2006).

Based on the above, the lack of inhibitory control in ADHD should not only be related to behavioral and cognitive impairments, but also to emotional disturbances, and although the deficit in emotional regulation is not currently one of the symptoms of ADHD diagnoses, various theoretical proposals suggest that it is a fundamental aspect of the disorder (Barkley, 2006).

Individuals with ADHD often have symptoms such as irritability, moodiness, low tolerance to frustration, and sudden and unpredictable changes associated with negative emotions such as anger and sadness (Sobanski et al., 2010), which could be explained by a deficit in emotional regulation, due to alterations in inhibitory control, as demonstrated by several studies which documented that individuals with ADHD not only suffer from attention difficulties, disorganization, hyperactivity and impulsivity, but also various emotional problems, such as emotional liability, excessive emotional reactivity, and irritability (Sobanski et al., 2010; Schoemaker et al., 2012; Arnett et al., 2013).

To Barkley (2006), emotional self-regulation is defined as a set of business processes that enable modular emotions and, upon receipt of a dysfunction, can lead to increased emotional responses to certain situations, as well as less empathy and less ability to regulate emotional states, hence the difficulties that individuals with ADHD have expressing emotions, a result of a primary dysfunction in the inhibitory control processes.

POST-TRAUMATIC STRESS DISORDER

Conceptualization, Prevalence, Comorbidity, and Clinical Criteria

According to the APA and the guidance provided in the DSM-5 (American Psychiatric Association [APA], 2013), PTSD is characterized as a psychiatric disorder, described as a categorical entity clinical order. It is currently classified as one of the disorders related to trauma and stress factors, and can occur in people who have experienced or witnessed a traumatic event such as a natural disaster, a serious accident, an act of terrorism, war or combat, violent personal assault or rape. PTSD is part of a real disorder that leads to short and long term involvement after having experienced or witnessed an event of great emotional impact (Bryant et al., 2011; Sard, 2011). Psychological distress following exposure to a traumatic or stressful events is variable. It has been shown that some people who have been exposed to a stressful or traumatic event do not exhibit clinical features related to PTSD or pathogenesis. This reveals a major contribution by modern science in relation to the existing biological predisposition in some individuals associated with a low susceptibility to this disorder, and therefore provides arguments that PTSD represents a specific phenotype associated with a failure to recover from the normal effects of trauma (Yehuda and LeDoux, 2007).

Regarding the prevalence of PTSD, the data tends to vary according to the diagnostic criteria used to define the disorder, the evaluation procedures implemented, the characteristics of the sample and the context in which the event occurred. All these factors must be considered when studying the phenomenon (Doctor et al., 2011). In the USA, the lifetime risk for PTSD, using the DSM-IV (American Psychiatric Association [APA], 1994) criteria, at the age of 75 years was 8.7% (American Psychiatric Association [APA], 2013). The annual prevalence among USA adults is about 3.5% (Kessler and Wang, 2008). The estimates reported in Europe and most of Asia, Africa and Latin America are lower, at a volume of 0.5–1.0% (Kessler et al., 2005). Although, different groups show different levels of exposure to traumatic events, the conditional probability for PTSD may also vary between different cultural groups when they develop a similar level of exposure. The PTSD rates are higher among veterans and other people whose profession presents a high risk of traumatic exposure (e.g., police, firefighters, emergency medical personnel). The highest rates (ranging from a third to more than half of those exposed) are among the survivors of rape, military combat, captivity and confinement and political or ethnic genocide (Chapman and Diaz-Arrastia, 2014). Classic reference studies have shown that traumatic events with a greater probability of causing a disorder for both men and women are: rape, war, aggression or witness of a murder, and suffering physical abuse in the early stages of life (Kessler et al., 2005; Ogle et al., 2013).

Individuals with PTSD are 80% more likely to have symptoms that meet diagnostic criteria for at least one other mental disorder (e.g., depression, bipolar disorder, anxiety or substance abuse disorders; de Jong et al., 2001; American Psychiatric Association [APA], 2013). Studies with military personnel and veterans reveal a joint incidence of PTSD and mild traumatic brain injury for almost 48% of cases (Chapman and Diaz-Arrastia, 2014). Similarly, there is considerable comorbidity between PTSD and a major neurocognitive disorder (Doctor et al., 2011; Maksimovskiy et al., 2014; Pagotto et al., 2015), including a high association between PTSD and a significant decline in physical and mental health (Blakeley and Jansen, 2013; Pacella et al., 2013). The essential feature for the start of a PTSD diagnosis is the appearance of symptoms after exposure to one or more traumatic events, either directly or indirectly experienced, such as witnessing something experienced by others. According to the DSM-5 (American Psychiatric Association [APA], 2013) criteria are applicable for adults, adolescents and children over 6 years of age, such as the presence of symptoms persisting for more than a month after experiencing the stressor event. The alteration leads to clinically significant distress or impairment in social, occupational or other important areas of functioning of the individual. The alteration cannot be attributed to the physiological effects of a substance (e.g., drugs, alcohol) or another medical condition (American Psychiatric Association [APA], 2013; Friedman, 2013).

Symptoms that form as a result of the traumatic experience are organized into categories: *Re-experiences or intrusions, Avoidance, Persistent negative alterations in ognition and mood,* and *Increased excitability* (Bryant et al., 2011; American Psychiatric Association [APA], 2013). Currently, there are criteria for children under 6 years in relation to the diagnosis of PTSD, as well as indications of clinical order as to the late expression of the disorder (Friedman et al., 2011; American Psychiatric Association [APA], 2013). Psychiatric indications are clear as to their non-linearity in the symptomatic expression in PTSD, as their presentation is varied, occurring specifically in many cases and in others displaying a combination of symptoms (Friedman, 2013). According to the literature, during the development and course of PTSD the symptoms usually begin within the first 3 months after the trauma, although there may be a delay of months, or even years, before the diagnostic criteria are met, which has been called "delayed expression" disorder (Greenberg et al., 2015). It must also specify if the individual experiences persistent dissociative symptoms (Friedman et al., 2011; American Psychiatric Association [APA], 2013). See **Table 2**.

Biological Bases in Post-traumatic Stress Disorder

Irregularities in the biological system involved in the response to stressful events largely lead to damages in the body, setting a pathological mechanism, compared to normal behavior (Yehuda and LeDoux, 2007; Skelton et al., 2012). Dysfunctions in the spinal sympathetic-adrenal-axis and the hypothalamic-pituitary-adrenal-cortical axis, neuroendocrine dysregulation in glutamatergic, noradrenergic, and serotonin systems result in an imbalance and consequently an increased vulnerability to developing PTSD (Pitman et al., 2012).

Studies using models of psychological stress to evaluate the function of the HPA axis revealed an exaggerated cortisol response and hypersecretion of CRH in the PTSD-state, as a result of physiological failures of the system (Dedovic et al., 2009; Sherin and Nemeroff, 2011; Pitman et al., 2012). Paradoxically, there is evidence showing low plasma cortisol levels and an increase in the negative feedback of the HPA axis under basal conditions (Pitman et al., 2012). The presence of low concentrations of cortisol in people who survive traumatic events is a fact that seems contrary to the idea that stress may be associated with elevated levels of cortisol. One explanation that can be made is that in the course of adaptation to trauma, low cortisol concentrations are detected first, reflecting a chronic adaptation of the HPA axis to stress.

Increased and persistent activation of CRH has also been associated with increased activity of the autonomic nervous system in PTSD victims, particularly in a group of women with a history of sexual abuse in childhood with symptoms of depression and anxiety (Heim et al., 2000). The increase in the negative feedback generated by the cortisol could offer an explanation to why the concentration of cortisol is low in the presence of elevated levels of CRH. Yehuda and LeDoux (2007) propose that chronic release of CRH produces an abnormal response by the pituitary gland. Since the number and sensitivity of lymphocytic glucocorticoid receptors is increased, the negative feedback is also increased, causing an attenuation of the cortisol. This increased negative feedback contrasts with the drop that occurs in depression, in which the chronic release of CRH causes decreased negative feedback leading to hypercortisolism and down-regulation of glucocorticoid receptors (Sherin and Nemeroff, 2011; Pitman et al., 2012). See **Figure 4**.

The hypothesis, which postulates that it exists because of chronic stress on the system, is based on the principle known as down-regulation of the GABAergic system, which leads to an excessive and constant activation of glutamate, which can induce long-term synaptic changes and therefore can damage the cognitive and emotional order. Equally important is the inhibition of GABAergic anomalies associated with cellular toxicity, which leads to high concentrations of harmful cell agents, and therefore a decrease in neuroplasticity, and in extreme cases, their death (Hasler et al., 2010; Sherin and Nemeroff, 2011; Pitman et al., 2012). Biochemical studies also reported a central noradrenergic dysfunction, associated with psychiatric symptoms of PTSD, indicating, in some cases, a noradrenergic hypersensitivity and a possible down-regulation of neural receptors that affect metabolic activity (Sherin and Nemeroff, 2011; Pitman et al., 2012; Yamamoto et al., 2013). The regulation of serotonin (5-HT) and consequently the release of corticosteroids under stressful events are positively associated with increased secretion of CRH and PTSD (Sherin and Nemeroff, 2011).

Neural Circuitry Alterations after Traumatic Events

Changes of the biological order, in most cases, lead to structural and functional flaws in several neural circuits after traumatic events (Bremner et al., 2008). The repercussions are evident in the set of clinical symptoms of the disorder (Suvak and Barrett, 2011). Affectations of anatomical and functional natures have been identified in the neurocircuits, especially in the medial PFC, hippocampus, and amygdala (Shin et al., 2006; Herringa et al., 2012). Similarly, cortical regions such as the insular cortex, anterior cingulate cortex, thalamus, and subcortical limbic structures have become important in understanding the anomalies present in PTSD (Herringa et al., 2012). Although, there is a high reproducibility in terms of deficits in classical structures of the human nervous system, there are also novel

TABLE 2 | Summary of specific criteria and symptoms for the diagnosis of PTSD (American Psychiatric Association [APA], 2013).

Re-experiences or intrusions (1/5)	
(1) Recurrent, involuntary, and intrusive distressing memories of the traumatic event(s).	(2) Recurrent distressing dreams in which the content and/or affect of the dream are related to the traumatic event(s).
(3) Dissociative reactions (e.g., flashbacks) in which the individual feels or acts as if the traumatic event(s) were recurring.	(4) Intense or prolonged psychological distress at exposure to internal or external cues that symbolize or resemble an aspect of the traumatic event(s).
(5) Marked physiological reactions to internal or external cues that symbolize or resemble an aspect of the traumatic event(s).	
Avoidance (1/2)	
(1) Avoidance or efforts to avoid distressing memories, thoughts or feelings about or closely associated with the traumatic event(s).	(2) Avoidance or efforts to avoid external reminders (people, places, conversations, activities, objects, situations) that arouse distressing memories, thoughts, or feelings about or closely associated with the traumatic event(s).
Persistent negative alterations in cognition and mood (2/7)	
(1) Inability to remember an important aspect of the traumatic event(s).	(2) Persistent and exaggerated negative beliefs or expectations about oneself, others, or the world.
(3) Persistent, distorted cognitions about the cause or consequences of the traumatic event(s) that lead the individual to blame himself/herself or others.	(4) Persistent negative emotional state.
(5) Markedly diminished interest or participation in significant activities.	(6) Feelings of detachment or estrangement from others.
(7) Persistent inability to experience positive emotions.	
Increased excitability (2/6)	
(1) Irritable behavior and angry outbursts (with little or no provocation) typically expressed as verbal or physical aggression toward people or objects.	(2) Reckless or self-destructive behavior.
(3) Hypervigilance.	(4) Exaggerated startle response.
(5) Problems with concentration.	(6) Sleep disturbance.

Applies to adults, adolescents and children over 6 years. The essential feature (PTSD) is the development of symptoms after exposure to one or more traumatic events. The duration of symptoms of disturbance should be more than 1 month. Dissociative symptoms should not be attributed to the physiological effects of a substance. (/): symptoms required for the category. The disturbance causes clinically significant distress or impairment in important social, occupational, or other areas of functioning.

reports in the scientific literature that reveal the complexity of the neurobiological mechanisms involved in the expression and development of psychopathology in PTSD (Herringa et al., 2012; Patel et al., 2012). There is no equality regarding variables such as study design, type of target population, biological technique, time of occurrence of the disorder, the expression of symptoms and its comorbidities with others, leading to absolute certainty of one single structure and a single key fault disorder (Etkin and Wager, 2007; Pitman et al., 2012).

The volume reduction in the hippocampus and hippocampal atrophy phenomenon detected in patients with chronic PTSD has been widely reported (Shin et al., 2006; Pitman et al., 2012). The most widespread hypothesis corresponds to a phenomenon of cytotoxicity and cell death, resulting from excessive stimulation of the system (Pitman et al., 2012). A decrease in hippocampal activation during symptomatic expression has also been reported, as well as in performing memory tasks involving a judgment of emotional valences (Sherin and Nemeroff, 2011). Conversely, changes in the system (5-HT) reach defined alterations in hippocampal increased activity and severity of symptoms in PTSD (Bremner, 2006; Bremner et al., 2008; Sherin and Nemeroff, 2011).

Amygdala deficits lead to flaws in the evaluation and regulation of biologically relevant threat signals. There is evidence of abnormalities in the functionality of the amygdala in PTSD, and increased startle response has been postulated to represent an increase in function (Bremner, 2006). Because of this, a large brain circuitry is involved in their functional ability, which is consequently committed to the ventromedial PFC and rostral anterior cingulate region (Sherin and Nemeroff, 2011; Pitman et al., 2012). Similarly, chronic PTSD has been correlated with a reduction in the dorsolateral prefrontal parietal gray matter and cingulate cortex (Pitman et al., 2012). The duration of the disorder has been analyzed as a direct proportion to the reduction in gray matter and the severity of the symptoms (Eckart et al., 2011; Chen et al., 2012; Pitman et al., 2012). Effects on the brain's medial diencephalic region, specifically the thalamus, by glutamatergic system failures have been associated with an expression of dissociative states in PTSD (Bremner et al., 2008). It is speculated that such dissociation occurs as a result of alterations in the thalamic transmission, which can be due either to a decrease in entries in the thalamus, which generates a suppression of emotional memories, or charging excessive noradrenergic input stimuli in the thalamus (O'Brien and Nutt, 1998).

Sartory et al. (2013) recently demonstrated a greater number of interconnected cortical areas involved in shaping the symptoms, specifically re-experiencing on a recurring basis. PTSD patients showed significant activation in the mid-line

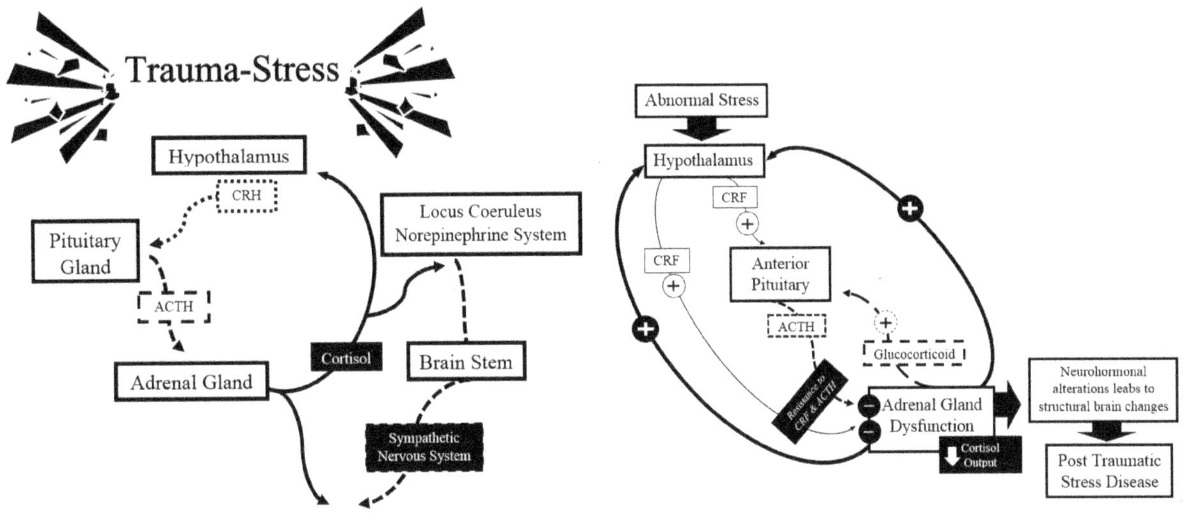

FIGURE 4 | Schematic summary of the classical model of neurobiology in the expression of PTSD: hypothalamic-pituitary-adrenal axis. Source: made by myself.

retrosplenial cortex and precuneus region in response to stimuli associated with the trauma. Likewise, a hyperarousal of the anterior cingulate gyrus was also evident as well as the bilateral amygdala and hypoactivation in sensory association areas, which could indicate that the attentional system required to meet the demand of a task is compromised by centralization of a traumatic memory, generating an associative learning bias due to its intrusive and disturbing connotations.

It is important to note that although research reveals a variety of structural and functional changes by neuroimaging evidence due to exposure to a traumatic event, these changes have been associated with the trauma and therefore care should be taken not to consider them as a cause-effect (Sherin and Nemeroff, 2011; Patel et al., 2012).

Genetic vulnerability, as well as the pre-existence of different abnormalities, are aspects that could be acting as a development risk factor of a symptomatic trauma or neurodegenerative pattern after the trauma (Miller and Sadeh, 2014). Knowledge of the genetic basis and neural pathways involved in the etiology and maintenance of the disorder allow better understanding from a clinical perspective (Suvak and Barrett, 2011; Pitman et al., 2012; Skelton et al., 2012).

Post-traumatic Stress Disorder and Inhibitory Control Dysfunction

According to the DSM-5 (American Psychiatric Association [APA], 2013), recurring memories of the event, avoidance of stimuli associated with the traumatic experience, diminished interest in significant activities, a constant state of hypervigilance, and attentional problems in terms of maintenance, form a pattern of information processing for the majority of PTSD cases.

The central components refer to neurobiological substrate irregularities involving an increased vulnerability in limbic and prefrontal regions, specifically during mnemonic, attentional, emotional and executive processing (Bonelli and Cummings, 2007; Pitman et al., 2012; Chen and Etkin, 2013).

Irregular functioning of inhibitory control, considering the properties of control and regulation, would lead to a permanent imbalance of the nervous system, as well as recurrent failures that would place the cognitive and emotional stability of the subject at risk (MacDonald et al., 2000; Gifford, 2002). The integrity of all executive capabilities provides benefits in terms of the strategy to direct attention and inhibit irrelevant stimuli, thus tending to best guarantee the achievement of a goal (Snyder et al., 2015). Failures in attentional efficiency of the executive control network, mainly in inhibiting interference and attentional failures, have been linked to a decreased ability to control voluntary actions in PTSD patients (Pacheco-Unguetti et al., 2011; Pechtel and Pizzagalli, 2011), as well as difficulties in developing efficient strategies to cope with potentially anxiety-inducing elements (Polak et al., 2012).

Inhibitory control is essential for the exercise of mental flexibility, control and impulsivity interference, WM, self-regulation of emotion and the capacity for analysis and synthesis of behavior (Aron, 2007; Diamond, 2013). An extensive network of frontostriatal circuits are affected in the inhibitory control of patients who have suffered traumatic experiences (Aupperle et al., 2012b; Pitman et al., 2012). Neuropsychological studies have documented anatomical and functional disorders associated with cognitive deficits in patients with PTSD, compared with controls (Bremner, 2006). Long-term effects have been identified in the memory domain for verbal information (McNally, 2006; Brewin, 2011) and visual memory (Marx et al., 2009), declarative memory (Samuelson, 2011), attention (Samuelson et al., 2006; Aupperle et al., 2012a), sustained attention (Vasterling et al., 2002), emotional processing (Milad et al., 2008), WM (Aupperle et al., 2012a), intelligence (Gilbertson et al., 2006), language and communication (McNally, 2006), learning (Samuelson et al., 2006), and processing speed (Samuelson et al., 2006). Disturbances in executive functioning are important to the large bias in cognitive activity in general (Pollak et al., 2010; Aupperle et al., 2012b).

Relationship between Attention Deficit Disorder/Hyperactivity and Post-traumatic Stress Disorder

The inhibitory control component of interest in this review lies mainly in its importance as a central aspect of EF (Banich, 2009; Diamond, 2013) and as a key mechanism that contributes significantly to the efficiency of the executive system in general (Aron, 2007; Banich, 2009). It is for this reason that the different components that make up the theory associated with EFs are initially highlighted, with special emphasis on inhibitory control.

The structural and functional abnormalities of both ADHD and PTSD are evident in a large and complex brain circuit that comprises frontal and medial areas, as well as the cingulate cortex and thalamus, the hippocampal formation and the amygdaloid complex (Bonelli and Cummings, 2007; Pitman et al., 2012; Etkin et al., 2013). This creates a permanent interest in their revision, seeking greater clarity of their underlying mechanisms, which can be a possible route in terms of objective biomarkers and its future use in the monitoring of each pathology.

On the other hand, endocrine factors and brain circuits are involved in the optimal functioning of inhibitory control, especially in the dorsal and ventral PFC, the supplementary motor area, anterior cingulate and parietal and occipital lobe. Such irregularities in the neural mechanisms are associated with the severity of the symptoms in both ADHD and PTSD, referring globally to deficits in attentional systems (Gifford, 2002; Rae et al., 2015).

Regarding the link between these two diagnostic entities, there is evidence suggesting comorbidity with prevalence estimates ranging from 12 to 37% (Adler et al., 2004). The comorbidity described is associated with problems in emotional modulation (arousal levels) that are common to both disorders (hyperarousal and hypoactivation; Harrington et al., 2012).

Adler et al. (2004) suggest that ADHD can become a risk factor that increases vulnerability to developing PTSD after exposure to a traumatic event, based on the finding that the patients with PTSD that they evaluated reported higher levels of ADHD in childhood compared to patients with other disorders.

A study by Koenen et al. (2007) showed patients were 50% more likely to experience psychological trauma if there was a history associated with hyperactivity problems, antisocial behavior, and irritability during childhood, compared to individuals with no such history.

Authors such as Adams (2010) have argued that experiencing traumatic events in childhood is strongly associated with development of psychiatric conditions for life, such as personality disorders, behavioral disorders, ADHD, depression, anxiety, substance abuse and PTSD; as well as developmental delay, impaired cognitive skills, learning difficulties, and even a lower IQ.

In 2000, Ford and collaborators revealed results that suggest that the presence of ADHD and Oppositional Defiant Disorder is more common in patients with a history of physical or sexual abuse, pointing to abuse as a significant risk factor for development of behavioral disorders.

Thus, ADHD during childhood increases exposure to trauma, including physical injuries, physical and sexual abuse, neglect, among others (Koenen et al., 2007; Ouyang et al., 2008). In addition, children who are exposed to traumatic events may be more vulnerable to experiencing an exacerbation of the symptoms of ADHD, such as those related to the regulation of impulses and physiological hyperarousal (Ford et al., 2000; Harrington et al., 2012).

The symptoms that reflect the overlap between ADHD and PTSD include irritability, excessive motor activity, learning disabilities, attention, the attentional shift and concentration difficulties, impulsive behavior, and exaggerated startle responses (Hervey et al., 2004; Daud and Rydelius, 2009), clearly demonstrating symptoms common to both disorders associated with EFs. Thus, alterations in the EFs due to ADHD may explain the high reporting of the disorder as a risk factor for developing PTSD, as suggested by several studies (Nigg et al., 2002; Martel and Nigg, 2006; Volkow et al., 2011).

Generally, according to Bernardi et al. (2012), high rates of impulsive behavior, inattentiveness, and alterations in inhibitory control in individuals with ADHD could provide explanations for the increased risk of trauma.

According to a study by Harrington et al. (2012), which used a confirmatory factor analysis to establish the level of correlation between ADHD and PTSD, the "lack of attention" in ADHD was identified as a factor associated moderately with symptoms of avoidance in the PTSD. Based on this result, the study authors explain that inattention in ADHD and avoidance symptoms in PTSD may reflect similar changes in cognitive control mechanisms, creating problems of distraction and disorganization in ADHD and difficulty in emotionally suppressing intrusive thoughts in PTSD, exposing possible associations between the two disorders related to alterations in inhibitory control.

Swick et al. (2013) evaluated the variability in RT as an indicator of executive dysfunction, specifically as it relates to difficulties in inhibitory control and excessive mental disorder in war veterans and controls, through the go/no go inhibition task, finding that individuals with PTSD had significantly greater variability in RT than the controls, suggesting that they are less successful in inhibiting appropriate responses; in addition, other symptoms such as attentional impulsivity are also present in individuals with ADHD. The findings of this study pointed to deficits in cognitive control processes, specifically top–down, which could contribute to the continuation of PTSD symptoms.

Greater RT variability in cognitive tasks has been associated with a greater propensity toward negative affect (Ode et al., 2011), among other conditions, for developmental disorders (Tamm et al., 2012) such as ADHD. In fact, the increased variability in RTs in ADHD is a highly replicable finding (Hervey et al., 2006; Swick et al., 2013; Tarantino et al., 2013). Among the various explanations for this increased RT variability are: deficits in sustained attention, problems processing time information, and difficulties in regulating behavior (Johnson et al., 2007; Tamm et al., 2012), resulting in a general marker of executive dysfunction (Ode et al., 2011).

However, it is not known whether deficiencies in the general cognitive mechanism such as top-down can account for similar deficits in several disorders, or whether different mechanisms are involved (Swick et al., 2013).

Based on the above, it could be argued that the cognitive, emotional and behavioral disfunctions that characterize both ADHD and PTSD may result from the overlapping of neural substrates.

GENERAL CONCLUSION

As a result of the review of literature associated with ADHD and PTSD, it can be said that these two clinical entities are characterized by a set of signs and symptoms that detail their particular neurobiology, thus allowing a better understanding for clinical management and behavioral aspects to be taken into account in the different diagnoses and future interventions.

Inhibitory control is a cognitive process that plays an important role in ADHD and PTSD; giving rise to the possibility that research generates experimental approaches where inhibitory control is associated with emotional components. In this regard, it would be possible to act on the "psychological distress" that leads these two disorders, especially regarding behavioral disturbances, threatening the adaptation of the affected subject to different contexts in which they operate, including comorbidity with various other mental disorders (Bonelli and Cummings, 2007; Etkin et al., 2013).

Current information on the link between ADHD and PTSD is inconclusive, which still allows for the development of knowledge and interest in its disclosure, primarily through the generation of new research.

On the other hand, continuing to generate associated research will undoubtedly provide a greater understanding as to the specificity of the neurobiological aspects present in both psychiatric conditions. In this sense, the following may be proposed: (1) Biomarker analysis and its future use in the monitoring of each pathology. Genetic and neurophysiological evidence can be integrated into the study of brain hemodynamics using fMRI, PET and SPECT techniques, for example, as well as EEG by monitoring spontaneous and induced electrical activity. Thus, we could better understand the physiological and cognitive mechanisms underlying these pathologic entities, generating new possibilities for clinical and experimental settings. (2) Use of neuropsychological assessment and neuroimaging in order to map the brain. It is vital to develop studies that record biological activity while simultaneously making assessments via cognitive tests (specifically frontal lobe assessment using EF tests). It would be more appropriate to combine traditional and ecological neuropsychological tools in order to obtain more reliable results. (3) Comorbidity and monitoring of the disorder. Given the explanations outlined in this review regarding the increased chance of individuals diagnosed with ADHD suffering from PTSD, is it possible to argue that ADHD worsens the outcome of PTSD, and can we therefore propose a comorbidity? If yes, this could be included in future diagnostic manuals to show the interaction between the two pathologies. Thus, it would contribute not only to the understanding and diagnosis of both diseases, but also to its monitoring at both the clinical and research levels.

Finally, it should be expected that the inclusion of technological tools in the diagnostic and intervention stage will allow better recreation of the scenarios of daily life, thus increasing understanding of rarely addressed cognitive and emotional strategies that are important in shaping ADHD and PTSD.

AUTHOR CONTRIBUTIONS

LM, EP, CS, MT, CT conceptualized and designed the work. LM, EP, CS drafted the work. LM, EP, CS, MT, CT critically revised and approved the manuscript.

REFERENCES

Adams, E. J. (2010). *Healing invisible wounds: Why Investing in Traumainformed Care for Children Makes Sense*. Washington, DC: Justice Policy Institute.

Adler, L. A., Kunz, M., Chua, H. C., Rotrosen, J., and Resnick, S. G. (2004). Attentiondeficit/hyperactivity disorder in adult patients with posttraumatic stress disorder (PTSD): Is ADHD a veulnerability factor? *J. Atten. Disord.* 8, 11–16. doi: 10.1177/108705470400800102

American Psychiatric Association [APA] (1994). *DSM-IV. Diagnostic and Statistical Manual of Mental Disorders*, 4th Edn. Washington, DC: Author.

American Psychiatric Association [APA] (2013). *DSM-5. Diagnostic and Statistical Manual of Mental Disorders*, 5th Edn. Washington, DC: Author.

Ardila, A. (2008). On the evolutionary origins of executive functions. *Brain Cogn.* 68, 92–99. doi: 10.1016/j.bandc.2008.03.003

Arnett, A. B., MacDonald, B., and Pennington, B. F. (2013). Cognitive and behavioral indicators of ADHD symptoms prior to school age. *J. Child Psychol. Psychiatry* 54, 1284–1294. doi: 10.1111/jcpp.12104

Arnsten, A. F., and Li, B. M. (2005). Neurobiology of executive functions: catecholamine influences on prefrontal cortical functions. *Biol. Psychiatry* 57, 1377–1384. doi: 10.1016/j.biopsych.2004.08.019

Arnsten, A. F., Steere, J. C., and Hunt, R. D. (1996). The contribution of alpha 2-noradrenergic mechanisms of prefrontal cortical cognitive function. Potential significance for attention deficit hyperactivity disorder. *Arch. Gen. Psychiatry* 53, 448–455. doi: 10.1001/archpsyc.1996.01830050084013

Aron, A. R. (2007). The neural basis of inhibition in cognitive control. *Neuroscientist* 13, 214–228. doi: 10.1177/1073858407299288

Aron, A. R., Robbins, T. W., and Poldrak, R. A. (2004). Inhibition and the right inferior frontal cortex. *Trends Cogn. Sci.* 8, 170–177. doi: 10.1016/j.tics.2004.02.010

Aupperle, R. L., Allard, C. B., Grimes, E. M., Simmons, A. N., Flagan, T., Behrooznia, M., et al. (2012a). Dorsolateral prefrontal cortex activation during emotional anticipation and neuropsychological performance in posttraumatic stress disorder. *Arch. Gen. Psychiatry* 69, 360–371. doi: 10.1001/archgenpsychiatry.2011.1539

Aupperle, R. L., Melrose, A. J., Stein, M. B., and Paulus, M. P. (2012b). Executive function and PTSD: disengaging from trauma. *Neuropharmacology* 62, 686–694. doi: 10.1016/j.neuropharm.2011.02.008

Banich, M. T. (2009). Executive function: the search for an integrated account. *Curr. Dir. Psychol. Sci.* 18, 89–94. doi: 10.1111/j.1467-8721.2009.01615.x

Barkley, R. A. (1997). Behavioral inhibition, sustained attention, and executive functions: constructing a unifying theory of ADHD. *Psychol. Bull.* 121, 65–94. doi: 10.1037/0033-2909.121.1.65

Barkley, R. A. (2006). "A theory of ADHD," in *Attention-Deficit Hyperactivity Disorder. A Handbook for Diagnosis and Treatment*, ed. R. A. Barkley (New York, NY: Guilford Press), 297–233.

Bernardi, S., Faraone, S. V., Cortese, S., Kerridge, B. T., Pallanti, S., Wang, S., et al. (2012). The lifetime impact of attention-deficit hyperactivity disorder: results from the national epidemiologic survey on alcohol and related conditions. *Psychol. Med.* 42, 875–887. doi: 10.1017/S003329171100153X

Biederman, J., Petty, C. R., Wozniak, J., Wilens, T. E., Fried, R., Doyle, A., et al. (2011). Impact of executive function deficits in youth with bipolar I disorder: a controlled study. *Psychiatry Res.* 186, 58–64. doi: 10.1016/j.psychres.2010.08.029

Blakeley, K., and Jansen, D. J. (2013). *Post-Traumatic Stress Disorder and Other Mental Health Problems in the Military: Oversight Issues for Congress*. Washington, DC: Congressional Research Service.

Bobb, A. J., Addington, A. M., Sidransky, E., Gornick, M. C., Lerch, J. P., Greenstein, D. K., et al. (2005). Support for association between ADHD and two candidate genes: NET1 and DRD1. *Am. J. Med. Genet. B Neuropsychiatr. Genet.* 134B, 67–72. doi: 10.1002/ajmg.b.30142

Bonelli, R., and Cummings, J. L. (2007). Frontal-subcortical circuitry and behavior. *Dialogues Clin. Neurosci.* 9, 141–151.

Boutros, N., Fraenkel, L., and Feingold, A. (2005). A four-step approach for developing diagnostic tests in psychiatry: EEG in ADHD as a test case. *J. Neuropsychiatry Clin. Neurosci.* 17, 455–464. doi: 10.1176/jnp.17.4.455

Bremner, J. D. (2006). The relationship between cognitive and brain changes in posttraumatic stress disorder. *Ann. N. Y. Acad. Sci.* 1071, 80–86. doi: 10.1196/annals.1364.008

Bremner, J. D., Elzinga, B., Schmahl, C., and Vermetten, E. (2008). Structural and functional plasticity of the human brain in posttraumatic stress disorder. *Prog. Brain Res.* 167, 171–186. doi: 10.1016/S0079-6123(07)67012-5

Brewin, C. R. (2011). The nature and significance of memory disturbance in posttraumatic stress disorder. *Annu. Rev. Clin. Psychol.* 7, 203–227. doi: 10.1146/annurev-clinpsy-032210-104544

Bruckmann, S., Hauk, D., Roessner, V., Resch, F., Freitag, C. M., Kammer, T., et al. (2012). Cortical inhibition in attention deficit hyperactivity disorder: new insights from the electroencephalographic response to transcranial magnetic stimulation. *Brain* 135, 2215–2230. doi: 10.1093/brain/aws071

Bryant, R. A., Friedman, M. J., Spiegel, D., Ursano, R., and Strain, J. (2011). A review of acute stress disorder in DSM-5. *Depress. Anxiety* 28, 802–817. doi: 10.1002/da.20737

Carlson, S. M., and Wang, T. (2007). Inhibitory control and emotion regulation in preschool children. *Cogn. Dev.* 22, 489–510. doi: 10.1016/j.cogdev.2007.08.002

Castellanos, F. X. (1997). Toward a pathophysiology of attention-deficit/hyperactivity disorder. *Clin. Pediatr.* 36, 381–393. doi: 10.1177/000992289703600702

Chamberlain, S. R., Robbins, T. W., Winder-Rhodes, S., Müller, U., Sahakian, B. J., Blackwell, A. D., et al. (2011). Translational approaches to frontostriatal dysfunction in attention-deficit/hyperactivity disorder using a computerized neuropsychological battery. *Biol. Psychiatry* 69, 1192–1203. doi: 10.1016/j.biopsych.2010.08.019

Chapman, J. C., and Diaz-Arrastia, R. (2014). Military traumatic brain injury: a review. *Alzheimers Dement.* 10, S97–S104. doi: 10.1016/j.jalz.2014.04.012

Chen, A. C., and Etkin, A. (2013). Hippocampal network connectivity and activation differentiates post-traumatic stress disorder from generalized anxiety disorder. *Neuropsychopharmacology* 38, 1889–1898. doi: 10.1038/npp.2013.122

Chen, Y., Fu, K., Feng, C., Tang, L., Zhang, J., Huan, Y., et al. (2012). Different regional gray matter loss in recent onset PTSD and non PTSD after a single prolonged trauma exposure. *PLoS ONE* 7:e48298. doi: 10.1371/journal.pone.0048298

Chung, H. J., Weyandt, L. L., and Swentosky, A. (2014). "The Physiology of executive functioning," in *Handbook of Executive Functioning*, eds S. Goldstein and J. A. Naglieri (New York, NY: Springer Science+Business Media), 13–27.

Collette, F., Hogge, M., Salmon, E., and Van der Linden, M. (2006). Exploration of the neural substrates of executive functioning by functional neuroimaging. *Neuroscience* 139, 209–221. doi: 10.1016/j.neuroscience.2005.05.035

Collette, F., Van der Linden, M., Delfiore, G., Degueldre, C., Luxen, A., and Salmon, E. (2001). The functional anatomy of inhibition processes investigated with the Hayling task. *Neuroimage* 14, 258–267. doi: 10.1006/nimg.2001.0846

Collins, A., and Koechlin, E. (2012). Reasoning, learning, and creativity: frontal lobe function and human decision-making. *PLoS Biol.* 10:e1001293. doi: 10.1371/journal.pbio.1001293

Comings, D. E. (2001). Clinical and molecular genetics of ADHD and Tourette syndrome. Two related polygenic disorders. *Ann. N. Y. Acad. Sci.* 931, 50–83. doi: 10.1111/j.1749-6632.2001.tb05773.x

Cortese, S., Kelly, C., Chabernaud, C., Proal, E., Di Martino, A., Milham, M. P., et al. (2012). Towards systems neuroscience of ADHD: a meta-analysis of 55 fMRI studies. *Am. J. Psychiatry* 169, 1–28. doi: 10.1176/appi.ajp.2012.11101521

Daud, A., and Rydelius, P. A. (2009). Comorbidity/overlapping between ADHD and PTSD in relation to IQ among children of traumatized/non-traumatized parents. *J. Atten. Disord.* 13, 188–196. doi: 10.1177/1087054708326271

de Jong, J. T., Komproe, I. H., Van Ommeren M., El Masri, M., Araya, M., Khaled, N., et al. (2001). Lifetime events and posttraumatic stress disorder in 4 postconflict settings. *JAMA* 286, 555–562. doi: 10.1001/jama.286.5.555

De La Fuente, A., Xia, S., Branch, C., and Li, X. (2013). A review of attention-deficit/hyperactivity disorder from the perspective of brain networks. *Front. Hum. Neurosci.* 7:192. doi: 10.3389/fnhum.2013.00192

Dedovic, K., Duchesne, A., Andrews, A., Engert, V., and Pruessner, J. C. (2009). The brain and the stress axis: the neural correlates of cortisol regulation in response to stress. *Neuroimage* 47, 864–871. doi: 10.1016/j.neuroimage.2009.05.074

Diamond, A. (2006). "The early development of executive functions," in *Lifespan Cognitive Mechanisms of Change*, eds E. Bialystok and F. Craik (New York, NY: Oxford University Press), 70–95.

Diamond, A. (2013). Executive functions. *Annu. Rev. Psychol.* 64, 135–168. doi: 10.1146/annurev-psych-113011-143750

Ditye, T., Jacobson, L., Walsh, V., and Lavidor, M. (2012). Modulating behavioral inhibition by tDCS combined with cognitive training. *Exp. Brain Res.* 219, 363–368. doi: 10.1007/s00221-012-3098-4

Doctor, J. N., Zoellner, L. A., and Feeny, N. C. (2011). Predictors of health-related quality-of-life utilities among persons with posttraumatic stress disorder. *Psychiatric Serv.* 62, 272–277. doi: 10.1176/appi.ps.62.3.272

Doyle, A. E. (2006). Executive functions in attention-deficit/hyperactivity disorder. *J. Clin. Psychiatry* 6, 21–26.

Eckart, C., Stoppel, C., Kaufmann, J., Tempelmann, C., Hinrichs, H., Elbert, T., et al. (2011). Structural alterations in lateral prefrontal, parietal and posterior midline regions of men with chronic posttraumatic stress disorder. *J. Psychiatry Neurosci.* 36, 176–186. doi: 10.1503/jpn.100010

Elliott, R. (2003). Executive functions and their disorders. *Br. Med. Bull.* 65, 49–59. doi: 10.1093/bmb/65.1.49

Etkin, A., Gyurak, A., and O'Hara, R. (2013). A neurobiological approach to the cognitive deficits of psychiatric disorders. *Dialogues Clin. Neurosci.* 15, 419–429. doi: 10.1016/j.jad.2005.11.006

Etkin, A., and Wager, T. D. (2007). Functional neuroimaging of anxiety: a meta-analysis of emotional processing in PTSD, social anxiety disorder, and specific phobia. *Am. J. Psychiatry* 164, 1476–1488. doi: 10.1176/appi.ajp.2007.070 30504

Ford, J. D., Racusin, R., Ellis, C. G., Daviss, W. B., Reiser, J., Fleischer, A., et al. (2000). Child maltreatment, other trauma exposure, and posttraumatic symptomatology among children with oppositional defiant and attention deficit hyperactivity disorders. *Child Maltreat.* 5, 205–217. doi: 10.1177/1077559500005003001

Friedman, M. J. (2013). Finalizing PTSD in DSM-5: getting here from there and where to go next. *J. Trauma Stress* 26, 548–556. doi: 10.1002/jts.21840

Friedman, M. J., Resick, P. A., Bryant, R. A., and Brewin, C. R. (2011). Considering PTSD for DSM-5. *Depress. Anxiety* 28, 750–769. doi: 10.1002/da.20767

Funahashi, S., and Andreau, J. M. (2013). Prefrontal cortex and neural mechanisms of executive function. *J. Physiol. Paris* 107, 471–482. doi: 10.1016/j.jphysparis.2013.05.001

Fuster, J. M. (2002). Frontal lobe and cognitive development. *J. Neurocytol.* 31, 373–385. doi: 10.1023/A:1024190429920

Fuster, J. M. (2008). *The Prefrontal Cortex.* London: Academic Press.

Gifford, A. (2002). Emotion and self-control. *J. Econ. Behav. Organ.* 49, 113–130. doi: 10.1016/S0167-2681(02)00061-6

Gilbertson, M. W., Paulus, L. A., Williston, S. K., Gurvits, T. V., Lasko, N. B., Pitman, R. K., et al. (2006). Neurocognitive function in monozygotic twins discordant for combat exposure: relationship to posttraumatic stress disorder. *J. Abnorm. Psychol.* 115, 484–495. doi: 10.1037/0021-843X.115.3.484

Greenberg, N., Brooks, S., and Dunn, R. (2015). Latest developments in post-traumatic stress disorder: diagnosis and treatment. *Br. Med. Bull.* 114, 147–155. doi: 10.1093/bmb/ldv014

Harrington, K. M., Miller, M. W., Wolf, E. J., Reardon, A. F., Ryabchenko, K. A., and Ofrat, S. (2012). Attention-deficit/hyperactivity disorder comorbidity in a sample of veterans with posttraumatic stress disorder. *Compr. Psychiatry* 53, 679–690. doi: 10.1016/j.comppsych.2011.12.001

Hart, H., Radua, J., Nakao, T., Mataix-Cols, D., and Rubia, K. (2013). Meta-analysis of functional magnetic resonance imaging studies of inhibition and attention in attention-deficit/hyperactivity disorder: exploring task-specific, stimulant medication, and age effects. *JAMA Psychiatry* 70, 185–198. doi: 10.1001/jamapsychiatry.2013.277

Hasler, G., Van der Veen, J. W., Grillon, C., Drevets, W. C., and Shen, J. (2010). Effect of acute psychological stress on prefrontal GABA concentration determined by proton magnetic resonance spectroscopy. *Am. J. Psychiatry* 167, 1226–1231. doi: 10.1176/appi.ajp.2010.09070994

Heim, C., Newport, D. J., Heit, S., Graham, Y. P., Wilcox, M., Bonsall, R., et al. (2000). Pituitary-adrenal and autonomic responses to stress in women after sexual and physical abuse in childhood. *JAMA* 284, 592–597. doi: 10.1001/jama.284.5.592

Herringa, R., Phillips, M., Almeida, J., Insana, S., and Germain, A. (2012). Post-traumatic stress symptoms correlate with smaller subgenual cingulate, caudate, and insula volumes in unmedicated combat veterans. *Psychiatry Res.* 203, 139–145. doi: 10.1016/j.pscychresns.2012.02.005

Hervey, A. S., Epstein, J. N., and Curry, J. F. (2004). Neuropsychology of adults with attention-deficit/hyperactivity disorder: a meta-analytic review. *Neuropsychology* 18, 485–503. doi: 10.1037/0894-4105

Hervey, A. S., Epstein, J. N., Curry, J. F., Tonev, S., Arnold, L. E., Conners, C. K., et al. (2006). Reaction time distribution analysis of neuropsychological performance in an ADHD sample. *Child Neuropsychol.* 12, 125–140. doi: 10.1080/09297040500499081

Hofmann, W., Schmeichel, B. J., and Baddeley, A. D. (2012). Executive functions and self-regulation. *Trends Cogn. Sci.* 16, 174–180. doi: 10.1016/j.tics.2012.01.006

Johnson, K. A., Kelly, S. P., Bellgrove, M. A., Barry, E., Cox, M., Gill, M., et al. (2007). Response variability in attention deficit hyperactivity disorder: evidence for neuropsychological heterogeneity. *Neuropsychologia* 45, 630–638. doi: 10.1016/j.neuropsychologia.2006.03.034

Jurado, M. B., and Rosselli, M. (2007). The elusive nature of executive functions: a review of our current understanding. *Neuropsychol. Rev.* 17, 213–233. doi: 10.1007/s11065-007-9040-z

Kane, M. J., Bleckley, M. K., Conway, A. R., and Engle, R. W. (2001). A controlled-attention view of working memory capacity. *J. Exp. Psychol. Gen.* 130, 169–183. doi: 10.1037/0096-3445.130.2.169

Kessler, R. C., Chiu, W. T., Demler, O., Merikangas, K. R., and Walters, E. E. (2005). Prevalence, severity, and comorbidity of 12-month DSM-IV disorders in the national comorbidity survey replication. *Arch. Gen. Psychiatry* 62, 617–627. doi: 10.1001/archpsyc.62.6.617

Kessler, R. C., and Wang, P. S. (2008). The descriptive epidemiology of commonly occurring mental disorders in the United States. *Annu. Rev. Public Health* 29, 115–129. doi: 10.1146/annurev.publhealth.29.020907.090847

Koenen, K. C., Moffitt, T. E., Poulton, R., Martin, J., and Caspi, A. (2007). Early childhood factors associated with the development of post-traumatic stress disorder: results form a longitudinal birth cohort. *Psychol. Med.* 37, 181–192. doi: 10.1017/S0033291706009019

Lange, K. W., Reichl, S., Lange, K. M., Tucha, L., and Tucha, O. (2010). The history of attention deficit hyperactivity disorder. *Atten. Defic. Hyperact. Disord.* 2, 241–255. doi: 10.1007/s12402-010-0045-8

Lundervold, A. J., Adolfsdottir, S., Halleland, H., Halmoy, A., Plessen, K., and Haavik, J. (2011). Attention network test in adults with ADHD—the impact of affective fluctuations. *Behav. Brain Funct.* 7, 27. doi: 10.1186/1744-9081-7-27

Lunt, L., Bramham, J., Morris, R. G., Bullock, P. R., Selway, R. P., Xenitidis, K., et al. (2012). Prefrontal cortex dysfunction and "jumping to conclusions": bias or deficit? *J. Neuropsychol.* 6, 65–78. doi: 10.1111/j.1748-6653.2011.02005.x

MacDonald, A. W., Cohen, J. D., Stenger, V. A., and Carter, C. S. (2000). Dissociating the role of the dorsolateral prefrontal and anterior cingulate cortex in cognitive control. *Science* 288, 1835–1838. doi: 10.1126/science.288.5472.1835

Maksimovskiy, A. L., McGlinchey, R. E., Fortier, C. B., Salat, D. H., Milberg, W. P., and Oscar-Berman, M. (2014). White matter and cognitive changes in veterans diagnosed with alcoholism and PTSD. *J. Alcohol. Drug Depend.* 2, 144. doi: 10.4172/2329-6488.1000144

Martel, M. M., and Nigg, J. T. (2006). Child ADHD and personality/temperament traits of reactive and effortful control, resiliency, and emotionality. *J. Child Psychol. Psychiatry* 47, 1175–1183. doi: 10.1111/j.1469-7610.2006.01629.x

Marvel, C. L., and Desmond, J. E. (2010). Functional topography of the cerebellum in verbal working memory. *Neuropsychol. Rev.* 20, 271–279. doi: 10.1007/s11065-010-9137-7

Marx, B. P., Doron-Lamarca, S., Proctor, S. P., and Vasterling, J. J. (2009). The influence of pre-deployment neurocognitive functioning on post-deployment PTSD symptom outcomes among Iraq-deployed Army soldiers. *J. Int. Neuropsychol. Soc.* 15, 840–852. doi: 10.1017/S13556177099 90488

McLoughlin, G., Palmer, J. A., Rijsdijk, F., and Makeig, S. (2014). Genetic overlap between evoked frontocentral theta-band phase variability, reaction time variability, and attention-deficit/hyperactivity disorder symptoms in a twin study. *Biol. Psychiatry* 75, 238–247. doi: 10.1016/j.biopsych.2013.07.020

McNally, R. J. (2006). Cognitive abnormalities in post-traumatic stress disorder. *Trends Cogn. Sci.* 10, 271–277. doi: 10.1016/j.tics.2006.04.00

Miller, M. W., and Sadeh, N. (2014). Traumatic stress, oxidative stress and posttraumatic stress disorder: neurodegeneration and the accelerated-aging hypothesis. *Mol. Psychiatry* 19, 1156–1162. doi: 10.1038/mp.2014.111

Milad, M. R., Orr, S. P., Lasko, N. B., Chang, Y., Rauch, S. L., and Pitman, R. K. (2008). Presence and acquired origin of reduced recall for fear extinction in PTSD: results of a twin study. *J. Psychiatr. Res.* 42, 515–520. doi: 10.1016/j.jpsychires.2008.01.017

Miyake, A., Friedman, N. P., Emerson, M. J., Witzki, A. H., Howerter, A., and Wager, T. D. (2000). The unity and diversity of executive functions and their contributions to complex "frontal lobe" tasks: a latent variable analysis. *Cogn. Psychol.* 41, 49–100. doi: 10.1006/cogp.1999.0734

Närhi, V., Lehto-Salo, P., Ahonen, T., and Marttunen, M. (2010). Neuropsychological subgroups of adolescents with conduct disorder. *Scand. J. Psychol.* 51, 278–284. doi: 10.1111/j.1467-9450.2009.00767.x

Nigg, J. T. (2001). Is ADHD an inhibitory disorder? *Psychol. Bull.* 127, 571–598. doi: 10.1037/0033-2909.127.5.571

Nigg, J. T., John, O. P., Blaskey, L. G., Huang-Pollock, C. L., Willcutt, E. G., Hinshaw, S. P., et al. (2002). Big five dimensions and ADHD symptoms: links between personality traits and clinical symptoms. *J. Pers. Soc. Psychol.* 83, 451–469. doi: 10.1037/0022-3514.83.2.451

O'Brien, M., and Nutt, D. (1998). Loss of consciousness and post-traumatic stress disorder: a clue to aetiology and treatment. *Br. J. Psychiatry* 173, 102–104. doi: 10.1192/bjp.173.2.102

Ode, S., Robinson, M. D., and Hanson, D. M. (2011). Cognitive-emotional dysfunction among noisy minds: predictions from individual differences in reaction time variability. *Cogn. Emot.* 25, 307–327. doi: 10.1080/02699931.2010.494387

Ogle, C. M., Rubin, D. C., Berntsen, D., and Siegler, L. C. (2013). The frequency and impact of exposure to potentially traumatic events over the life course. *Clin. Psychol. Sci.* 1, 426–434. doi: 10.1177/2167702613485076

Ouyang, L., Fang, X., Mercy, J., Perou, R., and Grosse, S. D. (2008). Attention-deficit/hyperactivity disorder symptoms and child maltreatment: a population based study. *J. Pediatr.* 153, 851–856. doi: 10.1016/j.jpeds.2008.06.002

Pacella, M. L., Hruska, B., and Delahanty, D. L. (2013). The physical health consequences of PTSD and PTSD symptoms: a meta-analytic review. *J. Anxiety Disord.* 27, 33–46. doi: 10.1016/j.janxdis.2012.08.004

Pacheco-Unguetti, A. P., Acosta, A., Marqués, E., and Lupiáñez, J. (2011). Alterations of the attentional networks in patients with anxiety disorders. *J. Anxiety Disord.* 25, 888–895. doi: 10.1016/j.janxdis.2011.04.010

Pagotto, L. F., Mendlowicz, M. V., Coutinho, E. S., Figueira, I., Luz, M. P., Araujo, A. X., et al. (2015). The impact of posttraumatic symptoms and comorbid mental disorders on the health-related quality of life in treatment-seeking PTSD patients. *Compr. Psychiatry* 58, 68–73. doi: 10.1016/j.comppsych.2015.01.002

Patel, R., Spreng, R. N., Shin, L. M., and Girard, T. A. (2012). Neurocircuitry models of posttraumatic stress disorder and beyond: a meta-analysis of functional neuroimaging studies. *Neurosci. Biobehav. Rev.* 36, 2130–2142. doi: 10.1016/j.neubiorev.2012.06.003

Pechtel, P., and Pizzagalli, D. A. (2011). Effects of early life stress on cognitive and affective function: an integrated review of human literature. *Psychopharmacology* 214, 55–70. doi: 10.1007/s00213-010-2009-2

Pitman, R. K., Rasmusson, A. M., Koenen, K. C., Shin, L. M., Orr, S. P., Gilbertson, M. W., et al. (2012). Biological studies of post-traumatic stress disorder. *Nat. Rev. Neurosci.* 13, 769–787. doi: 10.1038/nrn3339

Polak, A. R., Witteveen, A. B., Reitsma, J. B., and Olff, M. (2012). The role of executive function in posttraumatic stress disorder: a systematic review. *J. Affect. Disord.* 141, 11–21. doi: 10.1016/j.jad.2012.01.001

Pollak, S. D., Nelson, C. A., Schlaak, M. F., Roeber, B. J., Wewerka, S. S., Wiik, K. L., et al. (2010). Neurodevelopmental effects of early deprivation in post-institutionalized children. *Child Dev.* 81, 224–236. doi: 10.1111/j.1467-8624.2009.01391.x

Puentes-Rozo, P. J., Barceló-Martínez, E., and Pineda, D. A. (2008). Behavioural and neuropsychological characteristics of children of both sexes, between 6 and 11 years of age, with attention deficit hyperactivity disorder. *Rev. Neurol.* 47, 175–184.

Rae, C. L., Hughes, L. E., Anderson, M. C., and Rowe, J. B. (2015). The prefrontal cortex achieves inhibitory control by facilitating subcortical motor pathway connectivity. *J. Neurosci.* 35, 786–794. doi: 10.1523/JNEUROSCI.3093-13.2015

Ranby, K. W., Boynton, M. H., Kollins, S. H., McClernon, F. J., Yang, C., and Fuemmeler, B. F. (2012). Understanding the phenotypic structure of adult retrospective ADHD symptoms during childhood in the United States. *J. Clin. Child Adolesc. Psychol.* 41, 261–274. doi: 10.1080/15374416.2012.654465

Samuelson, K. W. (2011). Post-traumatic stress disorder and declarative memory functioning: a review. *Dialogues Clin. Neurosci.* 13, 346–351.

Samuelson, K. W., Metzler, T. J., Rothlind, J., Choucroun, G., Neylan, T. C., Lenoci, M., et al. (2006). Neuropsychological functioning in posttraumatic stress disorder and alcohol abuse. *Neuropsychology* 20, 716–726. doi: 10.1037/0894-4105.20.6.716

Sard, V. (2011). Developmental trauma, complex PTSD, and the current proposal of DSM-5. *Eur. J. Psychotraumatol.* 2, 5622. doi: 10.3402/ejpt.v2i0.5622

Sartory, G., Cwik, J., Knuppertz, H., Schürholt, B., Lebens, M., Seitz, R. J., et al. (2013). In search of the trauma memory: a meta-analysis of functional neuroimaging studies of symptom provocation in posttraumatic stress disorder (PTSD). *PLoS ONE* 8:e58150. doi: 10.1371/journal.pone.0058150

Schoemaker, K., Bunte, T., Wiebe, S. A., Andrews, K., Deković, M., and Matthys, W. (2012). Executive function deficits in preschool children with ADHD and DBD. *J. Child Psychol. Psychiatry* 53, 111–119. doi: 10.1111/j.1469-7610.2011.02468.x

Shen, H. I., Tsai, S. Y., and Duann, J. R. (2011). Inhibition control and error processing in children with attention deficit/hyperactivity disorder: an event-related potentials study. *Int. J. Psychophysiol.* 81, 1–11. doi: 10.1016/j.ijpsycho.2011.03.015

Sherin, J. E., and Nemeroff, C. B. (2011). Post-traumatic stress disorder: the neurobiological impact of psychological trauma. *Dialogues Clin. Neurosci.* 13, 263–278.

Shin, L. M., Rauch, S. L., and Pitman, R. K. (2006). Amygdala, medial prefrontal cortex, and hippocampal function in PTSD. *Ann. N. Y. Acad. Sci.* 1071, 67–79. doi: 10.1196/annals.1364.007

Singhal, A., Shafer, A. T., Russell, M., Gibson, B., Wang, L., Vohra, S., et al. (2012). Electrophysiological correlates of fearful and sad distraction on target processing in adolescents with attention deficit-hyperactivity symptoms and affective disorders. *Front. Integr. Neurosci.* 6:119. doi: 10.3389/fnint.2012.00119

Skelton, K., Ressler, K. J., Norrholm, S. D., Jovanovic, T., and Bradley-Davino, B. (2012). PTSD and gene variants: new pathways and new thinking. *Neuropharmacology* 62, 628–637. doi: 10.1016/j.neuropharm.2011.02.013

Snyder, H. R., Miyake, A., and Hankin, B. L. (2015). Advancing understanding of executive function impairments and psychopathology: bridging the gap between clinical and cognitive approaches. *Front. Psychol.* 6:328. doi: 10.3389/fpsyg.2015.00328

Sobanski, E., Banaschewski, T., Asherson, P., Buitelaar, J., Chen, W., Franke, B., et al. (2010). Emotional lability in children and adolescents with attention deficit/hyperactivity disorder (ADHD): clinical correlates and familial prevalence. *J. Child Psychol. Psychiatry* 51, 915–923. doi: 10.1111/j.1469-7610.2010.02217.x

Suvak, M. K., and Barrett, L. F. (2011). Considering PTSD from the perspective of brain processes: a psychological construction approach. *J. Trauma Stress* 24, 3–24. doi: 10.1002/jts.20618

Swick, D., Honzel, N., Larsen, J., and Ashley, V. (2013). Increased response variability as a marker of executive dysfunction in veterans with post-traumatic stress disorder. *Neuropsychologia* 51, 3033–3040. doi: 10.1016/j.neuropsychologia.2013.10.008

Tamm, L., Narad, M. E., Antonini, T. N., O'Brien, K. M., Hawk, L. W., and Epstein, J. N. (2012). Reaction time variability in ADHD: A Review. *Neurotherapeutics* 9, 500–508. doi: 10.1007/s13311-012-0138-5

Tarantino, V., Cutini, S., Mogentale, C., and Bisiacchi, P. S. (2013). Time-on-task in children with ADHD: an ex-Gaussian analysis. *J. Int. Neuropsychol. Soc.* 19, 820–828. doi: 10.1017/S1355617713000623

Vasterling, J. J., Duke, L. M., Brailey, K., Constans, J. I., Allain, A. N., and Sutker, P. B. (2002). Attention, learning, and memory performances and intellectual resources in Vietnam veterans: PTSD and no disorder comparisons. *Neuropsychology* 16, 5–14. doi: 10.1037/0894-4105.16.1.5

Volkow, N. D., Wang, G.-J., Newcorn, J. H., Kollins, S. H., Wigal, T. L., Telang, F., et al. (2011). Motivation deficit in ADHD is associated with dysfunction of the dopamine reward pathway. *Mol. Psychiatry* 16, 1147–1154. doi: 10.1038/mp.2010.97

Willcutt, E. G., Doyle, A. E., Nigg, J. T., Faraone, S. V., and Pennington, B. F. (2005). Validity of the executive function theory of attention-deficit/hyperactivity disorder: a meta-analytic review. *Biol. Psychiatry* 57, 1336–1346. doi: 10.1016/j.biopsych.2005.02.006

Yamamoto, K., Shinba, T., and Yoshii, M. (2013). Psychiatric symptoms of noradrenergic dysfunction: a pathophysiological view. *Psychiatry Clin. Neurosci.* 68, 1–20. doi: 10.1111/pcn.12126

Yehuda, R., and LeDoux, L. (2007). Response variation following trauma: a translational neuroscience approach to understanding PTSD. *Neuron* 56, 19–32. doi: 10.1016/j.neuron.2007.09.006

20

Working Memory Training and CBT Reduces Anxiety Symptoms and Attentional Biases to Threat

Julie A. Hadwin and Helen J. Richards*

Developmental Brain-Behaviour Laboratory, School of Psychology, University of Southampton, Southampton, UK

Edited by:
Rodrigo Grassi-Oliveira, Pontifical Catholic University of Rio Grande do Sul, Brazil

Reviewed by:
Elske Salemink, University of Amsterdam, Netherlands
Alexandre Luiz De Oliveira Serpa, São Francisco University, Brazil
Giuliano Emerenciano Ginani, Uniamérica, Brazil

***Correspondence:**
Julie A. Hadwin
jah7@soton.ac.uk

Research indicates that cognitive processes linked to the detection of threat stimuli are associated with poor attentional control, placing children and adolescents at increased risk for the development of anxious affect. The current study aimed to provide preliminary data to assess whether an intervention designed to improve attentional control (via working memory; WM) would lead to better performance in tests of WM and would be associated with positive changes in symptoms of trait and test anxiety, increased inhibitory control and reduced attention to threat. Forty adolescents aged 11–14 years who reported elevated anxiety and low attentional control were randomly allocated to a WM training or an active cognitive behavioural therapy (CBT) control group. Post intervention, WM training was associated with greater improvements (versus. CBT) in trained WM tasks. Both groups, however, reported fewer anxiety symptoms, demonstrated increased inhibitory control and a reduction in attentional biases to threat post intervention and these results were maintained at follow up. The study provides indicative evidence which suggests that WM training has similar benefits to a more traditional CBT intervention on reduced anxiety and attentional biases for threat. Future research should aim to replicate the findings in a large sample size and explore the broader impact of training on day-to-day functioning. In addition, further research is needed to identify which participants benefit most from different interventions (using baseline characteristics) on treatment compliance and outcome.

Keywords: anxiety, working memory, attentional control, intervention, attentional bias to threat, randomized control trial

INTRODUCTION

Research suggests that clinical levels of anxiety are experienced by 2–15% of children and adolescents (Rapee et al., 2009). Anxiety follows a chronic pathway through development and is associated with several negative outcomes including lowered attendance at school (Richards and Hadwin, 2011; Wood et al., 2012), educational underachievement (Owens et al., 2008), poor peer relationships (Asendorpf et al., 2008) and increased risk for further mental and physical health difficulties (Roza et al., 2003). Researchers recognize that increased recruitment of attentional processes linked to regions of the prefrontal cortex (PFC) are important in the regulation of negative affect (e.g., Banks et al., 2007; Hare et al., 2008; review by Graham and Milad, 2013). Theoretical frameworks of anxiety have increasingly focused on poor attentional control as one cognitive mechanism involved in the onset and maintenance of anxious affect (Eysenck and Calvo, 1992; Eysenck et al., 2007).

Cognitive theories aim to understand the nature and impact of anxiety-related impairments in attentional control on performance in cognitive tasks and on attention in daily life. Attentional Control Theory (Eysenck et al., 2007; Eysenck and Derakshan, 2011) for example, proposes that anxiety impacts core cognitive processes linked to inhibitory control (to resist interference from non-relevant distractors), set shifting (to move attention between relevant information or location) and updating information in WM (to remember and revise material for further processing). It suggests that the negative association between anxiety and cognition is most evident when attentional resources are directed toward external or internal threatening stimuli. Related theories similarly propose that elevated anxiety is associated with increased attention towards threat stimuli (e.g., Bar-Haim et al., 2007). Researchers have also argued that the allocation of attention to threat in anxiety leads to subsequent avoidance that works to help individuals regulate feelings of negative affect in the short term (Mogg and Bradley, 1998).

A substantial body of research has shown that children and adolescents with elevated anxiety rapidly focus attention on threat stimuli and demonstrate difficulties inhibiting task-irrelevant threat (Hare et al., 2008; Hadwin et al., 2009; Nightingale et al., 2010; Waters et al., 2012; review by Dudeney et al., 2015). Further research has found evidence of threat avoidance in childhood (Stirling et al., 2006) and adult anxiety (Horley et al., 2004). Attention processes associated with anxious affect have also been shown to predict anxiety over time in development. For example, poor attentional control at 6 years of age was associated with high stable and increasing anxiety trajectories across middle to late childhood (Duchesne et al., 2010). In addition, threat biases to angry (versus happy faces; as indicated in enhanced N170 amplitudes) were found to predict increased anxiety over time in children aged 5–7 years (O'Toole et al., 2013). Further studies have found that good attentional control moderates threat biases in anxiety. Susa et al. (2012), for example, found that a positive association between anxiety and attentional bias to threat was only evident in 9–14-year-old participants who reported low (versus high) levels of attentional control (see also Lonigan and Vasey, 2009 for similar results).

Attention bias modification (ABM) techniques were developed to reduce attentional biases to threat in anxiety using experimental paradigms that direct attention away from threatening stimuli or toward positive stimuli and where the overall aim is to reduce symptoms of anxious affect. Recent studies have found that ABM leads to reductions in attentional biases for threat and anxiety symptoms in children and adolescents (e.g., Rozenman et al., 2011; Eldar et al., 2012). For example, Eldar et al. (2012) conducted a randomised controlled trial (RCT) where participants aged 8–14 years completed four sessions of ABM (versus a placebo condition) over a 4 week period. The results showed reductions in attentional threat bias and clinician reported anxiety across the intervention period in the ABM (versus the placebo) group. Although significant reductions in parent and child report anxiety occurred across both groups. While a recent review outlined that further research is needed to understand the effectiveness of ABM in the reduction of anxiety (Lowther and Newman, 2014), studies have provided preliminary support for the development of interventions in children and adolescents to target anxiety symptoms via reduced attention to threat.

Further interventions have aimed to increase attentional control to reduce symptoms of psychopathology in development. These have largely focused on increasing WM capacity to impact inattention symptoms in children and adolescents diagnosed with attention deficit hyperactivity disorder (e.g., Beck et al., 2010; see review by Rabipour and Raz, 2012). WM is defined as a limited capacity system made up of the phonological loop, the visuospatial sketchpad (processing verbal versus visual and spatial information respectively), the central executive and the episodic buffer (suggested to act as an interface between current cognitive processing with information stored in long term memory; Baddeley, 2003). The central executive component of WM is proposed to form part of prefrontal processes that underpin attentional control (Baddeley, 2003; Kane and McVay, 2012). WM training has been linked to increased activation in prefrontal and parietal brain regions when completing WM tasks (Klingberg et al., 2002; Olesen et al., 2003; review by Bunge and Wright, 2007).

A recent review of training studies highlighted their utility in improving WM as well as attentional control more broadly (Jaeggi and Buschkuehl, 2014). Consistently, a recent meta-analysis reviewed 622 studies using one WM training programme (CogMed) and found evidence of moderate benefits (compared to passive control groups post intervention) and small to moderate benefits (between groups at follow-up) in WM capacity and inattention in daily life as reported by parents and teachers (Spencer-Smith and Klingberg, 2015[1]). Similarly, a meta-analysis of WM and executive function training more broadly (versus passive control groups) were reported to have beneficial effects in older adults on training tasks and wider executive attention (Karbach and Verhaeghen, 2014). Despite broadly positive outcomes for WM training, other reviews have highlighted some challenges within this literature linked to the longevity of effects and transfer to novel WM tasks or intelligence more broadly (Melby-Lervåg and Hulme, 2013).

Few studies have examined the impact of WM training on symptoms of negative affect. Owens et al. (2013) showed that WM training in adults who reported elevated symptoms of depression was associated with increased WM capacity (compared to a low level active control group). This improvement was reflected in greater event related potential (ERP) amplitudes as measured in contralateral delay activity following the intervention and where this component occurs around 300 ms after stimulus onset and is argued to reflect increased retention of remembered

[1]Note that a comment posted in the same journal and following the publication and re-analysis of data in this article argued that there was little evidence of WM training on positive change in daily life (Dovis et al., 2015).

items in visuospatial WM (see Ikkai et al., 2010). Consistent with this finding, an intervention study in 12- to 13-year-olds who were recognized to have social, emotional and behavioral difficulties demonstrated that a WM intervention (compared with a passive control group) increased performance in WM tasks and improved attentional control more broadly (as measured in a behavioral inhibition task). In addition, young people reported fewer symptoms of test anxiety following the intervention (Roughan and Hadwin, 2011). The possibility that a WM intervention can lower negative affect has significant implications for the development of translational research that increases attentional control to enable regulation of emotion and to allow individuals to meet goals in day-to-day life (see Bishop, 2007).

The current study aimed to provide preliminary data to test the proposition that interventions that work to increase attentional control (via improved WM) will have a positive effect on anxiety symptoms and attentional processes associated with negative affect (poor attentional control and attentional capture or avoidance of threat stimuli; Legerstee et al., 2010; Waters et al., 2012). Specifically, it assessed the impact of a WM intervention in adolescents who reported elevated anxiety symptoms and low attentional control. Previous work has reliably established that WM interventions show positive outcomes compared to passive control groups (review by Spencer-Smith and Klingberg, 2015). In addition, several researchers have highlighted that wait-list groups can overestimate treatment effects (e.g., Cunningham et al., 2013). Therefore, the current study compared a WM intervention to an active control group based on cognitive behavioural therapy (CBT); a widely accepted treatment of choice for anxiety (review by Cowart and Ollendick, 2010). Following previous research we anticipated that the CBT intervention would reduce anxiety symptoms in young people. We expected that the WM intervention should increase performance in WM tasks and that it would have a broader positive impact on key measures of attention (i.e., inhibitory control and attentional bias to threat), as well as feelings of anxious affect.

MATERIALS AND METHODS

Participants

Participants were 11–14 year olds from four secondary schools in the UK. One thousand, five hundred and sixty young people were invited to complete screening questionnaires and 640 individuals agreed to participate with parental consent. The only exclusion criterion was the documented presence of special educational needs, leading to the exclusion of 14 young people. Following exclusions and based on the screening inclusion criteria (see below), we identified and approached 146 young people who were eligible to take part and 40 individuals provided written assent and written parental consent to participate. Participants (mean age = 13 years, 0 months; 10 males; $N = 36$ White, $N = 1$ Asian and $N = 3$ Mixed Race.) were randomized to receive one of the two interventions. Appendix A in Supplementary Material outlines the flow of participants through each phase of the study.

Measures

Screening Measures

Participants completed two self-report questionnaires to assess anxiety and attentional control. Anxiety was measured using the 6-item generalized anxiety subscale from the Spence Children's Anxiety Scale (SCAS; Spence, 1998), with possible scores ranging from 0 to 18. Internal consistency in the screened sample was good ($\alpha = 0.84$). We screened attentional control using a 9-item questionnaire with possible scores ranging from 9 to 45; this measure included the seven items from the attention subscale on the Early Adolescent Temperament Questionnaire Revised (Ellis and Rothbart, 2001) and two additional items used to assess WM ability in a school or homework setting. The internal consistency of the scale in the screened sample was acceptable ($\alpha = 0.73$).

Individuals eligible to take part in the interventions scored above average (T-score > 50) on the anxiety questionnaire based on age and gender appropriate norms (scores of 6 or more for males and 7 or more for females) and scored at or below the median for the screened sample (Median = 31, $n = 640$) on the attentional control questionnaire. In the final sample, 27 participants scored in the 'elevated anxiety' range on the SCAS (T-score > 60, corresponding to scores of 9 or more) and 13 participants scored above average but below the elevated anxiety level (T-score > 50). The mean anxiety score in the screened sample ($n = 640$) was 5.79 ($SD = 3.92$, range = 0–18) and in the intervention group the mean was 11.15 ($SD = 3.52$, range = 6–17). Considering attentional control, respective means in the screened and the intervention samples were 5.32 ($SD = 5.32$, range = 15–44) and 26.50 ($SD = 26.50$, range = 20–31).

Outcome Measures

Outcome measures were completed at three time points: prior to the intervention (Time 1 - T1); within 3 weeks after the intervention (Time 2 - T2); between 3 and 4 months after the intervention (Time 3 - T3)[2] .

Working Memory

We measured near WM ability (tasks that were similar to taught tasks within the intervention) and distant WM ability (tasks that were not similar to taught tasks). Near tasks included a percentage correct composite score from the backward digit recall subtest and a modified (backward) version of the block recall subtest from the Working Memory Test Battery for Children (Pickering and Gathercole, 2001) to assess verbal and spatial WM, respectively. Participants heard a list of digits or saw a sequence of blocks of increasing length and were asked to repeat them in the reverse order.

Distant WM was assessed using the verbal and spatial versions of the computerized 2-n-back task (Shackman et al., 2006). In each task, an array of 34 letters was presented continuously for an entire block of trials. Each trial began with the appearance of a small square highlighting a subsection of the letters for 500 ms, followed by a 3500 ms interval in which the letter array was

[2]Participants also completed outcome measures for academic achievement, depression, and state and anxiety. The results associated with these measures were not a focus of the current paper and are therefore reported in Supplementary Analyses.

presented without the small square, followed immediately by the next trial. In the spatial task, participants pressed a button on each trial to indicate whether the location of the square was the same (matched trials) or different (mismatched trials) to the location of the square presented two trials earlier. In the verbal version, they indicated whether the type of letters inside the square was the same or different to the square presented two trials earlier. Each task included 18 matched trials and 54 mismatched trials. We calculated a composite score across tasks based on the percentage of accurate responses in the matched and mismatched trials.

Anxiety

The total score from the Revised Children's Manifest Anxiety Scale (RCMAS 2nd Edition; Reynolds and Richmond, 2008) was used to assess anxiety. The scale is made up of 40 items assessing physiological anxiety, worry and social anxiety. Participants answer each item with a yes/no response, generating possible scores from 0 to 40. The internal consistency for the total scale in the current sample was excellent ($\alpha = 0.90$, $n = 40$ at T1).

We used the total score from the Child Test Anxiety Scales to measure test anxiety (Wren and Benson, 2004). This scale includes 30 items to measure worry, physiological change and behaviors associated with taking tests. Participants are asked to indicate for each item (e.g., "I think most of my answers are wrong") whether they "almost never" (1), "some of the time" (2), "most of the time" (3) "to almost always" (4) show that behavior. The total score ranges from 30 to 120.

Inhibitory Control

Participants completed a computerized Stroop paradigm (Stroop, 1935) with 108 experimental trials. A trial consisted of a fixation cross for 500 ms, followed by a single word (BLUE, YELLOW, RED, or GREEN) or a horizontal string of Xs that disappeared upon response, followed by a blank screen for 1000 ms. The stimuli were typed in blue, yellow, red, or green font and participants pressed a button as quickly as possible to indicate the color of the font. There were three trial conditions presented with equal frequency and in a random order: (1) Congruent trials in which the word content and font color were matched; (2) Incongruent trials in which the word content and font color were mismatched; (3) Neutral trials in which participants were presented with a string of Xs in colored font. The dependent variable was an interference score in which mean RTs in the congruent condition were subtracted from mean RTs in the incongruent condition; positive scores indicate interference from incongruent information.

Attentional Bias to Threat

Participants completed a computerized dot probe task (MacLeod et al., 1986) consisting of 72 experimental trials. A trial started with a fixation cross for 500 ms, followed by a pair of faces presented for 500 ms, followed by a probe stimulus (two small dots) in the location of one of the previous faces until response, followed by a blank screen for 1000 ms. Participants indicated the orientation of the small dots (horizontal or vertical) as quickly as possible with a button press. The task included angry or neutral expressions portrayed by four models (two male, two female) from the NimStim set of facial expressions (Tottenham et al., 2009). The pair of faces in each trial was either angry-neutral (48 trials) or neutral-neutral (24 trials). There were three trial conditions that occurred with equal frequency and in a random order, where the probe replaced: (1) the angry face in angry-neutral pairs (congruent trials); (2) the neutral face in angry-neutral pairs (incongruent trials); (3) either of the faces in the neutral–neutral pairs (neutral trials). The dependent variable was an attentional bias score, calculated by subtracting the mean RT in the congruent condition from the mean RT in the incongruent condition; a positive score indicates a bias toward threat and a negative score indicates a bias away from threat. Scores that tend toward 0 indicate less interference from facial stimuli to meet task goals.

IQ

An estimate of full scale IQ was generated at T1 only using the matrix reasoning and vocabulary subtests from the Wechsler Abbreviated Scale of Intelligence (Wechsler, 1999). In the vocabulary subtest, the participant simultaneously hears and sees a word and is asked to explain its meaning. In the matrix reasoning subtest, participants are shown a matrix of visual stimuli with one piece missing; they are required to select the missing visual stimulus from five response options.

Interventions

Working Memory Training (Cogmed RM, Pearson)

Twenty participants were randomly allocated to the WM training, which consists of 25 sessions completed 5 days per week for 5 weeks; participants completing at least 20 sessions over 8 weeks are regarded as complying with training. Each 30–45 min session includes eight computerized tasks that require visuo-spatial or verbal WM. Each activity includes 15 trials and the difficulty level (number of items to be remembered) is adjusted trial-by-trial. The program generates an 'index of improvement' which provides a measure of the progress made on one verbal and one visuo-spatial task over the training period. Previous work indicates that the mean index of improvement for children aged 7–17 years is 27 ($SD = 13$; Cogmed Coaching Manual).

Thirteen participants (Mean age = 13 years, 0 months; two male) met criteria for training compliance, attending a mean of 22.77 sessions ($SD = 2.52$, Range = 20–25) and achieving a mean index of improvement of 22.62 ($SD = 14.18$, Range = 6–49). Seven participants (Mean age = 13 years, 1 month; two male) did not complete training due to low motivation, attending a mean of 7.00 sessions ($SD = 4.16$, range = 1–15). Completers and non-completers were compared on T1 measures and significant differences between groups were observed for IQ, $t(18) = 2.95$, $p = 0.009$; IQ scores were significantly greater in the completers ($M = 100.08$, $SD = 5.91$, range = 88–108) compared with the non-completers ($M = 92.29$, $SD = 5.02$; Range = 86–99).

FRIENDS for Life (Barrett, 2005)

Twenty participants were randomly allocated to the CBT intervention, which consisted of 10 one-hour sessions conducted twice per week for 5 weeks. The intervention followed a manual which incorporates small group activities on feelings, thoughts, relaxation techniques, problem solving and coping strategies. Nineteen participants (Mean age = 12 years, 11 months; six males) complied with training and attended a mean of 9.37 sessions ($SD = 0.83$, range = 8–10); one female participant did not comply with training due to scheduling difficulties and low attendance ($n = 4$ sessions).

Procedure

All aspects of the study were reviewed and approved by the internal university ethics and research governance procedures and complied with the ethical principles of the British Psychological Society. The screening questionnaires were administered in groups of 20–30 individuals during the school day supervised by teaching staff. Participants recruited into the interventions completed the outcome measures in two sessions during the school day at each time point. After completing T1 measures, participants were matched into pairs based on their RCMAS total anxiety scores. Using a computerized random number generator, one member of each pair was allocated to the WM group and the other member allocated to the CBT group by the second author who was blind to the identity or characteristics of the participants.

The WM training sessions were completed on a school or home computer; a trained Cogmed coach monitored progress following every completed session using the online system provided by Cogmed. The coach met with all participants who complied with training at least twice per week to provide motivation and feedback on progress. The CBT sessions were completed in small groups (4–6 individuals) in a classroom at school, led by a researcher trained to run the FRIENDS for Life program. Monetary reward were provided for both groups with £1 awarded for every session completed and an additional £5 awarded for participants completing all sessions.

Data Analysis

For each outcome measure (WM, anxiety, attentional control and attention to threat) we analyzed data between groups (WM, CBT) and over Time (T1, T2, T3) using repeated measures ANOVAs, where a group by time interaction would indicate a differential impact of the interventions over time. Exploratory data at T1 showed that IQ was correlated with WM scores ($r = 0.47$, $p = 0.01$ and $r = 0.37$, $p = 0.037$ for near and distant WM tasks respectively); therefore IQ was entered as a covariate in all WM analyses. For all analyses we report effect sizes and 95% confidence intervals around group means. The reported analyses are based on the participants who complied with training (completer analysis). For non-completers ($N = 8$), an intention-to-treat (ITT) analysis was also conducted for each outcome variable using the last-observation-carried-forward method (see Streiner, 2002). Five non-completers provided a full set of outcome measures at T1 only and the scores for these participants were carried forward to T2 and T3. Three non-completers provided outcome measures at all time points and these were used in the ITT analyses. All findings reported below for the completer analysis were replicated in the ITT analysis and these results are therefore not reported further. All statistical tests were two-tailed with an alpha level of 0.05.

RESULTS

Analyses were carried out to consider group differences in IQ and between IQ with outcome variables. There was no group difference in IQ ($t < 1$ and $p > 0.05$). **Table 1** presents the characteristics of the WM ($n = 13$) and CBT ($n = 19$) group at all three time points; there were no significant differences between the WM and CBT groups on any of the T1 measures in the completer or ITT samples (all $ts > 1.5$; $ps > 0.1$).

Training Effects

Working Memory (Near)

Analyses were carried out separately for the composite (spatial and verbal) WM near and distant scores. The repeated measures ANCOVA (controlling for IQ) on the percentage of trials correct in the near WM tasks showed a significant effect of group [$F(1,29) = 6.15$, $p = 0.019$, $\eta_p^2 = 0.18$][3] . The percentage of trials correct was higher in the WM group ($M = 55.16$, $SD = 8.73$, CI: 50.07 - 60.24) compared with the CBT group ($M = 47.14$, $SD = 10.43$, CI: 42.94 - 51.34). The main effect of time approached significance [$F(2,29) = 2.85$, $p = 0.066$, $\eta_p^2 = 0.09$], indicating a lower percentage of trials correct at T1 ($M = 47.16$, $SD = 8.99$, CI: 44.17 - 50.15) compared with T2 ($M = 52.72$, $SD = 12.81$, CI: 48.98 - 56.46) and T3 ($M = 53.56$, $SD = 11.89$, CI: 49.70 - 57.42) (T2 T3 ns.). The interaction between time and group was significant [$F(1,29) = 5.82$, $p = 0.005$, $\eta_p^2 = 0.17$], highlighting group differences at T2 ($M = 57.96$, $SD = 10.08$, CI:52.19 - 63.75 and $M = 47.47$, $SD = 12.50$, CI: 42.69 - 52.25 for the WM and CBT groups respectively) and T3 ($M = 58.58$, $SD = 10.53$, CI: 52.61 - 64.55 and $M = 48.54$, $SD = 10.98$, CI: 43.60 - 53.48 for the WM and CBT groups) respectively. The group difference at T1 (respective means: $M = 48.92$, $SD = 7.04$, CI: 44.29 - 53.54 and $M = 45.40$, $SD = 9.92$, CI: 41.58 - 49.23 was not significant; see **Figure 1**). Within group analyses for time were not significant for the WM group ($F < 2.5$, $p > 0.1$) or the CBT group ($F < 1$, $p > 0.1$).

Working Memory (Distant)

The repeated measures ANCOVA (controlling for IQ) on the percentage of trials correct in the distant WM tasks showed no main effect of group or time ($Fs < 1$, $p > 0.1$). In addition, the interaction between time and group was not significant ($F < 1.5$, $p > 0.1$); see **Figure 2**. The mean accuracy scores for the WM and CBT groups at T1, T2, and T3 were: 58.70, 68.61, 67.61, and 6.42, 64.41, 68.07; see **Figure 1**.

Anxiety Symptoms

For total anxiety symptoms the repeated measures ANOVA showed a main effect of time [$F(2,30) = 16.71$, $p < 0.001$, $\eta_p^2 = 0.36$], the mean anxiety scores at T2 ($M = 15.47$, $SD = 8.26$, CI: 12.83 - 18.84) and T3 ($M = 14.00$, $SD = 8.30$, CI:10.90 - 17.10) were significantly lower compared with T1 ($M = 19.96$, $SD = 31$, CI: 16.94-22.98) (T2 T3 ns following Bonferroni correction). There was no main effect of group and no interaction

[3]A *post hoc* power calculation for two independent samples and for a sample size of 13 for near WM tasks (related to mean T1T2 change in the WM group (mean = 9.29) versus the CBT group (mean = 1.90) indicated a power of 0.91.

TABLE 1 | Mean (SD) and range of working memory (WM) (% near and distant correct), anxiety symptoms, stroop interference score (ms), attentional bias score (ms) at measures at time 1 (T1- pre-intervention), time 2 (T2 – post-intervention) and time 3 (T3 – follow-up) in the WM and CBT groups.

	WM group**						CBT group#					
	T1		T2		T3		T1		T2		T3	
	M	*SD*	*M*	*SD*	*M*	*SD*	*M*	*SD*	*M*	*SD*	*M*	*SD*
Working memory tasks												
Near	49.39	7.04	58.69	10.08	58.97	10.53	45.07	9.91	46.97	12.49	48.27	10.98
Distant	59.40	17.37	69.41	14.93	68.37	15.27	59.94	10.16	63.86	13.16	67.54	14.60
Anxiety measures												
Trait anxiety	21.92	7.33	17.76	7.15	14.00	7.30	18.00	8.76	13.89	8.78	14.00	9.09
Test anxiety	74.54	15.14	70.77	19.25	61.77	19.00	74.37	19.13	68.79	19.42	70.79	24.11
Attention measures												
Interference*	97.55	19.46	57.13	16.86	57.39	14.87	85.96	16.54	66.83	37.51	42.76	12.64

	Both groups ($n = 32$)					
	T1		T2		T3	
Bias toward@	44.61	35.63	6.42	41.03	−24.46	−24.46
Bias away	−38.53	30.44	15.15	59.23	12.89	12.89

***N = 13 participants; #N = 19 participants, *interference scores indicate the RT (ms) differences between incongruent versus congruent trial (increased positive scores reflect greater interference) and N = 18 participants completed the stroop test in the CBT group because one participant reported color blindness. @Indicates bias toward threat and bias away from threat collapsed across groups.*

between group and time ($Fs < 2.5$, $p > 0.1$; see **Figure 2**). With respect to test anxiety, the analysis showed a main effect of time [$F(2,30) = 4.73$, $p = 0.012$, $\eta_p^2 = 0.14$], highlighting more reported symptoms of test anxiety at T1 ($M = 74.43$, $SD = 17.35$, CI: 67.97 – 80.93) compared with T3 ($M = 66.28$, $SD = 22.30$, CI: 58.12 – 74.44). There was no difference between T1 and T2 ($M = 69.78$, $SD = 19.06$, CI: 62.67 – 76.89) or T2 and T3 test anxiety scores. There was no main effect of group ($F < 1, p > 0.1$). The interaction between group and time approached significance [$F(2,30) = 2.45$, $p = 0.095$, $\eta_p^2 = 0.08$]; indicating that there were no significant differences between any time point for the CBT group. However, for the WM group, time differences were evident between T3 with both other time points (T1 T2 ns; see **Figure 2**).

Inhibitory Control

Task performance

A one way (stimulus type: congruent, incongruent, neutral) repeated measures ANOVA on RTs in the Stroop task at T1 revealed a typical congruency effect. There was a main effect of stimulus type [$F(1.36,40.81) = 36.60$, $p < 0.001$, $\eta_p^2 = 0.55$], where RTs were significantly longer in the incongruent condition ($M = 806.12$ ms, $SD = 133.13$, $CI = 757 – 854$) compared with the congruent ($M = 715.29$ ms, $SD = 106.42$, $CI = 676 – 754$, $p < 0.001$) and neutral conditions ($M = 741.87$ ms, $SD = 111.27$, $CI = 701 – 782$, $p < 0.001$). RTs in the congruent conditions were also significantly faster than the RTs in the neutral condition ($p < 0.001$).

The repeated measures ANOVA on interference scores revealed no significant main effect of group and no interaction between group and time ($Fs < 1$, all $ps > 0.1$). There was a main effect of time [$F(2,60) = 51$, $p = 0.003$, $\eta_p^2 = 0.18$] showing significantly higher interference scores at T1 ($M = 90.82$ ms, $SD = 69.25$, $CI = 65 – 116$) compared with T2 ($M = 62.76$, $SD = 59.99$, $CI = 41 – 85$) and T3 ($M = 48.90$ ms, $SD = 53.23$, $CI = 29 – 68$); see **Figure 3**.

Threat Bias

Task performance

A one way (probe position: congruent, incongruent, neutral) repeated measures ANOVA was conducted on RTs in the dot probe paradigm at T1 in order to understand baseline task performance. The results revealed no significant effect of probe position on RTs ($F < 1$, $p > 0.1$; congruent: $M = 715.71$ ms, $SD = 163.63$; incongruent: $M = 716.25$ ms, $SD = 163.42$; neutral: $M = 722.15$ ms, $SD = 162.57$).

Considering group differences and attentional bias to threat, the results showed no effect of group [$F(1,30) = 2.14$, $p = 0.12$, $\eta_p^2 = 0.02$]. In addition, there was no main effect of time and the interaction between time and group was not significant (in both cases $F < 1$ and $p > 0.1$). The respective mean bias scores (and SD) for threat for the WM and CBT intervention groups at each time point was 15.97, ($SD = 64.90$, $CI = -14.43$ – 46.37), 17.23 ($SD = 51.94$, $CI = -11.93$ – 46.38), −2.26 ($SD = 59.75$, $CI = -33.03$ – 28.51) and −10.01 ($SD = 44.65$, $CI = -35.16$ – 15.13), 6.85 ($SD = 51.17$, $CI = -17.27$ – 30.97), −6.24 ($SD = 50.39$, $CI = -31.70$ – 19.21). Further exploration of the T1 attentional bias scores showed that across the two intervention groups there were two types of participant at baseline; those that attended toward threat (bias score > 0, $n = 15$) and those that attended away from threat (bias score < 0, $n = 17$). Therefore, analyses were run separately for the two types of threat bias. Because sample sizes were small analyses

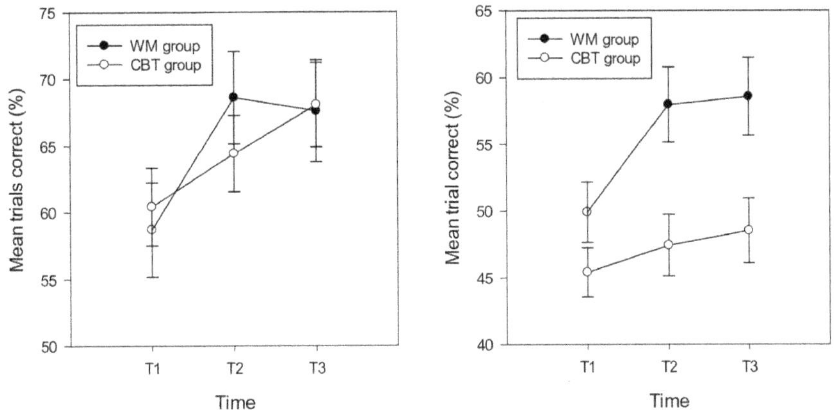

FIGURE 1 | Percentage of trials correct (and standard errors) in the near (right hand graph) and distant (left hand graph) working memory tasks in the WM and CBT intervention groups at each time point.

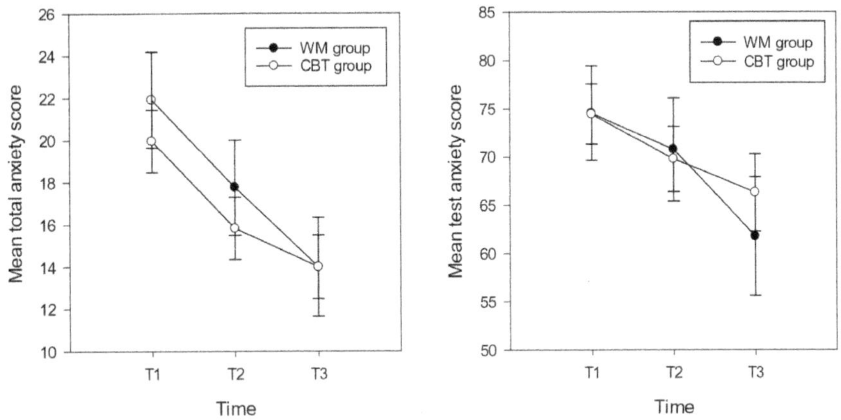

FIGURE 2 | Mean total anxiety scores (and standard errors) for total anxiety (left hand graph) and test anxiety (right hand graph) in the WM and CBT intervention groups at each time point.

were collapsed across groups to explore the effect of time on bias scores.[4]

For the participants who attended to threat at T1, the ANOVA revealed a main effect of time [$F(2,28) = 8.26$, $p = 0.002$, $\eta_p^2 = 0.37$], highlighting significantly higher bias scores at T1 ($M = 44.63$ ms, $SD = 35.64$, CI: 24.89 - 64.36) compared with T2 ($M = 6.42$, $SD = 41.03$, $p = 0.082$, CI:−16.29 - 29.14) and T3 ($M = -24.46$ ms, $SD = 52.96$, $p = 0.008$, CI: −53.78 - 4.68). Considering each time point separately, one sample t-tests showed a significant bias toward threat at T1 [$t(14) = 4.85$, $p < 0.001$], no bias at T2 ($t < 1$, $p > 0.1$) and a marginal trend for a bias away from threat at T3 [$t(14) = 1.79$, $p = 0.095$; see **Figure 3**]. For participants who attended away from threat at T1, the repeated measures ANOVA revealed a main effect of time [$F(2,32) = 6.75$, $p = 0.004$, $\eta_p^2 = 0.30$] with significantly higher (avoidant) bias scores at T1 ($M = -38.36$ ms, $SD = 34.44$, CI: −56.07 - −20.65) compared with T2 ($M = 15.16$, $SD = 59.24$, CI:−15.29 - 45.61) and T3 ($M = 12.88$ ms, $SD = 48.93$, CI:−12.28 - 38.03). One sample t-tests indicated that there was a significant bias away from threat for this group of participants at T1 [$t(16) = 4.59$, $p < 0.001$], and no bias at T2 or T3 ($ts < 1.5$, $p > 0.1$); see **Figure 3**.

DISCUSSION

The current study provides preliminary evidence to demonstrate reductions in self-report anxiety symptoms, anxiety-related cognitive biases for threat and increased inhibitory control following WM and CBT interventions for adolescents who reported elevated anxious affect and low attentional control. In addition, the WM group showed better performance post intervention on tasks similar to those that were trained, compared to the CBT group. The findings link to previous intervention studies which have found that adults with elevated depression symptoms benefitted from a WM intervention to

[4]Note that the addition of the group in both analyses did not change the main effect of time and in both cases the main effect of group and the interaction between group and time was not significant (all $Fs < 1$ and all $ps > 0.1$).

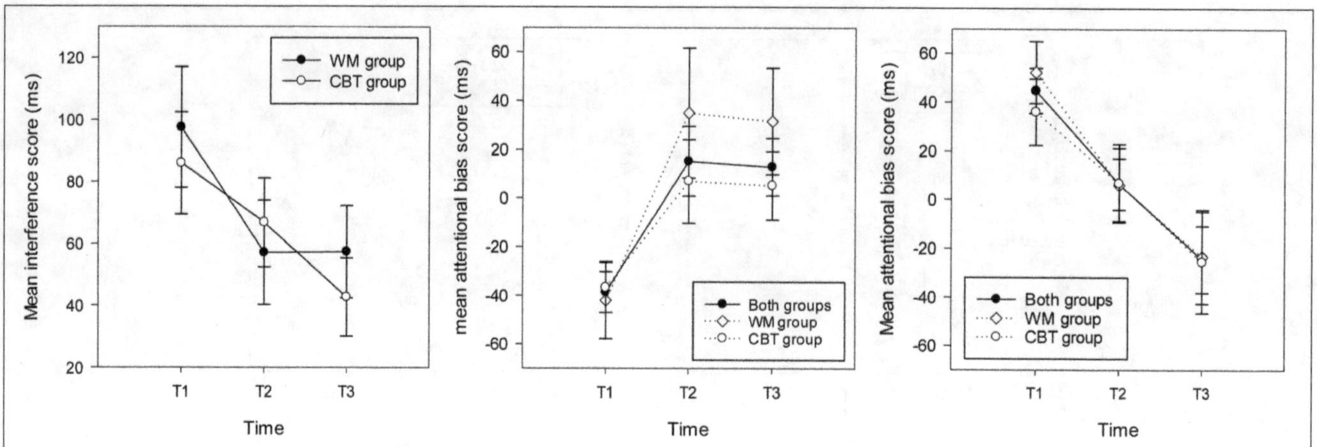

FIGURE 3 | Mean interference scores (and standard errors) in the stroop task (left hand graph) and attentional bias scores (and standard errors) in the WM group, the CBT and both groups combined for individuals attending toward threat (right hand graph) and away from threat (middle graph) at each time point.

show improved performance on WM tasks (Owens et al., 2013). In addition, they are consistent with research which has shown that young people with social and emotional behavioral difficulties who showed increased performance on WM tasks, better inhibitory control and fewer symptoms of test anxiety after completing a WM training intervention compared with a passive control group (Roughan and Hadwin, 2011). The current study extends previous research to show reduced attentional biases to threat following CBT and WM interventions. The findings fit with a broader literature highlighting the effectiveness of a WM training intervention on the reduction of symptoms associated with developmental psychopathology including inattention, hyperactivity and oppositional behavior (e.g., Klingberg et al., 2005; Beck et al., 2010).

Consistent with previous studies, the findings reported here showed reduced anxiety symptoms following a CBT intervention (e.g., Stallard et al., 2008). A recent meta-analysis highlighted that CBT is an effective treatment for anxiety reduction in children and adolescents compared to wait-list control groups (James et al., 2015). These authors noted, however, that few studies have compared CBT to active control groups receiving other forms of psychological intervention. The current study showed that the magnitude of the reduction in anxiety symptoms did not differ between the WM training and CBT intervention groups. They provide tentative evidence to suggest that attentional training could be a viable alternative or complementary intervention for children and adolescents with elevated anxious affect. Moreover, they fit with current studies suggesting that interventions that focus on attentional processes in anxiety might provide an important supplement to CBT and where this alternative approach could be most effective for individuals who are not responsive to more traditional treatment approaches (e.g., Bechor et al., 2014; review by Lowther and Newman, 2014).

The current study extends previous research to demonstrate that WM training and CBT led to increased inhibitory control post-intervention. In previous studies, wait-list control groups have shown relative stability in inhibitory control over a 3 months period (Roughan and Hadwin, 2011). Past research has not typically considered the impact of CBT on measures of attentional control. The current findings link to one study with adults with a clinical diagnosis of obsessive–compulsive disorder and who completed a CBT intervention. This group of adults showed cognitive deficits in set shifting, non-verbal memory and flexible behavior prior to treatment and these difficulties were no longer evident following CBT (Kuelz et al., 2006). In addition to improved inhibitory control, the current study found that across both groups adolescents showed reductions in attentional biases (characterized as biases toward or away from threat stimuli), indicating increased attention on task goals post intervention. This finding extends the previous literature (e.g., Waters et al., 2012) to indicate that reductions in attentional bias were not restricted to individuals completing CBT, but were also evident following a WM intervention.

Despite the growing emphasis on attentional control deficits in cognitive models of anxiety (e.g., Eysenck et al., 2007) and related research (Susa et al., 2012), the focus of recent interventions has been on modifying attentional biases to threat via ABM (e.g., Pérez-Edgar et al., 2014), rather than on improving attentional control more broadly. The results in the current study represent an important first step in the development of attention based interventions for adolescents who experience elevated anxiety. They suggest that biases for threat can be impacted via improved attentional control and in the absence of moderating attentional threat biases directly. Because improved attentional control and a reduction in threat biases was evident in both intervention groups, the results suggest that positive changes in anxiety symptoms can result from improved attentional control, as well as following more traditional CBT. Research with larger sample sizes would allow further examination of pathways to change via different interventions.

The proposition that increased attentional control (via WM training) can impact positively on anxiety symptoms is consistent with a broader literature that has highlighted the role of the PFC in emotional regulation (e.g., Davidson et al., 2000). It also links to related studies that have found a negative association between PFC activation with brain regions linked to fearful responding, including the amygdala (Etkin et al., 2006; Hare et al., 2008). For example, research has demonstrated that adults who report elevated anxiety show reduced ability to utilize attentional processes associated with the PFC (including the Anterior Cingulate Cortex and the lateral PFC) and where this pattern of activation is argued to maintain threat biases in anxiety (Öhman, 2005; reviews by Bishop, 2007).

Previous research also suggests that the reduction in anxiety symptoms following CBT has been associated with increased activation of the PFC and associated improvements in emotional regulation when completing cognitive tasks. One goal of CBT is positive re-framing (Cowart and Ollendick, 2010). The reduction in attention biases in the current study following CBT links to studies which have found that positive re-appraisal of negative stimuli is associated with increased activation in the PFC and reduced activation in the amygdala. For example, Ochsner et al. (2002) asked participants to attenuate emotional responses to negative picture stimuli (versus inspect them as they typically would). They showed that brain activation in the Dorsolateral PFC was associated with stimulus reappraisal and where this process was inversely linked to amygdala activation (Ochsner et al., 2002; see also Banks et al., 2007). Consistent with this finding, Maslowsky et al. (2010) showed that following a CBT intervention young adolescents with a primary diagnosis of generalized anxiety disorder showed increased activation in the right ventrolateral PFC and the authors argued that this activation reflected top-down regulation of negative emotion following treatment. To understand mechanisms of change, future research using WM and CBT interventions would benefit further from exploring neurocognitive change following treatment (e.g., Owens et al., 2013).

The current study had a number of further strengths. The inclusion of a 3-months follow-up assessment was important in highlighting that improvements on all outcome measures were maintained over an extended period of time. A further notable finding of the current study was to identify baseline characteristics associated with drop-out from the WM intervention. The results indicated that completion of the WM intervention was particularly challenging for individuals with lower IQ, raising the possibility that a reduction in the intensity of the intervention (i.e., the frequency and duration of sessions) could be beneficial for some young people. While this finding was important, the challenges associated with the WM group led to the attrition rate being higher than the CBT group. Although there were no differences on baseline measures between the individuals completing each intervention, we cannot rule out the possibility that the WM group represented a particularly motivated group who were able to overcome the challenges of the WM training (see Jaeggi and Buschkuehl, 2014). A further limitation in the current study was the absence of a wait-list control group. Previous research has consistently shown benefits of WM and CBT training versus passive control groups (James et al., 2015; Spencer-Smith and Klingberg, 2015) and researchers have argued that their inclusion can exaggerate treatment effects (Cunningham et al., 2013). However, the inclusion of a passive control group in the context of scoping trials does have some benefit in understanding the stability of outcome attentional measures over time and in the absence of an intervention. These limitations highlight the need for larger scale studies with increased sample sizes to account for high attrition rates and that include WM, active control and passive control groups.

One further difficulty in the current study was the lack of generalization of WM training to untrained WM tasks. A recent meta-analysis concluded that there was evidence of reliable near transfer effects on measures of verbal and visuospatial WM in the short term after training; however, there was no evidence of distant transfer effects on measures of cognitive ability or educational achievement (Melby-Lervåg and Hulme, 2013). It is possible that the current distant WM tasks utilized in the current study were not sensitive to differences between interventions, therefore, future research should aim to ensure that a range of untrained tasks is included in the evaluation of WM interventions. In addition, the current study focused on trait measurements of anxiety. And Supplementary Analysis revealed a mixed profile on outcomes linked to additional measures of negative affect and educational achievement. Though preliminary, they showed no effect of either intervention on self-report state anxiety, though some positive change in symptoms of depression and achievement scores in both groups. Consistent with theoretical accounts of anxiety, a recent review argued that state anxiety can moderate the impact of trait anxiety on attentional tasks, making it an important index of treatment outcome (Robinson et al., 2013). Moreover, it highlighted the complex association between anxiety and performance on WM tasks and where better performance can reflect increased individual effort and/or task cognitive load (see also Eysenck and Derakshan, 2011). Future research should aim to capture potential performance moderators using objective measures of effort and emotional regulation.

CONCLUSION

The current study outlines preliminary data which indicates that both WM and CBT interventions were effective in reducing anxiety symptoms in young people. While the study reflects a small sample size, its findings support the notion of a "proof of concept" in training WM (Gathercole et al., 2012) that indicate a broader positive impact on increased inhibitory control and attentional biases for threat. The novel findings should encourage the use of larger scale replication RCTs in clinical and educational settings that place greater emphasis on understanding the key mechanisms of change, as well the impact of baseline characteristics on attrition and treatment outcomes (Jaeggi and Buschkuehl, 2014).

AUTHOR CONTRIBUTIONS

Both authors made substantial, direct and intellectual contribution to the work, and approved it for publication.

ACKNOWLEDGMENTS

This research was supported by funding from Action Medical Research (award number SP4598). We would like to thank CogMed (Pearson) for access to training software and training and members of the Developmental Brain-Behaviour Laboratory at the University of Southampton for comments and advice on the development and analysis of this research. The current trial was registered and assigned an ISRCTN: http://www.isrctn.com/search?q=ISRCTN55164794

REFERENCES

Asendorpf, J. B., Denissen, J. J., and van Aken, M. A. (2008). Inhibited and aggressive preschool children at 23 years of age: personality and social transitions into adulthood. *Dev. Psychol.* 44, 997–1011. doi: 10.1037/0012-1649.44.4.997

Baddeley, A. D. (2003). Working memory: looking back and looking forward. *Nat. Rev. Neurosci.* 4, 829–839. doi: 10.1038/nrn1201

Banks, S. J., Eddy, K. T., Angstadt, M., Nathan, P. J., and Phan, K. L. (2007). Amygdala–frontal connectivity during emotion regulation. *Soc. Cogn. Affect. Neurosci.* 2, 303–312. doi: 10.1093/scan/nsm029

Bar-Haim, Y., Lamy, D., Pergamin, L., Bekermans-Kranenburg, M. J., and van IJzendoorn, M. H. (2007). Threat-related attentional bias in anxious and nonanxious individuals: a meta-analytic study. *Psychol. Bull.* 133, 1–24. doi: 10.1037/0033-2909/133.1.1

Barrett, P. (2005). *FRIENDS for Life: Workbook for Youth.* Bowen Hills: Australian Academic Press.

Bechor, M., Pettit, J. W., Silverman, W. K., Bar-Haim, Y., Abend, R., Pine, D. S., et al. (2014). Attention bias modification treatment for children with anxiety disorders who do not respond to cognitive behavioural therapy: a case series. *J. Anxiety Disord.* 28, 154–159. doi: 10.1016/j.janxdis.2013.09.001

Beck, S. J., Hanson, C. A., Puffenberger, S. S., Benninger, K. L., and Benninger, W. B. (2010). A controlled trial of working memory training for children and adolescents with ADHD. *J. Clin. Child Adolesc. Psychol.* 39, 825–836. doi: 10.1080/15374416.2010.517162

Bishop, S. J. (2007). Neurocognitive mechanisms of anxiety: an integrative account. *Trends Cogn. Neurosci.* 11, 307–316. doi: 10.1016/j.tics.2007.05.008

Bunge, S. A., and Wright, S. B. (2007). Neurodevelopmental changes in working memory and cognitive control. *Curr. Opin. Neurobiol.* 17, 243–250. doi: 10.1016/j.conb.2007.02.005

Cowart, M. J. W., and Ollendick, T. H. (2010). "Attentional biases in children: implications for treatment," in *Information Processing Biases and Anxiety: A Developmental Perspective*, eds J. A. Hadwin and A. P. Field (Chichester: Wiley-Blackwell), 297–319.

Cunningham, J. A., Kypri, K., and McCambridge, J. (2013). Exploratory randomized controlled trial evalutating the impact of a waiting list control design. *BMC Med. Res. Methodol.* 13:150. doi: 10.1186/1471-2288-13-150

Davidson, R. J., Jackson, D. C., and Kalin, N. H. (2000). Emotion, plasticity, context, and regulation: Perspectives from affective neuroscience. *Psychol. Bull.* 126, 890–909. doi: 10.1037/0033-2909.126.6.890

Dovis, S., Agelink van Rentergem, J., and Huizenga, H. M. (2015). Does cogmed working memory training really improve inattention in daily life? A reanalysis. *PLoS ONE* 10:e85992.

Duchesne, S., Larose, S., Vitaro, F., and Tremblay, R. E. (2010). Trajectories of anxiety in a population sample of children: clarifying the role of children's behavioral characteristics and maternal parenting. *Dev. Psychopathol.* 22, 361–373. doi: 10.1017/S0954579410000118

Dudeney, J., Sharpe, L., and Hunt, C. (2015). Attentional bias towards threatening stimuli in children with anxiety: a meta-analysis. *Clin. Psychol. Rev.* 40, 66–75. doi: 10.1016/j.cpr.2015.05.007

Eldar, S., Apter, A., Lotan, D., Edgar, K. P., Naim, R., Fox, N. A., et al. (2012). Attention bias modification treatment for pediatric anxiety disorders: a randomized controlled trial. *Am. J. Psychiatry* 169, 213–220. doi: 10.1176/appi.ajp.2011.11060886

Ellis, L. K., and Rothbart, M. K. (2001). Revision of the Early Adolescent Temperament Questionnaire. *Poster presented at the 2001 Biennial Meeting of the Society for Research in Child Development*, Minneapolis, MN.

Etkin, A., Egner, T., Peraza, D. M., Kandel, E. R., and Hirsch, J. (2006). Resolving emotional conflict: a role for the rostral anterior cingulate cortex in modulating activity in the amygdala. *Neuron* 51, 871–882. doi: 10.1016/j.neuron.2006.07.029

Eysenck, M. W., and Calvo, M. G. (1992). Anxiety and performance: the processing efficiency theory. *Cogn. Emot.* 6, 409–434. doi: 10.1080/02699939208409696

Eysenck, M. W., and Derakshan, N. (2011). New perspectives in attentional control theory. *Pers. Individ. Dif.* 50, 955–960. doi: 10.1016/j.paid.2010.08.019

Eysenck, M. W., Derakshan, N., Santos, R., and Calvo, M. G. (2007). Anxiety and cognitive performance: attentional control theory. *Emotion* 7, 336–353. doi: 10.1037/1528-3542.7.2.336

Gathercole, S. E., Dunning, D. L., and Holmes, J. (2012). Cogmed training: let's be realistic about intervention research. *J. Appl. Res. Mem. Cogn.* 1, 201–203. doi: 10.1016/j.jarmac.2012.06.003

Graham, B. M., and Milad, M. R. (2013). "Prefrontal cortex regulation of emotion and anxiety," in *Neurobiology of Mental Illness*, 4th Edn, eds D. S. Charney, P. Skar, J. D. Buxbaum, and E. J. Nestler (Oxford: Oxford University Press), 580–592.

Hadwin, J. A., Donnelly, N., Richards, A., French, C. C., and Patel, U. (2009). Childhood anxiety and attention to emotion faces in a modified Stroop task. *Br. J. Dev. Psychol.* 27, 487–494. doi: 10.1348/026151008X315503

Hare, T. A., Tottenham, N., Galvan, A., Voss, H. U., Glover, G. H., and Casey, B. J. (2008). Biological substrates of emotional reactivity in adolescence during a go-nogo task. *Biol. Psychiatry* 63, 927–934. doi: 10.1016/j.biopsych.2008.03.015

Horley, K., Williams, L. M., Gonsalvez, C., and Gordon, E. (2004). Face to face: visual scanpath evidence for abnormal processing of facial expressions in social phobia. *Psychiatry Res.* 127, 43–53. doi: 10.1016/j.psychres.2004.02.016

Ikkai, J., McCollough, A. W., and Vogel, E. K. (2010). Contralateral delay activity provides a neural measure of the number of representations in visual working memory. *J. Neurophysiol.* 103, 1963–1968. doi: 10.1152/jn.00978.2009

Jaeggi, S. M., and Buschkuehl, M. (2014). "Working memory training and transfer: theoretical and practical considerations," in *New Frontiers of Multidisciplinary Research in Steam-H*, ed. B. Toni (Cham: Springer International Publishing), 19–43.

James, A. C., James, G., Cowdrey, F. A., Soler, A., and Choke, A. (2015). *Cognitive Behavioural Therapy for Anxiety Disorders in Children and Adolescents.* Hoboken, NJ: John Wiley & Sons Ltd.

Kane, M. J., and McVay, J. C. (2012). What mind wandering reveals about executive-control abilities and failures. *Curr. Dir. Psychol. Sci.* 21, 348–354. doi: 10.1177/0963721412454875

Karbach, J., and Verhaeghen, P. (2014). Making working memory work: a meta-analysis of executive-control and working memory training in older adults. *Psychol. Sci.* 25, 2027–2037. doi: 10.1177/0956797614548725

Klingberg, T., Fernell, E., Olesen, P. J., Johnson, M., Gustafsson, P., Dahlstrom, K., et al. (2005). Computerized training of working memory in children with ADHD: a randomized controlled trial. *J. Am. Acad. Child Adolesc. Psychiatry* 44, 177–186. doi: 10.1097/00004583-200502000-00010

Klingberg, T., Forssberg, H., and Westerberg, H. (2002). Increased brain activity in frontal and parietal cortex underlies the development of visuospatial working memory capacity during childhood. *J. Cogn. Neurosci.* 14, 1–10. doi: 10.1162/089892902317205276

Kuelz, A. K., Riemann, D., Halsband, U., Vielhaber, K., Unterrainer, J., Kordon, A., et al. (2006). Neuropsychological impairment in obsessive compulsive disorder: improvement over the course of cognitive behavioral treatment. *J. Clin. Exp. Neuropsychol.* 28, 1273–1287. doi: 10.1080/13803390500507246

Legerstee, J. S., Tulen, J. H., Dierckx, B., Treffers, P. D., Verhulst, F. C., and Utens, E. M. (2010). CBT for childhood anxiety disorders: differential changes in selective attention between treatment responders and non-responders. *J. Child Psychol. Psychiatry* 51, 162–172. doi: 10.1111/j.1469-7610.2009.02143.x

Lonigan, C. J., and Vasey, M. W. (2009). Negative affectivity, effortful control, and attention to threat-relevant stimuli. *J. Abnorm. Child Psychol.* 37, 387–399. doi: 10.1007/s10802-008-9284-y

Lowther, H., and Newman, E. (2014). Attention bias modification (ABM) as a treatment for child and adolescent anxiety: a systematic review. *J. Affect. Disord.* 168, 125–135. doi: 10.1016/j.jad.2014.06.051

MacLeod, C., Mathews, A., and Tata, P. (1986). Attentional bias in emotional disorders. *J. Abnorm. Psychol.* 95, 15–20. doi: 10.1037/0021-843X.95.1.15

Maslowsky, J., Mogg, K., Bradley, B. P., McClure-Tone, E., Ernst, M., Pine, D. S., et al. (2010). A preliminary investigation of neural correlates of treatment in adolescents with generalized anxiety disorder. *J. Child Adolesc. Psychopharmacol.* 20, 105–111. doi: 10.1089/cap.2009.0049

Melby-Lervåg, M., and Hulme, C. (2013). Is working memory training effective? A meta-analytic review. *Dev. Psychol.* 49, 270–291. doi: 10.1037/a0028228

Mogg, K., and Bradley, B. P. (1998). A cognitive-motivational analysis of anxiety. *Behav. Res. Ther.* 36, 809–848. doi: 10.1016/S0005-7967(98)0g0063-1

Nightingale, Z. C., Field, A. P., and Kindt, M. (2010). "The emotional Stroop task in anxious children," in *Information Processing Biases and Anxiety: A Developmental Perspective*, eds J. A. Hadwin and A. P. Field (Chichester: Wiley-Blackwell), 47–75.

Ochsner, K. N., Bunge, S. A., Gross, J. J., and Gabrieli, J. D. E. (2002). Rethinking feelings: an fMRI study of the cognitive regulation of emotion. *J. Cogn. Neurosci.* 14, 1215–1229. doi: 10.1162/089892902760807212

Öhman, A. (2005). The role of the amygdala in human fear: automatic detection of threat. *Psychoneuroendocrinology* 30, 953–958. doi: 10.1016/j.psyneuen.2005.03.019

Olesen, P., Westerberg, H., and Klingberg, T. (2003). Increased prefrontal and parietal activity after training of working memory. *Nat. Neurosci.* 7, 75–79. doi: 10.1038/nn1165

O'Toole, L. J., DeCicco, J. M., Berthod, S., and Dennis, T. A. (2013). The N170 to angryfaces predicts anxiety in typically developing children over a two-year period. *Dev. Neurosci.* 38, 352–362. doi: 10.1080/87565641.2013.802321

Owens, M., Koster, E. H. W., and Derakshan, N. (2013). Improving attention control in dysphoria through cognitive training: transfer effects on working memory capacity and filtering efficiency. Psychophysiology 50, 297–307. doi: 10.1111/psyp.12010

Owens, M., Stevenson, J., Norgate, R., and Hadwin, J. A. (2008). Processing efficiency theory in children: working memory as a mediator between trait anxiety and academic performance. *Anxiety Stress Coping* 21, 417–430. doi: 10.1080/10615800701847823

Pérez-Edgar, K., Taber-Thomas, B., Auday, E., and Morales, S. (2014). Temperament and attention as core mechanisms in the early emergence of anxiety. *Contrib Hum Dev.* 26, 42–56. doi: 10.1159/000354350

Pickering, S., and Gathercole, S. (2001). *Working Memory Test Battery for Children (WMTB-C).* Harlow: Pearson Education Ltd.

Rabipour, S., and Raz, A. (2012). Training the brain: fact and fad in cognitive and behavioural remediation. *Brain Cogn.* 79, 159–179. doi: 10.1016/j.bandc.2012.02.006

Rapee, R. M., Schniering, C. A., and Hudson, J. L. (2009). Anxiety disorders during childhood and adolescence: origins and treatment. *Annu. Rev. Clin. Psychol.* 5, 311–341. doi: 10.1146/annurev.clinpsy.032408.153628

Reynolds, C. R., and Richmond, B. O. (2008). *Revised Children's Manifest Anxiety Scale*, 2nd Edn. North York, ON: Multi-Health Systems Inc.

Richards, H. J., and Hadwin, J. A. (2011). An exploration of the relationship between trait anxiety and school attendance in young people. *School Mental Health* 3, 236–244. doi: 10.1007/s12310-011-9054-9

Robinson, O. J., Vytal, K., Comwell, B. R., and Grillon, C. (2013). The impact of anxiety upon cognition: perspectives from human threat of shock studies. *Front. Hum. Neurosci.* 7:203. doi: 10.3389/fnhum.2013.00203

Roughan, L., and Hadwin, J. A. (2011). The impact of working memory training in young people with social, emotional and behavioural difficulties. *Learn. Individ. Dif.* 21, 759–764. doi: 10.1016/j.lindif.2011.07.011

Roza, S. J., Hofstra, M. B., Van Der Ende, J., and Verhulst, F. C. (2003). Stable prediction of mood and anxiety disorders based on behavioral and emotional problems in childhood: a 14-year follow-up during childhood, adolescence, and young adulthood. *Am. J. Psychiatry* 60, 2116–2121. doi: 10.1176/appi.ajp.160.12.2116

Rozenman, M., Weersing, V. R., and Amir, N. (2011). A case series of attention modification in clinically anxious youths. *Behav. Res. Ther.* 49, 324–330. doi: 10.1016/j.brat.2011.02.007

Shackman, A. J., Sarinopoulos, I., Maxwell, J. S., Pizzagalli, D. A., Lavric, A., and Davidson, R. J. (2006). Anxiety selectively disrupts visuospatial working memory. *Emotion* 6, 40–61. doi: 10.1037/1528-3542.6.1.40

Spence, S. H. (1998). A measure of anxiety symptoms among children. *Behav. Res. Ther.* 36, 545–566. doi: 10.1016/S0005-7967(98)00034-5

Spencer-Smith, M., and Klingberg, T. (2015). Benefits of a working memory training programme for inattention in daily life: a systematic review and metaanalysis. *PLoS ONE* 10:e0119522. doi: 10.1371/journal.pone.0119522

Stallard, P., Simpson, N., Anderson, S., and Goddard, M. (2008). The FRIENDS emotional health prevention programme: 12 month follow-up of a universal UK school based trial. *Eur. Child Adolesc. Psychiatry* 17, 283–289. doi: 10.1007/s00787-007-0665-5

Stirling, L. J., Eley, T. C., and Clark, D. M. (2006). Preliminary evidence for an association between social anxiety symptoms and avoidance of negative faces in school-age children. *J. Clin. Child Adolesc. Psychol.* 35, 440–445. doi: 10.1207/s15374424jccp3503_9

Streiner, D. L. (2002). The case of the missing data: methods of dealing with dropouts and other research vagaries. *Can. J. Psychiatry* 47, 68–75.

Stroop, J. R. (1935). Studies of interference in serial verbal reactions. *J. Exp. Psychol.* 18, 643–662. doi: 10.1037/h0054651

Susa, G., Pitica, I., Benga, O., and Miclea, M. (2012). The self regulatory effect of attentional control in modulating the relationship between attentional biases toward threat and anxiety symptoms in children. *Cogn. Emot.* 26, 1069–1083. doi: 10.1080/02699931.2011.638910

Tottenham, N., Tanaka, J. W., Leon, A. C., McCarry, T., Nurse, M., Hare, T. A., et al. (2009). The NimStim set of facial expressions: judgments from untrained research participants. *Psychiatry Res.* 168, 242–249. doi: 10.1016/j.psychres.2008.05.006

Waters, A. M., Mogg, K., and Bradley, B. P. (2012). Direction of threat attention bias predicts treatment outcome in anxious children receiving cognitive-behavioural therapy. *Behav. Res. Ther.* 50, 428–434. doi: 10.1016/j.brat.2012.03.006

Wechsler, D. (1999). *Wechsler Abbreviated Scale of Intelligence.* London: Pearson Ltd.

Wood, J. J., Lynne, S. D., Langer, D. A., Wood, P. A., Clark, S. L., Eddy, J. M., et al. (2012). School attendance problems, and youth psychopathology: structural cross-lagged regression models in three longitudinal datasets. *Child Dev.* 83, 351–366. doi: 10.1111/j.1467-8624.2011.01677.x

Wren, D. J., and Benson, J. (2004). Measuring test anxiety in children: scale development and internal construct validation. *Anxiety Stress Coping* 17, 227–240. doi: 10.1080/10615800412331292606

21

The Relationship between Sleep Complaints, Depression, and Executive Functions in Older Adults

Katie M. de Almondes[1], Mônica V. Costa[2], Leandro F. Malloy-Diniz[3] and Breno S. Diniz[4]*

[1] Group of Research Neuroscience Applied, Basic Process and Chronobiolog, Department of Psychology, Federal University of Rio Grande do Norte, Natal, Brazil, [2] Laboratory for Investigations in Clinical Neuroscience, School of Medicine, Federal University of Minas Gerais, Belo Horizonte, Brazil, [3] Department of Mental Health, School of Medicine, National Institute of Science & Technology Molecular Medicine, Federal University of Minas Gerais, Belo Horizonte, Brazil, [4] Department of Psychiatry and Behavioral Sciences, University of Texas Health Science Center at Houston, Houston, TX, USA

Edited by:
Roumen Kirov,
Bulgarian Academy of Sciences, Bulgaria

Reviewed by:
Timo Partonen,
National Institute for Health and Welfare, Finland
Roberto Monastero,
University of Palermo, Italy

****Correspondence:***
Katie M. de Almondes
katie.almondes@gmail.com

Aim: In this manuscript, we report data on the association between executive functions screened by Frontal Assessment Battery, Five Digit Test and Digit Span with self-reported depressive symptoms and sleep complaints in non-demented older adults.

Methods: A total sample of 95 non-demented older adults performed Geriatric Depression Scale short version, Frontal Assessment Battery, Five Digit Test, Digit Span, and clinical interview. We split participants in groups stratified by age according to: young-old (60–69 years of age), old-old (70–79 years), and oldest-old (>80 years) and compared these three groups on the sociodemographic characteristics and executive functions performance. We carried out Poisson regression with robust error variance to verify sleep complaints and depression effects on executive functions performance. Gender, age, years of formal education, use of antidepressants and of benzodiazepines were considered as confounding variables, taking into account executive functions as dependent and sleep complaints and depression as independent variables.

Results: Controlling the effect of age, gender, years of formal education, use of benzodiazepines and of antidepressants there was a significant influence of depression in motor programming, inhibitory control, and working memory. Individuals without depression show motor programming scores 68.4% higher, inhibitory control scores 3 times greater and working memory scores also 3 times greater than individuals without depression. There was a significant influence of sleep complaints in phonemic fluency, motor programming, inhibitory control, and working memory. Individuals without sleep complaints show phonemic fluency scores 2 times greater than, motor programming scores 85.9% higher, inhibitory control scores 3 times greater and working memory scores also 3 times greater than individuals without sleep complaints.

Conclusions: Sleep complaints are associated with phonemic fluency, motor programming, inhibitory control, and working memory impairment. Depression symptoms presence are associated with motor programming and working memory performances. Depression and sleep complaints interaction would determine worse phonemic fluency, inhibitory control and working memory cognitive performance than these two conditions alone.

Keywords: sleep, executive function, depression, geriatrics, mild cognitive impairment, older adults, neuropsychological tests

INTRODUCTION

Across the lifespan, sleep complaints are often comorbid with psychiatric disorders and are common in depression. Sleep has been studied extensively in this psychiatric disorder and were found objective, robust and relatively specific changes in sleep architecture related to neurobiology of depression (Benca and Peterson, 2008). On the present study, we provide a solid background for the importance of taking into account the interaction between cognition, sleep disorders, and depression among older adults.

During a depressive episode, cortical metabolic activity is increased in frontal areas, what impact sleep and cause subjective complaints of non-restorative sleep. In depressed patients, there is an imbalance of interaction between cholinergic and adrenergic mechanisms that promote abnormalities in sleep architecture (non-REM and REM). There are changes in non-REM sleep that result in excessive daytime sleepiness. Moreover, depressed patients exhibit cortisol and temperature desynchronization on advanced sleep phase (the expression of these rhythms appears earlier than expected) and on the sleep-wake cycle (Cajochen et al., 2001).

Processing speed (Bastien et al., 2003), executive functions such as switching, working memory, problem solving and inhibitory control (Nebes et al., 2009) and memory (Haimov et al., 2008), are associated with self-reported sleep complaints. Moreover, sleep disorders as self-reported change in sleep increases the risk of cognitive decline (Hahn et al., 2014).

Depression also increases susceptibility to cognitive decline and neurodegenerative dementia (Diniz et al., 2013), impact activities of daily living and patient quality of life, and rising health care costs. Among cognitive impairment associated with depression, executive function is the most prominent (Snyder, 2013), but deficits in processing speed (Jungwirth et al., 2011), spatial processing (Elderkin-Thompson et al., 2004), and verbal episodic memory (Nebes et al., 2000) are also found. They mediate decline in more complex functions such as attention, planning and problem solving. There is evidence of a close relationship between sleep loss, depression and cognition with effect sizes in "moderate range" (Lim and Dinges, 2010).

The aim of this study was to investigate the association between executive functions screened by Frontal Assessment Battery, Five Digit Test and Digit Span with comorbid self-reported depressive symptoms and sleep complaints in non-demented older adults. Overall, we hypothesized that sleep complaints and depression should be associated with executive functions impairment and that depression and sleep complaints interaction would determine a worse cognitive performance than these two conditions alone.

MATERIALS AND METHODS

Participants

We included a convenience sample of 95 older adults that were consecutively assessed at geriatric outpatient clinic at Belo Horizonte, Brazil between February 2011 and December 2015. These participants were visiting the clinic as a center of specialized geriatric treatments referred by other smaller primary care centers. The inclusion criteria were: age of 60 years or older. We excluded individuals that satisfied DSM-V and consensus criteria for dementia as NINCDS-ADRDA; individuals with major psychiatric comorbidities (e.g., bipolar disorder, schizophrenia, substance abuse); sensory disabilities that interfere with cognitive evaluation; neurodegenerative diseases of the central nervous system diagnosis (e.g., Parkinson's disease); clinical or historical evidence of transient ischemic attack or stroke or clinical instability. In the end, we have had a total of 175 participants. Of these 57 were excluded due to meet criteria for dementia due to Alzheimer's disease and 23 for dementia due to other etiologies such as frontotemporal and vascular dementia. Participants were instructed to perform tasks with the dominant hand. This study was approved by the local Ethics Committee (Belo Horizonte, MG) and all subjects agreed and signed the informed consent in accordance with the Declaration of Helsinki.

Neuropsychological Assessment

Neuropsychological assessments occurred between 08:00 a.m. and 05:00 p.m., then the time of day was not in a similar range for all the participants. There are evidence that cognitive performance may varies during the course of the day and reflect the level of alertness, which is determined by circadian rhythms (Schmidt et al., 2007). It is discussed that these findings can be attributed to underlying circadian and homeostatic factors. Different aspects of attention follow different time-of-day variations (Kraemer et al., 2000) and this bias was not controlled on the present study.

Diagnosis involved a clinical interview and a neuropsychological evaluation with a protocol previously validated for this population (de Paula et al., 2013a) composed by the following instruments: Mini Mental State Examination (MMSE) Brazilian version as a measure of general cognition; Clock Drawing Test as a measure of spatial processing, praxia, and executive functions; The Digit Span Task adapted from Wechsler Adult Intelligence Scale to assess short term memory; Corsi Blocks a measure of spatial short term memory; Semantic Verbal Fluency that measures the fluency component of the executive functions. Finally, Token Test-Short Version was used to assess language comprehension. Functional status was also assessed in the clinical interview using the caregivers' reports. Based on this evaluation, non-demented participants were invited for participation.

The MMSE were performed as a measure of general cognitive functioning and Activities of Daily Living (ADLs) inventory as a measure of functional status. Frontal Assessment Battery (FAB) Brazilian version was used to access executive functions. It presents a good validity for this population (de Paula et al., 2013b) and consists of six subtests which measures: Categorization, verbal fluency, motor programming, sensitivity to interference, inhibitory control, and environmental autonomy.

Depressive Symptoms Assessment

All the participants performed the short version (15-items) of the Geriatric Depression Scale (GDS-15) and we considered the cutoff 6 (non-case/case) to classify presence/absence of significant depressive symptoms. To minimize low education bias, the scale was applied orally and the questions were repeated if requested by the participant. Depressive symptoms assessment was conducted on the same date of neuropsychological assessment and participant were required to answer according to how he felt in "last few weeks."

Sleep and Pharmacological Assessment

Sleep complaints was evaluated qualitatively through of a clinical interview with self report of participants. It was required to participants if they had noticed sleep-related problems in recent months or weeks to date. The response was evaluated in "yes/no" and they also describe the sleep problems.

The use of drugs, including benzodiazepines, was assessed by patients' medical records. Pharmacological treatments were evaluated during the anamnesis. Patients and caregivers reported which drugs were used at that time, and based on these data the drugs were classified as antidepressants or benzodiazepines. In the database the names of the drugs were specified, the number of medications in use and dichotomous variables were created for use of hypnotics and antidepressants.

Statistical Procedures

Once our data distribution was predominantly non-parametric, the statistical procedures were performed by non-parametric tests. Sociodemographic description and neuropsychological tests were performed through Mann–Whitney *U*-test for continuous variables and by Chi-Square for dummies variables.

We split participants in groups stratified by age according to: young-old (60–69 years of age), old-old (70–79 years), and oldest-old (>80 years) and we compared these three groups on the sociodemographic characteristics and executive functions performance through Kruskal–Wallis Test.

We carried out Poisson regression with robust error variance (McCullagh and Nelder, 1983) to verify depression and sleep complaints effects on executive functions performance. Gender, age, years of formal education use of antidepressants and of benzodiazepines were considered as confounding variables, taking into account executive functions as dependent and depression and sleep complaints, as independent variables. These statistical procedures were performed using SPSS 21.0. and statistical significance was established at 0.05.

RESULTS

The demographic description and neuropsychological tests performance are shown in **Table 1** for Chi-square analysis and in **Table 2** for Mann–Whitney. A total of 95 non-demented older adults $(60–91 years ($M = 74$, $SD = 7$), predominantly low formal education ($M = 5$, $SD = 4$) were enrolled in this study. In this sample, 36% were depressed, 48% with sleep complaints, 14% in use of benzodiazepines, and 23% of antidepressants including 15 participants in use of selective serotonin reuptake inhibitors (SSRI) and 7 in use of tricyclic antidepressant (TCA) (**Table 1**). No significant differences between age ($U = 1128.00$, $p = 0.407$), education ($U = 1069.00$, $p = 0.273$) or proportion of men and women ($\chi^2 = 0.024$, $p = 0.524$) were found between patients with and without sleep complaints. There is no difference between performance on Mini Mental State Examination between two conditions ($U = 594.00$, $p = 0.756$), daily function activities ($\chi^2 = 0.437$, $p = 0.358$), FAB total score ($U = 1177.00$, $p = 0.623$), or use of benzodiazepines ($\chi^2 = 2.248$, $p = 0.113$). Differences in presence of significant depressive symptoms classified through GDS-15 cutoff between groups with and without sleep complaints are found ($\chi^2 = 16.429$, $p < 0.001$) with more patients with depression in the group with sleep complaints.

In **Tables 3, 4** we could see descriptive statistics between age groups for socio-demographic variables and results of group comparisons between executive functions performance among non-demented elderly stratified by age. There are significant differences on categorization between young-old (60–69 years of age) and oldest-old (>80 years) ($\chi^2 = 18.479$, $p = 0.046$). Phonemic verbal fluency performance is significantly different between young-old (60–69 years of age) and old-old (70–79 years) ($\chi^2 = 17.280$, $p = 0.019$). In relation to motor programming there are differences between young-old (60–69 years of age) and old-old (70–79 years) ($\chi^2 = 19.000$, $p = 0.031$) and between young-old (60–69 years of age) and oldest-old (>80 years) ($\chi^2 = 24.750$, $p = 0.003$). Otherwise, performance on inhibitory control is only significantly different between old-old (70–79 years) and oldest-old (>80 years) ($\chi^2 = 19.910$, $p = 0.006$). For FAB total score, performance is significantly different between young-old (60–69 years of age) and old-old (70–79 years) ($\chi^2 = 17.557$, $p = 0.032$) and young-old (60–69 years of age) and oldest-old (>80 years) ($\chi^2 = 32.250$, $p > 0.001$).

In **Table 5** we present the Poisson regression to verify depression and sleep complaints effects on executive functions performance. Controlling the effect of age, gender, years of formal education, use of benzodiazepines and of antidepressants sleep complaints are associated with cognitive impairment on phonemic fluency, motor programming, inhibitory control and working memory. Individuals without sleep complaints have FAB motor programming scores 85.9% higher, phonemic fluency scores twice as high as, inhibitory control scores three times as high as and Digit Span Backward scores three times as high as individuals with sleep complaints.

Depression complaints is associated with motor programming and working memory impairment. Individuals without depression symptoms have FAB motor programming 68.4% higher and Digit Span Backward scores three times as high as individuals with depression symptoms.

Individuals without use of benzodiazepines presents sensitivity to interference scores six times as high as individuals in use of benzodiazepines. However, the use is associated with an increase of 19.2% on phonemic fluency scores. Individuals in use of antidepressants have motor programming scores 39.2% higher than individuals with no use of antidepressants.

Interaction between sleep and depression complaints is associated with phonemic fluency, inhibitory control and working memory impairment. Those which showed these two types of symptoms presents FAB fluency subtest scores 56.6%, FAB inhibitory control subtest scores 75% and Digit

TABLE 1 | Results of Chi-square Tests on gender, use of benzodiazepines and use of antidepressants proportion for participants with and without sleep complaints.

	Total sample (%)	Sleep complaints (%)	With no sleep complaints (%)	Groups comparison between participants with sleep complaints and without sleep complaints	
				X^2	p
Gender[a]	62	73	77	0.332	0.564
Benzodiazepines[b]	12	20	10	2.248	0.134
Antidepressants[c]	22	32	15	3.644	0.056
Depression	31	57	17	16.266	<0.001

[a] *Proportion of women.*
[b] *Proportion of use.*
[c] *Proportion of use.*

TABLE 2 | Group comparisons between participants with sleep complaints and without sleep complaints.

	Total sample			Sleep complaints			Without sleep complaints			Groups comparisons		
	M	*SD*	Range	*M*	*SD*	Range	*M*	*SD*	Range	MW-U	*Z*	*p*
Age	74.46	7.355	58–91	73.80	7.654	58–90	75.08	6.990	62–91	1128	−0.829	0.407
Education	5.68	4.865	0–22	5.21	4.964	0–22	6.12	4.853	0–21	1069	−1.096	0.273
MMSE	25.67	3.078	15–30	25.08	4.041	15–30	25.87	2.419	21–30	594	−0.311	0.756
FAB	12.23	3.281	4–18	12.14	3.380	4–18	12.48	3.245	6–18	1177	−0.492	0.623
ADL	3.63	4.834	0–23	3.86	4.740	0–18	2.91	4.568	0–23	542	−1.201	0.23

Values are frequencies or Mean ± Standard Deviation (SD); FAB, Frontal Assessment Battery; MMSE, Mini-Mental State Examination; ADL, Activities of Daily Living; MW-U, Mann–Whitney U-Test; Z, difference between standard scores; p, significance level.

TABLE 3 | Descriptive statistics between age groups for socio-demographic variables.

	Total sample	Age groups		
Age ranges	**60–91**	**Young–old 60–69**	**Old–old 70–79**	**Oldest–old >80**
N	95	24	47	24
Age	74.49 ± 7.29	65.54 ± 2.637	74.62 ± 2.75	83.88 ± 3.180
SEX				
Men	29	5	16	8
Woman	66	19	31	16
EDUCATION				
Years of formal education	5.71 ± 4.89	7.142 ± 5.174	5.78 ± 5.133	4.08 ± 3.538
Illiteracy	7	2	3	2
Primary school	65	14	34	20
Secondary or Higher	23	8	10	2
Pfeffer scale	3.400 ± 4.648	4.230 ± 4.206	2.760 ± 3.940	4.050 ± 6.013
MMSE	25.591 ± 3.083	27 ± 2.221	25.588 ± 2.664	25.000 ± 3.293

Values are frequencies or Mean ± Standard Deviation (SD); MMSE, Mini Mental State Examination.

Span Backward scores 70.1% lower than individuals with no complaints.

Sociodemographic variables are also associated with executive functions performances. At each year added on age, FAB conceptualization scores decreases 1.9%, sensitivity to interference scores decreases 2.2%, inhibitory control scores decreases 3.6%, FAB total scores decreases 1.5% and errors on Five Digit Test cognitive flexibility task increases 3.5%. At each year added on formal education, FAB conceptualization scores increases 5.3%, phonemic verbal fluency scores increases 3.2%, motor programing scores increases 2.1%, FAB total scores increases 1.6% and Digit Span Backward scores increases 6.1%. Female individuals have FAB total scores 1.7% higher than the males (**Table 5**).

TABLE 4 | Results of group comparisons between executive functions performance among non-demented elderly stratified by age.

	Total sample	Age groups			Group comparisons		
		1—Young-Old	2—Old-Old	3—Oldest-Old	X^2	p	Differences between age groups
Age ranges	**60–91**	**60–69**	**70–79**	**>80**			
FAB (total score)	12.32 ± 3.294	14.33 ± 2.353	12.34 ± 3.171	10.54 ± 3.148	17.557	0.032	2 > 3
					32.250	<0.001	1 > 3
FAB—categorization	1.505 ± 1.071	1.958 ± 0.908	1.456 ± 1.110	1.208 ± 1.021	18.479	0.046	1 > 3
FAB—fonemic fluency	2.147 ± 0.989	2.625 ± 0.711	1.978 ± 1.022	2.083 ± 0.974	17.280	0.019	1 > 2
FAB—motor programming	1.726 ± 0.950	2.042 ± 0.806	1.782 ± 0.987	1.333 ± 0.917	19.000	0.031	1 > 2
					24.750	0.003	1 > 3
FAB—sensitivity to interference	2.357 ± 1.051	2.708 ± 0.751	2.326 ± 1.097	2.083 ± 1.176	2.988	0.131	–
FAB—inhibitory control	1.589 ± 1.180	2.000 ± 1.142	1.782 ± 1.153	0.875 ± 0.947	19.910	0.006	2 > 3
Five digit test inhibitory control	3.730 ± 5.535	2.940 ± 5.048	3.360 ± 5.709	5.110 ± 5.516	7.232	0.027	1 > 3
Five digit test cognitive flexibility	8.980 ± 8.611	7.330 ± 7.191	7.670 ± 7.680	12.860 ± 10.101	8.184	0.017	1 > 3
							2 > 3
Digit span backward	11.480 ± 9.573	13.920 ± 13.061	10.960 ± 8.565	10.570 ± 7.675	0.735	0.692	–

Values are frequencies or Mean ± Standard Deviation (SD); FAB, Frontal Assessment Battery.

DISCUSSION

Sleep complaints are associated with phonemic fluency, motor programming, inhibitory control, and working memory impairment. Depression symptoms presence are also associated with motor programming and working memory performances. Depression and sleep complaints interaction would determine phonemic fluency, inhibitory control, and working memory worse cognitive performances than these two conditions alone.

We found that depression is associated with less efficiency on motor programming. According to previous studies left dorsal prefrontal cortex and the right anterior cingulate cortex are more involved when subjects paid attention to the performance of a sequence of movements in comparison to automatic performance of this same task (Jueptner et al., 1997). Automatic aspects of motor performance are associated with subcortical structures, but sequential actions tasks with prefrontal networks (Fuster, 2001). It suggests that preparation of motor responses and learning of sequences of movements differs from an automatic condition and demands more from areas associated with executive function, which could be the same regions involved in depression. Studies of motor performance in depression corroborates these findings showing that cognitive difficulties increased with complexity of the tasks (Sabbe et al., 1996) and could be affected by pharmacological treatment (Mergl et al., 2007).

Long-term use of hypnotics may cause poor sleep quality (Vignola et al., 2000). It is also known that the use of benzodiazepines by older adults leads to cognitive decline (Glass et al., 2005). On the present study the use of benzodiazepines is associated with sensitivity to interference impairment. This is a component of executive functions related to selective attention measured by a task of conflicting instructions. Previous studies have also found association between attention and use of benzodiazepines (Barker et al., 2004) that could be due to inductive sedation effect (Chennu and Bekinschtein, 2012). Individuals in use of benzodiazepines showed phonemic fluency scores higher than individuals that are not in use of benzodiazepines. Considering that individuals without sleep complaints present phonemic fluency scores twice as high as those with sleep complaints, this may reflect the differences between those treated and untreated sleep disorders individuals. Those individuals treated probably have an improvement on fluency performance in comparison to untreated. Individuals in use of antidepressants also show motor programming scores higher than individuals with no use of antidepressants. Probably, this may reflect the differences between those treated and untreated individuals.

Deficits in verbal fluency are common finding after sleep loss, with reports of fewer words, and perseveration of incorrect responses, on tasks of verbal fluency (Harrison and Horne, 1998). These findings were not replicated in the study of (Tucker et al., 2010), but results have suggested an association between subjective sleep complaints and decline in phonemic fluency performance. Recently, McGregor and Alper (2015) showed that adults with sleep disorders were at a higher risk for language problems than healthy sleepers. The language problems typically co-occurred with problems of attention and executive function.

TABLE 5 | Effects of depression and sleep complaints on executive functions performance.

		Independent variables							
Dependent variables-neuropsychological assessment	**Parameters**	**Age (years)**	**Formal education (years)**	**Gender = Female**	**Depression**	**Sleep complaints**	**Use of benzodiaze-pines**	**Use of anti-depressants**	**Depression/Sleep complaints interaction**
FAB conceptualization	exp(β)	0.981	1.053	1.228	1.311	1.699	1.384	1.052	0.672
	p-value	0.036*	0.000*	0.147	0.607	0.334	0.398	0.802	0.486
FAB phonemic fluency	exp(β)	0.997	1.032	1.137	1.812	2.095	0.808	0.966	0.434
	p-value	0.657	0.000*	0.151	0.116	0.049*	0.016*	0.785	0.034*
FAB motor programming	exp(β)	0.987	1.021	1.274	1.684	1.859	1.141	1.392	0.605
	p-value	0.130	0.040*	0.061	0.014*	0.028	0.450	0.023*	0.112
FAB sensitivity to interference	exp(β)	0.978	1.000	0.934	1.662	1.610	6.509	0.975	0.578
	p-value	0.009*	0.984	0.517	0.137	0.175	0.040*	0.804	0.134
FAB inhibitory control	exp(β)	0.964	1.017	1.377	2.796	3.240	1.093	1.754	0.250
	P-value	0.006*	0.318	0.090	0.053*	0.036*	0.888	0.062	0.021*
FAB environmental autonomy	exp(β)	1.000	1.002	0.972	0.960	1.002	1.151	1.004	1.039
	p-value	0.581	0.252	0.115	0.239	0.885	0.133	0.856	0.246
FAB total score	exp(β)	0.985	1.016	1.125	1.036	1.168	1.087	1.092	0.843
	P-value	0.000*	0.002*	0.017*	0.709	0.094	0.290	0.125	0.136
Five digit test inhibitory control	exp(β)	1.033	0.963	0.727	0.887	1.026	0.666	0.970	0.950
	p-value	0.169	0.170	0.320	0.824	0.969	0.479	0.924	0.943
Five digit test cognitive flexibility	exp(β)	1.035	0.969	1.009	0.725	0.900	1.037	0.718	0.878
	p-value	0.009*	0.118	0.963	0.285	0.733	0.883	0.105	0.736
Digit span backward	exp(β)	0.994	1.061	1.025	3.467	3.438	1.071	0.991	0.299
	p-value	0.607	0.000*	0.873	0.000*	0.000*	0.771	0.959	0.001*

exp(β), exponentiated values of the coefficients; FAB, Frontal Assessment Battery.
**p-value < 0.05.*

The phonemic fluency is considered a complex task related to cognitive flexibility, sustained attention, inhibitory control, and semantic memory (Shao et al., 2014). All these processes for which sleep complaints determined lower scores are cognitive abilities controlled and can be considered executive functions, especially working memory and inhibitory control. Controlled processes as attention and working memory are linked to the functioning of frontal lobes (Alhola and Polo-Kantola, 2007). Whereas, the frontal areas are vulnerable to sleep disorders (Harrison et al., 2000), this can be associated with impairment in inhibitory control, working memory, and verbal fluency in individuals with sleep complaints. Another related issue is the developmental process of the executive functions. The functional apex of executive functions is reached during adulthood and from this point is expected to decline (Goh et al., 2013). The course of development these abilities are therefore associated with a curve in the inverted U shape, so such impairments are expected on older adults.

This sample was composed by low formal education older adults due to the characteristics of the origin country. Educational level is associated with cognitive decline (Ardila et al., 2000) and is considered a main factor throughout cognitive aging. Performance on FAB is influenced by formal education (Beato et al., 2012; de Paula et al., 2013a) age. In our sample formal education is associated with motor programming, FAB total scores increases, working memory, categorization, and phonemic verbal fluency. In young old percentile for illiterates is significantly different from university graduates (de Paula et al., 2013a). The scale validation study for this population (Beato et al., 2012) suggest four formal education tracks, with 50th percentile varying significantly according to the formal educational level.

The differences between age groups in performance on the FAB subtests are in agreement with previous studies which indicate a decline in executive functions over the years (Salthouse et al., 2003) even on healthy aging. Previous studies also found no age-related deficits specific to selective attention or task-switching location (Verhaeghen and Cerella, 2002). At each year added on age, conceptualization task scores decreases 1.9%, sensitivity to interference scores decreases 2.2%, inhibitory control scores decreases 3.6%, FAB total scores decreases 1.5%, and cognitive flexibility task errors increases 3.5%.

Finally, the study should be viewed in the light of these limitations: The pharmacological treatments as with antidepressants have not been completely controlled; convenience sample with inherent problems of selection. Outpatient clinic samples tend to present higher prevalence of cardiovascular diseases and other conditions increased by aging compared to the general population. Some confounders like these vascular risk factors or diseases were not controlled. The sleep evaluation of was not performed by a sleep specialist and the sleep quality evaluation depends on self report. It is known that depressed patients tend to overestimate or underestimate their sleep problems in self reports; The use of FAB to evaluate executive functions is also limited due to being a screening test and because items are evaluated on a scale between 0 and 3 points, which reduces the variation range. Additionally, Outpatient clinic samples tend to present higher prevalence of cardiovascular diseases and other conditions increased by aging compared to the general population. Some confounders like these vascular risk factors or diseases were not controlled.

Our findings suggest that depression and sleep are associated with impairment on executive functions in non-demented older adults, and that use of benzodiazepines and educational level are important variables. These data are important because executive functions are predictors of dementia in older adults.

AUTHOR CONTRIBUTIONS

All authors contributed and participated in the preparation of the article and all research steps: KMA contributed to the study on conception and design, on the statistical analysis, interpretation of data, wrote this article and approved the final version of the manuscript; MC contributed with acquisition of data, on supervising the geriatric assessment of the participants, on the statistical analysis, manuscript writing, and approved the final version of the manuscript; LM helped to design the study, on supervising the geriatric assessment of the participants, reviewed the statistical analysis and the manuscript and approved the final version of the manuscript; BD contributed to the study on conception and design, reviewed the statistical analysis and the manuscript, and approved the final version of the manuscript.

ACKNOWLEDGMENTS

The authors most warmly thank the study participants, Jenny de Andrade Faria and Laboratory of Clinical Neuroscience Investigations researchers involved in planning or carrying out the study.

REFERENCES

Alhola, P., and Polo-Kantola, P. (2007). Sleep deprivation: impact on cognitive performance. *Neuropsychiatr. Dis. Treat.* 3, 553.

Ardila, A., Ostrosky-Solis, F., Rosselli, M., and Gómez, C. (2000). Age-related cognitive decline during normal aging: the complex effect of education. *Arch. Clin. Neuropsychol.* 15, 495–513. doi: 10.1016/S0887-6177(99)00040-2

Barker, M. J., Greenwood, K. M., Jackson, M., and Crowe, S. F. (2004). Persistence of cognitive effects after withdrawal from long-term benzodiazepine use: a meta-analysis. *Arch. Clin. Neuropsychol.* 19, 437–454. doi: 10.1016/S0887-6177(03)00096-9

Bastien, C. H., Fortier-Brochu, É., Rioux, I., LeBlanc, M., Daley, M., and Morin, C. M. (2003). Cognitive performance and sleep quality in the elderly suffering from chronic insomnia: relationship between objective and subjective measures. *J. Psychosom. Res.* 54, 39–49. doi: 10.1016/S0022-3999(02)00544-5

Beato, R., Amaral-Carvalho, V., Guimarγes, H. C., Tumas, V., Souza, C. P., Oliveira, G. N. D., et al. (2012). Frontal assessment battery in a Brazilian sample of healthy controls: normative data. *Arq. Neuropsiquiatr.* 70, 278–280. doi: 10.1590/S0004-282X2012005000009

Benca, R. M., and Peterson, M. J. (2008). Insomnia and depression. *Sleep Med.* 9, S3–S9. doi: 10.1016/S1389-9457(08)70010-8

Cajochen, C., Knoblauch, V., Kräuchi, K., Renz, C., and Wirz-Justice, A. (2001). Dynamics of frontal EEG activity, sleepiness and body temperature under high and low sleep pressure. *Neuroreport* 12, 2277–2281. doi: 10.1097/00001756-200107200-00046

Chennu, S., and Bekinschtein, T. A. (2012). Arousal modulates auditory attention and awareness: insights from sleep, sedation, and disorders of consciousness. *Front. Psychol.* 5:65. doi: 10.3389/fpsyg.2012.00065

de Paula, J. J., Bertola, L., Ávila, R. T., Moreira, L., Coutinho, G., de Moraes, E. N., et al. (2013a). Clinical applicability and cutoff values for an unstructured neuropsychological assessment protocol for older adults with low formal education. *PLoS ONE* 8:e73167. doi: 10.1371/journal.pone.0073167

de Paula, J. J., Moura, S. M., Bocardi, M. B., Moraes, E. N., Malloy-Diniz, L. F., and Haase, V. G. (2013b). Screening for executive dysfunction with the Frontal Assessment Battery: psychometric properties analysis and representative normative data for Brazilian older adults. *Psicol. Pes.* 7, 89–98. doi: 10.5327/Z1982-1247201300010010

Diniz, B. S., Butters, M. A., Albert, S. M., Dew, M. A., and Reynolds, C. F. (2013). Late-life depression and risk of vascular dementia and Alzheimer's disease: systematic review and meta-analysis of community-based cohort studies. *Br. J. Psychiatry* 202, 329–335. doi: 10.1192/bjp.bp.112.118307

Elderkin-Thompson, V., Kumar, A., Mintz, J., Boone, K., Bahng, E., and Lavretsky, H. (2004). Executive dysfunction and visuospatial ability among depressed elders in a community setting. *Arch. Clin. Neuropsychol.* 19, 597–611. doi: 10.1016/j.acn.2003.08.009

Fuster, J. M. (2001). The prefrontal cortex—an update: time is of the essence. *Neuron* 30, 319–333. doi: 10.1016/S0896-6273(01)00285-9

Glass, J., Lanctôt, K. L., Herrmann, N., Sproule, B. A., and Busto, U. E. (2005). Sedative hypnotics in older people with insomnia: meta-analysis of risks and benefits. *BMJ* 331:1169. doi: 10.1136/bmj.38623.768588.47

Goh, J. O., Beason-Held, L. L., An, Y., Kraut, M. A., and Resnick, S. M. (2013). Frontal function and executive processing in older adults: process and region specific age-related longitudinal functional changes. *Neuroimage* 69, 43–50. doi: 10.1016/j.neuroimage.2012.12.026

Hahn, E. A., Wang, H. X., Andel, R., and Fratiglioni, L. (2014). A change in sleep pattern may predict Alzheimer disease. *Am. J. Geriatr. Psychiatry* 22, 1262–1271. doi: 10.1016/j.jagp.2013.04.015

Haimov, I., Hanuka, E., and Horowitz, Y. (2008). Chronic insomnia and cognitive functioning among older adults. *Behav. Sleep Med.* 6, 32–54. doi: 10.1080/15402000701796080

Harrison, Y., and Horne, J. (1998). Sleep loss impairs short and novel language tasks having a prefrontal focus. *J. Sleep Res.* 7, 95–100. doi: 10.1046/j.1365-2869.1998.00104.x

Harrison, Y., Horne, J. A., and Rothwell, A. (2000). Prefrontal neuropsychological effects of sleep deprivation in young adults–a model for healthy aging? *Sleep* 23, 1067–1073.

Jueptner, M., Stephan, K. M., Frith, C. D., Brooks, D. J., Frackowiak, R. S. J., and Passingham, R. E. (1997). Anatomy of motor learning. I. Frontal cortex and attention to action. *J. Neurophysiol.* 77, 1313–1324.

Jungwirth, S., Zehetmayer, S., Hinterberger, M., Kudrnovsky-Moser, S., Weissgram, S., Tragl, K. H., et al. (2011). The influence of depression on processing speed and executive function in nondemented subjects aged 75. *J. Int. Neuropsychol. Soc.* 17, 822–831. doi: 10.1017/S135561771100083X

Kraemer, S., Danker-Hopfe, H., Dorn, H., Schmidt, A., Ehlert, I., and Herrmann, W. M. (2000). Time-of-day variations of indicators of attention: performance, physiologic parameters, and self-assessment of sleepiness. *Biol. Psychiatry.* 48, 1069–1080. doi: 10.1016/S0006-3223(00)00908-2

Lim, J., and Dinges, D. F. (2010). A meta-analysis of the impact of short-term sleep deprivation on cognitive variables. *Psychol. Bull.* 136, 375. doi: 10.1037/a0018883

McCullagh, P., and Nelder, J. A. (1983). *Generalized Linear Models.* New York, NY; London: Chapman and Hall.

McGregor, K. K., and Alper, R. M. (2015). Sleep disorders as a risk to language learning and use. *EBP Briefs* 10, 1–21.

Mergl, R., Pogarell, O., Juckel, G., Rihl, J., Henkel, V., Frodl, T., et al. (2007). Hand-motor dysfunction in depression: characteristics and pharmacological effects. *Clin. EEG Neurosci.* 38, 82–88. doi: 10.1177/155005940703800210

Nebes, R. D., Butters, M. A., Mulsant, B. H., Pollock, B. G., Zmuda, M. D., Houck, P. R., et al. (2000). Decreased working memory and processing speed mediate cognitive impairment in geriatric depression. *Psychol. Med.* 30, 679–691. doi: 10.1017/S0033291799001968

Nebes, R. D., Buysse, D. J., Halligan, E. M., Houck, P. R., and Monk, T. H. (2009). Self-reported sleep quality predicts poor cognitive performance in healthy older adults. *J. Gerontol. B Psychol. Sci. Soc. Sci.* 64, 180–187. doi: 10.1093/geronb/gbn037

Sabbe, B., Hulstijn, W., Van Hoof, J., and Zitman, F. (1996). Fine motor retardation and depression. *J. Psychiatr. Res.* 30, 295–306. doi: 10.1016/0022-3956(96)00014-3

Salthouse, T. A., Atkinson, T. M., and Berish, D. E. (2003). Executive functioning as a potential mediator of age-related cognitive decline in normal adults. *J. Exp. Psychol. Gen.* 132:566. doi: 10.1037/0096-3445.132.4.566

Schmidt, C., Collette, F., Cajochen, C., and Peigneux, P. (2007). A time to think: circadian rhythms in human cognition. *Cogn. Neuropsychol.* 24, 755–789. doi: 10.1080/02643290701754158

Shao, Z., Janse, E., Visser, K., and Meyer, A. S. (2014). What do verbal fluency tasks measure? Predictors of verbal fluency performance in older adults. *Front. Psychol.* 5:772. doi: 10.3389/fpsyg.2014.00772

Snyder, H. R. (2013). Major depressive disorder is associated with broad impairments on neuropsychological measures of executive function: a meta-analysis and review. *Psychol. Bull.* 139, 81–132. doi: 10.1037/a0028727

Tucker, A. M., Whitney, P., Belenky, G., Hinson, J. M., and Van Dongen, H. P. (2010). Effects of sleep deprivation on dissociated components of executive functioning. *Sleep* 33, 47–57.

Verhaeghen, P., and Cerella, J. (2002). Aging, executive control, and attention: a review of meta-analyses. *Neurosci. Biobehav. Rev.* 26, 849–857. doi: 10.1016/S0149-7634(02)00071-4

Vignola, A., Lamoureux, C., Bastien, C. H., and Morin, C. M. (2000). Effects of chronic insomnia and use of benzodiazepines on daytime performance in older adults. *J. Gerontol. B Psychol. Sci. Soc. Sci.* 55, P54–P62.

22

Disentangling Working Memory Functioning in Mood States of Bipolar Disorder

Carolina Soraggi-Frez[1], *Flávia H. Santos*[2*], *Pedro B. Albuquerque*[2] *and Leandro F. Malloy-Diniz*[3]

[1] Department of Psychology, Faculty of Philosophy and Human Sciences, Federal University of Minas Gerais, Belo Horizonte, Brazil, [2] *School of Psychology (CIPsi), University of Minho, Braga, Portugal,* [3] *Department of Mental Health, National Science and Technology Institutes (INCT-MM), Federal University of Minas Gerais, Belo Horizonte, Brazil*

Edited by:
Amitai Abramovitch, Texas State University, USA

Reviewed by:
Hannah R. Snyder, Brandeis University, USA
Eyal Kalanthroff, Ben-Gurion University of the Negev, Israel

***Correspondence:**
Flávia H. Santos
flaviahs@psi.uminho.pt

Working memory (WM) deficits are often reported in patients with Bipolar Disorder (BD). However, it is not clear about the nature of these WM deficits (update or serial order processes) and their association with each BD states (euthymic, mania, and depressive). This review investigated the association between BD patient's states and the functioning of WM components. For this purpose, we carried out a systematic review fulfilling a search in the databases Medline, Scopus, SciELO, and Web of Science using specific terms in the abstracts of the articles that generated 212 outcomes in the restricted period from 2005 to 2016. Twenty-three papers were selected, completely read, and analyzed using PICOS strategy. The mood episodes predicted deficits in different components of WM in BD patients (the phonological loop or visuospatial sketchpad) and were associated with different WM processes (updating and serial recall). Lower cognitive scores persist even in remission of symptoms. This result suggests that WM deficit apparently is stage-independent in BD patients. Furthermore, findings suggest that the neutral point on Hedonic Detector component of WM could be maladjusted by BD.

Keywords: emotion, working memory, bipolar disorder, hedonic detector, mood states

INTRODUCTION

Bipolar Disorder (BD) is a severe and chronic disorder characterized by emotional and humoral dysregulation that leads to increased frequency of cognitive dysfunction and interpersonal problems (Chang et al., 2012). BD type I is characterized by one mania episode or rapid (daily) cycling episodes of mania and depression, preceded or followed by hypomanic or major depressive episodes, presenting euphoria and exaggerated behaviors such as glibness, greatness, flight of ideas, leading to social problems. In type II, at least one hypomanic episode alternates with depression phases, occurring less externalizing problems compared to mania episodes regarding to mood switching, interpersonal, and occupational problems (American Psychiatric Association, 2013). It has estimated that BD rank is the 17th cause of years lived with disability in Europe, accounting for 1.6% of the total (World Health Organization, 2016). In the United States 2.6% of adults are affected by BD (National Institute of Mental Health, 2011) and in developing countries like Brazil ~1% of the population are diagnosed with BD type I and II (Lima et al., 2005).

In addition to mood changes, patients with BD tend to show deficits in executive functions, verbal and visuospatial episodic memory, working memory (WM), verbal learning, information processing speed, sustained attention, and sensorimotor performance (Bora et al., 2009; Latalova et al., 2011; Lage et al., 2013; Loschiavo et al., 2013; Lee et al., 2014; Neves et al., 2014). Some studies have suggested more severe cognitive deficits in episodes of manic/mixed mood compared with depressive and euthymic episodes (Sweeney et al., 2000). Latalova et al. (2011) also observed that cognitive deficits tend to persist even in euthymic episodes, whereas, lower scores for verbal short-term memory and executive functions were found in both types of BD mood episodes, in tasks of WM, executive control, and verbal fluency. Some studies have shown that cognitive deficits observed in acute manic and depression episodes (Rubinsztein et al., 2000; Clark et al., 2001; Murphy, 2001), are also present in euthymic periods (van Gorp et al., 1998; Martinez-Aran et al., 2007; Wingo et al., 2009). Moreover, lower cognitive scores persist in visuospatial memory, verbal short and long-term memory, executive function, attention/processing speed, and WM, even after a long period of symptoms remission (van Gorp et al., 1998; Rubinsztein et al., 2000; Robinson et al., 2006; Martinez-Aran et al., 2007; Torres et al., 2007; McKenna et al., 2013; Ajilore et al., 2015). Besides that, first-episode BD is associated with widespread cognitive dysfunction (Lee et al., 2014), this result indicates cognitive deficits even in the earliest stages of disease and reinforces them as primary characters of BD. Symptoms of BD as anxiety and depression seem to reflect the malfunctioning of systems that provide a basis for action within a complex emotionally valenced world (Baddeley, 2013).

Among the cognitive deficits reported, WM seems to be relevant to understand the symptoms of BD. According to Miyake and Shah (1999) there are at least 10 diverse frameworks pointing different nature, structure, and functions of WM, which could diverge in terms of explanations of WM deficits. Then, it is important specifies some issues regarding this cognitive skill and its assessment that will be taken into account in the present paper. For instance, different tasks are considered measures of WM components: simple span tasks as measures of verbal and visuospatial storages, whereas, complex span tasks combine storage and attentional control (Baddeley, 1986). Currently, complex span tasks and n-back tasks are the most used WM measures (Miyake and Shah, 1999), since both require storing and maintain the information of a set of stimuli, and inhibiting interference of the signals recently presented (St Clair-Thompson and Gathercole, 2006). But there are dissimilarities, complex span tasks request keeping a serial order in mind at the same time of an ongoing cognitive task (Daneman and Merikle, 1996; Unsworth and Engle, 2007; Conway and Kovacs, 2013), while n-back tasks demand a constant updating of the relevant information (Kane et al., 2008; Wilhelm et al., 2013; Remoli and Santos, 2017). Apart from that, there are low correlations between n-back tasks and complex span tasks leading a conclusion that both evaluate different processes of WM (Kane et al., 2008; Redick and Lindsey, 2013), particularly concerning to the influence of emotional states (Ribeiro et al., submitted). A systematic review showed that different verbal WM capacities could be observed in studies that used mood induction before the completion of the task. While positive and negative stimuli seem to decrease the span task performance, no effects were found for n-back tasks (Ribeiro et al., submitted). In fact, negative mood induction can decrease WM performance during simple span and complex tasks (Spies et al., 1996; Santos et al., 2015; Soares, 2015).

In this review, WM is assumed to be a temporary information storage system that underpins the capacity for active thought by providing a cognitive workspace in which information may be temporarily maintained and manipulated (Baddeley, 2013). It is composed of multiple components, as the central executive, responsible for attentional control, and two subsidiary systems: the phonological loop and the visuospatial sketchpad, responsible for storing auditory-verbal and visual-spatial information, respectively (Baddeley et al., 2012). Subsequently, the episodic buffer was added to the initial WM model for integrating information from its multiple components with long-term memory (Baddeley, 2000). Previous studies indicated that when emotions and valenced thoughts are brought to WM they elicit somatic states (Bechara and Damasio, 2005), and the activation in brain emotional circuits, as conscious experience (LeDoux, 2000).

In fact, the connection of emotional states and working memory goes beyond the measurement instruments but in theoretical framework as well. For instance, the somatic marker hypothesis presented by Damasio et al. (1991) describes a mechanism for interaction between emotion and cognition in trial and decision-making processes (Bechara and Damasio, 2002, 2005; Bechara et al., 2005; Verdejo-García and Bechara, 2009). Damasio goes further by stating that the central executive component of working memory could be relevant in this process. As far as we know Baddeley's is the only model of WM explicitly addressing the capacity to temporary manipulate stored hedonic information. Baddeley proposed a new component, the Hedonic Detector which is understood as a neutral point that varies between positive and negative valences in response to environmental stimuli by establishing a mean value between stimulus and information retained in the WM to enable choices of future actions (Baddeley, 2007). It means that processing "hot" information (emotional content) disrupt the functioning of "cold" cognitive process, like core WM processes. Accounting this assumption, Baddeley et al. (2012) demonstrated that hedonic judgment of stimuli, such as words, pictures, and faces indeed could be influenced by the valence of an induced mood. Recently, different studies observed that mood induction procedures, e.g., listening valenced instrumental music while retrieving valenced autobiographical memories affect scores in WM tasks of health controls (e.g., Spachtholz et al., 2014; Allen et al., 2015). In this perspective, improper adjustment of the neutral point could be expressed by deficits to maintain, manipulate, and/or update information in WM. In the case of pathological affective episodes likewise in Bipolar Disorder (BD), the episodes itself could uncalibrated the hedonic detector.

Deficits in WM processing have been consistently reported in euthymic patients (MacQueen et al., 2005; Thompson et al., 2007; Daglas et al., 2015). Another study also observed that euthymic BD type I had worse performance on visuospatial tasks compared to healthy subjects (Farahmand et al., 2015). Although, there is no consensus in the literature, these findings suggest that deficits in WM could result from the intensification of emotional valences. In other words, the presence of WM deficits, could be considered a primary trace of BD, beyond state variables (Gruber et al., 2009; Kurtz and Gerraty, 2009). However, this particular issue remains controversial due to the diversity of methodologies used across the studies. In addition to the prevalence of within-subjects design, some authors rarely made the connection between theoretical models and cognitive tasks, limiting the comprehension about WM and their particular components.

In line with this argument, a review by Baddeley (2013) showed that in depressive patients negative mood influences hedonic judgment, explaining the trend of the negative perception of the situations in this clinical population. However, there is no significant evidence in respect to the influence of positive mood in hedonic detection system. Hypothetically, assuming that the neutral point in BD patients corresponds to euthymic phase, the exacerbated positive and negative valences would account for euphoric or depressed mood, respectively (Baddeley, 2007, 2013). As emotion in BD is deregulated, the study of this disorder seems to be necessary to understand the influence of improper adjustment of the hedonic detector neutral point in WM.

There are many meta-analyses which state significant neuropsychological deficits in euthymic bipolar patients (Robinson et al., 2006; Torres et al., 2007; Bora et al., 2009; Kurtz and Gerraty, 2009; Mann-Wrobel et al., 2011) and their relatives (Balanzá-Martínez et al., 2008; Arts et al., 2009; Bora et al., 2009). Most of these studies including working memory performance in bipolar patients Robinson et al. (2006), Torres et al. (2007), and Kurtz and Gerraty (2009) found that BD patients present deficits in measures of verbal working memory. In a recent review, Cullen et al. (2016) found similar results pointing that BD patients performed worse than controls in attention/working memory tasks. Bora et al. (2011) found evidences of verbal working memory deficits both in Type I and II bipolar patients. These deficits are found even in BD's relatives suggesting that these deficits are potential endophenotypes in Bipolar disorder; (Balanzá-Martínez et al., 2008; Arts et al., 2009) found evidences of worse performance in verbal working memory tasks in both BD's patients and relatives. Nonetheless these WM deficits are heterogeneous and seems to be affected by both demographic (e.g., educational level) and clinical aspects of the disorder (e.g., number of episodes) (Arts et al., 2009; Kurtz and Gerraty, 2009).

More recently, some studies using meta-analytical methodology addressed specific cognitive deficit in the bipolar patient as in theory of mind (Bora et al., 2016), social cognition (Samamé et al., 2015), and verbal fluency (Raucher-Chéné et al., 2017). Nonetheless, we did not found studies focusing in working memory deficits in bipolar disorder patients. Most of systematic review consider working memory in comparison to another cognitive functioning and some of than considered these deficits together with another executive functioning component (Robinson et al., 2006; Torres et al., 2007) and even attentional functioning (Cullen et al., 2016). Therefore, the purposes of this study are (i) to update the knowledge of working memory deficits including recent published data about working memory deficits in bipolar patients; (ii) analyze if BD patients show WM deficits, contrasting studies that used complex span tasks and n-back tasks; (iii) to investigate if different BD mood episodes predict different patterns of WM functioning, analyzing its components in each mood phase. The primary hypothesis of the present review is that working memory deficits are worsened during active phases of the disorder but remains in euthymic patients.

METHODS

This study is a descriptive and informative systematic review of the literature about the association between BD patient's states and the functioning of WM components. We used the instructions of Cochrane Foundation (Higgins and Green, 2011) to ensure the presentation of comprehensive and unbiased data. The following questions were asked to guide the review: Do patients diagnosed with BD have deficits in working memory? Are specific states of BD (mania, hypomania, depression, and euthymic) related to changes in working memory processes, such as updating and serial recall?

After the definition of the guiding questions, the following steps were taken: setting and collection of studies in databases; critical evaluation of studies, data selection and analysis, presentation, and interpretation of results (Bento, 2014).

All articles indexed in MEDLINE, Scopus, SciELO, and web of Science search databases that used, at least, one WM task in patients with BD, during a specified mood episode were included. Papers with available abstracts and written in Portuguese, English, or Spanish were considered.

Selected articles evaluated the WM in adult patients with BD, aged from 18 to 65 years old, and published until 15st July 2016. Literature reviews, case studies, and studies that referred to psychological or pharmacological interventions were excluded. Research and selection of manuscripts were done by the first author (CSF) and reviewed by the second author (FHS), with agreement between them.

For searches in databases, the terms "*transtorno bipolar,*" "*memória operatória,*" and "*emoção*"; "*trastorno bipolar,*" "*memoria operativa,*" *and* "*emoción*"; and "bipolar disorder," "working memory," and "emotion" were used. We found 55 papers in MEDLINE, 63 in Scopus, 1 in Scielo, and 95 in Web of Science in the first search until 15th July 2016. No studies were found in Portuguese and only one study was written in Spanish.

Among the 214 papers identified, 34 were repeated, and 20 were found in more than two databases. Based on the abstract reading, from the 160 remaining studies 25 papers were selected and 135 were excluded, due to the presented criteria: (1) 16 did not use WM tasks; (2) 42 referred to literature reviews; (3) 27 had samples whose participants were under 18- or over 65-years old; (4) eight evaluated the effectiveness of psychological or pharmacological interventions; (5) three were animal sample studies; (6) 39 had undiagnosed BD participants.

Twenty-five articles were thoroughly analyzed, being excluded two studies for the following reasons: (1) the lack of contrast between WM measures and non-social domains, which were used only as demographic control measures; (2) absence of description about the measures of WM and other cognitive domains in this session. As a result, 23 papers were discussed in this review (**Figure 1**).

Since most studies were methodologically unrelated to each other, carry out a meta-analysis in the present state of art would be premature, therefore we opted to systematically organize the selected articles hoping that this effort will provide new insights for researchers in order to advance in this field. Therefore, the current systematic review structured the analyses focused on the three main working memory processes (maintenance, manipulation, and updating), in respective modalities (verbal or non-verbal). The fundamental aspects of the papers were organized using the PICOS strategy, an acronym that represents the initials of the items: Population, Intervention (procedure), Comparison, Outcome, and Study Design (Bento, 2014). In this way, we used the following topics: population, type of intervention, methodological design, evaluated variables or expected results, and study design (**Table 1**). Based on these items

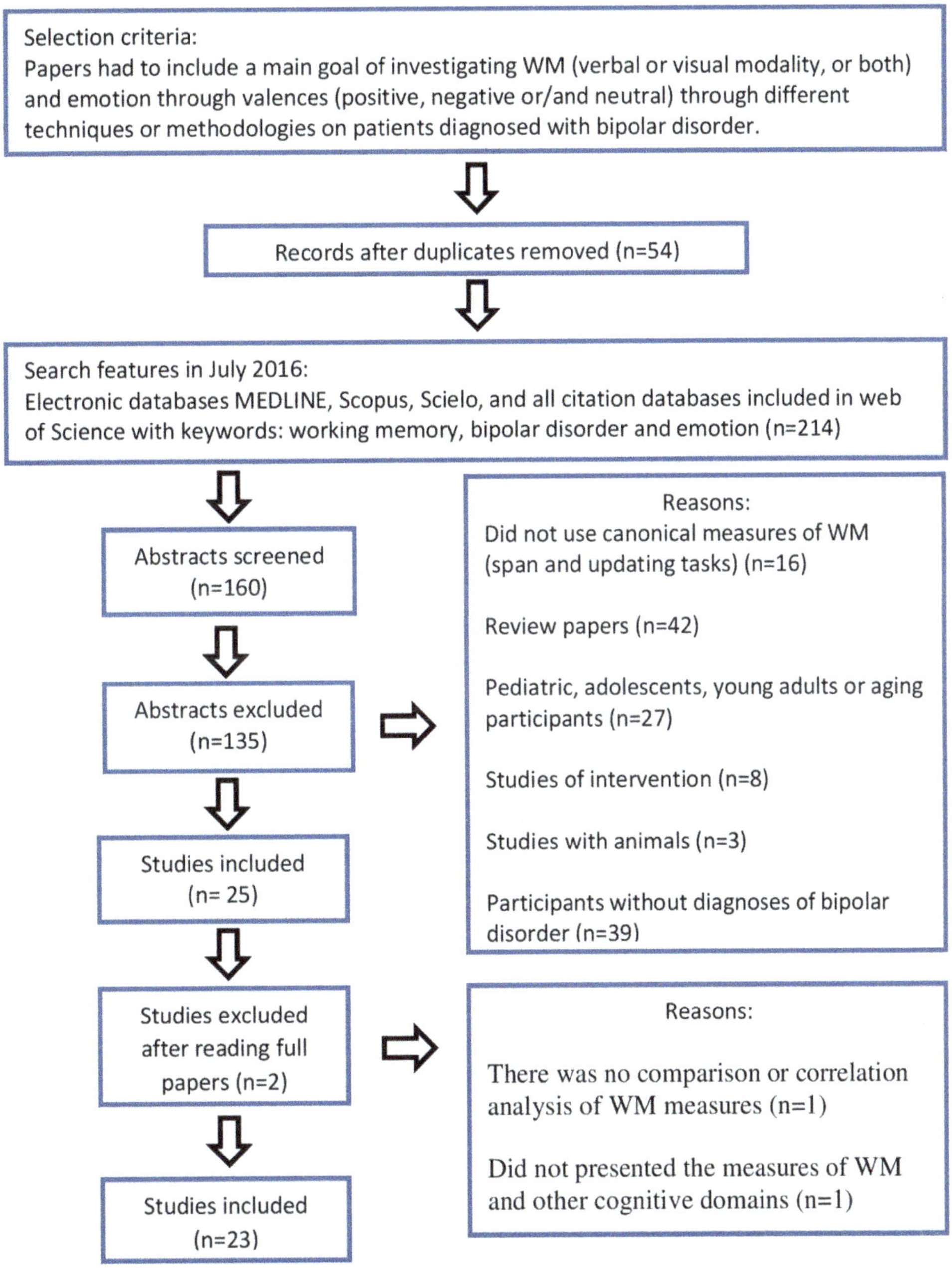

FIGURE 1 | Flowchart of search criteria and articles included in this review. WM, working memory.

TABLE 1 | Summary of selected articles with have investigated WM performance in BD subjects.

Article	Population	Intervention	Comparison	Outcome	Study design
Liu et al., 2010	*N* = 14 BD I, mean age 35.6 (10.9); *N* = 13 BD II, mean age 35.1 (9.8); *N* = 21 controls, mean age 38.3 (11.9)	Neuropsychological and behavioral assessment combined with physiological parameters	Cerebral white matter patterns and cognitive functioning correlation between groups	BD I: alterations in the right hemisphere. BD II: lower scores associated with cognitive and emotional processes. Brain alterations correlated with deficits of WM and executive function in both subtypes	Quantitative cross-sectional study
Bertocci et al., 2011	*N* = 23 unipolar depression (UD), mean age 29.74 (8.22); *N* = 18 BD I in depressive phase, mean age 31.94 (8.54); *N* = 16 controls, mean age 32.76 (6.50)	Neuropsychological and behavioral assessment combined with physiological parameters	Brain monitoring using fMRI during the tasks	Higher activity of dAMCC in UD, controls and BD I groups were found during 2-back neutral faces tasks	Quantitative cross-sectional study
Deckersbach et al., 2008	*N* = 9 BD I in moderated depressive phase, mean age 27.6 (2.8); *N* = 17 controls, mean age 25.6 (5.9)	Neuropsychological and behavioral assessment combined with physiological parameters	Sadness state induction using autobiographical memory and brain monitoring using fMRI during the tasks	BD I: greater activation in the left DLPFC and dACC in sadness condition	Prospective
Lee et al., 2013−1	*N* = 68 euthymic BD, mean age 43.9 (10.6); *N* = 38 schizophrenia in remission, mean age 44.7 (9.1); *N* = 36 controls, mean age 41.4 (9.9)	Neuropsychological and behavioral assessment	Social cognitive performance among clinical sample subgroups and controls	No significant difference in social cognitive performance between BD and control groups	Quantitative cross-sectional study
Lee et al., 2013−2	Same as Lee et al., 2013−1	Same as Lee et al., 2013−1	Social and nonsocial cognitive patterns among clinical groups	BD group had similar performance to controls in all areas. BD: more nonsocial than social deficit. Schizophrenia showed the opposite pattern	Same as Lee et al., 2013−1
Lee et al., 2013−3	*N* = 68 euthymic BD, mean age 43.9 (10.6); *N* = 38 schizophrenia in remission, mean age 44.7 (9.1)	Same as Lee et al., 2013−1	Comparison of social and nonsocial cognitive performance inter-clinical groups	Schizophrenia: more social cognitive deficits. BD: more nonsocial cognitive deficits	Idem
Levy et al., 2011	*N* = 82 euthymic BD I: 22 readmitted to the hospital, mean age 39.9 (12.7); 60 outpatient care, mean age 38.4 (11.6)	Neuropsychological and behavioral assessment	Mood state and cognitive performance before discharge and after 3 months inter-groups	Readmitted group: severe mood episodes and lower scores for executive function, attention and WM, visual and verbal episodic memory performance	Cohort prospective study
Miguélez-Pan et al., 2014	*N* = 31 euthymic BD, mean age 41.3 (11.1); *N* = 25 controls, mean age 40.40 (9.7)	Neuropsychological and behavioral assessment	Descriptive analysis of executive and functional profile and comparison of results inter-groups	BD: worse performance in flexibility, plan implementing, set-shifting and verbal fluency. No significant differences in WM	Descriptive cross-sectional study
Pomarol-Clotet et al., 2014	*N* = 38 BD I in mania state, mean age 39.74 (11.3); *N* = 38 BD in depression state - 32 BD I and 6 BD II - mean age 39.89 (10.39); 38 euthymic BD I, mean age 40 (8.7); *N* = 38 controls, mean age 39.68 (8.8)	Neuropsychological and behavioral assessment combined with physiological parameters	Brain monitoring using fMRI during cognitive the tasks in different mood phases	BD patients in depressive and manic phases showed worse performance in WM and lower activation in prefrontal dorsolateral and parietal cortex compared to controls; also in parietal cortex comparing to euthymic group. Mania group reported lower activation in left prefrontal dorsolateral cortex than euthymic group	Quantitative cross-sectional study
Roiser et al., 2009	*N* = 49 BD unmedicated in depression, majority BD II, mean age 33.6 (8.9); *N* = 55 controls, mean age 34.9 (8.1)	Neuropsychological and behavioral assessment combined with physiological parameters	Cognitive deficit inter-groups	BD: lower scores for short-term spatial memory, decision-making and insensitivity to negative feedback but not inattention, visual episodic memory and WM deficits	Quantitative cross-sectional study

(Continued)

TABLE 1 | Continued

Article	Population	Intervention	Comparison	Outcome	Study design
Thermenos et al., 2010	$N = 19$ euthymic BD, mean age 41.1 (3.1), $N = 18$ relatives without psychiatric diagnoses—RELs—mean age 36.6 (2.6); $N = 19$ controls, mean age 39.2 (2.7)	Neuropsychological and behavioral assessment combined with physiological parameters	Brain monitoring using fMRI during the tasks	BD and RELs: alterations in frontopolar cortex and insula during WM task. Correlations between brain activity, mood and WM	Quantitative cross-sectional study
Barrett et al., 2008	$N = 26$ euthymic. BD type I, mean age 52.50 (14.17); BD type II, mean age 41.43 (9.06); $N = 26$ controls, mean age 49.75 (13.11)	Neuropsychological and behavioral assessment	Cognitive deficit inter-groups and gender; cognitive performance intra-individual correlation	BD: greater visuospatial WM and verbal fluency low score. Deficits were more detectable in men compared to women, but both had similar number of errors	Quantitative cross-sectional study
Bauer et al., 2015	$N = 90$ euthymic BD, mean age 35.18 (1.3): 59 BD I, 28 BD II, 3 BD not specified; $N = 56$ controls, mean age 36.17 (1.9)	Neuropsychological and behavioral assessment	Cognitive deficit inter-groups and intra-individual correlation	BD: no affective short-term memory and verbal fluency deficit. No significant difference in WM	Quantitative cross-sectional study
Dittman et al., 2008	$N = 74$ euthymic BD—52 BD I and 23 BD II—mean age 42.52 (12.23); $N = 42$ controls, mean age 43.02 (12.75)	Neuropsychological and behavioral assessment combined with physiological parameters	Level of homocystein inter-groups and cognitive performance and level of homocystein intra-individual correlation	BD: deficit in all cognitive tasks, including WM deficits	Quantitative cross-sectional study
Drapier et al., 2008	$N = 20$ BD I, mean age 42.7 (10.4); $N = 20$ relatives without substitute TAB for BD, mean age 43 (13.8); $N = 20$ controls, mean age 41.9 (11.6)	Neuropsychological and behavioral assessment combined with physiological parameters	Brain monitoring using fMRI during the tasks	BD: lower WM scores compared to control and relative groups. BD and relative groups: more prefrontal cortex activity	Quantitative cross-sectional study
Fleck et al., 2005	$N = 26$ BD I hospitalized in mania/ mixed + psychotic symptoms, mean age 28 (7); $N = 23$ euthymic BD outpatient care, mean age 28 (7); $N = 28$ controls, mean age 28 (9)	Neuropsychological and behavioral assessment	Cognitive performance, reaction time and sensitivity perceptual correlation inter-groups	Manic BD group showed recognition effectiveness and directed-forgetting effectiveness deficit. The BD group needed more effort to encode information	Quantitative cross-sectional study
Gruber et al., 2013	$N = 29$ euthymic BD I, mean age 30.28 (8.7); $N = 29$ major depression in remission, mean age 31.32 (11.32); $N = 30$ controls, mean age 31.45 (9.3).	Neuropsychological and behavioral assessment.	Negative and positive mood maintainability capacity; and WM correlation inter-groups	BD I: affective WM deficit compared to other groups. No difference between euthymic and control groups	Quantitative cross-sectional study
Malhi et al., 2007	$N = 10$ euthymic BD I, mean age 32.4 (10.8); $N = 10$ controls, mean age 31.7 (11.9)	Neuropsychological and behavioral assessment combined with physiological parameters	Brain monitoring using fMRI during the tasks on different mood valences	Control group: increased activation in medial prefrontal cortex, medial frontal cortex and right parahippocampal gyrus during positive and negative valences induction. No difference in reaction time and accuracy	Quantitative cross-sectional study
Mullin et al., 2012	$N = 22$ euthymic BD I, mean age 31.68 (8.9); $N = 19$ controls, mean age 32.54 (6.5)	Neuropsychological and behavioral assessment combined with physiological parameters	Brain monitoring using fMRI during the tasks	BD: (i) less activation in dorsolateral prefrontal cortex, dACC, and parietal cortex without emotional distractors; (ii) increased amygdala and striatum activity before negative stimuli; and (iii) greater connection activity in dACC and amygdala after positive stimuli	Quantitative cross-sectional study
Russo et al., 2014	$N = 64$ euthymic BD—77% BD I, 14% BD II and 9.4% not specified—mean age 41.2 (10.5); $N = 109$ controls, mean age 37.9 (11.6)	Neuropsychological and behavioral assessment	Mood state, temperament and cognition inter-groups and intra-individual correlation	BD: positive correlation in level of cyclotimia and irritability with information processing, WM, reasoning and problem solving	Quantitative cross-sectional study

(Continued)

TABLE 1 | Continued

Article	Population	Intervention	Comparison	Outcome	Study design
Thompson et al., 2007	$N = 50$ euthymic BD—44 BD I and 6 BD II—mean age 44.42 (8.6); $N = 57$ controls, mean age 44.86 (9.2).	Neuropsychological and behavioral assessment	Cognitive deficit inter-groups	BD: lower scores in Backward Digit Span. No difference in recognition task, visuospatial WM, Forward Digit Span and executive processes (verbal fluency; visual attention) between groups	Quantitative cross-sectional study
Muhtadie and Johnson, 2015	$N = 27$ euthymic BD I, mean age 35.63 (12.5); $N = 24$ controls, mean age 30.42 (11)	Neuropsychological and behavioral assessment combined with physiological parameters	Autonomic physiology and emotional reactions monitoring during the task	BD: high levels of emotional (anxiety) and autonomic (cardiovascular) reactivity, which were positively correlated	Quantitative cross-sectional study
Gvirts et al., 2015	$N = 30$ BD mildly affective symptoms, 26 BD I, 4 BD II, mean age 41.93 (12.94); $N = 32$ Borderline Personality Disorder (BPD), mean age 29.01 (9.28); matching a healthy control group	Neuropsychological and behavioral assessment	Cognitive performance inter-groups and correlation between sustained attention and cognitive measures	BD: deficits in strategy formation and planning execution time comparing to other groups; poorer utilization of strategy in the SWM task comparing to BPD. BPD: deficit in planning in comparison to all groups; in problem-solving comparing to controls. BD and BPD: deficits in sustained attention	Quantitative cross-sectional study
Sabater et al., 2016	$N = 73$ euthymic BD: 29 in lithium monotherapy (L), mean age 24.3 (9.3); 28 lithium + anticonvulsants (LA), mean age 26.8 (10.8); 16 in anticonvulsant therapy (A), mean age 28.6 (12.1); $N = 25$ controls	Neuropsychological and behavioral assessment	Comparison of cognitive performance between groups	BD-L: preserved short-term auditory memory, long-term memory, and attention. BD-A: worse performance in short-term visual memory, WM, and several executive functions. All BD patients: poorly in processing speed, resistance to interference, and emotion recognition	Quantitative cross-sectional study
McCormack et al., 2015	$N = 99$ high genetic risk (AR relatives), mean age 22.0 (4.5); $N = 52$ BD higher mood severity symptoms, 27 BD I, 25 BD II, mean age 24.6 (3.8); $N = 78$ controls, mean age 22.4 (3.9)	Neuropsychological and behavioral assessment	Comparison of cognitive performance between groups	AR: verbal reasoning and affective response inhibition deficits. BD: deficits in attention. Neither AR nor BD patients showed lower scores for general intellectual ability, WM, visuospatial or language ability. Only the BD participants showed impaired emotion recognition	Quantitative cross-sectional study

BD, Bipolar disorder; WM, working memory; REL, relatives; dAMCC, dorsal anterior midcingulate cortex; DLPFC, left dorsolateral prefrontal cortex; dACC, dorsal anterior cingulate cortex; fMRI, functional magnetic resonance imaging.

we could discuss them into three sessions: "Cognitive deficits and neurobiological correlates in BD patients," "Different patterns of cognitive processes in each mood phase," and "Relationship among WM and other clinical features." The first two items addressed clearly the objectives that motivated the present study and the final session account for other findings observed in the selected articles.

RESULTS

The *SCImago Journal* & *Country Rank* was used as an indicator of visibility in scientific domains by ranking the journals in which papers were published. The ranking for psychology, neuroscience, and medicine areas in the last 7 years were considered. Twenty-one studies were published in Q1 journals (Fleck et al., 2005; Malhi et al., 2007; Thompson et al., 2007; Barrett et al., 2008; Deckersbach et al., 2008; Drapier et al., 2008; Roiser et al., 2009; Liu et al., 2010; Thermenos et al., 2010; Bertocci et al., 2011; Levy et al., 2011; Mullin et al., 2012; Gruber et al., 2013; Lee et al., 2013; Pomarol-Clotet et al., 2014; Russo et al., 2014; Bauer et al., 2015; Gvirts et al., 2015; McCormack et al., 2015; Muhtadie and Johnson, 2015; Sabater et al., 2016), one in Q2 journal (Miguélez-Pan et al., 2014), and one in Q3 journal (Dittman et al., 2008). These quartiles also indicated that the majority of selected studies were published in higher impact factor journals.

According to the publication period of the selected articles, the first research of a direct association between emotions and WM in BD patients was performed by Fleck et al. (2005). The other studies were published in the following periods. The research studies have been mostly carried out in America, with eleven studies in the United States, eight in Europe, four of them in Asia.

Considering the first topic of analysis, most studies participants were subjects of both gender, except articles by Bertocci et al. (2011), Deckersbach et al. (2008), Malhi et al. (2007), and Thermenos et al. (2010) that only studied women. There were higher prevalence of studies with euthymic phase of BD samples, but three studies considered only depressive episodes in BD subjects (Deckersbach et al., 2008; Roiser et al., 2009; Bertocci et al., 2011). Furthermore, one paper compared a manic/psychotic symptoms group with a euthymic population (Fleck et al., 2005) and another one assessed three groups: mania, depression, and euthymic (Pomarol-Clotet et al., 2014). Articles by Liu et al. (2010) and McCormack et al. (2015) did not characterize explicitly the sample mood despite presented scores of symptoms scales and the study by Gvirts et al. (2015) comprised two subgroups with regard to affective symptoms: asymptomatic and mildly symptomatic patients. Regarding the subtypes of BD, 13 studies used BD I and II mixed groups, nine studies analyzed only BD type I subjects, and one paper compared BD type I, type II, and control groups (Liu et al., 2010).

Most studies evaluated the sample in just one mood episode in BD. Euthymic patients were predominant in the samples (Malhi et al., 2007; Barrett et al., 2008; Dittman et al., 2008; Drapier et al., 2008; Thermenos et al., 2010; Levy et al., 2011; Mullin et al., 2012; Gruber et al., 2013; Lee et al., 2013; Miguélez-Pan et al., 2014; Russo et al., 2014; Bauer et al., 2015; Muhtadie and Johnson, 2015; Sabater et al., 2016), few studies evaluated depressions phases of BD (Deckersbach et al., 2008; Roiser et al., 2009; Bertocci et al., 2011) and only one compared the performance in manic and euthymic episodes in relation to health controls (Fleck et al., 2005). All studies have used between-groups comparison, and only article by Pomarol-Clotet et al. (2014) also had a within-participants design and evaluated the same patients in three characteristics mood phases of BD.

Regarding the intervention, all studies used cognitive tests and self-reported mood scales. Seven studies (Malhi et al., 2007; Deckersbach et al., 2008; Drapier et al., 2008; Thermenos et al., 2010; Bertocci et al., 2011; Mullin et al., 2012; Pomarol-Clotet et al., 2014) also applied functional magnetic resonance imaging (fMRI) to measure brain activity. In relation to the cognitive instruments, 16 studies used span tasks (Malhi et al., 2007; Thompson et al., 2007; Barrett et al., 2008; Dittman et al., 2008; Roiser et al., 2009; Liu et al., 2010; Levy et al., 2011; Gruber et al., 2013; Lee et al., 2013; Miguélez-Pan et al., 2014; Russo et al., 2014; Bauer et al., 2015; Gvirts et al., 2015; McCormack et al., 2015; Muhtadie and Johnson, 2015; Sabater et al., 2016), and six studies chose n-back tasks (Deckersbach et al., 2008; Drapier et al., 2008; Thermenos et al., 2010; Bertocci et al., 2011; Mullin et al., 2012; Pomarol-Clotet et al., 2014), with two of them using the modified EFNBACK instrument. Only one article used a supra span task, the yes/no recognition memory test, based in verbal directed-forgetting paradigm. For the evaluation of mood symptoms, the most used instruments were: Young Mania Rating Scale (YMRS) for mania symptoms (Fleck et al., 2005; Malhi et al., 2007; Thompson et al., 2007; Barrett et al., 2008; Deckersbach et al., 2008; Dittman et al., 2008; Liu et al., 2010; Bertocci et al., 2011; Levy et al., 2011; Mullin et al., 2012; Gruber et al., 2013; Lee et al., 2013; Miguélez-Pan et al., 2014; Pomarol-Clotet et al., 2014; Bauer et al., 2015; Gvirts et al., 2015; McCormack et al., 2015; Sabater et al., 2016); Hamilton Depression Rating Scales (Fleck et al., 2005; Malhi et al., 2007; Thompson et al., 2007; Barrett et al., 2008; Deckersbach et al., 2008; Dittman et al., 2008; Liu et al., 2010; Bertocci et al., 2011; Mullin et al., 2012; Lee et al., 2013; Miguélez-Pan et al., 2014; Pomarol-Clotet et al., 2014; Russo et al., 2014; Gvirts et al., 2015; Sabater et al., 2016), Montgomery Åsberg Depression Rating Scale (Malhi et al., 2007; Roiser et al., 2009; Liu et al., 2010; Bauer et al., 2015; McCormack et al., 2015), and Beck Depression Inventory (Malhi et al., 2007; Thompson et al., 2007; Drapier et al., 2008; Muhtadie and Johnson, 2015) for depressive symptoms (**Table 2**).

Methodologies of selected studies were characterized by the comparison of cognitive variables and mood episodes between clinical and control groups. Seven articles carried just a comparison of cognitive profile between groups (Fleck et al., 2005; Thermenos et al., 2010; Levy et al., 2011; Miguélez-Pan et al., 2014; Pomarol-Clotet et al., 2014; McCormack et al., 2015; Sabater et al., 2016). In addition, eight studies evaluated correlation between variables, such as cognitive pattern and brain activation pattern (Liu et al., 2010), gender and cognitive pattern (Barrett et al., 2008), functionality, and cognition (Bauer et al., 2015), homocysteine levels and cognitive performance (Dittman

TABLE 2 | Summary of WM tasks, cognitive tests, behavioral, and physiological measures used in the selected articles.

Article	Working memory tasks	Cognitive tests	Behavioral measures	Physiological measures
Liu et al., 2010	Word retrieval test from Wechsler Memory Scale-III	Wisconsin Card Sorting Test (WCST); Test for Attention Performance (version 1.02)	Young Mania Rating Scale (YMRS), 17-item Hamilton Rating Scale for Depression (HAM-D-17), Montgomery Åsberg Depression Rating Scale (MADRS)	Fractional anisotropy (FA)
Bertocci et al., 2011	N-back (EFNBACK) task	–	HAM-D-25; YMRS	Functional magnetic resonance imaging (fMRI)
Deckersbach et al., 2008	N-back task	–	HAM-D; YMRS	fMRI
Lee et al., 2013	MATRICS Consensus Cognitive Battery (MCCB)	Facial affect recognition task; Mayer-Salovey-Caruso Emotional Intelligence Test (MSCEIT); Empathic accuracy task; The Awareness of Social Inference Test, Part III (TASIT); Self-referential memory task	HAM-D; YMRS	–
Levy et al., 2011	Digit Span subtest from the Wechsler Adult Intelligence Scale—Third Edition	Trail Making Test (TMT); Controlled Oral Word Association Test (COWAT); Stroop Color-Word Interference Test; WCST; Wechsler Abbreviated Scale of Intelligence (WASI); Letter and Symbol Cancellation Task; California Verbal Learning Test II—Short Form; Logical Memory from Wechsler Memory Scale-R; Rey Complex Figure test (RCFT)	Beck Depression Inventory (BDI-II); YMRS.	–
Miguélez-Pan et al., 2014	WAIS-III Digits Forward; WAIS-III Digits Backward subtest	Token Test (TT); WAIS-III Vocabulary subtest; WCST-64; WAIS-III Similarities subtest; TMT; Tower of London-Drexel University; FAS; Five Point Test (5PT); Stroop Color and Word Test; Frontal Assessment Battery (FAB)	Global Assessment of Functioning (GAF); HAM-D; YMRS	–
Pomarol-Clotet et al., 2014	N-back task	–	YMRS; HAM-D	fMRI
Roiser et al., 2009	Cambridge Neuropsychological Test Automated Battery (CANTAB): Spatial Span, Spatial Working Memory test (SWM)	CANTAB: Intra-dimensional/Extra-dimensional Set-Shifting (ID/ED), Spatial Recognition Memory, Pattern Recognition Memory; Delayed Match to Sample, Rapid Visual Information Processing (RVIP), Cambridge Gamble task, Affective Go/No-go test (AGN), Probabilistic Reversal Learning	MADRS; Inventory of Depressive Symptomatology	–
Thermenos et al., 2010	Two-Back Working Memory Task	Control CPT-X Task; Vocabulary and Block Design subtests of the WAIS-R; reading subtest of the WRAT-R	Profile of Mood States (POMS)	fMRI
Barrett et al., 2008	CANTAB: SWM	CANTAB: Stocking of Cambridge test (SoC); (ID/ED); Set-Shifting task	HAM-D; YMRS	–
Bauer et al., 2015	Cognition in Affective Disorders (BAC-A): Digit Sequencing Task	BAC-A: Token Motor Task, Symbol Coding, List Learning, Category In-stances, Controlled Oral Word Association Test (F and S-words), Tower of London, Emotion Inhibition Test, affective auditory verbal learning test	GAF; MADRS; YMRS	–
Dittman et al., 2008	Wechsler Adult Intelligence Scale III (WAIS-III): Letter-Number Sequencing Subtest (LNST)	TMT; Repeatable Battery for the Assessment of Neuropsychological Status Form A (RBANS)	HAM-D; YMRS	–

(Continued)

TABLE 2 | Continued

Article	Working memory tasks	Cognitive tests	Behavioral measures	Physiological measures
Drapier et al., 2008	N-back working memory task	Baseline attention task	BDI; Altman Self-Rated Mania Scale (ASRM)	fMRI
Fleck et al., 2005	Yes/no recognition memory tests	CPT	YMRS; HAM-D; Scale for the Assessment of Positive Symptoms (SAPS)	–
Gruber et al., 2013	Wechsler Adult Intelligence Scale-Fourth Edition (WAIS-IV): LNST; Affective Working Memory Task	Shipley Institute of Living Scale (SILS)	YMRS; Inventory of Depressive Symptomatology-Clinician Rating (IDS-C)	–
Malhi et al., 2007	Delayed-response working memory paradigm based on the Sternberg memory task	Extracted visual stimuli of Lang Affective Norms for English Words (ANEW) database	HAM-D-17; YMRS; MADRS; GAF; BDI	fMRI task with implicit affective content
Mullin et al., 2012	EFNBACK	–	HAM-D-25; YMRS	fMRI
Russo et al., 2014	MCCB	–	TEMPS-A; HAM-D; Clinician Administered Rating Scale for Mania (CARS-M)	–
Thompson et al., 2007	Digits Forwards; Backwards Digit Span	Self-Ordered Pointing Task –modified version (SOPT); CANTAB; Executive functions and WM tasks: Stroop, initial letter; FAS, TMT	HAM-D; YMRS; BDI ASRM	–
Muhtadie and Johnson, 2015	Automated Symmetry Span Task	–	Self-Reported Emotions; BDI–SF; ARSM	Cardiovascular Physiology
Gvirts et al., 2015	CANTAB: SWM	CANTAB: RVIP, CANTAB's version of the Tower of London task (ToL), ID/ED	HAM-D-17, YMRS, GAF; clinical global impression (CGI)	–
Sabater et al., 2016	Wechsler Memory Scale-Revised (WMSR)	WAIS-III, digit span; TMT-A and B; RCFT; WCST; Tower of Hanoi (TOH-4); Stroop color word test; FAB; Copy RCFT; Eye Test	Visual Analog Scale and the Spanish Version of the Chinese Polarity Inventory; HAM-D; YMRS; CGI-BP	–
McCormack et al., 2015	RBANS; WAIS-III: digit span task and letter–number sequencing tasks	Wechsler Abbreviated Scale of Intelligence; RBANS subscales; CANTAB: ID/ED, SoC, AGN; Ekman 60-Faces emotion recognition test; Awareness of Social Inference Test -A	Family Interview for Genetic Studies (FIGS); Kiddie Schedule for Affective Disorders and Schizophrenia for School-Aged Children – Bipolar Disorder version (K-SADS-BP); K-SADS (WASH-U-KSADS); Diagnostic Interview for Genetic Studies (DIGS); MADRS; Bipolar Depression Rating Scale (BDRS); YMRS; Children's Depression Inventory (CDI)	–

References of the instruments cited in the Table are available on the original articles.

et al., 2008), reaction time and perceptual sensitivity (Fleck et al., 2005), humor and WM (Gruber et al., 2013; Russo et al., 2014), and cognitive pattern (Gvirts et al., 2015). Two of the seven fMRI studies stand out, one described brain activation in different mood phases of BD (Pomarol-Clotet et al., 2014) and the other assessed brain effect of mood induction (Malhi et al., 2007). The article by Muhtadie and Johnson (2015) differ from others because combined evaluation of autonomic variables during WM performance (**Table 1**).

The results showed different brain patterns activity during the performance of WM tests. Most of the neuroimaging studies used n-back tasks to evaluate WM processing. Studies that chose the n-back paradigm found low left dorsal anterior midcingulate cortex (dAMCC) activation in depressive phase of BD type I group (Bertocci et al., 2011), low dorsolateral prefrontal and parietal cortex activation in depression and manic phases (Pomarol-Clotet et al., 2014), and low activity of dorsolateral prefrontal cortex, dorsal anterior cingulate cortex (dACC) and parietal cortex in euthymic group (Mullin et al., 2012). However, some studies have shown conflicting results, as greater prefrontal cortex activation in BD patients and their relatives (Drapier et al., 2008) as well as increased dorsolateral prefrontal cortex and dAMCC activity in episodes of depressed mood (Deckersbach et al., 2008). Low activations in prefrontal cortex in span tasks studies were also confirmed (Malhi et al., 2007; Liu et al., 2010; Thermenos et al., 2010). Article by Liu et al. (2010) indicated that BD type I subjects tend to show lateralized alterations in the right brain hemisphere, while BD type II presented more distributed deficits. In addition, BD patients and their relatives showed frontopolar cortex and insula brain alterations (Thermenos et al., 2010) and euthymic BD subjects exposed to positive and negative valences reported less activation in medial prefrontal cortex, medial frontal cortex, and right parahippocampal gyros (Malhi et al., 2007).

Regarding the cognitive performance of participants in WM tasks, 11 studies demonstrated lower performance in BD patients compared to control groups. Three studies involving processing of visuospatial information (Fleck et al., 2005; Barrett et al., 2008; Gvirts et al., 2015); six papers concerning auditory verbal processing (Dittman et al., 2008; Levy et al., 2011; Gruber et al., 2013; Lee et al., 2013; Pomarol-Clotet et al., 2014; Sabater et al., 2016); and one article studying updating of visuospatial information (Drapier et al., 2008). Concerning effect sizes reported on such articles we decided to analyze mean effect size on studies that produced lower scores for working memory performance. This descriptive analysis showed an average effect size of 0.39 to studies that involved processing of visuospatial information; and 0.41 to the papers concerning auditory verbal processing. The only paper that used measures of updating visuospatial information presented a effect size of 0.33. We can conclude that all the average effect sizes are low (Cohen, 1988). There are also nine papers (Malhi et al., 2007; Deckersbach et al., 2008; Drapier et al., 2008; Liu et al., 2010; Thermenos et al., 2010; Bertocci et al., 2011; Mullin et al., 2012; Pomarol-Clotet et al., 2014; Muhtadie and Johnson, 2015) that reported a variety of neurobiological changes in BD patients (e.g., prefrontal cortex activation or dorsal anterior cingulate cortex; see **Table 3**).

However, four studies found no difference between groups (Roiser et al., 2009; Miguélez-Pan et al., 2014; Bauer et al., 2015; McCormack et al., 2015). Article by Pomarol-Clotet et al. (2014) distinguished cognitive profiles according to the mood phases of patients, showing that manic or depressive episodes in BD reported worse performance in WM tasks compared with euthymic and controls groups. However, WM deficits (Thompson et al., 2007; Drapier et al., 2008) and other cognitive low scores can also be observed in euthymic phase, for example, visuospatial WM (Barrett et al., 2008), short-term non-affective memory (Bauer et al., 2015), unsocial cognition (Lee et al., 2013), flexibility, plan implementing, set-shifting (Miguélez-Pan et al., 2014), processing speed, resistance to interference and emotion recognition (Sabater et al., 2016), and verbal fluency (Barrett et al., 2008; Miguélez-Pan et al., 2014; Bauer et al., 2015). In addition, WM performance was associated with cyclothymic levels and irritability in euthymic episodes (Russo et al., 2014; **Table 3**).

Euthymic patients during conducted span tasks showed deficits in several WM components, such as auditory information updating (Thompson et al., 2007), simultaneous processing of visuospatial information (Barrett et al., 2008), and processing of auditory-verbal information (Thompson et al., 2007; Dittman et al., 2008; Levy et al., 2011; Gruber et al., 2013; Lee et al., 2013). BD type I patients also reported lower scores for updating visuospatial information during the n-back task (Drapier et al., 2008).

Some researches of euthymic samples used auditory-verbal complex span tasks (Miguélez-Pan et al., 2014; Bauer et al., 2015; Sabater et al., 2016). Nevertheless, clinical groups performed similarly to controls in processing auditory information (Miguélez-Pan et al., 2014; Bauer et al., 2015). Article by Roiser et al. (2009) also did not found deficits to perform a visuospatial span task in depressive episodes in BD patients during washout of psychotropic medications.

A prevalence of quantitative cross-sectional methodology experiment designs were characterized in selected articles (Fleck et al., 2005; Malhi et al., 2007; Thompson et al., 2007; Barrett et al., 2008; Dittman et al., 2008; Drapier et al., 2008; Roiser et al., 2009; Liu et al., 2010; Thermenos et al., 2010; Bertocci et al., 2011; Mullin et al., 2012; Gruber et al., 2013; Lee et al., 2013; Pomarol-Clotet et al., 2014; Russo et al., 2014; Bauer et al., 2015; Gvirts et al., 2015; McCormack et al., 2015; Muhtadie and Johnson, 2015; Sabater et al., 2016). Only three studies used other experimental designs, such as cohort study (Levy et al., 2011), descriptive study (Miguélez-Pan et al., 2014), and prospective study (Deckersbach et al., 2008) (**Table 1**).

DISCUSSION

The aims of the present systematic review were (i) update the knowledge about working memory deficits in BD; (ii) to analyze if BD patients show WM low scores, contrasting studies that used complex span tasks and n-back tasks, and (iii) to investigate if different BD mood episodes could predict different patterns of cognitive processes based on the WM components of the

TABLE 3 | Summary of WM performance and neurobiological changes in BD subjects in selected articles categorized according WM processes and modalities.

Article	Performance in WM tasks	WM processes and modalities	Effect size	Neurobiological alterations
Barrett et al., 2008	↓	Processing of visuospatial information	0.58 (r)	–
Fleck et al., 2005	↓	Processing of visuospatial information	0.23 (η)	–
Gvirts et al., 2015	↓	Processing of visuospatial information	0.21 (d)	–
Muhtadie and Johnson, 2015	–	Processing of visuospatial information	0.76 (d)	Autonomic changes associated with emotional reactivity during cognitive tasks
Roiser et al., 2009	=	Processing of visuospatial information	−0.16 (d)	–
Russo et al., 2014	WM performance was associated with cyclothymic levels and irritability in euthymic episodes	Processing of visuospatial and auditory-verbal information	0.54 (r)	–
Bauer et al., 2015	=	Processing of auditory-verbal information	–	–
Dittman et al., 2008	↓	Processing of auditory-verbal information	0.41 (d)	–
Gruber et al., 2013	↓	Processing of auditory-verbal information	0.26 (η)	–
Lee et al., 2013	↓	Processing of auditory-verbal information	0.61 (η)	–
Lee et al., 2013	↓	Processing of auditory-verbal information	0.61 (η)	–
Levy et al., 2011	↓	Processing of auditory-verbal information	0.56 (d)	–
Liu et al., 2010	–	Processing of auditory-verbal information	–	BD I: lateralized changes in the right hemisphere and more cognitivedeficits. BD II: more distributed deficits associated with cognitive and emotional processes
McCormack et al., 2015	=	Processing of auditory-verbal information	–	–
Miguélez-Pan et al., 2014	=	Processing of auditory-verbal information	−0.29 (d)	–
Sabater et al., 2016	↓ BD patients in anticonvulsant therapy	Processing of auditory-verbal information	0.16 (η)	–
Thompson et al., 2007	↓	↓ auditory information updating/ ↓ processing of auditory-verbal information	0.39 (d)	–
Bertocci et al., 2011	–	Updating visuospatial information	0.75 (d)	↓ dAMCC activation with neutral stimuli in depressive episodes
Deckersbach et al., 2008	–	Updating visuospatial information	0.07 (d)	↑ DLPFC and dACC activation when negative valence stimuli were presented
			0.03 (r)	
Drapier et al., 2008	↓	Updating visuospatial information	0.33 (η)	↓ prefrontal cortex activation
Malhi et al., 2007	–	Updating visuospatial information	–	↓ prefrontal cortex activation
Mullin et al., 2012	–	Updating visuospatial information	–	↓ prefrontal cortex activation
Pomarol-Clotet et al., 2014	↓ manic and depressive episodes	Updating visuospatial information	–	Parietal alterations in manic and depressive episodes
Thermenos et al., 2010	–	Updating visuospatial information	1.05 and 1.33 (d)	Frontopolar cortex and insula alterations brain

WM, working memory; dACC, dorsal anterior cingulate cortex; dAMCC, left dorsal anterior midcingulate cortex; DLPFC, left dorsolateral prefrontal cortex; BD, bipolar disorder; d, Cohen's d; n, Eta-squared; r, Pearson's correlation; =, no significant differences.

tasks in each mood phase. Considering the first objective our study found similar results to previous systematic review and meta-analyses pointing to working memory deficits in Bipolar patients (Robinson et al., 2006; Torres et al., 2007; Kurtz and Gerraty, 2009; Bora et al., 2011; Mann-Wrobel et al., 2011). Most of these reviews pointed to verbal working memory deficits in BD (Robinson et al., 2006; Torres et al., 2007; Kurtz and Gerraty, 2009). These findings could be explained by the fact that those reviews considered only digit span measures. In our review, we included both verbal and visuospatial working memory measures. In agreement with previous reviews, we found that both verbal and visuospatial working memory are impaired in BD (Bora et al., 2011; Mann-Wrobel et al., 2011).

Considering objective (ii) and (iii) they were respectively presented in Sections Introduction and Methods. This review seems to be necessary because individual results of studies are confusing, due to the fact that there are three emotional phases in BD (euthymic, euphoric, and depressed) and different WM mental operations (serial recall and update), which are expressed in at least two different modalities (phonological and visuospatial) (**Table 4**). For this purpose, after the selection of the articles according to the inclusion and exclusion criteria, a systematic review was carried out. Twenty-three studies in the restricted period 2005–2016 were found using different approaches as cognitive, behavioral, neuroimaging, and measures of autonomic responses. The study also convey the possibility of

TABLE 4 | Summary of mental WM operations and phonological and visuospatial modalities in three emotional phases in BD presented in the selected articles.

Modality/task	Euthymic	Depressive	Manic
Verbal n-back	–	–	–
Visuospatial n-back	Malhi et al., 2007; Drapier et al., 2008; Mullin et al., 2012	Deckersbach et al., 2008; Pomarol-Clotet et al., 2014	Pomarol-Clotet et al., 2014
Verbal span	Thompson et al., 2007; Dittman et al., 2008; Levy et al., 2011; Gruber et al., 2013; Lee et al., 2013; Sabater et al., 2016[a]	–	–
Visuospatial span	Fleck et al., 2005[b]; Barrett et al., 2008; Gvirts et al., 2015[c]	–	–

[a] *BD anticonvulsant therapy.*
[b] *Supra span task.*
[c] *Mildly affective symptoms.*

Bipolar Disorder as model for the study of the new component of WM, the Hedonic Detector, for this reason the relationship among WM and other clinical features in the final section.

Cognitive Deficits and Neurobiological Correlates in BD Patients

Regarding the first aim of this review, statistically significant differences in WM performance between groups were found in most studies (Fleck et al., 2005; Thompson et al., 2007; Barrett et al., 2008; Deckersbach et al., 2008; Dittman et al., 2008; Drapier et al., 2008; Levy et al., 2011; Gruber et al., 2013; Lee et al., 2013; Pomarol-Clotet et al., 2014; Gvirts et al., 2015; Sabater et al., 2016). These results confirm that BD patients tend to have lower WM performance (MacQueen et al., 2005; Thompson et al., 2007; Lee et al., 2014; Daglas et al., 2015). According to our review both modalities are disrupted, deficits in auditory-verbal information processing were reported in six selected articles (Thompson et al., 2007; Dittman et al., 2008; Levy et al., 2011; Gruber et al., 2013; Lee et al., 2013; Sabater et al., 2016) and visuospatial low scores in five other studies (Fleck et al., 2005; Barrett et al., 2008; Drapier et al., 2008; Pomarol-Clotet et al., 2014; Gvirts et al., 2015). Our analysis also showed that the effect sizes of the studies that reported deficit on BD patients on several measures of working memory were small, either on updating or maintenance measures. These effect sizes were 0.33, 0.39, and 0.41, respectively, for updating visuospatial information, processing of visuospatial information, and processing of auditory verbal information. Together with results reported on the papers that showed neurobiological changes of BD patients during the experiments, these results clearly conclude that BD affects both working memory performance and brain functioning.

According to a recent meta-analysis, there is no consensus in the literature defining if cognitive deficits are somatic markers or a consequence of mood episodes in BD (Daglas et al., 2015). Previous researches have shown that information processing, visual episodic memory, and verbal WM deficit were associated with clinical expressions of BD, since it was not observed in first-degree relatives. Therefore, these cognitive lower performances in BD were not associated with genetic susceptibility (Bora et al., 2009). A review by Boland and Alloy (2013) showed that sleep disruption present in BD patients can also be either a predisposing factor or worsening neurocognitive deficits throughout the illness course, resulting in sustained functional deficit, despite the remission of mood symptoms.

Other studies also claimed that the level of neuropsychological deficits in BD was influenced by anti-psychotics and mood stabilizers (Donaldson et al., 2003; Savitz et al., 2008), weakening the hypothesis of WM as a somatic marker of BD. Most studies in the present review used medicated samples, except the article by Roiser et al. (2009) that apparently did this variable. Although, the participants were taking psychotropic medication during assessments, most of the studies of euthymic samples reported significant WM deficits (Thompson et al., 2007; Barrett et al., 2008; Dittman et al., 2008; Drapier et al., 2008; Levy et al., 2011; Gruber et al., 2013; Lee et al., 2013). Then, at least in these cases, results do not satisfy the state-independence criterion mentioned by some authors as a key factor in assessing potential endophenotypes of BD (Hasler et al., 2006). Also, the results suggested that WM can be a susceptibility biomarker in BD patients rather than a state-dependent variable of the disorder (Gruber et al., 2009; Kurtz and Gerraty, 2009).

Despite neurobiological correlates of WM are not clearly elucidated in literature, there is evidence of the association between neuropsychological and morphological factors in BD, which support WM deficits as a possible endophenotype of BD (Glahn et al., 2010). Based on 12 studies, a meta-analysis conducted by Lee et al. (2014) showed generalized neuropsychological deficits since the first episode of the disorder. In theory, patients with BD due to the constant changes in both emotional valences; would have an uncalibrated Hedonic Detector. Consequently it would cause deficits in WM as predicted in Baddeley's model (Baddeley, 2007). Besides, in the current review, some studies observed social cognitive deficits affecting emotional response, which is an indirect evidence of dysfunctional Hedonic Detector.

Although, assessing WM deficits in people at high genetic risk of developing BD had not been an objective of this study, it was observed that some authors considered heritability (Drapier et al., 2008; Thermenos et al., 2010; McCormack et al., 2015). Relatives without psychiatric diagnoses did not report significant deficits in WM, but they showed lower scores for verbal reasoning and affective response inhibition (McCormack et al., 2015). In contrast, relatives as BD patients also showed alterations in prefrontal cortex activity and insula during WM task (Drapier et al., 2008; Thermenos et al., 2010). These results show that WM deficits are not only state variables, but seem to be primary character of the disease (Gruber et al., 2009; Kurtz and Gerraty, 2009).

However, based on the reviewed articles there is insufficient data to conclude that WM deficits are present since the onset of disease. Only one study considered population between 18 and 25 years old and it did not show lower WM scores in BD patients (McCormack et al., 2015). Among the eight researches that studied sample aged ranging from 26 to 35 years, three articles showed deficits in WM (Fleck et al., 2005; Gruber et al., 2013; Sabater et al., 2016) and four described neurocognitive deficits in BD patients (Malhi et al., 2007; Deckersbach et al., 2008; Bertocci et al., 2011; Mullin et al., 2012). Ten out of fourteen studies found poor WM performance or other neuropsychological deficits in middle age sample (Thompson et al., 2007; Barrett et al., 2008; Dittman et al., 2008; Drapier et al., 2008; Liu et al., 2010; Thermenos et al., 2010; Levy et al., 2011; Lee et al., 2013; Pomarol-Clotet et al., 2014; Gvirts et al., 2015). There was no study with sample above fifty six years old.

Different Patterns of Cognitive Processes in Each Mood Phase

The second objective of this review was to investigate if diverse BD mood would predict a different WM pattern. Updating deficits of visuospatial information were found in depressive BD patients assessed by n-back tasks (Deckersbach et al., 2008; Pomarol-Clotet et al., 2014) and in mania phases (Pomarol-Clotet et al., 2014). Despite WM alterations have been reported during mood episodes of BD, it is suggested that deficits in WM persist during remission of symptoms (MacQueen et al., 2005; Thompson et al., 2007; Daglas et al., 2015; Farahmand et al., 2015).

According to neurophysiological studies in euthymic phases of BD, patients presented lower prefrontal cortex activation during visuospatial n-back tasks (Malhi et al., 2007; Drapier et al., 2008; Mullin et al., 2012). Mullin et al. (2012), for example, found lower dorsal anterior cingulate cortex (dACC) activity during EFNBACK task with neutral stimuli. In addition, depressive episodes in BD patients showed lower left dorsal anterior midcingulate cortex (dAMCC) activation during visuospatial n-back task with neutral stimuli (Bertocci et al., 2011). In contrast, a different brain activation pattern was reported during n-back tasks with emotional auditory-verbal stimuli. Such as greater left dorsolateral prefrontal cortex (DLPFC) and dACC activation were found when negative valence stimuli were presented (Deckersbach et al., 2008). Therefore, it was suggested that updating was influenced by emotional factors.

According to processing efficiency theory (Eysenck and Calvo, 1992), high levels of anxiety reduce the efficiency of cognitive processing, specifically the central executive of the WM system (Derakshan et al., 2009), confirming the influence of emotions on updating. Besides there are three major control functions of the central executive: inhibition, shifting, and updating (Miyake et al., 2000), study by Eysenck et al. (2007), based on attentional control theory showed that anxiety impairs two major functions of the central executive: negative attentional control (inhibition function) and positive attentional control (shifting function).

In addition, to the decrease activation in dorsolateral prefrontal cortex, parietal alterations in manic, and depressive episodes of BD patients were reported during visuospatial tasks (Pomarol-Clotet et al., 2014). Even in euthymic patients the brain activation pattern varied depending on the mood valences (Malhi et al., 2007). Thus, there was more activity in dACC and amygdala regions over negative valences and a greater connection between dACC and amygdala regions in positive valences (Mullin et al., 2012). It is consistent with the Somatic Marker hypothesis that supports physiological influence on emotional responses through the central executive (Damasio et al., 1991; Damasio, 1998). It was also verified the existence of autonomic changes associated with emotional reactivity during cognitive tasks (Muhtadie and Johnson, 2015). Then, by inference it seems that Hedonic Detector is also affected in WM tasks requiring information updating.

Remarkably, few studies assessed WM performance in more than one mood episode (Fleck et al., 2005; Pomarol-Clotet et al., 2014). Only four papers carried out mood induction prior performing tasks (Malhi et al., 2007; Deckersbach et al., 2008; Bertocci et al., 2011; Mullin et al., 2012) and just the research of autonomic response used a verbal stressor during the test (Muhtadie and Johnson, 2015). In this way, it is difficult to generalize the results for the second objective of this review. In addition, many studies selected BD I patients samples (Fleck et al., 2005; Malhi et al., 2007; Deckersbach et al., 2008; Drapier et al., 2008; Bertocci et al., 2011; Levy et al., 2011; Mullin et al., 2012; Gruber et al., 2013), and few studies assessed BD II subjects. Most papers did not differentiate subtypes of the disorder.

Despite Baddeley's model is the most commonly used theory in WM researches (Malhi et al., 2007; Thompson et al., 2007; Barrett et al., 2008; Dittman et al., 2008; Roiser et al., 2009; Liu et al., 2010; Levy et al., 2011; Gruber et al., 2013; Lee et al., 2013; Miguélez-Pan et al., 2014; Russo et al., 2014; Bauer et al., 2015; Muhtadie and Johnson, 2015), the discrepancies between studies may be explained by the new appearance neuroscience technologies that demand designed tasks such as n-back tasks (Deckersbach et al., 2008; Drapier et al., 2008) to investigate state-based models (D'Esposito, 2007). It appears that authors rarely made the connection between theoretical models and cognitive tasks. Then, despite the fact of some studies confirmed emotion and WM association in depressive or manic BD patients (Malhi et al., 2007; Deckersbach et al., 2008; Mullin et al., 2012; Pomarol-Clotet et al., 2014; Muhtadie and Johnson, 2015), the Hedonic Detector component was not considered in these selected articles of this review.

Once n-back tasks and complex span tasks apparently evaluate different processes (Ribeiro et al., submitted; Kane et al., 2007), WM researches should consider the differences between tasks and how they affect the result explanations (Redick and Lindsey, 2013; Remoli and Santos, 2017). That seems to be crucial for explaining the outcomes and for the replication of future studies (Ribeiro et al., submitted). Further restriction of this review is that diagnoses of BD suffered some changes from DSM-IV (American Psychiatric Association, 2000) to DSM-V (American Psychiatric Association, 2013). This fact could lead some methodological differences in selected studies. However, it was not the purpose of this work to analyze diagnoses differences of BD.

Relationship among WM and other Clinical Features

Only article by Liu et al. (2010) compared BD I and BD II subjects. They showed that neural activation patterns were different between subgroups of the disorder during auditory-verbal information processing tasks. BD type I patients reported lateralized changes in the right hemisphere and more cognitive deficits while BD type II subjects revealed more distributed lower performance associated with cognitive and emotional processes.

In addition to this other evidence suggest that BD I and II patients present different neuropathological substrates in terms of the loss of bundle coherence or the disruption of fiber tracts (Liu et al., 2010), BD type I and II also exhibit heterogeneous clinical presentations and cognitive functions. Besides BD I patients manifested more cognitive dysfunction in verbal learning, recall, recognition, and set-shifting compared to bipolar II patients (Simonsen et al., 2008), it has been suggested that both suicide and attempted suicide are more common in BD II disorder than in BD I disorder (Jamison, 2000; Rihmer and Kiss, 2002; Hawton et al., 2005).

Article by Levy et al. (2011) showed that BD I patients readmitted to the hospital after 3-month had more psychotic episodes, lower level of global functionality, severe mood episodes, and lower scores for executive function, attention, and WM, visual, and verbal episodic memory performance comparing to outpatients care. While WM low score in BD type I samples were suggested in some studies (Drapier et al., 2008; Levy et al., 2011; Pomarol-Clotet et al., 2014), WM deficits were not found in the majority of BD II sample (Roiser et al., 2009). BD I hospitalized in mania/mixed with psychotic symptoms group also reported lower scores for recognition effectiveness and directed-forgetting effectiveness than expected (Fleck et al., 2005).

Although, epidemiological studies with non-clinical populations have suggested psychotic experiences as a predictor of suicidal behavior (Nishida et al., 2010; DeVylder et al., 2015) and study by Finseth et al. (2012) showed that suicidal attempt are more common in patients with mood disorders with psychotic features, this has not been a consensus in all studies. Besides psychotic symptoms are more common in BD type I patients, a recent study by Gesi et al. (2016) showed that psychotic features, as evaluated upon the presence of delusions or hallucinations, are not associated with suicidality among subjects with BD I, suggesting that suicide behavior is more common in BD type II disorder.

It is important to note that anxiety (Derakshan et al., 2009) and even mood (Derakshan et al., 2009) could modulate cognitive performance as, for example, attentional control. Future studies should address the role of mood states and even positive and negative emotions in working memory in BD patients to explore the role of hedonic detector.

Emotional States and Working Memory: Hedonic Detector and Its Implication to Cognition in Mood Disorders

In fact, the connection between emotional states and working memory plays a role in the measurement instruments and in theoretical framework as well. For instance, the Somatic Marker hypothesis presented by Damasio et al. (1991) describes a mechanism for interaction between emotion and cognition in trial processes and decision-making (Bechara and Damasio, 2002, 2005; Bechara et al., 2005; Verdejo-García and Bechara, 2009). Damasio even states that the executive component of WM could be relevant in this process. Baddeley's model of WM explicitly addressed the interference of emotions in WM information processing, by its new component, the Hedonic Detector (Baddeley, 2007). The Hedonic Detector works as a neutral point that varies between positive and negative valences in response to environmental stimuli. It establishes a mean value between stimulus and information retained in the WM to enable choices of future actions (Baddeley, 2007). In this perspective, improper adjustment of the neutral point could enhance the appearance of pathological affective episodes, for instance, the Bipolar Disorder (BD).

Deficits in WM processing have been consistently reported in euthymic patients (MacQueen et al., 2005; Thompson et al., 2007; Daglas et al., 2015). Another study also observed that euthymic BD type I had worse performance on visuospatial tasks compared to healthy subjects (Farahmand et al., 2015). Although, there is no consensus in the literature, these findings suggest that lower performance in WM could result in the intensification of emotional valences. In other words, the presence of WM deficits, could be considered a primary trace of BD, beyond state variables (Gruber et al., 2009; Kurtz and Gerraty, 2009). However, this particular issue remains controversial due to the diversity of methodologies used across the studies. Apart from the prevalence of within-subjects design, studies rarely made the connection between theoretical models and cognitive tasks, hindering the comprehension about WM components.

In line with this argument, a review by Baddeley (2013) showed that in depressive patients negative mood influences hedonic judgment, explaining the trend of the negative perception of the situations in this clinical population. However, there is no significant evidence in respect to the influence of positive mood in hedonic detection system. Hypothetically, assuming that the neutral point in BD patients corresponds to euthymic phase, the exacerbated positive and negative valences would account for euphoric or depressed mood, respectively (Baddeley, 2007, 2013). As emotion in BD is deregulated, the study of this disorder seems to be necessary to understand the influence of improper adjustment of the Hedonic Detector neutral point in WM.

CONCLUSION

In conclusion, BD mood episodes were associated with both WM processes (updating and serial recall), cognitive lower performance persist even in remission of symptoms. This evidence suggests that BD patients have deficits in monitoring content in WM. But the data at this point is so different across studies that it does not seem prudent to generalize conclusions. Considering that WM deficit apparently is stage-independent in BD patients (Gruber et al., 2009; Kurtz and Gerraty, 2009), future studies should evaluate the convergence of Damasio's Somatic Marker hypotheses and Baddeley's Hedonic Detector in BD. In other words, how the neutral point is deregulated by the interaction between environmental stimuli and mood episodes and affect WM processes.

AUTHOR CONTRIBUTIONS

Conception or design of the work: CS and FS. Data collection: CS. Data analysis and interpretation: CS and FS. Drafting the article: CS, FS, PA, and LM. Critical revision of the article: FS, PA, and LM. Final approval of the version to be published: CS, FS, PA, and LM. Agreement to be accountable for all aspects of the work in ensuring that questions related to the accuracy or integrity of any part of the work are appropriately investigated and resolved: CS, FS, PA, and LM.

REFERENCES

Ajilore, O., Vizueta, N., Walshaw, P., Zhan, L., Leow, A., and Altshuler, L. L. (2015). Connectome signatures of neurocognitive abnormalities in euthymic bipolar I disorder. *J. Psychiatr. Res.* 68, 37–44. doi: 10.1016/j.jpsychires.2015.05.017

Allen, D. N., Bello, D. T., and Thaler, N. S. (2015). Neurocognitive predictors of performance-based functional capacity in bipolar disorder. *J. Neuropsychol.* 9, 159–171. doi: 10.1111/jnp.12042

American Psychiatric Association (2013). *Diagnostic and Statistical Manual of Mental Disorders, 5th Edn.* Washington, DC: American Psychiatric Association.

Arts, B., Jabben, N., Krabbendam, L., and van Os, J. (2009). Meta-analyses of cognitive functioning in euthymic bipolar patients and their first-degree relatives - correction. *Psychol. Med.* 39, 525. doi: 10.1017/S0033291708004972

American Psychiatric Association (2000). *Diagnostic and Statistical Manual of Mental Disorders (DSM-IV).* Arlington, TX: Springer; American Psychiatric Association.

Baddeley, A. (2013). Working memory and emotion: ruminations on a theory of depression. *Rev. Gen. Psychol.* 17, 20–27. doi: 10.1037/a0030029

Baddeley, A., Banse, R., Huang, Y.-M., and Page, M. (2012). Working memory and emotion: detecting the hedonic detector. *J. Cogn. Psychol.* 24, 6–16. doi: 10.1080/20445911.2011.613820

Baddeley, A. D. (1986). *Working Memory.* Oxford: Clarendon Press.

Baddeley, A. D. (2000). The episodic buffer: a new component of working memory? *Trends Cogn. Sci.* 4, 417–423. doi: 10.1016/S1364-6613(00)01538-2

Baddeley, A. D. (2007). *Working Memory, Thought and Action.* Oxford: Oxford University Press.

Balanzá-Martínez, V., Rubio, C., Selva-Vera, G., Martinez-Aran, A., Sánchez-Moreno, J., Salazar-Fraile, J., et al. (2008). Neurocognitive endophenotypes (endophenocognitypes) from studies of relatives of bipolar disorder subjects: a systematic review. *Neurosci. Biobehav. Rev.* 32, 1426–1438. doi: 10.1016/j.neubiorev.2008.05.019

Barrett, S. L., Kelly, C., Bell, R., and King, D. J. (2008). Gender influences the detection of spatial working memory deficits in bipolar disorder. *Bipolar Disord.* 10, 647–654. doi: 10.1111/j.1399-5618.2008.00592.x

Bauer, I. E., Keefe, R. S. E., Sanches, M., Suchting, R., Green, C. E., and Soares, J. C. (2015). Evaluation of cognitive function in bipolar disorder using the Brief Assessment of Cognition in Affective Disorders (BAC-A). *J. Psychiatr. Res.* 60, 81–86. doi: 10.1016/j.jpsychires.2014.10.002

Bechara, A., and Damasio, A. R. (2005). The somatic marker hypothesis: a neural theory of economic decision. *Games Econ. Behav.* 52, 336–372. doi: 10.1016/j.geb.2004.06.010

Bechara, A., and Damasio, H. (2002). Decision-making and addiction (part I): impaired activation of somatic states in substance dependent individuals when pondering decisions with negative future consequences. *Neuropsychologia* 40, 1675–1689. doi: 10.1016/S0028-3932(02)00015-5

Bechara, A., Damasio, H., Tranel, D., and Damasio, A. R. (2005). The Iowa Gambling task and the somatic marker hypothesis: some questions and answers. *Trends Cogn. Sci.* 9, 159–162. doi: 10.1016/j.tics.2005.02.002

Bento, T. (2014). Revisões sistemáticas em desporto e saúde: orientações para o planeamento, elaboração, redação e avaliação. *Motricidade* 10, 107–123. doi: 10.6063/motricidade.10(2).3699

Bertocci, M. A., Bebko, G. M., Mullin, B. C., Langenecker, S. A., Ladouceur, C. D., Almeida, J. R. C., et al. (2011). Abnormal anterior cingulate cortical activity during emotional n-back task performance distinguishes bipolar from unipolar depressed females. *Psychol. Med.* 42, 1417–1428. doi: 10.1017/S003329171100242X

Boland, E. M., and Alloy, L. B. (2013). Sleep disturbance and cognitive deficits in bipolar disorder: toward an integrated examination of disorder maintenance and functional impairment. *Clin. Psychol. Rev.* 33, 33–44. doi: 10.1016/j.cpr.2012.10.001

Bora, E., Bartholomeusz, C., and Pantelis, C. (2016). Meta-analysis of Theory of Mind (ToM) impairment in bipolar disorder. *Psychol. Med.* 46, 253–264. doi: 10.1017/S0033291715001993

Bora, E., Yucel, M., and Pantelis, C. (2009). Cognitive endophenotypes of bipolar disorder: a meta-analysis of neuropsychological deficits in euthymic patients and their first-degree relatives. *J. Affect. Disord.* 113, 1–20. doi: 10.1016/j.jad.2008.06.009

Bora, E., Yücel, M., Pantelis, C., and Berk, M. (2011). Meta-analytic review of neurocognition in bipolar II disorder. *Acta Psychiatr. Scand.* 123, 165–174. doi: 10.1111/j.1600-0447.2010.01638.x

Chang, Y.-H., Chen, S.-L., Lee, S.-Y., Hsu, Y.-W., Wu, J. Y.-W., Chen, S.-H., et al. (2012). Neuropsychological functions in bipolar disorders I and II with and without comorbid alcohol dependence. *Prog. Neuro Psychopharmacol. Biol. Psychiatry* 37, 211–216. doi: 10.1016/j.pnpbp.2012.01.015

Clark, L., Iversen, S. D., and Goodwin, G. M. (2001). A neuropsychological investigation of prefrontal cortex involvement in acute mania. *Am. J. Psychiatry* 158, 1605–1611. doi: 10.1176/appi.ajp.158.10.1605

Cohen, J. (1988). *Statistical Power Analysis for the Behavioral Sciences, 2nd Edn.* Hillsdale, NJ: Lawrence Erbaum.

Conway, A. R. A., and Kovacs, K. (2013). Individual differences in intelligence and working memory. *Psychol. Learn. Motiv.* 233–270. doi: 10.1016/B978-0-12-407237-4.00007-4

Cullen, B., Ward, J., Graham, N. A., Deary, I. J., Pell, J. P., Smith, D. J., et al. (2016). Prevalence and correlates of cognitive impairment in euthymic adults with bipolar disorder: a systematic review. *J. Affect. Disord.* 205, 165–181. doi: 10.1016/j.jad.2016.06.063

Daglas, R., Yücel, M., Cotton, S., Allott, K., Hetrick, S., and Berk, M. (2015). Cognitive impairment in first-episode mania: a systematic review of the evidence in the acute and remission phases of the illness. *Int. J. Bipolar Disord.* 3:9. doi: 10.1186/s40345-015-0024-2

Damasio, A. R. (1998). The somatic marker hypothesis and the possible functions of the prefrontal cortex. *Prefrontal Cortex Exec. Cogn. Funct.* 351, 36–50. doi: 10.1093/acprof:oso/9780198524410.003.0004

Damasio, A. R., Tranel, D., and Damasio, H. (1991). "Somatic markers and the guidance of behaviour: theory and preliminary testing," in *Frontal Lobe Function and Dysfunction*, eds H. S. Levin, H. M. Eisenberg, and A. L. Benton (New York, NY: Oxford University Press), 217–229.

Daneman, M., and Merikle, P. M. (1996). Working memory and language comprehension: a meta-analysis. *Psychon. Bull. Rev.* 3, 422–433. doi: 10.3758/BF03214546

Deckersbach, T., Rauch, S. L., Buhlmann, U., Ostacher, M. J., Beucke, J.-C., Nierenberg, A. A., et al. (2008). An fMRI investigation of working memory and sadness in females with bipolar disorder: a brief report. *Bipolar Disord.* 10, 928–942. doi: 10.1111/j.1399-5618.2008.00633.x

Derakshan, N., Smyth, S., and Eysenck, M. W. (2009). Effects of state anxiety on performance using a task-switching paradigm: an investigation of attentional control theory. *Psychon. Bull. Rev.* 16, 1112–1117. doi: 10.3758/PBR.16.6.1112

D'Esposito, M. (2007). From cognitive to neural models of working memory. *Philos. Trans. R. Soc. B.* 362, 761–772. doi: 10.1098/rstb.2007.2086

DeVylder, J. E., Thompson, E., Reeves, G., and Schiffman, J. (2015). Psychotic experiences as indicators of suicidal ideation in a non-clinical college sample. *Psychiatry Res.* 226, 489–493. doi: 10.1016/j.psychres.2015.02.007

Dittman, S., Seemuller, F., Grunze, H. C., Schwarz, M. J., Zach, J., Fast, K., et al. (2008). The impact of homocysteine levels on cognition in euthymic bipolar patients. *J. Clin. Psychiatry* 69, 899–906. doi: 10.4088/JCP.v69n0603

Donaldson, S., Goldstein, L. H., Landau, S., Raymont, V., and Frangou, S. (2003). The maudsley bipolar disorder project. *J. Clin. Psychiatry* 64, 86–93. doi: 10.4088/JCP.v64n0116

Drapier, D., Surguladze, S., Marshall, N., Schulze, K., Fern, A., Hall, M.-H., et al. (2008). Genetic liability for bipolar disorder is characterized by excess frontal activation in response to a working memory task. *Biol. Psychiatry* 64, 513–520. doi: 10.1016/j.biopsych.2008.04.038

Eysenck, M. W., and Calvo, M. G. (1992). Anxiety and performance: the processing efficiency theory. *Cogn. Emot.* 6, 409–434. doi: 10.1080/02699939208409696

Eysenck, M. W., Derakshan, N., Santos, R., and Calvo, M. G. (2007). Anxiety and cognitive performance: attentional control theory. *Emotion* 7, 336–353. doi: 10.1037/1528-3542.7.2.336

Farahmand, Z., Tehrani-Doost, M., Amini, H., Mohammadi, A., Mirzaei, M., and Mohamadzadeh, A. (2015). Working memory and response inhibition in patients with bipolar I disorder during euthymic period. *Iran. J. Psychiatry Behav. Sci.* 9:e209. doi: 10.17795/ijpbs209

Finseth, P. I., Morken, G., Andreassen, O. A., Malt, U. F., and Vaaler, A. E. (2012). Risk factors related to lifetime suicide attempts in acutely admitted bipolar disorder inpatients. *Bipolar Disord.* 14, 727–734. doi: 10.1111/bdi.12004

Fleck, D. E., Shear, P. K., and Strakowski, S. M. (2005). Processing efficiency and directed forgetting in bipolar disorder. *J. Int. Neuropsychol. Soc.* 11, 871–880. doi: 10.1017/s1355617705051027

Gesi, C., Carmassi, C., Miniati, M., Benvenuti, A., Massimetti, G., and Dell'Osso, L. (2016). Psychotic spectrum symptoms across the lifespan are related to lifetime suicidality among 147 patients with bipolar I or major depressive disorder. *Ann. Gen. Psychiatry* 15:15. doi: 10.1186/s12991-016-0101-7

Glahn, D. C., Almasy, L., Barguil, M., Hare, E., Peralta, J. M., Kent, J. W., et al. (2010). Neurocognitive endophenotypes for bipolar disorder identified in multiplex multigenerational families. *Arch. Gen. Psychiatry* 67, 168. doi: 10.1001/archgenpsychiatry.2009.184

Gruber, J., Purcell, A. L., Perna, M. J., and Mikels, J. A. (2013). Letting go of the bad: deficit in maintaining negative, but not positive, emotion in bipolar disorder. *Emotion* 13, 168–175. doi: 10.1037/a0029381

Gruber, O., Tost, H., Henseler, I., Schmael, C., Scherk, H., Ende, G., et al. (2009). Pathological amygdala activation during working memory performance: evidence for a pathophysiological trait marker in bipolar affective disorder. *Hum. Brain Mapp.* 31, 115–125 doi: 10.1002/hbm.20849

Gvirts, H. Z., Braw, Y., Harari, H., Lozin, M., Bloch, Y., Fefer, K., et al. (2015). Executive dysfunction in bipolar disorder and borderline personality disorder. *Euro. Psychiatry* 30, 959–964. doi: 10.1016/j.eurpsy.2014.12.009

Hasler, G., Drevets, W. C., Gould, T. D., Gottesman, I. I., and Manji, H. K. (2006). Toward constructing an endophenotype strategy for bipolar disorders. *Biol. Psychiatry* 60, 93–105. doi: 10.1016/j.biopsych.2005.11.006

Hawton, K., Sutton, L., Haw, C., Sinclair, J., and Harriss, L. (2005). Suicide and attempted suicide in bipolar disorder: a systematic review of risk factors. *J. Clin. Psychiatry* 66, 693–704.

Higgins, J. P. T., and Green, S. (eds.). (2011). *Cochrane Handbook for Systematic Reviews of Interventions. The Cochrane Collaboration, 2011*, Version 5. 1. 0. Available online at: http://handbook.cochrane.org

Jamison, K. R. (2000). Suicide and bipolar disorder. *J. Clin. Psychiatry* 61(Suppl. 9), 47–51.

Kane, M. J., Conway, A. R. A., Hambrick, D. Z., and Engle, R. W. (2008). Variation in working memory capacity as variation in executive attention and control. *Variation Work. Mem.* 1, 21–48. doi: 10.1093/acprof:oso/9780195168648.003.0002

Kane, M. J., Conway, A. R., Miura, T. K., and Colflesh, G. J. H. (2007). Working memory, attention control, and the n-back task: a question of construct validity. *J. Exp. Psychol. Learn. Mem. Cogn.* 33, 615–622. doi: 10.1037/0278-7393.33.3.615

Kurtz, M. M., and Gerraty, R. T. (2009). A meta-analytic investigation of neurocognitive deficits in bipolar illness: profile and effects of clinical state. *Neuropsychology* 23, 551–562. doi: 10.1037/a0016277

Lage, G. M., Malloy-Diniz, L. F., Neves, F. S., Gallo, L. G., Valentini, A. S., and Corrêa, H. (2013). A kinematic analysis of manual aiming control on euthymic bipolar disorder. *Psychiatry Res.* 208, 140–144. doi: 10.1016/j.psychres.2012.09.046

Latalova, K., Prasko, J., Diveky, T., and Velartova, H. (2011). Cognitive impairment in bipolar disorder. *Biomed. Papers* 155, 19–26. doi: 10.5507/bp.155.2011.003

LeDoux, J. E. (2000). Emotion circuits in the brain. *Ann. Rev. Neurosci.* 23, 155–184. doi: 10.1146/annurev.neuro.23.1.155

Lee, J., Altshuler, L., Glahn, D. C., Miklowitz, D. J., Ochsner, K., and Green, M. F. (2013). Social and nonsocial cognition in bipolar disorder and schizophrenia: relative levels of impairment. *Am. J. Psychiatry* 170, 334–341. doi: 10.1176/appi.ajp.2012.12040490

Lee, R. S., Hermens, D. F., Scott, J., Redoblado-Hodge, M. A., Naismith, S. L., Lagopoulos, J., et al. (2014). A meta-analysis of neuropsychological functioning in first-episode bipolar disorders. *J. Psychiatr. Res.* 57, 1–11. doi: 10.1016/j.jpsychires.2014.06.019

Levy, B., Medina, A. M., Manove, E., and Weiss, R. D. (2011). The characteristics of a discrete mood episode, neuro-cognitive impairment and re-hospitalization in bipolar disorder. *J. Psychiatr. Res.* 45, 1048–1054. doi: 10.1016/j.jpsychires.2011.01.005

Lima, M., Tassi, J., Novo, I., and Mari, J. (2005). Epidemiologia do transtorno bipolar. *Arch. Clin. Psychiatry*32, 15–20. doi: 10.1590/s0101-60832005000700003

Liu, J.-X., Chen, Y.-S., Hsieh, J.-C., Su, T.-P., Yeh, T.-C., and Chen, L.-F. (2010). Differences in white matter abnormalities between bipolar I and II disorders. *J. Affect. Disord.* 127, 309–315. doi: 10.1016/j.jad.2010.05.026

Loschiavo, F., Sedyiama, C. Y., Neves, F. S., Corrêa, H., Malloy-Diniz, L., and Bateman, A. (2013). Clinical application of DEX-R for patients with bipolar disorder type I and II. *Clin. Neuropsychiatry* 10, 86–94.

MacQueen, G. M., Hajek, T., and Alda, M. (2005). The phenotypes of bipolar disorder: relevance for genetic investigations. *Mol. Psychiatry* 10, 811–826. doi: 10.1038/sj.mp.4001701

Malhi, G. S., Lagopoulos, J., Owen, A. M., Ivanovski, B., Shnier, R., and Sachdev, P. (2007). Reduced activation to implicit affect induction in euthymic bipolar patients: an fMRI study. *J. Affect. Disord.* 97, 109–122. doi: 10.1016/j.jad.2006.06.005

Mann-Wrobel, M. C., Carreno, J. T., and Dickinson, D. (2011). Meta-analysis of neuropsychological functioning in euthymic bipolar disorder: an update and investigation of moderator variables. *Bipolar Disord.* 13, 334–342. doi: 10.1111/j.1399-5618.2011.00935.x

Martinez-Aran, A., Vieta, E., Torrent, C., Sanchez-Moreno, J., Goikolea, J., Salamero, M., et al. (2007). Functional outcome in bipolar disorder: the role of clinical and cognitive factors. *Bipolar Disord.* 9, 103–113. doi: 10.1111/j.1399-5618.2007.00327.x

McCormack, C., Green, M. J., Rowland, J. E., Roberts, G., Frankland, A., Hadzi-Pavlovic, D., et al. (2015). Neuropsychological and social cognitive function in young people at genetic risk of bipolar disorder. *Psychol. Med.* 46, 745–758. doi: 10.1017/S0033291715002147

McKenna, B. S., Sutherland, A. N., Legenkaya, A. P., and Eyler, L. T. (2013). Abnormalities of brain response during encoding into verbal working memory among euthymic patients with bipolar disorder. *Bipolar Disord.* 16, 289–299. doi: 10.1111/bdi.12126

Miguélez-Pan, M., Pousa, E., Cobo, J., and Duño, R. (2014). Cognitive executive performance influences functional outcome in euthymic type I bipolar disorderoutpatients. *Psicothema* 26, 166–173. doi: 10.7334/psicothema2013.111

Miyake, A., Friedman, N. P., Emerson, M. J., Witzki, A. H., Howerter, A., and Wager, T. D. (2000). The unity and diversity of executive functions and their contributions to complex "frontal lobe" tasks: a latent variable analysis. *Cogn. Psychol.* 41, 49–100. doi: 10.1006/cogp.1999.0734

Miyake, A., and Shah, P. (eds.). (1999). *Models of Working Memory: Mechanisms of Active Maintenance and Executive Control, 1st Edn.* New York, NY: Cambridge University Press.

Muhtadie, L., and Johnson, S. L. (2015). Threat sensitivity in bipolar disorder. *J. Abnorm. Psychol.* 124, 93–101. doi: 10.1037/a0038065

Mullin, B. C., Perlman, S. B., Versace, A., de Almeida, J. R. C., LaBarbara, E. J., Klein, C., et al. (2012). An fMRI study of attentional control in the context of emotional distracters in euthymic adults with bipolar disorder. *Psychiatry Res.* 201, 196–205. doi: 10.1016/j.pscychresns.2011.09.002

Murphy, F. C. (2001). Neuropsychology of bipolar disorder. *Br. J. Psychiatry* 178, 120s–127s. doi: 10.1192/bjp.178.41.s120

National Institute of Mental Health (2011). *Fact Sheeton Bipolar Disorder.* Available online at: https://www.nimh.nih.gov/health/statistics/prevalence/bipolar-disorder-among-adults.shtml (Accessed February 15, 2016).

Neves, M. C., Albuquerque, M. R., Neves, F. S., Lage, G. M., Malloy-Diniz, L., Nicolato, R., et al. (2014). Sensorimotor performance in euthymic bipolar disorder: the MPraxis (PennCNP) analysis. *Rev. Bras. Psiquiatr.* 36, 248–250. doi: 10.1590/1516-4446-2013-1243

Nishida, A., Sasaki, T., Nishimura, Y., Tanii, H., Hara, N., Inoue, K., et al. (2010). Psychotic-like experiences are associated with suicidal feelings and deliberate self-harm behaviors in adolescents aged 12–15 years. *Acta Psychiatr. Scand.* 121, 301–307. doi: 10.1111/j.1600-0447.2009.01439.x

Pomarol-Clotet, E., Alonso-Lana, S., Moro, N., Sarro, S., Bonnin, M. C., Goikolea, J. M., et al. (2014). Brain functional changes across the different phases of bipolar disorder. *Br. J. Psychiatry* 206, 136–144. doi: 10.1192/bjp.bp.114.152033

Raucher-Chéné, D., Achim, A. M., Kaladjian, A., and Besche-Richard, C. (2017). Verbal fluency in bipolar disorders: a systematic review and meta-analysis. *J. Affect. Disord.* 207, 359–366. doi: 10.1016/j.jad.2016.09.039

Redick, T. S., and Lindsey, D. R. B. (2013). Complex span and n-back measures of working memory: a meta-analysis. *Psychon. Bull. Rev.* 20, 1102–1113. doi: 10.3758/s13423-013-0453-9

Remoli, T. C., and Santos, F. H. (2017). Interactions between working memory and creativity: a systematic review. *Psicol. Estud.* 22, 53–65. doi: 10.4025/psicolestud.v22i1.32518

Rihmer, Z., and Kiss, K. (2002). Bipolar disorder and suicidal behavior. *Bipolar Disord.* 4(Suppl 1), 21–25. doi: 10.1034/j.1399-5618.4.s1.3.x

Robinson, L. J., Thompson, J. M., Gallagher, P., Goswami, U., Young, A. H., Ferrier, I. N., et al. (2006). A meta-analysis of cognitive deficits in euthymic patients with bipolar disorder. *J. Affect. Disord.* 93, 105–115. doi: 10.1016/j.jad.2006.02.016

Roiser, J. P., Cannon, D. M., Gandhi, S. K., Tavares, J. T., Erickson, K., Wood, S., et al. (2009). Hot and cold cognition in unmedicated depressed subjects with bipolar disorder. *Bipolar Disord.* 11, 178–189. doi: 10.1111/j.1399-5618.2009.00669.x

Rubinsztein, J. S., Michael, A., Paykel, E. S., and Sahakian, B. J. (2000). Cognitive impairment in remission in bipolar affective disorder. *Psychol. Med.* 30, 1025–1036. doi: 10.1017/S0033291799002664

Russo, M., Mahon, K., Shanahan, M., Ramjas, E., Solon, C., Braga, R. J., et al. (2014). Affective temperaments and neurocognitive functioning in bipolar disorder. *J. Affect. Disord.* 169, 51–56. doi: 10.1016/j.jad.2014.07.038

Sabater, A., García-Blanco, A. C., Verdet, H. M., Sierra, P., Ribes, J., Villar, I., et al. (2016). Comparative neurocognitive effects of lithium and anticonvulsants in long-term stable bipolar patients. *J. Affect. Disord.* 190, 34–40. doi: 10.1016/j.jad.2015.10.008

Samamé, C., Martino, D. J., and Strejilevich, S. A. (2015). An individual task meta-analysis of social cognition in euthymic bipolar disorders. *J. Affect. Disord.* 173, 146–153. doi: 10.1016/j.jad.2014.10.055

Santos, F. H., Soares, R. F. G., and Albuquerque, P. B. (2015). "How emotions modulate working memory capacity?," in *Poster Presented at the 19th Conference of the European Society for Cognitive Psychology* (Paphos: ESCOP).

Savitz, J. B., van der Merwe, L., Stein, D. J., Solms, M., and Ramesar, R. S. (2008). Neuropsychological task performance in bipolar spectrum illness: genetics, alcohol abuse, medication and childhood trauma. *Bipolar Disord.* 10, 479–494. doi: 10.1111/j.1399-5618.2008.00591.x

Simonsen, C., Sundet, K., Vaskinn, A., Birkenaes, A. B., Engh, J. A., Hansen, C. F., et al. (2008). Neurocognitive profiles in bipolar I and bipolar II disorder: differences in pattern and magnitude of dysfunction. *Bipolar Disord.* 10, 245–255. doi: 10.1111/j.1399-5618.2007.00492.x

Soares, R. F. G. (2015). *Influência da Indução de Emoções Positivas e Negativas na Memória Operatória.* Braga: Universidade do Minho.

Spachtholz, P., Kuhbandner, C., and Pekrun, R. (2014). Negative affect improves the quality of memories: trading capacity for precision in sensory and working memory. *J. Exp. Psychol.* 143, 1450–1456. doi: 10.1037/xge0000012

Spies, K., Heese, F. W., and Hunimitzsch, C. (1996). Mood and capacity in Baddeley's model of human memory. *Z. Psychol.* 204, 367–381.

St Clair-Thompson, H. L., and Gathercole, S. E. (2006). Executive functions and achievements in school: shifting, updating, inhibition, and working memory. *Q. J. Exp. Psychol.* 59, 745–759. doi: 10.1080/17470210500162854

Sweeney, J. A., Kmiec, J. A., and Kupfer, D. J. (2000). Neuropsychologic impairments in bipolar and unipolar mood disorders on the CANTAB neurocognitive battery. *Biol. Psychiatry* 48, 674–684. doi: 10.1016/S0006-3223(00)00910-0

Thermenos, H. W., Goldstein, J. M., Milanovic, S. M., Whitfield-Gabrieli, S., Makris, N., LaViolette, P., et al. (2010). An fMRI study of working memory in persons with bipolar disorder or at genetic risk for bipolar disorder. *Am. J. Med. Genet. B. Neuropsychiatr. Genet.* 153B, 120–131. doi: 10.1002/ajmg.b.30964

Thompson, J. M., Gray, J. M., Hughes, J. H., Watson, S., Young, A. H., and Nicol Ferrier, I. (2007). Impaired working memory monitoring in euthymic bipolar patients. *Bipolar Disord.* 9, 478–489. doi: 10.1111/j.1399-5618.2007.00470.x

Torres, I. J., Boudreau, V. G., and Yatham, L. N. (2007). Neuropsychological functioning in euthymic bipolar disorder: a meta-analysis. *Acta Psychiatr. Scand.* 116, 17–26. doi: 10.1111/j.1600-0447.2007.01055.x

Unsworth, N., and Engle, R. W. (2007). The nature of individual differences in working memory capacity: active maintenance in primary memory and controlled search from secondary memory. *Psychol. Rev.* 114, 104–132. doi: 10.1037/0033-295X.114.1.104

van Gorp, W. G., Altshuler, L., Theberge, D. C., Wilkins, J., and Dixon, W. (1998). Cognitive impairment in euthymic bipolar patients with and without prior alcohol dependence. *Arch. Gen. Psychiatry* 55:41. doi: 10.1001/archpsyc.55.1.41

Verdejo-García, A., and Bechara, A. (2009). A somatic-marker theory of addiction. *Neuropharmacology* 56(Suppl. 1), 48–62. doi: 10.1016/j.neuropharm.2008.07.035

Wilhelm, O., Hildebrandt, A., and Oberauer, K. (2013). What is working memory capacity, and how can we measure it? *Front. Psychol.* 4:433. doi: 10.3389/fpsyg.2013.00433

Wingo, A. P., Harvey, P. D., and Baldessarini, R. J. (2009). Neurocognitive impairment in bipolar disorder patients: functional implications. *Bipolar Disord.* 11, 113–125. doi: 10.1111/j.1399-5618.2009.00665.x

World Health Organization (2016). *Regional Office for Europe.* Available online at: http://www.euro.who.int/en/health-topics/noncommunicable-diseases/mental-health/data-and-statistics (Accessed November 7, 2016).

23

The Geriatric Forensic Psychiatry Rotation at University of Chicago: Utilization and Educational Benefit of a Subspecialty Rotation in Psychiatric Residency Training

Carolyn Shima[1,2], Sanford Finkel[1,2], Deborah Spitz[1,2] and Amanda I. Goldstein[3]*

[1] The University of Chicago, Chicago, IL, United States, [2] University of Chicago Medicine, Chicago, IL, United States, [3] University of California, Los Angeles, Los Angeles, CA, United States

Edited by:
Natalie L. Denburg,
The University of Iowa, United States

Reviewed by:
Kathleen Coen Buckwalter,
The University of Iowa, United States
Mark Reed Nathanson,
Columbia University, United States

***Correspondence:**
Carolyn Shima
carolyn.shima@uchospitals.edu

Ten years ago, the University of Chicago Department of Psychiatry and Behavioral Neuroscience established a geriatric forensic psychiatry rotation for 4th-year psychiatry residents as one option in a required experience in forensic psychiatry. The rotation's primary emphasis was to learn about cases of testamentary capacity and undue influence. The program was supervised by a senior faculty member, an experienced clinician who was board-certified in Geriatric Psychiatry.

Results: Over the past decade, three of the 11 residents have pursued career paths in forensic psychiatry, while another has become a geriatric psychiatrist. More than half of the respondents have pursued geriatric and/or forensic work following their graduations, and all believe that what they learned in the rotation applied to their general practice work. All 11 indicated that the rotation increased their interest in and understanding of forensic work. Ten "strongly agreed" that the geriatric forensic psychiatry rotation was a valuable learning experience; one "agreed." On average, trainees worked on 4.64 forensic cases over the course of the rotation and attended 2–3 trials or depositions. Over the last 3 years of the program, all three of the participating residents have chosen to complete a forensic fellowship following the rotation.

Conclusion: Residents affirm that a geriatric forensic psychiatry rotation is a valuable learning experience, one that has utility after their graduation. The University of Chicago Department of Psychiatry and Behavioral Neuroscience is committed to continuing this rotation as an important part of their forensic experience in resident education and to encourage more interest in the area of geriatric psychiatry.

Keywords: testamentary capacity, undue influence, forensic psychiatry, training, geriatric psychiatry and aging, psychiatry training programs

INTRODUCTION

There are many specialized clinical and educational experiences offered within psychiatry residency programs in the United States and Canada, the content of which may depend in part on departmental expertise, priorities, and orientation, as well as on geography and resident interest. Some of these educational experiences are well established, while others are relatively new; some involve all residents in a program, while others are elective and appeal to only some residents each year; some have been studied, while others, unstudied, remain important experiences within residency programs. A handful of such specialized programs are presented each year at the annual meeting of AADPRT, the American Association of Directors of Psychiatric Residency Training, and serve as models for similar programs at other sites. The University of Chicago has crafted one such training program, focused on geriatric forensic psychiatry. In our review of the literature, we did not find any examples of similar studied rotations focusing on the intersection between geriatric and forensic psychiatry.

Over the last 10 years, the American Board of Psychiatry and Neurology reports issuing 17,189 board certifications for the specialty of Psychiatry. Of those, there were 694 board certifications for forensic psychiatry and 733 for geriatric psychiatry. Forensic and geriatric psychiatry continue to be less represented in residency education in specialized training experiences in comparison to the more common rotations for residents of consult-liaison psychiatry, child and adolescent psychiatry, and addictions psychiatry. The University of Chicago, like many programs, provides residents with the opportunity to observe, assist, or write a shadow report on at least one forensic case during their residency training. At many institutions, this is the only forensic opportunity available to residents. The University of Chicago has crafted a more robust training experience to allow interested residents a hands-on, one-on-one training experience focused specifically in these two frequently overlooked divisions of psychiatry.

Ten years ago, the University of Chicago Department of Psychiatry and Behavioral Neuroscience established a specialized training experience to increase resident knowledge and experience in geriatric and forensic psychiatry. The rotation has never been formally assessed as to its impact on learning or residency experience. The rotation's primary emphasis was on exposing residents to cases of testamentary capacity and undue influence in geriatric forensic psychiatry. The program was supervised by a senior faculty member, an experienced psychiatrist with over 30 years experience as an expert witness, and national recognition in the area of geriatric forensics.

The intersection of geriatric and forensic psychiatry occurs most frequently in cases of testamentary capacity in which a person's ability to knowingly and purposefully execute a will comes into question. Challenges to executed wills occur most commonly after the testator has expired and so the majority of testamentary capacity cases occur when a personal evaluation of the testator is no longer possible. As a result, particular expertise in the evaluation of medical records, evaluation of suspicious circumstances surrounding a will, and evaluation of family dynamics becomes particularly important. When the validity of a will is in question, many testamentary capacity cases also raise the concern for undue influence, or an allegation that a beneficiary has exerted coercive or excessive influence to override the testator's wishes in executing a will. Our senior faculty member focuses on testamentary capacity and undue influence cases in his work, and so the majority of the geriatric forensic rotation consists of residents observing and assisting in these two challenging yet common case topics.

Residents rotated over the course of an entire year in their PGY-4 training year. During the year, residents met with the senior faculty member at least weekly to discuss and participate in his ongoing gero-forensic case-work. Residents discussed geriatric forensic cases and issues, reviewed methodology and literature, assisted with deposition preparation and research, and were given the opportunity to participate in attorney meetings regarding legal cases in which the faculty member was engaged as an expert witness. Residents were also given the opportunity to travel to observe depositions and expert witness testimony at trial on the cases they followed.

Forensic topics of discussion and learning included forensic report writing, expert witness testimony, biological/psychiatric/legal determinants of testamentary capacity, biological/psychiatric/legal determinants of undue influence, evaluation of family dynamics and relationships, ethics in forensic psychiatry, private practice management, retainer agreements, and managing attorney expectations. Geriatric topics of discussion and learning included neuro-cognitive disorders and dementias, cognitive testing methods, evaluating medical records, health conditions specific to the geriatric population, pharmacological management in geriatric patients, and psychosis/delirium in the geriatric population.

In this study, we aimed to measure the utilization of the rotation, experience of residents, and educational benefit to residents who completed the year-long elective specialized training experience.

METHODS

Graduates of the University of Chicago Psychiatry Residency Program who had completed the Geriatric Forensic Psychiatry Rotation between 2011 and 2019 were invited by email to fill out a survey regarding their experiences on the rotation, educational benefit, and attitudes toward the geriatric forensic psychiatry rotation. The survey was completed by 11 of the 12 graduates. Responses were voluntary and anonymous. Written informed consent was obtained from participants. The survey was designed using REDCap and consisted of 30 questions. Question format consisted of Likert scales, slider questions, forced-choice (yes/no) responses, numerical responses, and narrative comments. Information obtained included both qualitative and quantitative data regarding the educational experience as well as details of post-graduation geriatric and forensic psychiatry practice.

Ten Likert scale questions were scored on a scale of strongly agree, agree, disagree, or strongly disagree. They consisted of the following:

1. I will be likely to pursue forensic work in the future, or I have pursued forensic work since completing the rotation.
2. The geriatric forensic psychiatry rotation gave me a better understanding of forensic psychiatry.
3. The geriatric forensic psychiatry rotation gave me a better understanding of geriatric psychiatry.

4. I feel knowledgeable in the topic of undue influence.
5. I feel knowledgeable in the topic of testamentary capacity.
6. I feel knowledgeable in the topic of insane delusions.
7. I feel the geriatric forensic psychiatry rotation was a valuable learning experience.
8. The geriatric forensic psychiatry rotation increased my interest in forensic psychiatry.
9. The geriatric forensic psychiatry rotation provided me with a clear understanding of expert witness testimony.
10. The geriatric forensic psychiatry rotation educated me about court procedure.

Participants were then asked to answer five slider scale questions ranking their knowledge prior to and following the rotation on a scale from 0 to 100. The questions consisted of the following:

1. How knowledgeable did you feel about forensic psychiatry prior to the rotation?
2. How knowledgeable did you feel about forensic psychiatry after the rotation?
3. How knowledgeable did you feel about geriatric psychiatry prior to the rotation?
4. How knowledgeable did you feel about geriatric psychiatry after the rotation?
5. [If a fellowship was pursued after the rotation] How prepared did you feel by the geriatric forensic rotation?

Participants were then asked to provide a numerical response to the following questions. A space for comments was provided.

1. How many depositions did you observe over the course of your rotation?
2. How many cases did you work on over the course of your rotation?
3. How many instances of expert witness testimony did you observe at trial or deposition?
4. How many meetings with attorneys did you participate in over the course of your rotation?
5. How often did you meet with the supervising faculty?
6. Approximately how many hours/week did you dedicate to this rotation?

Finally, participants were asked to answer yes/no questions with a space for comments, and a few short answer questions.

1. Have you pursued forensic or geriatric work in your career?
2. Since graduating, have you worked with geriatric patients?
3. Since graduating, have you taken on any forensic cases?
4. Did you do a fellowship in geriatrics or forensics?
5. Was (the time spent per week on the rotation) sufficient to have a full experience?
6. Are there things you learned that apply to your general practice work? Please explain.
7. Are there any specific vignettes or information that stand out for you? Please explain.
8. What was your favorite part of the experience?
9. What was your least favorite part of the experience?

RESULTS

The 11 graduates dedicated an average of 4.09 h per week to the Geriatric Forensic Psychiatry Rotation. Nine participants (82%) met with the senior faculty member at least once a week throughout the year-long rotation. On average, residents focused on 5.00 forensic cases (range 2–12) over the year. Along with the senior faculty member, residents participated in an average of 4.64 (range 1–14) attorney meetings. The average number of occurrences of expert witness testimony observed at depositions and/or trials was 2.64 (range 1–6).

On a scale from 0 to 100, where 0 indicated "not knowledgeable at all" and 100 indicated "extremely knowledgeable," participants felt their knowledge about forensic psychiatry increased by 44.28 points on the scale after the rotation (**Table 1**). Similarly, participants felt their knowledge about geriatric psychiatry increased by 31.63 points on the scale after the rotation. The majority of graduates (72%) felt they knew less about forensics than geriatrics prior to the rotation.

The 11 graduates were unanimous that the rotation provided education on court procedure and an understanding of expert witness testimony. Ten graduates (91%) felt knowledgeable on the topics of testamentary capacity and insane delusions at the time of the survey. Nine graduates (82%) felt knowledgeable on the topic of undue influence at the time of the survey. Eight participants "strongly agreed" and three "agreed" that the rotation increased their interest in forensic psychiatry. Ten participants "strongly agreed" and one "agreed" that the rotation was a valuable learning experience.

Eight participants "agreed" or "strongly agreed" that they are likely to pursue or have already pursued forensic work following graduation (**Figure 1**). Three of the 11 participants (27%) will complete or have completed a fellowship in forensic psychiatry by 2020. Eight graduates (72%) have worked with geriatric patients, and one of these graduates specializes in geriatric psychiatry. All 11 participants (100%) believed that what they learned during the rotation was applicable to their general practice work.

Over the last 3 years of the program, all three of the participating residents have chosen to complete a forensic fellowship following the rotation. One prior graduate reported that they did not complete a forensic fellowship, but actively work on forensic cases in their current practice. Seven of the eleven participants indicated that they have worked with geriatric patients since their graduation, and one reported they planned to after their graduation. One participant commented that they had more exposure to civil forensic work during the rotation than they had during their entire fellowship year. Participants

TABLE 1 | Knowledge of forensic and geriatric psychiatry on a 100-point scale before and after the rotation.

	Knowledge of forensic psychiatry	Knowledge of geriatric psychiatry
Prior to the rotation	31.27	40.55
After the rotation	75.55	72.18
Knowledge gained	44.28	31.63

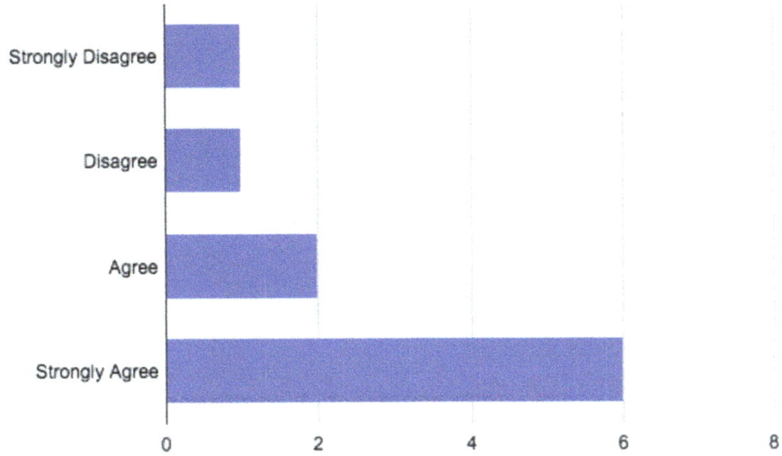

FIGURE 1 | Participant response of whether they are likely to pursue/have pursued forensic work following the rotation.

also reported specific learning which has been useful in their general practice, such as knowledge about "cognitive screening," "teamwork," "the writing of concise clinical progress notes to improve patient care," and psychiatric "ethics." One participant wrote that due to the rotation, "The knowledge of ways in which elderly can be taken advantage of and what to watch out for is something that is on my mind with patients daily." There were no negative comments regarding the content or experience of the rotation.

DISCUSSION

In our examination of the utilization, experience of residents, and educational benefit of this specialized training experience in geriatric forensic psychiatry, we found resident response to be overwhelmingly positive. The fact that at least one fourth-year psychiatric resident has chosen this elective experience each year underscores the popularity and worthwhileness of this rotation. Particularly interesting is the recent increase in participants choosing careers and fellowships in forensic psychiatry in the most recent 3 years. While the overall content and supervision approach has not changed much over the last decade, we hypothesize that word-of-mouth from senior to junior residents has increased the appeal of this rotation for residents contemplating forensic careers. It has also become more common for residents to seek fellowship training in psychiatry over the last 10 years nationwide, and forensic psychiatry has been gaining popularity in sub-specialty choice. The comments and responses from residents were highly favorable, and there was not a single negative comment regarding the content or benefit of the rotation. We would like to recognize the limitations of our study, particularly that some residents were asked to recall experiences that occurred many years ago, introducing recall bias to our conclusions. For the future, it may be helpful to provide this survey immediately following the rotation, and to provide additional questions regarding what lead to a choice of forensic or geriatric work in future practice.

To further characterize the types of cases and learning which occurred during this valuable rotation, we will discuss some of the main topics covered in education and some examples of the case-work. The following represent some of the cases and issues that have been highlighted in this rotation.

From a *biological* perspective, there are a range of medical conditions that are not commonly seen but have relevance to the issues of testamentary capacity and/or undue influence. A few examples:

1. The case of multisystem atrophy, an illness with profound physical effects, but with few cognitive deficits. Some of the children in the case asserted that their father lacked capacity and was unduly influenced. Discovery demonstrated father's intact capacity and lack of susceptibility to undue influence, and the case settled favorably to the defense.
2. The case of a patient with Castleman's disease, which led to severe fatigue, weight loss, and debilitation. The jury ruled that this woman was competent to execute a will but was vulnerable to undue influence.
3. The case of a 98-year-old woman who changed her will after a TIA. The judge ruled that she had the capacity to do so.

Other cases include mesothelioma, progressive supranuclear palsy, cancer with metastasis to the brain, and corticobasal degeneration. Further, multiple cases involve patients with delirium (Liptzin et al., 2010) or deathbed wills (Peisah et al., 2014).

Other *psychiatric and neurological* conditions:

1. A range of dementing illnesses (Major Neurocognitive Disorders) (DSM-5, 2013), which include Alzheimer's disease, Frontotemporal dementia, Lewy Body dementia, Posterior Cerebral Atrophy, Traumatic Brain Injury, and Parkinson's disease.

2. The case of a man with a diagnosis of schizophrenia, paranoid type, who believed that God was ordering him to poison the drinking water for his cattle so that they would die, but who otherwise fulfilled the criteria for possessing testamentary capacity.
3. The case of a severely depressed 89-year-old man, fearful of losing his caregiver, and thereby agreeing to leave her his estate.

Inasmuch as expert work generally requires arriving at a diagnosis, it is important to note that the DSM-5 must be interpreted broadly. For example, in a narrow sense, an illness such as Frontotemporal dementia requires cognitive testing and neuroimaging, even if the patient presents with advanced symptomatology, and clinical judgment is sufficient to establish a diagnosis. In such a situation, it is important to note that the DSM-5, more generally, does allow for clinical expertise to transcend the specific listed criteria.

Psychological and psychosocial considerations:

1. The most common litigation posits siblings in which one or more are provided a larger portion of the parent's estate.
2. The second most frequently experienced litigation involves second (or third) spouses against children of prior marriages.
3. Indicia of undue influence are common in the elderly, especially sequestration and dependency (Peisah et al., 2009), and so a close examination of the indicia and how these fit into the larger picture of the medical records and family dynamics becomes important.
4. Another frequent element is the interpretation of neuropsychological testing: for many elderly, particularly those with medical illnesses, the multi-hour testing results in gradually declining performance. Moreover, many of the tasks are unfamiliar and may result in poor results because of lack of motivation. Thus, conclusions are best interpreted in the context of the person's medical and psychiatric condition and motivation.

Medico-legal considerations:

Although courts generally allow experts to opine on susceptibility to undue influence, there is a lack of judicial consensus as to whether the expert can provide an opinion on undue influence. During this 10-year experience, on two occasions, courts in one state allowed the expert to testify on the ultimate question of undue influence, whereas subsequently a third court did not.

Older people often are exposed to painful "arrows," such as illnesses, loss of spouses and friends, and financial setbacks. These are internal arrows and often unavoidable. As clinicians, we are repeatedly called upon to address these problems and help our patients. Undue influence represents an external arrow in which a perpetrator creates a situation which results in pain and suffering for the individual. As such, the problem is an extension of the clinical problems which we encounter on a regular basis.

CONCLUSION

The geriatric forensic psychiatry rotation at the University of Chicago is a unique experience. While many other programs have developed niche experiences for residents to learn about particular areas of psychiatric practice, we did not find any published evidence that a similar program exists at other institutions. Universities tend to create these experiences in areas in which they have an especially robust clinical focus or faculty with particular expertise.

The results of the survey demonstrate that participants found the geriatric forensic psychiatry rotation to be successful in its aims of educating residents on the interface of forensic psychiatry and geriatric psychiatry, and the related issues of testamentary capacity and undue influence; giving them experience in these fields and interesting them in related careers.

AUTHOR CONTRIBUTIONS

CS provided coordination, contributed to the Introduction, Methods, Discussion, Conclusion, and Results sections, and managed survey administration and creation of survey. SF contributed to the survey development, wrote the Discussion section, and contributed to the editing. DS wrote the Introduction section, contributed to the survey participant/survey creation, and editing. AG assisted with survey creation/administration/dissemination, contributed to the Results and Methods sections, and editing.

REFERENCES

Liptzin, B., Peisah, C., Shulman, K., and Finkel, S. (2010). Testamentary capacity and delirium. *Int. Psychogeriatr.* 22, 950–956. doi: 10.1017/S1041610210000712

Peisah, C., Finkel, S. I., Reisberg, B., Shulman, K., Melding, P., Luxenberg, J., et al. (2009). The wills of older people: Risk factors for undue influence. *Int. Psychogeriatr.* 21, 7–15. doi: 10.1017/S1041610208008120

Peisah, C., Luxenberg, J., Liptzin, B., Wand, A. P., Shulman, K., and Finkel, S. (2014). Deathbed wills: Assessing testamentary capacity in the dying patient. *Int. Psychogeriatr.* 26, 209–216. doi: 10.1017/S1041610213001774

Permissions

All chapters in this book were first published in EFPD&CEPBSS, by Frontiers; hereby published with permission under the Creative Commons Attribution License or equivalent. Every chapter published in this book has been scrutinized by our experts. Their significance has been extensively debated. The topics covered herein carry significant findings which will fuel the growth of the discipline. They may even be implemented as practical applications or may be referred to as a beginning point for another development.

The contributors of this book come from diverse backgrounds, making this book a truly international effort. This book will bring forth new frontiers with its revolutionizing research information and detailed analysis of the nascent developments around the world.

We would like to thank all the contributing authors for lending their expertise to make the book truly unique. They have played a crucial role in the development of this book. Without their invaluable contributions this book wouldn't have been possible. They have made vital efforts to compile up to date information on the varied aspects of this subject to make this book a valuable addition to the collection of many professionals and students.

This book was conceptualized with the vision of imparting up-to-date information and advanced data in this field. To ensure the same, a matchless editorial board was set up. Every individual on the board went through rigorous rounds of assessment to prove their worth. After which they invested a large part of their time researching and compiling the most relevant data for our readers.

The editorial board has been involved in producing this book since its inception. They have spent rigorous hours researching and exploring the diverse topics which have resulted in the successful publishing of this book. They have passed on their knowledge of decades through this book. To expedite this challenging task, the publisher supported the team at every step. A small team of assistant editors was also appointed to further simplify the editing procedure and attain best results for the readers.

Apart from the editorial board, the designing team has also invested a significant amount of their time in understanding the subject and creating the most relevant covers. They scrutinized every image to scout for the most suitable representation of the subject and create an appropriate cover for the book.

The publishing team has been an ardent support to the editorial, designing and production team. Their endless efforts to recruit the best for this project, has resulted in the accomplishment of this book. They are a veteran in the field of academics and their pool of knowledge is as vast as their experience in printing. Their expertise and guidance has proved useful at every step. Their uncompromising quality standards have made this book an exceptional effort. Their encouragement from time to time has been an inspiration for everyone.

The publisher and the editorial board hope that this book will prove to be a valuable piece of knowledge for researchers, students, practitioners and scholars across the globe.

List of Contributors

Daniel D. Hutto
Faculty of Law, Humanities and the Arts, School of Humanities and Social Inquiry, University of Wollongong, Wollongong, NSW, Australia

Judith C. L. M. Duijkers
Centre of Excellence for Korsakoff and Alcohol Related Cognitive Dysfunctions/Addiction Care, Vincent van Gogh Institute for Psychiatry, Venray, Netherlands, Behavioural Science Institute, Radboud University Nijmegen, Nijmegen, Netherlands

Constance Th. W. M. Vissers
Behavioural Science Institute, Radboud University Nijmegen, Nijmegen, Netherlands
Kentalis Academy, Royal Dutch Kentalis, Sint-Michielsgestel, Netherlands

Jos I. M. Egger
Behavioural Science Institute, Radboud University Nijmegen, Nijmegen, Netherlands
Centre of Excellence for Neuropsychiatry, Vincent van Gogh Institute for Psychiatry, Venray, Netherlands
Donders Institute for Brain, Cognition and Behaviour, Radboud University Nijmegen, Nijmegen, Netherlands
Pompe Institute for Forensic Psychiatry, Pro Persona, Nijmegen, Netherlands

William Bechtel
Department of Philosophy and Center for Circadian Biology, University of California San Diego, San Diego, CA, USA

Cristina Y. N. Sediyama
Faculty of Medicine, Federal University of Minas Gerais, Belo Horizonte, Brazil

Ricardo Moura
Department of Basic Psychological Processes, Institute of Psychology, University of Brasília, Brasília, Brazil

Marina S. Garcia and Fernando S. Neves
Molecular Medicine Department at Federal University of Minas Gerais - INCT, Federal University of Minas Gerais, Belo Horizonte, Brazil

Antonio G. da Silva
Latin American Psychiatry Society, Porto University, Porto, Portugal

Carolina Soraggi
Department of Psychology, Federal University of Minas Gerais, Belo Horizonte, Brazil

Maicon R. Albuquerque
Department of Sports, Federal University of Minas Gerais, Belo Horizonte, Brazil

Setephen P. Whiteside
Mayo Clinic, Rochester, MN, USA

Leandro F. Malloy-Diniz
Molecular Medicine Department at Federal University of Minas Gerais - INCT, Federal University of Minas Gerais, Belo Horizonte, Brazil
Brazilian Society of Dual Pathology, Ilumina Neurosciences and Mental Health, Belo Horizonte, Brazil

Dan J. Stein
MRC Unit on Anxiety and Stress Disorders, Department of Psychiatry, Groote Schuur Hospital, University of Cape Town, Cape Town, South Africa

Judy Illes
National Core for Neuroethics, Division of Neurology, Department of Medicine, University of British Columbia, Vancouver, BC, Canada

Gerald Young
York University, Toronto, ON, Canada

Raphael van Riel
Philosophy, Philipps-University Marburg, Marburg, Germany
Philosophy, University Duisburg-Essen, Essen, Germany

Nadine Dijkstra
Donders Institute for Brain, Cognition and Behavior, Radboud University Nijmegen, Nijmegen, Netherlands

Leon de Bruin
Department of Philosophy, VU University Amsterdam, Amsterdam, Netherlands

Wandersonia Medeiros
Laboratory of Cognitive Sciences and Perception-Laboratory of Mental Health, Education and Psychometric, Universidade Federal da Paraíba, Paraíba, Brazil

Nelson Torro-Alves
Postgraduate Program in Cognitive Neuroscience and Behaviour, Laboratory of Cognitive Sciences and Perception, Universidade Federal da Paraíba, Paraíba, Brazil

Leandro F. Malloy-Diniz
ILUMINA Neurosciences, LINC-INCT, Universidade Federal de Minas Gerais, Belo Horizonte, Brazil

Carla M. Minervino
Postgraduate Program in Cognitive Neuroscience and Behaviour, Laboratory of Mental Health, Education and Psychometric, Universidade Federal da Paraíba, Paraíba, Brazil

Victor Gijsbers
Institute for Philosophy, Universiteit Leiden, Leiden, Netherlands

Ingeborg Warnke, Alex Gamma, Maria Buadze, Roman Schleifer, Carlos Canela and Michael Liebrenz
Department of Forensic Psychiatry, Institute of Forensic Medicine, University of Bern, Bern, Switzerland

Bernd Strebel
Department of Psychosomatic Medicine, Protestant Hospital Hagen-Haspe, Hagen, Germany

Tamás Tényi
Department of Psychiatry and Psychotherapy, University of Pécs, Pécs, Hungary

Wulf Rössler
Department of Psychiatry, Psychotherapy and Psychosomatics, Psychiatric Hospital, University of Zurich, Zurich, Switzerland
Laboratory of Neuroscience (LIM 27), Institute of Psychiatry, University of São Paulo, São Paulo, Brazil
Department of Psychiatry and Psychotherapy, Charité University of Medicine, Berlin, Germany

Nicolas Rüsch
Department of Psychiatry II, University of Ulm and Bezirkskrankenhaus Günzburg, Ulm, Germany

Amrei Wittwer
Collegium Helveticum, University of Zurich and Swiss Federal Institute of Technology, Zurich, Switzerland

Lea M. Hulka
Experimental and Clinical Pharmacopsychology, Department of Psychiatry, Psychotherapy, and Psychosomatics, Psychiatric Hospital, University of Zurich, Zurich, Switzerland
Center for Addictive Disorders, Department of Psychiatry, Psychotherapy, and Psychosomatics, Psychiatric Hospital, University of Zurich, Zurich, Switzerland

Hans R. Heinimann
Future Resilient Systems, Singapore-ETH Centre, Singapore, Singapore
Department of Environmental Systems Science, ETH Zurich, Zurich, Switzerland

Matthias Vonmoos
Experimental and Clinical Pharmacopsychology, Department of Psychiatry, Psychotherapy, and Psychosomatics, Psychiatric Hospital, University of Zurich, Zurich, Switzerland

Boris B. Quednow
Experimental and Clinical Pharmacopsychology, Department of Psychiatry, Psychotherapy, and Psychosomatics, Psychiatric Hospital, University of Zurich, Zurich, Switzerland
Neuroscience Center Zurich, University of Zurich and Swiss Federal Institute of Technology Zurich, Zurich, Switzerland

Rafika Zebdi
Laboratoire EvaCliPsy (EA CLIPSYD 4430), Université Paris Ouest Nanterre La Défense, Nanterre, France

Louise Goyet
Laboratoire Paragraphe (EA 349), Université Paris 8 Vincennes-Saint-Denis, Saint-Denis, France

Charlotte Pinabiaux
Laboratoire CHArt (EA 4004), Université Paris Ouest Nanterre La Défense, Nanterre, France

Bahia Guellaï
Laboratoire Ethologie, Cognition, Développement, Université Paris Ouest Nanterre La Défense, Nanterre, France

Barbara Berger, Tamas Minarik and Paul Sauseng
Department of Psychology, Biological Psychology, Ludwig-Maximilians University, Munich, Germany

Birgit Griesmayr
Department of Psychology, University of Salzburg, Salzburg, Austria

Renate Stelzig-Schoeler and Wolfgang Aichhorn
University Clinic for Psychiatry and Psychotherapy, Christian-Doppler-Clinic, Paracelsus-Medical Private University, Salzburg, Austria

Tim Thornton
College of Health and Wellbeing, University of Central Lancashire, Preston, UK

Leonardo Caixeta
Bipolar Disorder Unit, Hospital das Clínicas, School of Medicine, Federal University of Goiás, Goiania, Brazil,
Unit of Neuropsychiatry, Neuropsychology and Behavior Neurology (UNCO), Federal University of Goiás, Goiania, Brazil

Vânia L. D. Soares, Renata T. Vieira, Cândida D. Soares and Sandra B. Ferreira
Unit of Neuropsychiatry, Neuropsychology and Behavior Neurology (UNCO), Federal University of Goiás, Goiania, Brazil

Victor Caixeta
Bipolar Disorder Unit, Hospital das Clínicas, School of Medicine, Federal University of Goiás, Goiania, Brazil

Tales A. Aversi-Ferreira
Federal University of Alfenas, Alfenas, Brazil,
System Emotional Science, School of Medicine and Pharmaceutical Sciences, University of Toyama, Toyama, Japan

Erin E. Venza, Sandra B. Chapman, Jennifer E. Zientz and Jeffrey S. Spence
Center for BrainHealth, The University of Texas at Dallas, Dallas, TX, USA

Sina Aslan
Center for BrainHealth, The University of Texas at Dallas, Dallas, TX, USA,
Advance MRI, LLC, Frisco, TX, USA

David L. Tyler
Private Practice, Dallas, TX, USA

Bruno Kluwe-Schiavon
Experimentelle und Klinische Pharmakopsychologie, Psychiatrische Universitätsklinik Zürich, Zürich, Switzerland
Developmental Cognitive Neuroscience Lab, Graduate Program in Psychology, Pontifical Catholic University of Rio Grande do Sul (PUCRS), Porto Alegre, Brazil

Thiago W. Viola
Developmental Cognitive Neuroscience Lab, Graduate Program in Pediatrics and Child Health, Pontifical Catholic University of Rio Grande do Sul (PUCRS), Porto Alegre, Brazil

Breno Sanvicente-Vieira
Developmental Cognitive Neuroscience Lab, Graduate Program in Psychology, Pontifical Catholic University of Rio Grande do Sul (PUCRS), Porto Alegre, Brazil

Leandro F. Malloy-Diniz
Department of Mental Health, School of Medicine, Federal University of Minas Gerais, Belo Horizonte, Brazil
LUMINA Neurosciences and Mental Health Institute, Belo Horizonte, Brazil

Rodrigo Grassi-Oliveira
Developmental Cognitive Neuroscience Lab, Graduate Program in Psychology, Pontifical Catholic University of Rio Grande do Sul (PUCRS), Porto Alegre, Brazil
Developmental Cognitive Neuroscience Lab, Graduate Program in Pediatrics and Child Health, Pontifical Catholic University of Rio Grande do Sul (PUCRS), Porto Alegre, Brazil

Lía Martínez and Maria C. H. Tavares
Laboratory of Neurosciences and Behavior, Department of Physiological Sciences, University of Brasilia, Brasilia, Brazil

Edward Prada
Laboratory of Neurosciences and Behavior, Department of Physiological Sciences, University of Brasilia, Brasilia, Brazil
Faculty of Psychology, Social Sciences Department, Universidad Pontificia Bolivariana Seccional Bucaramanga, Bucaramanga, Colombia

Corina Satler
Faculty of Ceilandia, University of Brasilia, Brasilia, Brazil

Carlos Tomaz
Laboratory of Neurosciences and Behavior, Department of Physiological Sciences, University of Brasilia, Brasilia, Brazil,
Neuroscience Research Program, University CEUMA, São Luis, Brazil

Julie A. Hadwin and Helen J. Richards
Developmental Brain-Behaviour Laboratory, School of Psychology, University of Southampton, Southampton, UK

Katie M. de Almondes
Group of Research Neuroscience Applied, Basic Process and Chronobiolog, Department of Psychology, Federal University of Rio Grande do Norte, Natal, Brazil

Mônica V. Costa
Laboratory for Investigations in Clinical Neuroscience, School of Medicine, Federal University of Minas Gerais, Belo Horizonte, Brazil

Leandro F. Malloy-Diniz
Department of Mental Health, School of Medicine, National Institute of Science & Technology Molecular Medicine, Federal University of Minas Gerais, Belo Horizonte, Brazil

Breno S. Diniz
Department of Psychiatry and Behavioral Sciences, University of Texas Health Science Center at Houston, Houston, TX, USA

Carolina Soraggi-Frez
Department of Psychology, Faculty of Philosophy and Human Sciences, Federal University of Minas Gerais, Belo Horizonte, Brazil

Flávia H. Santos and Pedro B. Albuquerque
School of Psychology (CIPsi), University of Minho, Braga, Portugal

Leandro F. Malloy-Diniz
Department of Mental Health, National Science and Technology Institutes (INCT-MM), Federal University of Minas Gerais, Belo Horizonte, Brazil

Carolyn Shima, Sanford Finkel and Deborah Spitz
The University of Chicago, Chicago, IL, United States, University of Chicago Medicine, Chicago, IL, United States

Amanda I. Goldstein
University of California, Los Angeles, Los Angeles, CA, United States

Index

A

Alcohol Use Disorder, 13, 15, 20

Amygdala, 26, 174, 185-187, 192, 201-203, 217, 225, 228

Anxiety Disorders, 18, 59, 64, 121-122, 124-125, 164, 182, 192, 202-203

Attentional Bias to Threat, 193-196, 198

Attentional Control, 125, 170, 193-195, 197, 199-200, 202-203, 213, 225-226, 228-229

B

Balloon Analogue Risk Task, 117

Bipolar Disorder, 13, 15, 18-20, 22-24, 32-33, 36, 150, 154-155, 158-161, 164-165, 184, 218, 221, 223-224, 227-229

Brain Oscillations, 127

C

Causal Mechanisms, 37-38, 52, 146

Cerebellum, 26, 183, 191

Cerebral Blood Flow, 155-156, 161, 164-165

Circadian Mechanism, 23, 25-26, 28-29

Circadian Rhythms, 22-30, 211

Clusters, 42-51, 54, 60, 159

Cognitive Control, 7, 14, 20, 71, 79, 126, 135, 138-139, 161-162, 164, 166-168, 170, 175, 177, 179, 183, 188-189, 191, 202

Cognitive Flexibility, 78-80, 83-84, 122-124, 126, 167-170, 172, 175, 179, 207-210

Cognitive Neuroscience, 1, 5-7, 68-76, 78, 86, 149, 164, 166

Cognitive Training, 155-157, 160-165, 190, 203

Comorbidity, 13, 15, 20-21, 55, 125, 154, 181, 184, 188-191

Cortex, 26, 72, 76, 84-85, 111, 119, 121, 124-125, 128-129, 131, 137-140, 156, 161-162, 164-165, 167-169, 176-177, 179, 185-193, 201-202, 208, 211, 216-218, 222-225, 227

Counterfactual Incompatibility, 87-88, 94-95

Counterfactuals, 87, 93, 95-96

Cultural Formulation, 60-61, 63

Cumulative Lifetime Consumption, 110, 116

D

Dichotomy, 40, 52, 67, 84-85, 170

Digit Span Backward, 80-82, 206-209

Disunity of Science, 76, 87, 89, 95

Drug Dealer, 14

Drug Dependence, 110, 120

Dual-diagnosis, 13-15, 18-19

E

Emotional Salience, 170-172, 174

Endophenotypes, 38, 151, 154, 214, 224, 227-228

Explanatory Pluralism, 87-90, 95-96

F

Frontal Networks, 155

Fronto-parietal Network, 127, 131, 140

G

Global Mental Health, 37-40

I

Impulsive Behavior Scale, 32-33, 35-36

Impulsivity, 19, 32-36, 72, 76, 110, 119-120, 175-176, 179-182, 184, 187-188

Inferior Frontal Gyrus, 155, 161

Inhibitory Control, 15, 17-20, 78-80, 83, 111, 123-124, 150-151, 153-154, 164, 167, 170, 172, 174-175, 178-184, 187-190, 192-194, 196, 198-201, 204-210

Insula, 191, 217, 222-224

Iowa Gambling Task, 16-17, 21, 78, 80, 82, 85-86, 120

L

Lithium, 24, 26, 28, 30-31, 157, 163, 218, 229

M

Mechanistic Explanations, 22, 29

Mental Disorder, 1-3, 13, 39, 41, 43-45, 47-51, 54, 56-57, 59-62, 64-68, 99, 188, 203

Micro-environmental Factors, 122-123

Mood Disorders, 22-24, 26-29, 31, 33, 68, 181, 226, 229

Mood Mechanisms, 23, 28-29

N

Narrative Therapy, 1, 11

Negative Feelings, 14, 203

Neuroethics, 37, 39

Neuroplasticity, 92-93, 96, 118, 157, 160, 164, 168, 185

Neuropsychology, 4, 20, 32, 125, 149-152, 165-168, 177-178, 191-192, 228-229

Neuroscientist, 94-95, 189

Neurotransmitters, 22, 26, 30

Neutral Stimuli, 223, 225

Norepinephrine, 24, 26, 92-94, 183

Nucleus Accumbens, 26

P

Parenting, 121, 123-124, 126, 202

Phenomenology, 6, 53, 57, 60, 63-64, 68

Philosophy of Cognitive Science, 1, 4-5

Philosophy of Mind, 1-2, 12, 70, 93

Philosophy of Psychiatry, 1, 68, 144
Posttraumatic Stress Disorder, 41, 45, 54-55, 57, 86, 122, 125, 189-192
Problem Solving, 84, 123, 158-160, 169-170, 172, 175, 179, 197, 205, 217
Psychiatric Classification, 56, 65
Psychological Disorders, 121-122
Psychometric, 32-33, 35-36, 78, 211
Psychostimulant Addiction, 118, 120

R
Randomized Lottery Task, 110, 112
Risk-prone Behavior, 115-116, 118

S
Schizophrenia, 13-21, 61, 66, 79, 111, 124, 127-130, 135, 137-140, 144, 149, 164-165, 170, 176-177, 181, 205, 216, 221, 228, 234
Scientism, 37-39, 52, 54, 68
Skepticism, 37-39, 41, 51-52, 54, 98
Social Construction, 56, 59, 61, 63-64, 68
Substance Use Disorder, 13, 15, 18, 20-21

U
Unity Of Science, 87-90, 95-96, 142, 149

V
Visuospatial Sketchpad, 194, 212-213

W
Working Memory, 16-19, 21, 78-81, 84, 111-117, 121-123, 127-130, 132, 150-153, 158, 165, 167-170, 173-177, 179, 191, 193, 195-199, 202-206, 210-215, 218, 226-229

www.ingramcontent.com/pod-product-compliance
Lightning Source LLC
LaVergne TN
LVHW061512220926
848485LV00017B/880